Genetic Predisposition to Cancer

Genetic Predisposition to Cancer

Edited by

Rosalind A. Eeles

Senior Lecturer and Honorary Consultant in Cancer Genetics and
Clinical Oncology, Institute of Cancer Research and Royal Marsden
Hospital, Surrey, UK

Bruce A. J. Ponder

Director, CRC Human Cancer Genetics Research Group, University of
Cambridge, UK

Douglas F. Easton

Director, CRC Genetic Epidemiology Unit, University of Cambridge, UK

Alan Horwich

Director of Clinical Research, Academic Unit of Radiotherapy and Oncology,
Institute of Cancer Research and Royal Marsden Hospital, Surrey, UK

With a Foreword by

Gordon McVie

Cancer Research Campaign, London, UK

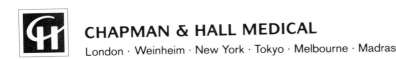

CHAPMAN & HALL MEDICAL
London · Weinheim · New York · Tokyo · Melbourne · Madras

Published by Chapman & Hall, 2–6 Boundary Row, London SE1 8HN, UK

Chapman & Hall, 2–6 Boundary Row, London SE1 8HN, UK

Chapman & Hall GmbH, Pappelallee 3, 69469 Weinheim, Germany

Chapman & Hall USA, 115 Fifth Avenue, New York, NY 10003, USA

Chapman & Hall Japan, ITP-Japan, Kyowa Building, 3F, 2–2–1 Hirakawacho, Chiyoda-ku, Tokyo 102, Japan

Chapman & Hall Australia, 102 Dodds Street, South Melbourne, Victoria 3205, Australia

Chapman & Hall India, R. Seshadri, 32 Second Main Road, CIT East. Madras 600 035, India

First edition 1996

© 1996 Chapman & Hall

Typeset in 10/12 Palatino by Photoprint, Torquay, Devon
Printed in Great Britain at The Alden Press, Oxford

ISBN 0 412 56580 3

A catalogue record for this book is available from the British Library

Library of Congress Catalog Card Number

Contents

Contents

Contents

Contents

Contents

Contributors

Dr Colin F. Arlett
MRC Cell Mutation Unit
University of Sussex
Falmer
Brighton BN1 9RR UK

Dr P. Biggs
CRC Institute of Cancer Studies
The University of Birmingham
Medical School
Birmingham B15 2TJ UK

Dr Jillian M. Birch
CRC Paediatric and Familial Cancer
   Research Group
Royal Manchester Children's Hospital
Manchester M27 4HA

Dr P. J. Byrd
CRC Laboratories
Department of Cancer Studies
The University of Birmingham Medical
   School
Birmingham B15 2TJ UK

Professor D. Timothy Bishop
ICRF Genetic Epidemiology Laboratory
Ashley Wing
St James's University Hospital
Beckett Street
Leeds LS9 7TF UK

Dr Lisa Cannon–Albright
Department of Internal Medicine
University of Utah
391 Chipeta Way
Suite D2
Salt Lake City
Utah 84108 USA

Professor Jocelyn Chamberlain
Cancer Screening Evaluation Unit
Institute of Cancer Research
Section of Epidemiology
D Block
Cotswold Road
Sutton
Surrey SM2 5NG UK

Dr Colin Cooper
CRC Section of Molecular Carcinogenesis
Institute of Cancer Research
Haddow Laboratory
15 Cotswold Road
Sutton
Surrey SM2 5NG UK

Professor John K Cowell
Department of Neurosciences, NC30
Cleveland Clinic Foundation
Research Institute
9500 Euclid Avenue
Cleveland
Ohio 44195 USA

Contributors

Mr Timothy I. Davidson
University College of London
Medical School
67–73 Riding House Street
London W1P 7LD UK

Dr Malcolm G. Dunlop
MRC Human Genetics Unit
Western General Hospital
Crewe Road
Edingurgh EH4 2XU UK

Dr Douglas F. Easton
CRC Genetic Epidemiology Unit
Department of Community Medicine
Institute of Public Health
University of Cambridge
University Forvie Site
Robinson Way
Cambridge CB2 2SR UK

Dr Rosalind A. Eeles
CRC Academic Unit of Radiotherapy and
    CRC Section of Molecular Carcinogenesis
Institute of Cancer Research and Royal
    Marsden Hospital
Downs Road
Sutton
Surrey SM2 5PT UK

Dr D. Gareth R. Evans
CRC Department of Cancer Genetics
Paterson Institute for Cancer Research
Christie Hospital
Manchester M20 9BX UK

Dr Peter A. Farndon
University Department of Clinical Genetics
Birmingham Maternity Hospital
Edgbaston
Birmingham B15 2TG UK

Dr Susan M. Farrington
MRC Human Genetics Unit
Western General Hospital
Crewe Road
Edingurgh EH4 2XU UK

Ms Deborah Ford
The Institute of Cancer Research
CRC Section of Epidemiology
Block D
15 Cotswold Road
Sutton
Surrey SM2 5NG UK

Dr David E. Goldgar
Department of Medical Informatics
University of Utah
391 Chipeta Way
Salt Lake City
Utah 84108 USA

Dr Alisa M. Goldstein
Genetic Epidemiology Branch
Department of Health and Human Services
National Cancer Institute
Executive Plaza North, Room 439
Bethesda
Maryland 20892 USA

Dr Nigel R. Hall
ICRF Genetic Epidemiology Laboratory
St James's University Hospital
Beckett Street
Leeds LS9 7TF UK

Professor Rodney Harris
Department of Medical Genetics
St Mary's Hospital
Manchester M13 0JH UK

Dr D. Hernandez
CRC Laboratories
Department of Cancer Studies
The University of Birmingham Medical
    School
Birmingham B15 2TJ UK

Dr Richard S. Houlston
CRC Section of Epidemiology
Block D, Institute of Cancer Research
Sutton
Surrey SM2 5NG UK

Dr Susan M. Huson
Department of Clinical Genetics
The Churchill Hospital
Oxford OX3 7LJ UK

Dr Kathryn M. Kash
The Strang Cancer Prevention Center
428 East 72nd Street Ste. 900
New York NY 10021 USA

Professor Alan R. Lehmann
MRC Cell Mutation Unit
University of Sussex
Falmer
Brighton BN1 9RR UK

Dr Christopher G. Mathew
Regional DNA Laboratory
Division of Medical and Molecular Genetics
Guy's Hospital
St Thomas' Street
London SE1 9RT UK

Dr C.M. McConville
CRC Laboratories
Department of Cancer Studies
The University of Birmingham Medical
    School
Birmingham B15 2TJ UK

Dr Victoria A. Murday
Clinical Genetics Unit
Jenner Wing
St George's Hospital Medical School
Cranmer Terrace
London SW17 0RE UK

Dr Mary E.R. O'Brien
Division of Medicine
Royal Marsden Hospital
Downs Road
Sutton
Surrey SM2 5PT UK

Dr Helen Patterson
CRC Section of Molecular Carcinogenesis
Institute of Cancer Research
Haddow Laboratory
15 Cotswold Road
Sutton, Surrey SM2 5NG UK

Professor Julian Peto
CRC Section of Epidemiology
Block D, Institute of Cancer Research
Sutton
Surrey SM2 5NG UK

Professor Bruce A.J. Ponder
CRC Human Cancer Genetics Research
    Group
Department of Pathology
University of Cambridge
Tennis Court Road
Cambridge CB2 1QP UK

Dr Trevor J. Powles
Division of Medicine
Royal Marsden Hospital
Downs Road
Sutton
Surrey SM2 5PT UK

Dr Kathryn Pritchard-Jones
Department of Paediatric Oncology
Royal Marsden Hospital and Institute of
    Cancer Research
Downs Road
Sutton
Surrey SM2 5PT UK

Mr Nigel P.M. Sacks
Consultant Surgeon and Head of The
    Breast Unit
St George's Hospital
Blackshaw Road
London SW17 0QT UK

Dr D. Scott
Paterson Institute of Cancer Research
Christie Hospital NHS Trust
Manchester M20 9BX UK

Contributors

Dr Thomas A. Sellers
Division of Epidemiology
School of Public Health and Institute of
   Human Genetics
University of Minnesota
1300 South Second Street
Suite 300
Minneapolis MN 55454 USA

Dr M. Stacey
CRC Laboratories
Department of Cancer Studies
The University of Birmingham Medical
   School
Birmingham B15 2TJ UK

Dr Michael R. Stratton
The Institute of Cancer Research and
   The Royal Marsden Hospital
Section of Epidemiology
Block D 15 Cotswold Road
Sutton
Surrey SM2 5NG UK

Dr A.M.R. Taylor
CRC Laboratories
Department of Cancer Studies
The University of Birmingham Medical
   School
Birmingham B15 2TJ UK

Dr Margaret A. Tucker
Genetic Epidemiology Branch
Department of Health and Human
   Services
National Cancer Institute
Executive Plaza North, Room 439
Bethesda Maryland 20892 USA

Dr C.G. Woods
The Murdoch Institute
Royal Children's Hospital
Melbourne, Victoria
Australia

Foreword

It is a personal pleasure to commend this superlative text to medical students, doctors, and scientists involved in the business of cancer. From cloning to counselling, the text comprehensively covers the field of cancer genetics as it impacts on the revolution occurring in today's medicine. Genes and genetic diseases are not the sole prerogative of oncology, but it is important to note that much of the technology which has facilitated the recent exponential surge of genetic research emanated from cancer scientists. Cancer doctors have also been at the forefront of translating this research to the clinical context.

Of necessity some of the book produces a snapshot – there will be more genes cloned in the time from writing to publication. However, the principles involved in the search for genes are acutely relevant, as are the ways in which they facilitate the selection of high risk individuals, the opportunities and the expectations they generate for screening and early diagnosis for the measurement of risk, and for explanation, reassurance and counselling of the 'potential patient' and the actual cancer sufferer.

Down the line it is likely that gene manipulation and restoration will offer new avenues for prevention and therapy. Five years ago the Cancer Research Campaign declared inherited predisposition to cancer as its top priority for investment. The editors of the book have all been key parties to the evolution of that strategy and quite appropriately are accounting for their work in this splendid book. The contributors are all authorities in their fields and they have delivered readable, understandable and relevant copy. The undergraduate embarking on medicine five years ago did not need to be equipped with this book. The undergraduate starting now will not be able to cope without it. Practising graduates in medicine will have experienced severe discomfort of late, challenged by the media and their patients to explain the business of genetic predisposition. This book will help them personalize the risk and discuss wider ethical questions ranging from insurance to employment and, most critically, consequences for other family members. This is an extremely complex but exciting and fast moving area where the opportunities of real improvement towards cancer prevention are there to be grasped, so this book is a timely contribution to the transmission of 'state of the art' thinking. With five significant cancer genes cloned in the last five years, the time to cloning is ever shortening. So, the next quinquennium should see a further increase in the knowledge of relevant cancer genes and hopefully the application of that knowledge in the clinic. The second edition of this text will need to appear before the end of the quinquennium.

Professor J. Gordon McVie

Preface

Genetic predisposition to cancer is an area which will impinge upon the practice of most clinicians managing cancer patients and their relatives in the near future. Until about 5 years ago, the study of genetic predisposition to cancer was largely confined to the rarer cancer family syndromes where one of the features of the genetic syndrome is predisposition to cancer development. However, it has long been recognized that most common types of cancer also show a tendency to run in families. Now, with the revolutionary advances in molecular genetics technology, many of the genes causing this inherited predisposition to cancer are being identified. Although the proportion of cases arising as a result of high-risk dominant genes may be small, the absolute numbers of cancer cases due to a genetic predisposition may be very large. These individuals need to be identified because they are at a markedly higher cancer risk than the general population and could be targeted for prevention and early detection strategies. Often the cancers in these individuals occur at a young age with attendant morbidity, not only for the affected individual, but also for their young dependents.

The aim of this book is to aquaint the clinician with the current status of this rapidly moving field. It covers the area from first principles, and then each chapter is expanded to provide a comprehensive review of the area. The first section covers the background genetics and molecular biology. This is followed by accounts of the rarer cancer family syndromes and then sections on the common cancers. The management options are discussed and the methods of genetic screening are described. Although this area of cancer care opens up the opportunity to identify those at a high risk of cancer so attempts can be made to prevent the disease; there are ethical and psychosocial issues which are also discussed.

We hope that this book will be of interest and use to clinicians and those in allied specialties who work with cancer patients and their families.

R. Eeles
B. Ponder
D. Easton
A. Horwich

Part One

Basic Principles

Chapter 1

Genetic predisposition to cancer: an introduction

D. TIMOTHY BISHOP

1.1 INTRODUCTION

Evidence that inherited susceptibility plays a role in the risk of malignancy comes from three separate sources. These observations are that:

1. In some syndromes which are rare in the general population but which are clearly genetically determined, there is a dramatically increased risk of cancer in gene carriers over and above that of the general population. Often these syndromes predispose to cancers which are rare outside this context and the cancers are diagnosed at atypically young ages.
2. Occasionally, families are found which contain a number of cases of 'common' cancers and the number of such cases in these families far exceeds that predicted by population rates. Again, many of these families exhibit cancers at noticeably young ages.
3. On a population level there is an increased risk of cancer to relatives of cancer cases; in many cases the relatives are at increased risk of the same cancer although relatives may also be at increased risk of other cancers.

To make this list more precise by defining 'rare' versus 'common' is not necessary, since there would doubtless be counter-examples to these 'rules'; the list is intended only as a guide to the types and informativeness of the observations. Each of these three categories requires further detail but broadly we can say that the role of genetic susceptibility is clearest in (1) and least clear in (3). In the first category, rare inherited syndromes have been recognized where genetic predisposition is obviously the major determinant; this conclusion follows simply by examining the occurrence of disease in relatives of cases and observing the precise genetic relationships among affected family members. Almost by definition these syndromes must be rare since it is the unusual occurrence of multiple cases in the same family that brings the syndrome to our attention. The observations from category (2) suggest that some small percentage of the common cancers may be directly due to genetic factors. Finally, in

Genetic Predisposition to Cancer. Edited by R.A. Eeles, B.A.J. Ponder, D.F. Easton and A. Horwich. Published in 1996 by Chapman & Hall, London.
0 412 56580 3

category (3), family aggregation alone could be attributable to genes shared by family members, exposure to the same risk factors or the interactive effects of the two. The biological interpretation of these increased risks of cancer in relatives is a matter of current intense speculation.

Syndromes from the first category above indicate the occurrence of genetic mutations which may produce a very high cancer risk in a carrier. When we translate this into a public health perspective, very few of the general public will carry the mutation; the rarity of such families indicates that the mutation(s) explain only a fraction of 1% of all cancers. At the other extreme, the third category of observation leaves open the possibility that genes could play a role in the majority of cancer incidence. The net result is that while we can elaborate (at least to some extent) on the mechanisms of inherited susceptibility, overall it is impossible to say with any justification at present the magnitude of the effect of inherited susceptibility, i.e. to say the proportion of each cancer that is directly attributable to inherited susceptibility.

1.1.1 RARE SYNDROMES

Many rare syndromes predispose to cancer. In his catalogue of inherited disorders McKusick [1] lists several hundred which feature cancer susceptibility. We recognize that these syndromes are due to a mutated gene or genes because relatives are observed to have the same syndrome, even though this syndrome is rare in the general population. In these syndromes, the precise genetic relationships of affected relatives to each other form a recognizable 'pattern' which is a signature for the mode of action of the responsible gene. For instance, some rare syndromes have the following readily recognizable expression: the disease is transmitted vertically through the pedigree from one generation to the next

and on average 50% of the children of an affected parent will themselves become affected, though the number of affected children in each family will vary (some will have none affected, some will have all). This pattern is characteristic of an 'autosomal dominant gene'; by this we mean that a gene which is present in aberrant form (a 'mutation') is associated with a high risk of disease and that it is 'autosomal' to indicate that males and females can carry and transmit the mutation to both sons and daughters and 'dominant' to indicate only a single copy of this mutation is necessary to produce this high risk of disease [2]. As an example of such a syndrome, Figure 1.1 shows pedigrees in which family members suffer from the syndrome 'familial polyposis coli' which is one such dominant syndrome [3]. These were identified by Lockhart–Mummery [4] and used as the basis of his assessment that inheritance played a role in susceptibility to cancer in some families.

In many instances, these syndromes were identified because they lead to malignancies which are 'rare' in the general population and so the observation of the same malignancy in close relatives is particularly noticeable. For instance, while childhood retinoblastoma is the most common malignant ocular tumour, it affects only 1 in 20 000 children [5]. However, in familial retinoblastoma due to inherited susceptibility about 90% of mutation carriers develop a tumour, so in such families approximately 45% of children of parental carriers of the mutation will develop retinoblastoma (one-half will inherit the mutation and of these 90% will develop retinoblastoma). Multiple endocrine neoplasia type 2A, another dominant syndrome, is characterized by predisposition to medullary thyroid carcinoma and phaeochromocytoma [6]. The phaeochromocytomas develop in approximately one-half of the patients and about 10% of the lesions become malignant. Again, the rarity of the tumours in the

FAMILY 1

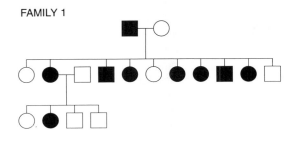

FAMILY 2

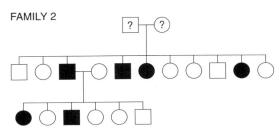

Fig. 1.1 Families originally published by Lockhart-Mummery [4] with familial polyposis. These pedigrees are shown as evidence that cancer has a hereditary component. The family is read as follows: males are represented by squares, females by circles. A solid symbol represents a family member with polyposis, while open symbols represent unaffected family members. Horizontal lines connecting a male and female symbol indicate that these two are the parents of the offspring who are vertically below them in the pedigree. This syndrome shows the 'classic' features of a dominant gene, in that affected individuals in each generation are affected and on average one-half of the offspring of affected individuals are themselves affected.

general population and the recognition of the way in which risk is transmitted through families provides clear evidence for a genetic aetiology.

In other cases, there are other phenotypes associated with the syndrome which are particularly overt. The recognizable feature of the syndromes may itself be the indirect reason for susceptibility to malignancy. For instance, in familial adenomatous polyposis,

a dominantly inherited disorder (Figure 1.1), carriers develop hundreds or even thousands of adenomas in the bowel [3]. These are apparent from the second decade of life and increase in number and size until eventually the large bowel is removed. Adenomas are thought to be the precursor lesion of most, if not all, colorectal cancers and carriers develop colorectal cancer, on average, during their fifth decade of life. Estimates of the prevalence of polyposis vary widely but, in one of the most respected studies, Bülow [7] calculated that the carrier frequency is 1 in 8000 at birth.

A final class of syndromes should be mentioned. These are characterized by the instability of chromosomes in cell cultures derived from affected individuals. Such syndromes are 'recessively inherited syndromes' and also have a recognizable pattern of expression within families. Typically, brothers or sisters of cases are at risk of the syndrome (indeed one-quarter of them on average will have the same syndrome) while parents and offspring essentially never express it because it is recessive [2, 8]. An example of such a syndrome is ataxia telangiectasia (AT) which is an autosomal recessive disorder which has a frequency of about 1 in 40 000 [8]. Individuals with the recessive phenotype (i.e. who are homozygotes for the *AT* gene) have a 10–20% chance of developing malignancy. Often, these malignancies are lymphoma or leukaemia, although there are increased risks later in life for epithelial carcinoma (see Chapter 9).

1.1.2 RARE FAMILIES SHOWING AGGREGATION TO COMMON CANCERS

Since cancer is a common disease affecting one in three people in their lifetime, one would expect to find families which have several cases of 'common' cancers, which must occur by chance alone. However, in some families, the excess is particularly noticeable, especially if the onset occurs early in life (as compared with the cancer incidence in the general population) or if bilateral tumours of paired organs are frequently reported in family members. Observations have shown an 'unusual' combination of cancers, the particular configuration of cancer cases being extremely rare under the age and sex-specific rates of the general population. The identification of a number of such families which show similar characteristics in terms of the spectrum of cancers recognized and the ages at which the cancers occur suggests a 'syndrome'. In some families, members seem to be predisposed to malignancies at the same site, while in others susceptibility applies to a number of different sites. The two cancers that have received the most interest in this area are breast cancer and colorectal cancer.

(a) Breast cancer

For breast cancer, examination shows at least two types of family; in some, female gene carriers are at high risk (approaching 100% over a lifetime) of breast or ovarian cancer [9–11] while in others, only breast cancer is observed [12, 13]. There is still a debate as to whether such families truly represent a separate syndrome or whether susceptibility is to both breast and ovarian cancer but, by chance, no female relatives have developed ovarian cancer [14]. Susceptibility is again due to a rare autosomal dominant mutation. Figure 1.2 shows a family studied because of the occurrence of early-onset breast cancer as well as ovarian cancer identifiable as a dominant inheritance; the interpretation of the pattern of disease within the family is complicated by the inability to identify those males who also carry the high-risk mutation. In this family, as with many similar families, the risk of breast cancer is noticeable at young ages so

that many such cancers are diagnosed before the age of 45

(b) Colorectal cancer

For colorectal cancer, the work of Dr Henry Lynch and colleagues is particularly notable, although many have made similar observations. Lynch obtained detailed family history information of cancer and followed 'interesting' leads. Many of these searches lead to publications reporting extensive families which showed evidence of dominantly inherited susceptibility to cancer extending over many generations [15, 16]. Of course, many of the distant relatives within the families were unaware of each other's disease state or even of the existence of such distant relatives; this provides further evidence that genetic factors play a major role and not environmental factors alone. Following families with a family history of colorectal cancer sometimes not only led to identifying previously unrecognized familial polyposis families, but also to the observation of numerous families with none of the characteristic phenotypic features of polyposis but in which the average age of onset of colorectal cancer was similar. Observation of a large number of such families led Lynch to propose two characteristic patterns [16]. In the first, labelled Lynch syndrome I, predisposition is to colorectal cancer alone, while in Lynch syndrome II, predisposition is predominantly to colorectal cancer and endometrial cancer, although authors differ in their opinion as to the other cancers included in the definition. The generic term for both syndromes is 'hereditary non-polyposis colorectal cancer' (HNPCC), acknowledging the lack of the usual phenotypic marker associated with polyposis. Lynch syndrome II is also often termed 'cancer family syndrome'. The progress in our understanding of the genetics of colorectal cancer has recently been

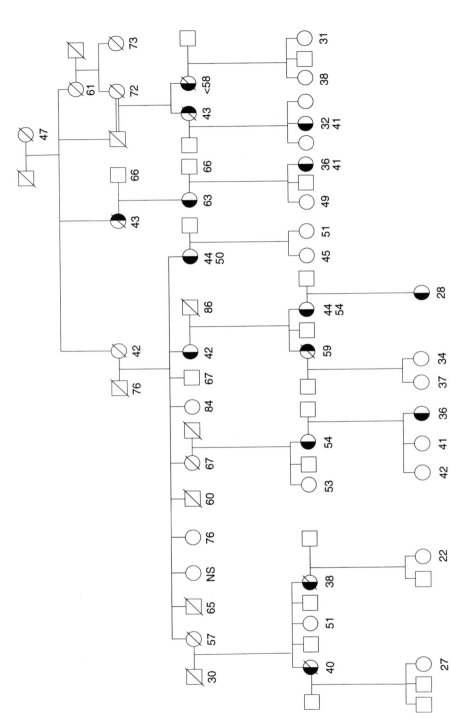

Fig. 1.2 A family with hereditary predisposition to breast and ovarian cancer. Although breast cancer is 'common' in the general population, this family shows early onset and evidence of bilateral breast disease. If it is taken into account that men will only rarely develop breast cancer and considered that women with either breast or ovarian cancer are showing evidence of carrying the gene, then once again this family shows evidence of dominantly inherited susceptibility. Shading of the left half of the female (circle) symbol implies that the woman developed breast cancer, while shading of the right half of the symbol implies ovarian cancer. The age (years) at diagnosis of the cancer, the current age or the age at death are recorded under the pedigree symbols. A diagonal line across the symbol denotes a deceased individual. Note that although the symbols for male, female and deceased are standardized, the meaning of types of shading varies and should therefore be explained with each pedigree.

reviewed by Menko [17] and is also discussed in Chapters 20 and 21.

1.1.3 POPULATION STUDIES

Analytical epidemiological studies of cancer often involve the interviewing of cases with particular tumour and age and sex-matched controls. The same questions are asked of the cases and the controls and the answers of the two groups compared. A significant difference in the distribution of responses may suggest that the focus of the questions is involved in the disease process either as a risk factor or as a reflection of the disease state. Many of these studies have considered the question of family history by asking if 'the patient has a relative with the same tumour'. Often attention is focused on first-degree relatives (parents, brothers and sisters, children) and the presence of a first-degree relative with the tumour is noted. A person has a positive family history if one or more of the relatives has been diagnosed previously with a tumour at the defined site.

For cancer, the majority of such studies have indeed shown that cases more frequently have a positive family history than controls and often the ratio of positive family histories is between two and four (although there are notable exceptions outside this range) [18, 19]. An alternative way of thinking about this ratio is to interpret it as the increased risk to relatives of cases as compared with relatives of controls; strictly speaking the equivalence of these two interpretations is not always exact, but for the examples considered here, the similarity is sufficient.

Several conclusions can be made for the common cancers. First, the absolute risk of cancer in the relative of a case is inversely proportional to the age of onset of the interviewed case. Thus, the earlier the age of onset of that case, the higher is the age-specific risk observed in the relatives. For cases diagnosed around the median age of onset of cancer or later, the increased risk to the relatives is usually minimal. For instance, in the Cancer and Steroid Hormone Study (CASH) performed in the USA during the early 1980s, almost 5000 women diagnosed with breast cancer before the age of 55 years were interviewed about their family history of cancer [20, 21]. The risk of breast cancer before the age of 60 years in the relatives of breast cancer cases was 16% if the case was diagnosed before age 30 years, 10% if diagnosed between 30 and 39, 6% if diagnosed between 40 and 49, and 4% if diagnosed between 50 and 54. For comparison, the risk of breast cancer is 3% by age 60 in the general population. Second, the risk to relatives of cases depends upon the number of cases diagnosed in the family to date. Specifically, a family with two affected first-degree relatives leads to a considerably larger risk than when only one first-degree relative is affected. For instance, again in the CASH study, the risk up to age 50 years to sisters of cases diagnosed before age 55 years who also had an affected mother was estimated to be 12%, as compared with 3% if their mother were unaffected, and 1.5% if there were no affected relative.

1.2 IDENTIFYING GENES ASSOCIATED WITH RISK OF CANCER

There are two approaches to identifying the specific genes that predispose to cancer. The first, and simplest approach is possible when a known gene is considered to be a likely candidate for being cancer-predisposing. This gene can then be sequenced in both affected ('cases') and unaffected individuals ('controls'); then, if mutations predicted to alter gene functions are shown to occur more frequently in cases than controls, this suggests that the candidate gene is actually involved in susceptibility. Logically this approach is exactly analogous to determining the exposure of cases and controls to other putative risk factors, except that in this case, the risk factor is intrinsic to the individual. Practically, this approach is often not feasible unless mutations are easy to detect because of the resources required for sequencing on a large scale; however, in theory the approach is straightforward.

In the largest such study performed to date, cases of stomach cancer were blood-typed for the ABO system, as were a large number of controls. Cases were more likely to have blood type 'A' as compared with controls, suggesting that the ABO blood group is associated with a small but significantly increased risk of stomach cancer [22]; the risk of gastric cancer is about 25% higher for individuals who are blood type 'A' as compared with blood type 'O'.

The second approach is applicable when there are no clues as to the particular chromosome on which the disease gene lies. This is called genetic linkage (see also Chapter 2). The approach is based on the knowledge that genes which are closely physically located on the same chromosome ('linked') are inherited together from one generation to the next, while genes located on separate chromosomes will be inherited independently. So, if a disease gene is located adjacent to another known gene whose presence can be readily identified, one is aware of the genetic location of the disease gene. This is ascertained by noting the inheritance pattern of known genes or genetic markers and their correlation with disease status i.e. the phenotype. If a known gene or marker is inherited or segregates with the cancer cases more frequently than would be expected by chance, the marker or known gene and disease gene are linked. This approach has been enhanced greatly over the last 10 years with the identification of thousands of DNA sequences (some of which are part of genes, most of which are not) which have now been characterized so the degree of variation among the general population for that sequence is known,

as is the genetic location; such sequences are termed 'DNA markers' [23]. By screening large numbers of DNA markers until one or more which co-segregates with the disease is identified, we continue to identify regions in which the disease gene does not lie until one in which it does lie is found. Such approaches are resource-intensive and require the collection of DNA from families with multiple cases of cancer, as well as the typing of a large number of such markers. Molecular techniques involving the identification of genes adjacent to these DNA markers are subsequently applied to identify the precise gene involved. (For further details, see Chapter 2.)

Tables 1.1 and 1.2 show some of the progress made in terms of identifying the crucial genes for some of the rare syndromes and those associated with common cancer. As these tables show, while these genes collectively are rare, they are associated with increased risk of cancer, often at a variety of sites.

1.3 MECHANISM OF ACTION OF PREDISPOSING GENES

For many of the syndromes described on pages 10, 11, the genes have been mapped so that their chromosomal location is known with great precision, and in many cases these genes have been cloned. The identification of such genes has been important scientifically because mechanisms of carcinogenesis have been elaborated with the insights gained from the study of these syndromes. For instance, retinoblastoma and familial polyposis represent mutations in tumour suppressor genes, genes which have the responsibility within the cell for suppressing growth or cellular proliferation at inappropriate times [47, 48]. Mutations within these genes are thought to inactivate them so that less restricted cellular proliferation follows. In contrast, multiple endocrine neoplasia

Genetic predisposition to cancer: an introduction

Table 1.1 Some of the 'rare' syndromes associated with an increased risk of malignancy and their mode of inheritance

Syndrome	Neoplasia or malignancy	Risk (%)[1]	Frequency[2]	Mode[3]	Chromosomal location	Reference
Neurofibromatosis type 1	Plexiform		1/3000	D	17q	[24]
	Neurofibroma	<4				[25]
	Optic glioma	<15				
Familial polyposis coli	Bowel cancer	≈100	1/8000	D	5q21	[26]
	Cancer of duodenum	NA				[27]
						[28]
Von Hippel–Lindau	Cerebellar		1/35000	D	3p	[29]
	haemangioblastoma	84				
	Retinal angioma	70				
	Renal cell carcinoma	69				
Ataxia telangiectasia	Lymphoma	60	1/40000	R	11q22-q23	[30]
	Leukaemia	27				
Multiple endocrine neoplasia type 2A	Medullary carcinoma of thyroid	NA	NA	D	10q11.2	[31]
						[32]
	Phaeochromocytoma	50				[33]

[1] Lifetime risk of neoplasia or cancer.
[2] The estimated population frequency at birth of individuals with this syndrome.
[3] Mode of inheritance is classified as 'autosomal dominant' (D) or 'autosomal recessive' (R).
NA, not available.

type 2A is caused by a mutation in a proto-oncogene, a class of genes which plays a role in normal cellular growth and differentiation [47]. In the mutated form, they act as 'accelerators' to the process; that is, cells are 'pushed' to divide in an unconstrained way.

A further term should be introduced; we define 'familial' tumours as those that arise in the context of an inherited syndrome while 'sporadic' tumours occur in individuals with no such striking family history. Germline mutations (which cause the syndromes) are rare in the germline or blood DNA in the general population, but a remarkable observation made over the last 10 years is that sporadic tumours often have somatic changes in the same genes as those involved in germline mutations in familial tumours. That is, only the cells involved in a developing tumour in sporadic cases show mutations in these genes while the remainder of the cells of the individual contain the normal

sequence. For instance, somatic changes of the APC gene (mutations in which cause familial polyposis coli) are found in more than 60% of all colorectal carcinomas [49]. Most tumours arise because of these mutations or alterations of crucial genes rather than because of the germline mutations, but in many cases it is the determination of the critical genes for the inherited syndromes that has pinpointed the genes important in the development of sporadic tumours. Detailed studies of colorectal tumours have shown that mutations in proto-oncogenes as well as tumour suppressor genes are required for the development of a cancer from normal mucosa [50].

Finally, genes which affect the ability of a cell to repair damage are natural candidates for being involved in tumour development [51]. Two such genes have recently been shown to be responsible for many families with HNPCC (Table 1.2). Failure to repair

Table 1.2 Syndromes associated with increased risk of malignancy where the major site associated with the syndrome is a 'common' cancer. For none of these sites is there currently a precise estimate as to the frequency. The references refer only to the mapping and cloning of the genes, or the estimation of penetrance associated with the mutations. Some sites are associated with multiple syndromes

Reference name	Malignancies	Risk of cancer (%)[1]	Chromosomal location	Gene name	Reference
Melanoma	Melanoma	65[2]	9p13-p22	*MLM*	[34, 35] [36]
Breast/ovary cancer syndrome	Breast	85	17q21	*BRCA1*	[37] [14]
	Ovary	63			
	Colon	× 4.1			
	Prostate	× 3.3			
HNPCC	Colon and endometrium	75–90	2p	*hMSH2*	[38] [39] [40] [41]
			3p	*hMLH1*	[42] [43] [44] [41]
Muir–Torré syndrome	As HNPCC with skin lesions		2p	*hMSH2*	[45] (see also HNPCC references)
Li Fraumeni syndrome	Brain tumours Early-onset breast cancer sarcomas		17p	*TP53*	[46]

[1] The risk is either the 'lifetime risk', as quoted in the referenced articles, or the 'risk to age 70 years' in those studies which have performed detailed age-specific calculations, or the increased relative risk (RR) associated with that site (× RR). Where possible a per site risk is given; in the absence of such figures a 'syndrome' penetrance estimate is provided.

[2] Risk to age 80 years.

damage to DNA allows the development of tumours with more serious damage and hence the evolution of a cancer in that clone of cells. In this case, the genes are involved in 'mismatch repair'; that is, the recognition that the two strands of DNA do not have their usual complementary sequences.

1.4 COLORECTAL CANCER AS AN EXAMPLE

For some cancers, the three categories of observations outlined at the beginning of the chapter have been made. In this section, we focus on colorectal cancer, since evidence of predisposition can be made at each level. We have already described how some people have a germline mutation in the *APC* gene resulting in the proliferation of adenomatous polyps throughout the colon. This syndrome, termed 'familial adenomatous polyposis', is a rare autosomal dominant disease with a carrier frequency for the mutation of 1 in 8000 individuals [7]. In a recent survey of colorectal cancer cases diagnosed under the age of 45 years, four out of 80 such cases were found to

11

be the result of familial polyposis coli (N.R. Hall, personal communication). Of course, this number is much lower than would be true if surgery were not generally performed on patients with polyposis to remove the majority of the at-risk colon.

A second syndrome which predisposes to colorectal cancer is hereditary non-polyposis colorectal (HNPCC; discussed earlier). Recent linkage analysis has shown that there are at least two genes implicated, mutations in either of which can produce HNPCC. One of these genes has been shown to lie on chromosome 2 and the other on chromosome 3. These two genes have been cloned and are involved in DNA repair, so mutations in them are presumably important because such cells are unable to repair DNA damage efficiently. Genetic analysis suggests that in the majority of families with HNPCC, the condition is due to mutations in one or the other of these genes, however, the proportion of all colorectal cancer cases which arise in the context of this syndrome is unknown. In a survey of 523 cases of colorectal cancer, diagnosed at any age, St John *et al.*[52] (also D.J.B. St John, personal communication) identified four families with apparent evidence of HNPCC through a detailed examination of the family history of cancer occurrence in relatives of index cases. They conclude that this syndrome accounts for perhaps 1% of all colorectal cancer. This estimate may be a little on the low side since, by chance, families with a mutation in one of the HNPCC genes may not have produced a sufficient number of colorectal cancer cases to be identified in this way.

While these two syndromes are associated with highly increased risks of colorectal cancer, as can be estimated from population studies, together they account for probably only 2–3% of all colorectal cancer cases. Many studies have shown that overall relatives of colorectal cases have an increased risk of cancer at the same site [53, 54]. In a recent study performed by St John *et al.* [52], cancers diagnosed in family members were verified as far as possible through medical and pathological records. Examination of the risk of colorectal cancer in relatives showed that relatives had a 2.4-fold increased risk of colorectal cancer as compared with the general population. The risks for first-degree relatives (parents and brothers and sisters) of cases were similarly elevated and the risk of colorectal cancer depended upon the age of onset of the interviewed case. Relatives of cases diagnosed before the age of 45 years had a lifetime risk of colorectal cancer of 7% (to age 70 years) while relatives of cases diagnosed after the age of 65 years had a lifetime risk of 4%. Hence, there is clear evidence that colorectal cancer still aggregates in families over and above these two syndromes.

This familial aggregation of 'common' colorectal cancer could be due to inherited susceptibility, but the mechanism would be different from that presented by these two syndromes. The syndromes described previously are clearly due to rare mutations which have a major effect on risk of colorectal cancer; observation of families suggests that the lifetime risk of cancer when someone has one of these mutations approaches 100%. These risks seen in relatives of 'common' colorectal cancer cases could be consistent with a more frequent mutation which had a more moderate effect on cancer risk. One gene which is thought to be a candidate for playing a role in such a susceptibility is the *GSTM1* gene. Cytosolic glutathione S-transferases (GSTs) catalyse the conjugation of glutathione to a variety of electrophilic compounds, including carcinogens, and one of the four classes of this gene family is termed the mu family [55]. Because of their function, these genes are good candidates for cancer-predisposition genes. In a recent survey, colorectal cancer cases were shown to have a different distribution of GSTM1 genotypes than random controls [56]. This distinction was most noticeable when only cases with tumours of the proximal colon were considered. The figures would suggest that carriers of a common GSTM1 type would have a 1.5-fold increased risk of colorectal cancer and that about 40% of the general population would have this common type. On this basis, almost 60% of all colorectal cancers would occur in this increased risk group. If the results of this study are confirmed then this will represent a gene which contributes to 'common' colorectal cancer rather than the rare syndromes. Of course, interaction with the appropriate environmental exposures must be important within this class of genes.

1.5 SUMMARY

In this chapter, we have attempted to elaborate some of the concepts of inherited susceptibility to cancer. The majority of these issues will be discussed in greater detail throughout the book. Broadly, we can say that the three types of observations implicate genetic factors as a source of susceptibility for cancer: the first is the rare or very rare syndromes which are clearly due to genetic factors. Overall, these account for a trivial proportion of all cancers in the general population, but within the few families that have such a syndrome the impact is, of course, immense since parents not only worry about their own health (and ability to look after their children) but are also concerned about having passed on the critical gene to their children [31]. One of the immediate effects of identifying the critical gene for a syndrome is to allow the family member to have the choice knowing their genetic status. While this does not of course alleviate any problems, it can allow targeted screening of at-risk family members.

We have also learned over the last few years of the role of inherited predisposition to the common cancers, particularly breast, ovarian and bowel cancer. There is – and will be – long-running debate about the importance of genes for such syndromes in terms of the proportion of all cancer that is directly attributable to such predisposition. Finally, the evidence that relatives of cases of a particular cancer have an increased risk of the same cancer suggests that genetic susceptibility could play a role in a large proportion of all cancers. The speculation is that, unlike the rare syndromes associated with a high risk of cancer and for which there is no evidence that manipulation of other environmental exposures could affect the occurrence of cancer, some form of modification may be relevant for individuals with a modestly increased genetically determined risk of cancer.

REFERENCES

1. McKusick, V.A., Francomano, C.A. and Antonarakis, S.E. (1992) *Mendelian Inheritance in Man: Catalogs of Autosomal Dominant, Autosomal Recessive, and X-linked Phenotypes*, 10th edn, Johns Hopkins University Press, Baltimore.
2. Fraser Roberts, J.A. and Pembrey, M.E. (1985) *An Introduction to Medical Genetics*, 8th edn, Oxford University Press, Oxford.
3. Northover, J.M.A. and Murday, V.A. (1989) Familial colorectal cancer and familial adenomatous polyposis. *Baillière's Clin. Gastroenterol.*, **3**(3), 613.
4. Lockhart-Mummery, P. (1925) Cancer and heredity. *Lancet*, **i**, 427–9.
5. Vogel, F. (1979) Genetics of retinoblastoma. *Hum. Genet.*, **52**, 1–54.
6. Larsson, C. and Nordenskjöld, M. (1990) Multiple endocrine neoplasia. *Cancer Surv.*, **9**, 703–23.
7. Bülow, S. (1987) Familial and polyposis coli. A clinical and epidemiological study. *Dan. Med. Bull.*, **34**, 1–15.
8. Hodgson, S.V. and Maher, E.R. (1993) *A Practical Guide to Human Cancer Genetics*, Cambridge University Press, Cambridge.

9. Gardner, E.J. and Stephens, F.E. (1950) Breast cancer in one family group. *Am. J. Hum. Genet.*, **2**, 30–40.

10. Fraumeni, J.F., Grundy, G.W., Creagan, E.T. and Everson, R.B. (1975) Six families prone to ovarian cancer. *Cancer*, **36**(2), 364–9.

11. Lynch, H.T., Harris, R.E., Guirgis, H.A., Maloney, K.M., Carmody, L.L. and Lynch, J.F. (1978) Familial association of breast/ovarian cancer. *Cancer*, **41**, 1543–9.

12. Lynch, H.T. and Watson, P. (1990) Early age at breast cancer onset – a genetic and oncologic perspective. *Am. J. Epidemiol.*, **131**(6), 984–6.

13. Lynch, H.T., Watson, P., Conway, T.A. and Lynch, J.F. (1990) Clinical/genetic features in hereditary breast cancer. *Breast Cancer Res. Treat.*, **15**(2), 63–71.

14. Ford, D., Easton, D.F., Bishop, D.T., Narod, S.A., Goldgar, D.E. and the Breast Cancer Linkage Consortium (1994) Risks of cancer in BRCA1-mutation carriers. *Lancet*, **343**, 692–5.

15. Lynch, H.T., Rozen, P., Schuelke, G.S. *et al.* (1984) Hereditary colorectal cancer review: colonic polyposis and nonpolyposis colonic cancer (Lynch Syndrome I and II). *Surv. Dig. Dis.*, **2**, 244–60.

16. Lynch, H.T., Watson, P., Kriegler, M. *et al.* (1988) Differential diagnosis of hereditary nonpolyposis colorectal cancer (Lynch syndrome I and Lynch syndrome II). *Dis. Colon Rectum*, **31**(5), 372–7.

17. Menko, F.H. (1993) *Genetics of Colorectal Cancer for Clinical Practice*, Kluwer, Dordrecht, The Netherlands.

18. Cannon-Albright, L.A., Bishop, D.T., Godgar, G. and Skolnick, M.H. (1991) Genetic predisposition to cancer, in *Important Advances in Oncology*, (eds V.T. DeVita, S. Hellman and S.A. Rosenberg) Lippincott, USA pp. 39–55.

19. Easton, D. and Peto, J. (1990) The contribution of inherited predisposition to cancer incidence. *Cancer Surv.*, **9**(3), 395–416.

20. Claus, E.B., Risch, N.J. and Thompson, W.D. (1990) Age at onset as an indicator of familial risk of breast cancer. *Am. J. Epidemiol.*, **131**, 961–72.

21. Claus, E.B., Risch, N. and Thompson, W.D. (1991) Genetic analysis of breast cancer in the Cancer and Steroid Hormone study. *Am. J. Hum. Genet.*, **48**(2), 232–42.

22. Clarke, C.A. (1961) Blood groups and disease, in *Progress in Medical Genetics*, (ed. A.G. Steinberg), Vol. 1, Grune and Stratton, New York, pp. 81–119.

23. Botstein, D., White, R., Skolnick, M. and Davis, R. (1980) Construction of a genomic linkage map in man using restriction fragment length polymorphisms. *Am. J. Hum. Genet.*, **32**(3), 314–31.

24. Huson, S.M., Compston, D.A.S. and Harper, P.S. (1989) A genetic study of von Recklinghausen neurofibromatosis in South East Wales. II Guidelines for genetic counselling. *J. Med. Genet.*, **26**(11), 712–21.

25. Lewis, R.A., Riccardi, V.M., Gerson, L.P., Whitford, R. and Axelson, K. A. (1984) Von Recklinghausen neurofibromatosis: II. Incidence of optic-nerve gliomata. *Ophthalmology*, **91**, 929–35.

26. Alm, T. and Licznerski, G. (1973) The intestinal polyposes. *Clin. Gastroenterol.*, **2**(3), 577–602.

27. Bodmer, W.F., Bailey, C.J., Bodmer, J. *et al.* (1987) Localization of the gene for familial adenomatous polyposis on chromosome 5. *Nature*, **328**, 614–16.

28. Groden, J., Thliveris, A., Samowitz, W. *et al.* (1991) Identification and characterization of the familial adenomatous polyposis coli gene. *Cell*, **66**, 589–600.

29. Maher, E.R. (1991) Genetic mechanisms in von Hippel–Lindau disease. *Lancet*, **337**, 1478–9.

30. Johnson, J.A. (1989) Ataxia telangiectasia and other α-fetoprotein-associated disorders, in *Genetic Epidemiology of Cancer*, (eds H.T. Lynch and T. Hirayama) CRC Press, Boca Raton, pp. 145–7.

31. Eng, C., Stratton, M., Ponder, B., *et al.* (1994) Familial cancer syndromes. *Lancet*, **343**, 709–13.

32. Saad, M.F., Ordonez, N.G., Rashid, R.K. *et al.* (1984) Medullary carcinoma of the thyroid. A study of the clinical features and prognostic factors in 161 patients. *Medicine*, **63**(6), 319–39.

33. Mulligan, L.M., Knole, J.B.J., Healey, C.S. *et al.* (1993) Germ-line mutations of the RET proto-oncogene in multiple endocrine neoplasia type 2A. *Nature*, **363**, 458–60.

34. Cannon-Albright, L.A., Goldgar, D.E., Meyer, L.J. *et al.* (1992) Assignment of a locus for familial melanoma, MLM, to chromosome 9p13–p22. *Science*, **258**, 1148–52.

35. Cannon-Albright, L.A., McWhorter, W.P., Meyer, L.J. *et al.* (1993) Penetrance and expressivity of the chromosome 9p melanoma susceptibility gene. *Am. J. Hum. Genet.*, **53**(3)Suppl, 171.

36. Nancarrow, D.J., Mann, G.J., Holland, E.A. *et al.* (1993) Confirmation of chromosome 9p linkage in familial melanoma. *Am. J. Hum. Genet.*, **53**(4), 936–42.

37. Easton, D.F., Bishop, D.T., Ford, D., Crockford, G.P. and the Breast Cancer Linkage Consortium (1993) Genetic linkage analysis in familial breast and ovarian cancer: results from 214 families. *Am. J. Hum. Genet.*, **52**(4), 678–701.

38. Peltomäki, P., Aaltonen, L.A., Sistonen, P. *et al.* (1993) Genetic mapping of a locus predisposing to human colorectal cancer. *Science*, **260**, 810–12.

39. Fishel, R., Lescoe, M.K., Rao, M.R.S. *et al.* (1993) The human mutator gene homolog *MSH2* and its association with hereditary nonpolyposis colon cancer. *Cell*, **75**, 1027–38.

40. Leach, F.S., Nicolaides, N.C., Papadopoulos, N. *et al.* (1993) Mutations of a mutS homolog in hereditary nonpolyposis colorectal cancer. *Cell*, **75**, 1215–25.

41. Anderson, D.E. (1980) An inherited form of large bowel cancer. Muir's syndrome. *Cancer*, **45**(suppl. 5), 1103–7.

42. Lindblom, A., Tannergård, P., Werelius, B. and Nordenskjöld, M. (1993) Genetic mapping of a second locus predisposing to hereditary non-polyposis colon cancer. *Nature Genet.*, **5**(3), 279–82.

43. Bronner, C.E., Baker, S.M. Morrison, P.T. *et al.* (1994) Mutation in the DNA mismatch repair gene homologue hMLH1 is associated with hereditary non-polyposis colon cancer. *Nature*, **358**, 258–61.

44. Papadopoulos, N., Nicolaides, N.C., Wei, Y.-F. *et al.* (1994) Mutation of a mutL homolog in hereditary colon cancer. *Science*, **263**, 1625–9.

45. Hall, N.R., Murday, V.A., Chapman, P. *et al.* (1994) Genetic linkage in Muir–Torre syndrome to the same chromosomal region as cancer family syndrome. *Eur. J. Cancer*, **30A**(2), 180–2.

46. Malkin, D., Li, F.P., Strong, L.C. *et al.* (1990) Germ Line p53 mutations in a familial syndrome of breast cancer, sarcomas, and other neoplasms. *Science*, **250**, 1233–8.

47. Teich, N.M. (1991) Oncogenes and cancer, in *Introduction to the Cellular and Molecular Biology of Cancer*, 2nd edn, (eds L.M. Franks and N.M. Teich), Oxford University Press, Oxford, pp. 230–68.

48. Ponder, B. (1988) Gene losses in human tumours. *Nature*, **335**, 400–2.

49. Wyllie, A.H., Ashton-Rickardt, P., Dunlop, M.G. *et al.* (1990) Status of the APC gene in familial and sporadic colorectal tumours as determined by closely flanking markers, in *Hereditary Colorectal Cancer*, (eds J. Utsunomiya and H.T. Lynch), Springer-Verlag, Tokyo, pp. 453–6.

50. Vogelstein, B., Fearon, E.R., Hamilton, S.R. *et al.* (1988) Genetic alterations in colorectal tumour development. *N. Engl. J. Med.*, **319**(9), 525–32.

51. Bodmer, W.F., Bishop, D.T. and Karran, P. (1994) Genetic steps in colorectal cancer. *Nature Genet.*, **6**(4), 217–19

52. St John, D.J.B., McDermott, F.T., Hopper, J.L., Debney, E.A., Johnson, W.R. and Hughes, E.S.R. (1993) Cancer risk in relatives of patients with common colorectal-cancer. *Ann. Intern. Med.* **118**(10), 785–90.

53. Anderson, D.E. (1980) Risk in families of patients with colon cancer, in *Colorectal Cancer: Prevention, Epidemiology and Screening*, (eds S. Winawer, D. Schottenfeld and P. Sherlock) Raven Press, New York, pp. 109–15.

54. Bishop, D.T. and Thomas, H.J.W. (1990) The genetics of colorectal cancer. *Cancer Surv.* **9**(4), 585–604.

55. Wolf, C.R. (1990) Metabolic factors in cancer susceptibility. *Cancer Surv.*, **9**(3), 437–4.

56. Zhong, S., Wyllie, A.H., Barnes, D., Wolf, C.R. and Spurr, N.K. (1993) Relationship between the GSTM1 genetic polymorphism and susceptibility to bladder, breast and colon cancer. *Carcinogenesis*, **14**(9), 1821–4.

Chapter 2

From families to chromosomes: genetic linkage, and other methods for finding cancer-predisposition genes

DOUGLAS F. EASTON

2.1 INTRODUCTION

The past decade has seen rapid progress towards the mapping and identification of genes involved in inherited predisposition to cancer. Before 1987 no genes conferring a high inherited risk of cancer had been identified or even localized; at that time the only genetic loci known to be involved in cancer predisposition were the HLA system, where certain HLA haplotypes were known to predispose to Hodgkin's disease [1] and to nasopharyngeal cancer [2], and the ABO blood group, where stomach cancer had been shown to be slightly more common in individuals with group A [3]. All of these associations are, however, quite weak. This situation was transformed in the 1980s by the development of techniques for typing DNA polymorphisms which could be used for linkage analysis [4]. In 1987 the genes for familial adenomatous polyposis [5] and multiple endocrine neoplasia [6, 7] were first localized, and since then genes for all the major 'inherited cancer syndromes' (that is, those rare syndromes where evidence for Mendelian inheritance was apparent from clinical studies) have now been either identified or at least mapped precisely within the human genome (see Chapter 1). Genetic linkage analysis has been the major technique by which these genes have been initially localized, although in some cases there were cytogenetic clues as to the location.

More recently, genetic linkage studies have successfully localized a number of genes responsible for predisposition to common cancers, where the evidence for a single major gene was previously more equivocal. These include two genes responsible for

Genetic Predisposition to Cancer. Edited by R.A. Eeles, B.A.J. Ponder, D.F. Easton and A. Horwich. Published in 1996 by Chapman & Hall, London.
0 412 56580 3

colon cancer (or HNPCC) families [8, 9], the *MTS*1 gene on chromosome 9p responsible for familial melanoma [10] and the *BRCA*1 and *BRCA*2 genes on chromosomes 17q and 13q, respectively, responsible for familial breast and ovarian cancer [11, 12]. In all of these cases mapping by linkage has already led to identification of the gene itself by positional cloning (see Chapter 3).

In addition to being the first step in positional cloning of disease genes, genetic linkage analysis has several other uses in complex disorders such as common cancers. Perhaps most importantly, it provides conclusive evidence that certain families with a high risk of disease are due to genetic susceptibility. (Although evidence of major genetic effects can be strongly suggested by anecdotal high-risk families or segregation analyses, neither of these is definitive.) Secondly, it can provide information on the model of susceptibility underlying the disease, for example whether the gene acts in a dominant or recessive fashion, and provide an estimate of penetrance (see page 32). Once one gene is localized by linkage analysis, it becomes possible to evaluate whether there is evidence for genetic heterogeneity (i.e. the gene is only responsible for the high risk of disease in a subset of families) and, hence, whether there are other disease genes to be mapped. It may also be possible to define more precisely the phenotype associated with different susceptibility genes. For example, following the linkage of certain early-onset breast cancer families to chromosome 17q [11], it became clear that this gene (*BRCA*1) was responsible for most families with a high risk of both breast and ovarian cancer, but a lower proportion of breast cancer families without ovarian cancer [13, 14]. Similarly, the high risk of male breast cancer in certain breast cancer families has been shown to be due (at least in part) to the *BRCA*2 gene on chromosome 13q but not

the *BRCA*1 gene [12, 15]. Finally, linkage analysis can be an important aid to genetic counselling, since it enables gene carriers and non-carriers in linked families to be identified with a high degree of certainty.

In this chapter we describe the general principles of linkage analysis, examine some of the particular difficulties in using linkage analysis to find cancer susceptibility genes, and examine some alternative methods for finding disease genes. For a fuller treatment of the statistical methods, the reader should refer to the textbook by Terwilliger and Ott [16]. This chapter is primarily aimed at non-statisticians, and the number of equations has been kept to a minimum. Those that are included (for example on pp. 20–22) can be ignored without losing the meaning of the chapter. Some other statistical derivations are given as footnotes which can again be ignored by non-mathematical readers.

2.2 GENERAL PRINCIPLES OF LINKAGE ANALYSIS

The concept of genetic linkage was first recognized by Mendel, who noted that certain characteristics of his experimental plants tended to be co-inherited. The explanation for this phenomenon became clear once it was recognized that chromosomes contain the genetic material; two traits were linked if and only if the corresponding genes reside close together on the same chromosome. Loci which are located some distance apart on the same chromosome need not be co-inherited, due to the process of recombination or cross-over which occurs at meiosis. In humans there are typically one or two cross-over events on each chromosome per meiosis, with about 30 cross-overs in total over the human genome, but the actual positions of the cross-overs vary from one meiosis to another. The probability that a recombination occurs between two loci is

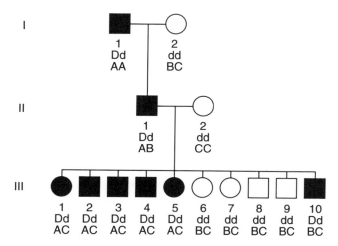

Fig. 2.1 An example of linkage analysis in an experimental backcross. D denotes the disease-causing allele at the disease locus, and d the normal allele. A, B and C are alleles at the marker locus.

known as the **recombination fraction**, usually represented by θ. Thus θ=0 indicates that no recombinations ever occur between the two loci, i.e. they are completely (or 'tightly' linked), as would occur if the two loci are very close together. At the other extreme θ=1/2 indicates that the two loci segregate independently, i.e. they are unlinked; this would occur if the two loci are far apart on the same chromosome, or on different chromosomes. Thus the recombination fraction θ is a measure of distance between two loci, with θ increasing as the two loci become further apart. The distance over which the probability of recombination is 1% is known as one **centimorgan** (cM). Since the total physical length of the 22 human autosomes is about 3 billion base pairs, 1 cM equates, on average, to about 1 million bases (1 Mb). However, the genetic distance is not related linearly to physical distance, since there are known regions of high and low recombination per unit physical distance. In particular, centromeres are known to be regions of low recombination, whereas the telomereric regions tend to exhibit high recombination rates. The rate of recombination differs

between male and female meioses; overall the female recombination rate is higher but the pattern across each chromosome differs between the sexes and there are regions where the male recombination rate is higher.

2.3 STATISTICAL ANALYSIS OF LINKAGE DATA

In experimental systems, the results of an experiment examining the genetic linkage between two Mendelian traits can be summarized straightforwardly in terms of the numbers of recombinant and non-recombinant events in informative backcrosses. Figure 2.1 illustrates a simple example in which there are ten informative meioses, generating the ten offspring of individual II-1. In nine of the meioses, alleles from the disease locus and the marker locus are co-inherited (D with A, d with B); in the tenth, generating individual III-10, the disease and marker alleles are not co-inherited, since individual III-10 gets the disease allele D from her affected father but the marker allele (B) on the opposite chromosome. Thus, a recombination between the disease gene and the marker has occurred. The estimated recombination fraction between the marker and disease loci is therefore $\theta = 1/10$. The probability of such a low rate of recombination occurring by chance if the two loci are unlinked is $11/2^{10}$ (a simple one-tailed probability from a binomial distribution, the same as the probability of obtaining zero or one tail in ten tosses of a coin), or about 0.01, indicating strong but not overwhelming evidence of linkage. Note that the test for linkage is a one-tailed test, because linkage implies values of θ less than $1/2$ – values of θ greater than $1/2$ have no biological interpretation.

Most linkage analyses in human pedigrees are, unfortunately, not this simple. Most human disease pedigrees are not simple back-crosses and, moreover, one must also be able to allow for complexities in the disease such as incomplete penetrance (where not all genetically susceptible individuals become affected) and sporadic cases (i.e. disease occurring in individuals who are not gene carriers), and other complications such as individuals being untyped. The standard method for analysing linkage data in humans, which can handle all these complexities, is known as the LOD score method, first proposed by Morton [17]. The LOD score method is based on the following function:

$$LOD(\theta) = \log_{10}[L(\theta)/L(1/2)]$$

Here $L(\theta)$ is the likelihood or probability of the observed pattern of marker and disease phenotypes within the family, given a recombination fraction θ between the disease and marker loci. $LOD(\theta)$ is thus the logarithm to base 10 of the ratio of the probability of the observed data given linkage at a certain

recombination fraction θ to the corresponding probability in the absence of linkage (where θ is $1/2$, or, more informally, the 'logarithm of the odds' in favour of linkage). The values of $LOD(\theta)$ for different values of θ are usually known as LOD scores; below we give some examples of LOD scores computations in simple situations. First we note three important properties of LOD scores which explain why they are so useful for summarising linkage evidence. These are:

1. Summing LOD scores across families. LOD scores can be added up across families. Thus if for example linkage data is available for two families with the same disease, and the LOD scores are $LOD_1(\theta)$ for family 1 and $LOD_2(\theta)$ for family 2, then the LOD scores for the two families combined, for different values of θ, are $LOD_1(\theta) + LOD_2(\theta)$. (This is a consequence of LODs being a logarithm of probabilities. **Probabilities** of independent events can be **multiplied** to give their combined probability, so **logarithms** of probabilities can be **added**.)

2. Estimating the recombination fraction. The value of θ between 0 and $\frac{1}{2}$ at which $LOD(\theta)$ takes its maximum value provides a good estimate of the recombination fraction. (In statistical jargon, it is the maximum likelihood estimate and hence, given a sufficiently large amount of data, will provide an unbiased estimate with the smallest possible standard error.) LOD scores can also be used to construct confidence intervals for the recombination fraction[1].

3. The maximum LOD score as a test of linkage. The maximum value of $LOD(\theta)$ over different values of θ can be used as the basis of a statistical test of linkage. The

---

[1] These are given to those values of θ for which $LOD(\theta)$ is within some value k of its maximum. According to standard statistical theory 95% confidence limits are given by $k=3.84/2\log_e 10$, or 0.83; however, it is (unfortunately) also common to see confidence limits based on $k=1$ (called 1-LOD confidence limits) quoted.

conventional critical value in linkage studies by genomic search is a maximum LOD score of 3.0. This corresponds, approximately, to a *P*-value of about 0.0001.[1] The reason for using such a low significance level is that the prior probability of linkage to any given marker is low – in a typical genomic search several hundred markers might be typed, almost all of which would be unlinked. A LOD score of 3.0 in fact corresponds to a probability of about 9% that any marker tested on a given dataset would be positive by chance. (The appropriate threshold for a 5% genome-wide false positive rate is a LOD score of 3.3 [18].) However, like any significance test this threshold is only a guide. If one is testing linkage to a marker which is tightly linked to a strong candidate susceptibility gene then a lower positive LOD score (say 2.0) could be quite convincing. On the other hand, many linkage analyses in complex diseases make use of multiple analyses and demand a higher threshold (see pp. 29–30).

It is important to note that these *P*-values are not necessarily a good approximation in small samples [19]. For example, a LOD score of 3 can be obtained using 10 scorable phase known meiosis, if all 10 are consistent with linkage, which would occur by chance with probability $1/2^{10}$ or about 1 in 1000. If necessary 'exact' *P*-values can be obtained by simulation [20].

2.4 EXAMPLE OF LOD SCORE CALCULATIONS

Figure 2.2 illustrates some examples of LOD score calculations in simple families. In Figure 2.2(a), the disease is assumed to be due to a rare autosomal dominant gene with complete penetrance (i.e. all individuals with the gene develop the disease). Individual II-1 receives allele A from her affected parent; therefore the disease gene, if it is on the same chromosome as the marker, must be on the same chromosome as the A allele rather than the B allele in individual II-1. We describe individual II-1 as being of known phase, since the chromosome on which the mutated disease gene lies is determined. The three affected children of II-1 all receive the A allele from II-1, whereas the two unaffected children receive the B allele, that is all five meioses are 'consistent' with linkage. The LOD score for this family is then:

$$\text{LOD}(\theta) = \log_{10}\{[(1/2)^5(1-\theta)^5]/[(1/2)^5(1/2)^5]\}$$
$$= 5\log_{10}(1-\theta) + 5\log_{10}2$$

This maximizes at $\theta=0$, with a maximum LOD score of $5\log_{10}2$, or about 1.5. Thus the best estimate of θ is 0, as expected.

In Figure 2.2(b), the marker segregation is identical except that affected individual III-5 receives the B allele; thus a recombination must have occurred in between the disease gene and the marker at meiosis. The probability of one recombinant meiosis and four non-recombinant meioses, given a recombination fraction θ, is $5\theta(1-\theta)^4$, so the LOD score is

$$\text{LOD}(\theta) = \log_{10}\{[5\theta(1-\theta)^4]/[5(1/2)^5]\}$$
$$= \log_{10}\theta + 4\log_{10}(1-\theta) + 5\log_{10}2$$

This maximizes at $\theta=0.2$, with a maximum LOD score of about 0.42.

In general, in a family with n children where the phase is known, and where r of

---

[1] In standard statistical terminology, the maximum LOD score is a log-likelihood ratio statistic, so that in large samples the statistical significance of the maximum LOD score can be derived by referring $2(\log_e 10)\text{LOD}(\theta)$ to a chi-squared distribution on 1 degree of freedom. Thus a LOD score of 3 corresponds to $\chi^2_1=13.82$, or a one-tailed *P*-value of about 0.0001.

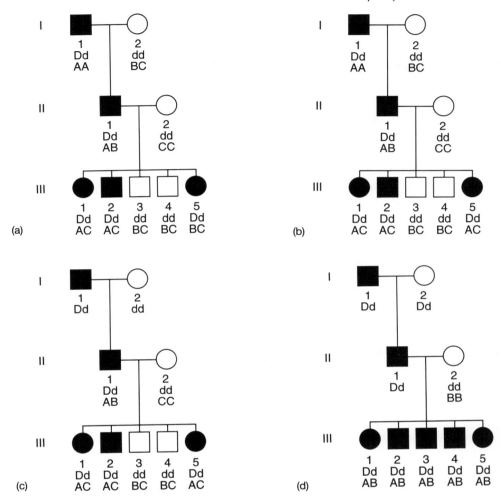

Fig. 2.2 (a–d) Some simple examples of linkage analysis. D denotes the disease causing allele at the disease locus, and d the normal allele. A, B and C are alleles at the marker locus.

the children are recombinant, the LOD score is:

$$\text{LOD}(\theta) = \log_{10}\{[\theta^{r}(1-\theta)^{n-r}]/[(1/2)^{n}]\}$$

$$= r\log_{10}\theta + (n-r)\log_{10}(1-\theta) + n\log_{10}2$$

with the maximum LOD score occurring at $\theta = r/n$.

In Figure 2.2(c) all five children in generation III are again consistent with linkage. However, their affected grandparent I–1 is not typed, so it is not known whether the mutated disease gene in individual II-1 is on the same chromosome as the A allele or the B allele – each of these possibilities is, a priori, equally likely; in this case individual II-1 is said to be of unknown phase. The LOD score computation must take account of both these possibilities:

$$\text{LOD}(\theta) = \log_{10}\{[(1/2)\theta^{5} + (1/2)(1-\theta)^{5}]/[(1/2)^{5}]\}$$

$$= \log_{10}[\theta^{5}+(1-\theta)^{5}]+4\log_{10}2$$

21

This maximizes at θ=0 but with a maximum LOD score of 1.2. The effect of the phase being unknown is therefore to reduce the overall informativeness of the family, in this case by one meiosis.

In Figure 2.2(d), individual II-1 is untyped. Suppose the marker is known to have just two alleles A and B. Given the marker typings in her offspring, her genotype at the marker locus must be either A-A or A-B; the probabilities of these two possibilities will depend on the frequencies of the A and B alleles in the population from which she is descended. A priori, the probabilities of an individual having genotypes A-A, A-B or B-B are p_A^2, $2p_Ap_B$ and p_B^2 respectively, where p_A and p_B are the population frequencies of alleles A and B.[1] The LOD score is then of the form:

$$LOD(\theta) = \log_{10}\{[p_A^2+p_Ap_B((1-\theta)^5+\theta^5)]/$$
$$[p_A^2+2p_Ap_B(1/2)^5]\}$$

If $p_1=0.2$ say, then the maximum LOD score would be 0.60 at θ=0. If however, p_A were small, say 0.001, the maximum LOD score would increase to 1.2, the same as in Figure 2.2(c). (This, of course, is because if A is rare, the affected parent II-1 almost certainly has genotype A-B and is therefore informative for this marker.) Thus, as one would expect, the fact that the marker is less than fully informative substantially reduces the informativeness of the family.

Finally, suppose the penetrance of the disorder is incomplete. Then in the example in Figure 2.2(a) say, the LOD score will be:

$$LOD(\theta) = \log_{10}\{(1/2)(1-\theta)^3((1-t)\theta+t(1-\theta))^2$$
$$+(1/2)\theta^3(t\theta+(1-t)(1-\theta))^2]/(\tfrac{1}{2})^5\}$$

where t is the penetrance. If $t=0.5$ say, the maximum LOD score would be 0.60 at θ=0.0.

Thus, again, the reduced penetrance decreases the informativeness of the family.

2.5 NOTES ON LOD SCORE CALCULATIONS

The computation of LOD scores by hand in the way outlined in the previous section becomes impractical for large pedigrees, particularly with complications such as missing typings and incomplete penetrance. Fortunately a number of efficient computer algorithms exist for computing LOD scores in general pedigrees. Of these by far the most widely used is the LINKAGE program developed by Lathrop *et al.* [21]. This is an extremely flexible program, allowing one to handle markers with any number of alleles, disease genes with penetrances which can vary between individuals according to covariates such as age and sex, and even quantitative trait loci. The same computations can be carried out in other programs such as MENDEL [22].

To facilitate combining the data between families, it is usual to report LOD scores in the form of a table giving LOD scores at standard recombination fractions; the usual values of the recombination fraction are 0.001, 0.01, 0.05, 0.1, 0.2, 0.3 and 0.4. Table 2.1 gives an example of a LOD score table summarizing evidence for linkage between 15 breast and/or ovarian cancer and the marker D17S588 on chromosome 17q [23]. Even though none of the families has substantial evidence for linkage on its own, the overall evidence for linkage is strong, a result confirmed by other studies [13].

One final point about LOD score calculations. The computed LOD scores do not depend at all on the process by which the disease families came to be selected for study. Thus it does not matter that families with, for example, five affected siblings, might be extremely rare. It is perfectly legitimate (and usually essential) to select such families from

---

[1] These probabilities are strictly only appropriate for a random mating population, when the allele frequencies are said to be in Hardy–Weinberg equilibrium [16], but this assumption is usually satisfactory in linkage analysis.

Table 2.1 Two-point LOD scores for 11 Edinburgh breast–ovarian cancer families, for linkage between the marker D17S588 and the disease. (From [23].)

Family identifier	Recombination fraction				
	0.0	0.05	0.1	0.2	0.3
37	0.51	0.43	0.36	0.21	0.10
1	−0.81	0.22	0.21	0.21	0.07
11	2.08	1.85	1.60	1.11	0.63
2000	0.66	0.58	0.54	0.49	0.32
16	0.68	0.60	0.51	0.32	0.17
33	0.24	0.21	0.17	0.11	0.05
2	0.39	0.70	0.72	0.57	0.33
3	0.58	0.48	0.38	0.20	0.08
1021	−0.06	−0.05	−0.04	−0.02	−0.01
30	0.30	0.24	0.19	0.11	0.05
84	−0.06	−0.05	−0.05	−0.03	−0.01
Total	4.51	5.21	4.59	3.28	1.78

a larger sample of families in order to increase the informativeness of the study; the recombination estimates and significance levels based on the maximum LOD score will remain valid.

2.6 TYPES OF GENETIC MARKER AND LABORATORY TECHNIQUES

Before 1983 very few important genes causing inherited diseases had been mapped to a particular chromosomal region. The reason for this was simply that very few genetic markers were available with which to detect linkage. The most important breakthrough in mapping disease genes came in the late 1970s with the realization that single base pair DNA polymorphisms could be recognized by restriction enzymes and resolved by electrophoresis, using a technique known as Southern blotting [24]. This revolutionized the field by providing a much larger class of polymorphisms which were numerous throughout the genome. These restriction fragment length polymorphisms (or RFLPs) became the basis of many successful linkage studies in Mendelian disorders, including

cancer syndromes such as familial adenomatous polyposis [5].

Another major advance has been the development of DNA polymorphisms based on repetitive sequences. These were first recognized by Jeffreys *et al.* [25], who noted that certain short DNA sequences were tandemly repeated and that the number of repeats was often highly variable between individuals. The variation in these 'minisatellite' polymorphisms (also known as variable number of tandem repeats or VNTRs) can also be detected by electrophoresis. The great advantage of these polymorphisms over RFLPs is that they are usually much more polymorphic. Almost all RFLPs have just two alleles and are often not particularly informative; for example, if an affected individual is homozygous for the marker, all their offspring are uninformative for linkage. In contrast, the 'minisatellite' polymorphisms often have large numbers of alleles so that most individuals are heterozygous, making the marker much more informative for linkage.

The next important advance was the identification of dinucleotide 'microsatellite' polymorphisms by Weber and May [26]. These are based on repeats of dinucleotide sequences, most frequently repeated runs of the bases CA, or $(CA)_n$. Such sequences are extremely frequent throughout the genome; there are estimated to be 50 000–100 000 in total. Most sequences with at least 10 repeats are polymorphic, and many have ten or more alleles. Many other simple tandem repeat markers (or STRs) have also been identified, for example based on tri- or tetranucleotide repeats (e.g. $(GATA)_n$). These longer repeats are often easier to resolve on an electrophoresis gel than dinucleotide repeats due to the larger differences in size between adjacent alleles. STR polymorphisms have now become the markers of choice in linkage searches.

The standard method for typing these markers relies on using the polymerase chain reaction (PCR) to amplify the repeat, using primers based on unique DNA sequences either side of the repetitive sequence [27]. The alleles can be resolved by radiolabelling one of the primers, running the PCR product down a electrophoretic gel and autoradiographing, although methods for fluorescent labelling (which avoids the use of radioactivity) are now becoming standard.

Another major advantage of these markers is that, because they use the PCR, they can be typed using very small quantities of DNA. In particular, they have been typed successfully using DNA extracted from stored pathological sections of tumour and normal tissue. This is particularly useful in cancer families since it enables the markers to be typed on material from dead affected individuals [27].

An area of technology which could make an important impact in the future is the development of techniques for looking directly at similarities or differences in genomic sequences between individuals in pedigrees (known as representational difference analysis [28] or genomic mismatch scanning [29]). These techniques could enable disease genes to be localized rapidly without the need for typing large numbers of polymorphic markers.

2.7 MULTIPOINT LINKAGE ANALYSIS

Once a disease gene has been localized to a chromosomal region by linkage analysis, a more precise localization can usually be obtained by typing a series of markers in the region. This process is illustrated in Figure 2.3. In this example, the disease cosegregates with markers B and C, but not with marker A. Individual III-3 receives the A2 allele from her affected parent, whereas her affected siblings receive the A1 allele. This single observation suggests strongly that the disease gene (if located in the region of these markers) must be below marker A. If the disease gene were above A, at least two

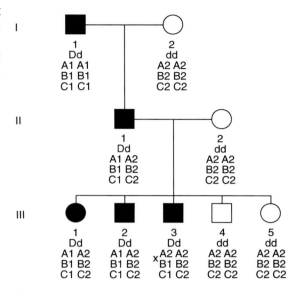

Fig. 2.3 The principle of multipoint linkage analysis. A, B and C denote linked marker loci in chromosomal order ABC, each with alleles 1 and 2. D and d denote the disease causing and normal alleles respectively at the disease locus. 'x' indicates the recombination event.

recombination events would be required to explain the markers' alleles inherited by individual III-3, which is unlikely in a small chromosomal region; whereas if the disease gene were below A only a single recombination is required, a far more likely explanation given that the markers are relatively close together. This process can be formalized into **multipoint linkage analysis**, in which LOD scores can be computed for different locations of the disease based on the segregation of the disease and a number of marker loci. A number of programs including LINKAGE are able to carry out such computations. The results of such analyses are often presented in terms of a graph of LOD score against position along the chromosome. An example of such an analysis is given in Figure 2.4, which is taken from the linkage analysis of breast–ovarian cancer families with the 17q

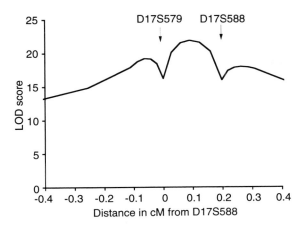

Fig. 2.4 Multipoint LOD scores in 57 breast–ovarian cancer families, for linkage between the markers D17S588, D17S579 and breast or ovarian cancer [13].

markers D17S588 and D17S579 conducted by the Breast Cancer Linkage Consortium [13]. The maximum LOD score is 20.79, which is obtained at a location between the two markers. This analysis therefore not only provides strong evidence of linkage to this region but also provides a more precise indication of location than is possible with analyses involving a single marker; the maximum LOD scores in the intervals proximal to D17S250 and distal to D17S588 are substantially lower (16.88 and 18.86) and therefore less likely. The evidence in favour of a particular location is usually expressed in terms of the 'relative odds' of a particular order, defined as the ratio of the antilogarithms of the maximum LOD score with the disease gene at the best location and the maximum LOD score in other possible intervals. In this example, the 'odds' in favour of a location between D17S588 and D17S250 are 86:1 over a location distal to D17S588 and 8050:1 over a location proximal to D17S250. A detailed discussion of the precise significance of these ratios is beyond the scope of this chapter, but odds of 1000:1 or greater are

conventionally regarded as conclusive [16]. Unfortunately, the computational difficulty of such analyses increases dramatically as the number of loci increases, particularly in complex disease pedigrees, so that formal multipoint analyses is usually not computationally feasible with more than three marker loci and a disease locus. Even then, it is often necessary in complex pedigrees to reduce the numbers of alleles at the marker loci to as few as possible by recoding alleles [30]. Currently, various Monte Carlo methods for solving these difficulties are under development, such as sequential imputation [31] and Monte Carlo Markov Chains based on Gibbs sampling [32], but none is yet in widespread use.

Individuals such as III–3 in Fig. 2.3 who show recombination with some markers in the region but not others are often described as 'critical recombinants'; identifying them often is a key process in localizing the gene to a small interval. Unless the disease is fully penetrant, the recombinant must occur in an affected individual (or in an obligate gene carrier) to be totally convincing, since an unaffected individual may or may not be a gene carrier. Even an affected individual in a linked family does not provide completely definitive localizing information in cancer families, since they may be a sporadic case. In this regard, phenotypic features of the case may be helpful in determining whether the case is likely to be a sporadic; for example, the familial risk of breast cancer is strongly related to age at onset [33] so that in a breast cancer family, a case diagnosed at age 35 would be unlikely to be a sporadic case whereas a 75-year-old case would have a substantial probability of being sporadic. A woman with both breast and ovarian cancer or a male with breast cancer would be very unlikely to be sporadic since such cases are so rare in the general population.

Another important step interpreting these critical recombinants is 'haplotyping' the marker alleles in the family correctly, that is, assigning the alleles for a number of different markers on the same chromosome to the correct copy of the chromosome. In the example given, there is no ambiguity, but often several configurations of haplotypes are possible and these may lead to different interpretations of critical recombinants. Haplotyping can usually be done by eye, although various algorithms for assigning marker haplotypes have been developed which are helpful if the number of markers is large. Haplotyping closely linked markers is helpful for identifying data errors, which will often be revealed as unlikely multiple recombinants.

Another related technique is to compare marker haplotypes between different linked families. If the disease gene is thought to be rare, it is quite likely that different families carry the same ancestral mutation. This is particularly likely if one is studying families from an isolated population. Since there may be a large number of meioses between different families the region shared between different families could be quite small, allowing precise localization of the disease gene, as occurred in the case of diastrophic dysplasia in Finland [34].

In addition to localizing disease loci, multipoint linkage analysis is used extensively to construct linkage 'maps' of genetic markers, which define the order of and distance between genetic markers on each chromosome. These maps are extremely valuable in determining suitable markers to type in genomic linkage searches for disease loci, and as a basis for multipoint analyses of a disease locus relative to several marker loci. These maps are mainly constructed using marker typings on large reference families, notably those collected by the CEPH (Centre d'Etude du Polymorphisme Humaine) collaboration; many hundreds of markers have been placed on such maps [35].

2.8 GENETIC HETEROGENEITY

In the linkage calculations discussed above we assumed implicitly that all families were due to the same gene. However, many genetic diseases, including inherited cancer syndromes, can result from mutations in more than one gene, a situation known as genetic heterogeneity. Genetic heterogeneity introduces a major complication in linkage analyses, since in any given set of families the disease may be linked to one locus in some families and to a second locus in other families. A genetic marker linked to the first locus will then give evidence for linkage (i.e. positive LOD scores) in some families and evidence against linkage (negative LOD scores) in others, so that adding up the LOD scores from different families is not so helpful. (In fact, the maximum LOD score across all families is still expected to be positive, so that one should still detect linkage given a sufficiently large sample size, but the best estimate of θ will be larger than the true value.)

2.8.1 ESTIMATING THE PROPORTION OF FAMILIES DUE TO A PARTICULAR GENE

It is tempting to deal with the situation of apparent genetic heterogeneity by combining only the positive LOD scores, discarding those families with evidence against linkage. This type of analysis, however – which is analogous to excluding non-responders in clinical trials – is to be avoided as the maximum LOD score is uninterpretable. The most widespread (legitimate) method for incorporating genetic heterogeneity into linkage analysis is the **admixture** model of Smith [36]. Under this model we assume that some proportion α of all families are due to the locus of interest, the remaining proportion $1-\alpha$ being due to some other gene(s). Suppose we have a collection of n families with

Table 2.2 LOD scores between D2S123 and the disease in 10 HNPCC families. (From [36].)

Family identifier	Recombination fraction					
	0.0	0.01	0.05	0.10	0.20	0.3
L4	2.73	2.78	2.66	2.12	1.37	0.61
L7	−2.60	−2.61	−2.24	−1.48	−0.64	−0.24
L8	1.74	1.70	1.54	1.33	0.94	0.56
L621	2.64	2.60	2.43	2.18	1.60	0.94
L1933	0.29	0.30	0.34	0.35	0.30	0.18
L2516	−1.29	−1.08	−0.62	−0.33	−0.10	−0.04
L3106	−0.26	−0.16	0.09	0.25	0.31	0.20
L3427	−1.21	−1.11	−0.79	−0.52	−0.19	−0.03
B1	−1.97	−1.79	−1.30	−0.92	−0.45	−0.19
B2	−1.02	−0.82	−0.46	−0.27	−0.10	−0.05
Total	−0.99	0.24	1.77	3.25	3.79	2.70

linkage data, and the LOD score for family i, assuming that the disease is linked in this family at recombination fraction θ is $LOD_i(\theta)$. Then one can construct a LOD score for the set of families under the assumption of heterogeneity, depending on both α and θ.[1] Maximizing this LOD score provides estimates of both α and θ, together with a test for heterogeneity.

The effects of genetic heterogeneity are neatly illustrated by data from a recent study of HNPCC families [37]. Table 2.2 shows LOD scores for linkage to the marker D2S123 in 10 families. The maximum total LOD score is 3.79, maximizing at a recombination fraction of 0.20. However, inspection of the LOD scores in some of the families (such as L7) show strong evidence against linkage. Using the admixture model, the maximum LOD score under heterogeneity is 4.92 at $\theta=0.01$, with $\alpha=0.41$ (i.e. an estimated 41% of families are

due to a gene on chromosome 2p). The test statistic for heterogeneity is $\chi^2_1=5.16$, which corresponds to a P-value of about 0.01. This is much closer to the truth, since families positive for linkage to chromosome 2p have been shown to be due to germline mutations in the MSH2 gene, which is about 2cM from D2S123 [38]. Thus neglecting genetic heterogeneity gives an exaggerated estimate of the recombination fraction. In fact, a number of the families with evidence against linkage to 2p have been shown to be due to the MLH1 gene on chromosome 3p [38].

Once evidence of heterogeneity has been established, the admixture model can be used to determine the probability that any given family is linked, given their linkage result (the so-called, posterior probability).[2]

For some disorders it is possible to define a useful subdivision of families on the basis of the observed clinical phenotypes, which may reflect the action of distinct genes. For example, selecting breast cancer families on the basis of the presence of male cases defines a set of families likely to be linked to BRCA2 [12]. In this case it will be more powerful to test for linkage by summing LOD scores within these phenotypic subsets rather than by using the admixture method.

In practice, detection of genetic heterogeneity can be quite difficult using data on a single linked marker, unless the families are quite large. The reason for this is that recombination between the disease and the marker in a small family could indicate a recombination event in a linked family or an unlinked family, so that it is difficult to

[1] This is given by [37]:
$$LOD(\alpha,\theta) = \log_{10}\{\alpha L(\theta|\text{linked})+(1-\alpha)L(\theta|\text{unlinked})\}/L(\tfrac{1}{2})$$
$$= \log_{10}\{(1-\alpha) + \alpha 10^{LOD_i(\theta)}\}$$
Maximizing $LOD(\alpha,\theta)$ over α and θ provides estimates for these parameters, and a statistical test of heterogeneity is provided by calculating the statistic:
$$\chi^2 = 2\log_{10}e\{LOD(\hat{\alpha},\hat{\theta})-LOD(1,\bar{\theta})\}$$
In this formula $LOD(\hat{\alpha},\hat{\theta})$ is the maximum heterogeneity LOD score, and $LOD(1,\bar{\theta})$ is the maximum LOD score under homogeneity. Since this is again a log-likelihood ratio statistic, its significance is determined by comparison with a chi-squared distribution on 1 degree of freedom.
[2] This posterior probability is given by: $P_i = \alpha 10^{LOD_i(\theta)}/[(1-\alpha) + \alpha 10^{LOD_i(\theta)}]$

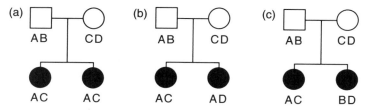

Fig. 2.5 The principle of affected sib pair analysis. A, B, C and D represent marker allele or haplotypes. A pair of affected siblings may share two haplotypes, as in (a), one haplotype, as in (b), or zero haplotypes, as in (c). These outcomes have probabilities 1/4, 1/2 and 1/4 respectively if the marker is unlinked to any disease causing gene. Deviation from these probabilities provides evidence for linkage.

distinguish tight linkage in a small proportion of families from loose linkage in a high proportion. (In statistical jargon, α and θ are confounded.) However, it is usually possible to get much clearer evidence for or against heterogeneity with multipoint linkage [39]. This is because a multipoint analysis can determine a particular interval in which the gene lies (effectively restricting the possible range of the recombination fraction), so that strong evidence against linkage in a particular family may be obtained if affected individuals in the family do not share a haplotype across the interval in which the gene must lie.

Although these statistical methods are helpful for detecting and estimating genetic heterogeneity, they cannot take away the fact that power of any given set of families to detect linkage can be much lower under genetic heterogeneity than under homogeneity. To take a simple example, for a disorder caused by a single dominant gene, five families each with three fully informative phase unknown meioses could be sufficient to detect linkage, assuming a highly polymorphic marker tightly linked to the disease gene. If instead the disorder can be caused by either of two genes of equal frequency, then on average 22 such families will be required to detect linkage. This can be particularly serious for families with few affected individuals, so in general it is better to collect a few large families than many small families if one suspects genetic heterogeneity (see section 2.11).

2.9 NON-PARAMETRIC METHODS OF LINKAGE ANALYSIS

One of the perceived disadvantages of classical linkage analysis, using LOD scores, is that performing the calculations requires one to specify in advance the precise genetic model underlying the disease, i.e. whether the gene is dominant or recessive, the gene frequency and penetrance and the rate of sporadic cases. These parameters are usually known, at best, very imprecisely and, at worst, not at all. Fortunately, as discussed below, mis-specification of the genetic model does not usually lead to a serious loss of power. Nevertheless, it is unsatisfactory for the results of a linkage analysis to be dependent on an arbitrary choice of genetic model. For this reason, many authors have considered methods for linkage analysis which do not depend on specifying a particular model. These methods depend on counting marker alleles, or haplotypes, between affected relatives, for example affected sibling pairs. The principle is illustrated in Figure 2.5. At any locus, the two affected siblings may share either two, one or zero of the haplotypes they inherit from their parents. If the locus is unlinked to any disease susceptibility gene, the probabilities of sharing two, one or zero haplotypes based on Mendelian segregation are 1/4, 1/2 and 1/4. On the other hand, if the marker locus is linked to a disease susceptibility locus, these probabilities will differ from the values under no linkage. Therefore, evidence for linkage in a series of affected sibling pairs can be assessed by testing whether the proportions sharing two, one or zero haplotypes identical by descent differ significantly from the proportions expected given no linkage (for a recent discussion of efficient tests for detecting linkage in sibling pairs see [40]). This principle can easily be extended to other types of affected relative pair, such as uncle–nephew or cousin pairs [41, 42]. The method has also been extended to families with more than two affected relatives by Weeks and Lange [43]; their method, which counts allele sharing between all possible pairs of affected relatives, is known as the Affected Pedigree Member or APM method.

2.10 PITFALLS IN LINKAGE ANALYSIS

Although the LOD score method of linkage analysis is an extremely powerful and flexible technique, it does have some drawbacks. The first is purely a presentational one. A table of LOD scores in a paper disguises the raw data and can be difficult to interpret; one cannot tell at a glance, for example, how many recombinant and non-recombinant affected individuals there are. Ideally these raw data should be conveyed by displaying the actual pedigrees with marker typings but this is not always practical. One compromise is to present, in addition to the LOD scores, a summary of the sharing of marker alleles (or haplotypes) between affected individuals.

A second difficulty with the LOD score method is that the method requires one to specify the exact genetic model, including gene frequency, degree of dominance, and penetrances (possibly age and sex specific), whereas in practice these will not be known with any certainty. In some cases population-based family studies can be used to provide at least rough estimates of the genetic parameters, using segregation analyses. Unfortunately, such analyses have only been possible

for a few cancers. Moreover, the results of such segregation analyses may not apply to high-risk families selected for linkage analysis.

Fortunately, both theoretical studies and practical experience have shown that linkage analysis is fairly robust to mis-specifying the genetic model. It can be shown that assuming the wrong genetic model has no effect on the type I error rate, that is, the probability of obtaining any specified maximum LOD score (e.g. greater than 3) when there is in fact no linkage. It is also true that, at least for two-point linkage analysis, the power to detect linkage is not seriously impaired by mis-specifying the disease parameters. In particular, mis-specifying the penetrance is known to have relatively little effect on the overall maximum LOD score, although it will result in a biased estimate of the recombination fraction [44]. The LOD score is also fairly insensitive to the assumed disease gene frequency. A more serious error is mis-specifying the degree of dominance (i.e. specifying a dominant model instead of a recessive model or vice-versa), which can lead to a serious loss of power [45]. For this reason LOD scores should be computed under both dominant and recessive models if there is any doubt as to which is correct.

Multipoint linkage analysis is less robust to mis-specifying the genetic model than two-point analysis. In two-point linkage analysis, mis-specification of the model will lead to a biased estimate of the recombination fraction but little change in the maximum LOD score, but with multipoint analysis the recombination fraction is not free to vary in the same way; this can lead to linkage being erroneously rejected from the whole region. Risch and Giuffra [45] have suggested that this difficulty can be overcome by assuming a common disease gene frequency (for example 0.05 for a dominant gene or 0.20 for a recessive gene).

Although the LOD score method is robust to mis-specification of the disease model, the same is not true of the marker allele frequencies. Allele frequencies have no impact on linkage analysis if all the relevant individuals can be typed, but this is rarely possible in cancer families. Mis-specifying marker allele frequencies can then easily lead to spurious evidence for linkage, if affected individuals share (by chance) a marker allele which is common in the population, but the allele is assumed incorrectly to be rare [46]. Ironically, this problem has become worse with the introduction of microsatellite markers. Although these markers can have a dozen or more alleles, it is typical for one or two alleles to be relatively common in the general population (occasionally 50% or more). Since allele sizes may only vary by two base pairs, it is fairly easy to misread a common allele for a rare one. A further complication is that allele frequencies may vary substantially between populations. Fortunately, with the density of polymorphic markers now available, it should always be possible to resolve the problem of unknown allele frequencies by typing a number of markers in the region and developing haplotypes. With a haplotype of four or five microsatellite markers, for example, it becomes unlikely that any observed haplotype would have a frequency of more than 10%. However, one should always be cautious of positive linkage results generated on the basis of a single marker.

The other common way in which a high probability of type I errors can be generated is by using multiple phenotypic endpoints. This can lead to a serious multiple testing problem. This type of problem has been much more in evidence in psychiatric genetics (for example, schizophrenia) where there are many ways of defining the disease, than in cancer, where the disease of interest is usually well defined. However, it could become an issue in the future if one were attempting to conduct linkage studies in families with many different types of cancer.

One rather common example of multiple testing is performing linkage analysis over a range of penetrance estimates, when the penetrance has not been previously estimated. In this case an appropriate correction can be made by increasing the LOD score threshold [47].

2.11 DESIGN CONSIDERATIONS

Now that highly polymorphic markers spanning the entire genome are available, the main limitation in any linkage search is the availability of a sufficiently large set of informative families. The important question, therefore, in designing a linkage search is what constitutes a large enough sample of informative families.

For a simple rare Mendelian disorder, such as familial adenomatous polyposis, the ideal family is clear, namely a family with as many affected individuals as possible. (The number of unaffected individuals does not have much impact on the power to detect linkage, unless the penetrance is near complete.) This is particularly important if there is genetic heterogeneity. The power to detect linkage using any given set of families can be estimated by simulation, using programs such as SLINK [48] or SIMLINK [49]. Power calculations are often expressed most simply in terms of the expected LOD score (or ELOD) which will be generated by a given set of families, perhaps under a range of alternative models and types of marker. One can then gauge under what circumstances a LOD score of 3, for example, is likely to be achieved.

Most common cancers are not of course Mendelian. However, population-based segregation analyses have suggested that at least some of common cancers do contain a subpopulation caused by a relatively rare autosomal dominant gene conferring a high risk; these include breast, colon, ovarian, prostate and lung cancer. In order to detect these high-risk genes one needs to identify those families which are most likely to be segregating the high-risk gene; this again implies families with as many affected individuals as possible. For

Table 2.3 Sample size requirements for various types of family and various genetic models (number of families required to give an expected LOD score of 3.0,[1] assuming a highly polymorphic marker tightly linked to the disease locus

	One gene				Two genes[2]			
	Familial relative risk				Familial relative risk			
	3		2		3		2	
Dominant gene								
Gene frequency	0.001	0.05	0.001	0.05	0.001	0.05	0.001	0.1
Risk ratio	50.2	21.1	34.8	10.0	34.8	10.0	24.4	6.1
Family structure of affecteds								
Affected sib pair	57	56	106	104	244	239	439	424
Three affected sibs	11	25	13	37	52	123	61	185
Four affected sibs	6	18	7	25	27	97	30	132
Avuncular pair	53	53	122	125	219	222	495	499
(e.g. uncle–nephew)								
Cousin pair	48	49	128	131	182	185	491	493
Sib pair + affected pair	17	42	20	75	74	200	90	337
Recessive gene								
Gene frequency	0.01	0.2	0.01	0.2	0.01	0.2	0.01	0.2
Risk ratio	289	26.0	203	14.7	203	14.7	143	9.3
Family structure of affecteds								
Sib pair	13	26	23	45	51	100	88	175
Three sibs	3	15	3	19	10	61	11	83
Four sibs	1	15	1	18	6	61	6	73

[1] Strictly, the appropriate LOD score threshold under heterogeneity is >3, but 3 is used for simplicity.
[2] Genes acting additively on disease risk (as in a genetic heterogeneity model). These sample size estimates assume two genes each with identical gene frequencies and penetrances. If the two genes have different models (e.g. a rare gene and a common gene) the relative efficiencies of different family structures may be very different [51].

many of these cancers one should also try to select families with many early onset cases (e.g. in the case of breast cancer, cases diagnosed below age 50), since family studies suggest that these are more likely to be due to a high-risk gene than later onset cases.

At the opposite extreme from using large families is the affected relative pair design (i.e. two affected individuals per family). The power to detect linkage using a set of affected relative pairs is relatively straightforward to evaluate. If disease susceptibility is due to a single dominant gene, then the power to detect linkage depends only on the observed familial relative risk to first-degree relatives of affected individuals [41]. For example, if the observed familial relative risk is three-fold, then about 60 affected sibling pairs would be required to detect linkage with 50% power and a significance level of 0.0001 (equivalent to a LOD score of 3), assuming that a highly polymorphic marker tightly linked to the disease locus is available. Sample sizes required in some other situations, including families with three or four affected individuals, are illustrated in Table 2.3. If the disease is due to a recessive gene, the power to detect linkage is dependent on the familial relative risk to both parents and siblings of affected individuals [41]. If disease susceptibility is the result of more than one gene, the power to detect linkage depends on the contribution to the familial risk made by each locus [41]. It also depends on how the different loci interact, for example whether they act additively or multiplicatively (epistasis) on disease risk. Some examples of the effect of heterogeneity on the power of affected relative pairs are given in Table 2.3.

The major limitation of the relative pair approach is that the sample sizes required to detect linkage increase rapidly if the familial relative risk due to the gene reduces below about 2. Unfortunately, the overall familial relative risks for most common cancers is only about 2 [50], with some notable exceptions such as testis cancer and thyroid cancer. A simple affected relative pair design is thus unlikely to detect susceptibility genes unless one gene is responsible for most of the familial risk. A more promising approach is to select the relative pairs based on a subset of cases with a higher familial risk. For example, the familial relative risks for several common cancers such as prostate, breast and colon are much higher at young ages [50], so it makes sense to select relative pairs with early-onset disease.

The optimal linkage designs for detecting relatively common low penetrance genes are not as clear as for rare high penetrance genes. As shown in Table 2.3, families with three or four cases are almost always more powerful than affected pairs. However, families with large numbers of affected individuals may be less efficient in this case for two reasons. First, because the disease gene is common; families with many affected members could be segregating more than one copy of the disease susceptibility allele. This could make the family uninformative for linkage if the transmitting parent were homozygous at the disease locus. Second, if the disease can also be caused by a rare high penetrance gene or genes, families with many affecteds are probably due to the high-risk gene. Easton and Goldgar [51] found that affected sib trios are a good strategy for detecting low penetrance genes across a wide range of models.

2.12 ESTIMATING PENETRANCE

It is not always appreciated that, once linkage has been established, marker data in linked families can provide useful estimates of model parameters such as penetrance. This is true even though the families may have been ascertained on the basis of a large number of affected individuals. Suppose for example that the disease is due to a rare dominant gene with uncertain penetrance. If the penetrance is high, most carriers will be affected so the proportion of unaffected relatives who carry the marker allele linked to the disease will be low. Conversely, if the penetrance is low, the proportion of unaffected siblings carrying the linked allele will approach 50%. This approach can be formalized into a procedure for estimating penetrance by maximizing the LOD score over possible penetrances [52] (sometimes referred to as the MOD score method [45]). However, one word of caution: many inherited disorders show variation in penetrance between families. The maximum LOD score approach is necessarily based on large families used for linkage, which will be the families due to the mutations with the highest penetrance. If there is variable penetrance, therefore, the method will provide an estimate relevant to the families with high penetrance, rather than an average penetrance over all possible mutations. A similar approach of comparing LOD scores can be used to distinguish between different modes of inheritance, such as dominant and recessive [53].

2.13 PREDICTIVE TESTING

Another important application of genetic linkage is predictive testing in high-risk families, that is, determining whether a given individual in a family carries the disease causing mutation for the purposes of counselling and management, by observing whether or not the individual carries the marker haplotype linked to the disease. Predictive testing has been used widely in some of the inherited cancer syndromes, and to some extent in common cancer syndromes such as *BRCA*1. Given the genetic heterogeneity underlying most inherited cancers, testing on the basis of linkage is only reliable in large families where the evidence for linkage is unequivocal; for smaller families reliable testing is only possible once the disease causing mutation has been identified (see Chapter 26).

2.14 USE OF LOSS OF HETEROZYGOSITY DATA IN TUMOURS

Many of the genes causing inherited cancer syndromes are known to be tumour suppressor genes, in which the inherited mutation is inactivating. In order for tumours to develop in susceptible individuals, the other homologous copy of the gene must also be lost or inactivated, usually by mitotic recombination or non disjunction (see Chapter 4); in contrast, sporadic tumours may require somatic inactivation of both copies. This model was first proposed in a famous paper by Knudson [54] to explain inherited and sporadic retinoblastoma, and subsequently confirmed for retinoblastoma by Cavanee *et al.* [55], and later for a number of other inherited cancers. Inactivation of one copy of the gene can often be detected by observing loss of heterozygosity in tumour material with polymorphic markers near the disease locus, and loss of heterozygosity in tumours can therefore provide clues to the locations for tumour suppressor genes. An important consequence of the Knudson model is that if the susceptibility gene acts as a tumour suppressor gene then any loss of heterozygosity in high families due to the gene must affect the wild-type (non-susceptible) chromosome. This has been observed, for example, in the case of *BRCA*1 [56]. This non-random loss of heterozygosity in tumours can be used as an adjunct to increase the power of linkage studies [57]. The gain in power can be considerable, particularly in the case of small families such as affected relative pairs [58].

2.15 PHENOTYPIC MARKERS

Another approach to the problem of detecting cancer susceptibility genes conferring only a moderate risk is to attempt to identify phenotypes associated with cancer risk which are themselves heritable. Many potential examples of such 'phenotypic markers' of susceptibility have been proposed. These include in particular a number of phenotypes which are precursors of cancer, such as adenomatous polyps of the large bowel, which are known precursors of colorectal cancer [59], and atypic melanocytic naevi or large numbers of benign naevi, which are associated with a high risk of melanoma [60]. Other promising phenotypes include abnormal sensitivity to ionising radiation [61] and abnormal patterns of TP53 protein staining [62], both of which could be measured *in vitro*.

The rationale for using these phenotypic markers in place of cancer in linkage studies is that the penetrance of a predisposing gene for the precursor trait is presumably likely to be higher than the cancer risk, and moreover it will be expressed at an earlier age (perhaps at all ages). It may also be possible to score the phenotype on a continuous scale, as in the case of naevi. These factors might enable one to collect much more informative pedigrees than are possible based on a cancer phenotype.

Despite this, very little use has been made to date of such precursor phenotypes for linkage analysis, though this may change as most of the obvious cancer syndromes have now been mapped and linkage analysis based on cancer as a phenotype becomes more problematic. The major drawback of the phenotypic markers is that the genetics of these phenotypes are not necessarily simple. For example, segregation analysis of the large Utah naevus dataset suggests strongly that benign naevi have a large inherited component but that this is almost certainly polygenic [63, 64]. For a phenotype to be really effective for mapping studies, one would wish to observe some evidence of a Mendelian component. Another problem with many of the phenotypes proposed to date is that they are not easy to measure and there may be substantial interobserver variability.

2.16 ASSOCIATION STUDIES

A number of disease susceptibility loci have been identified through direct testing of candidates, looking for associations between particular alleles and disease by comparing allele frequencies in affected individuals and matched controls. The many associations between particular HLA types and disease were identified in this way, though some have subsequently been confirmed by linkage. In cancer the most notable recent example of a susceptibility locus identified through association studies rather than linkage is the HRAS1 minisatellite locus, where certain alleles appear to be associated with a modest increased risk of a wide range of cancers [65].

In these allelic associations the observed high-risk allele need not be a disease-causing mutation itself. A much more likely cause of the association is **linkage disequilibrium**. If there are a relatively small number of founder disease-causing mutations, then the disease will be associated with any marker alleles which were present on the founder chromosomes, provided that the marker is tightly linked to the disease locus. The key here is tightly linked; for loosely linked markers, the effects of linkage disequilibrium will disappear within a few generations of the founding mutation [66].

Allelic association studies have a major advantage over linkage studies in terms of collection of material, in that they can be performed on series of unrelated cases and controls, which are usually much easier to obtain than multiple case families needed for linkage analysis. Moreover, allelic association studies can detect genetic effects which would be undetectable in any linkage study. For example, suppose a particular allele has a population frequency of 5% and causes a two-fold risk of cancer. This effect could be detected with a sample size of about 190 cases and matched controls, with 50% power and a significance level of 0.0001 (roughly equivalent to getting a LOD score of 3). To detect the same effect by linkage would require about 22 000 affected sibling pairs, even assuming no genetic heterogeneity! Of course, if one is only observing a polymorphism in linkage disequilibrium with the disease causing mutation then the effects would be smaller, but nevertheless the range of detectable effects is potentially much greater using an association study.

The difficulty with the candidate gene approach is, of course, identifying worthwhile candidate genes to test. Given the low prior probability that any particular gene is involved in susceptibility, one would need strong reasons for selecting particular genes to test. A much more feasible approach would be to test polymorphic loci across the genome, analogous to a genomic linkage search. The difficulty here is that, as mentioned above, linkage disequilibrium decays rapidly over time except for very tightly linked loci. Therefore, a genomic search using an allelic association approach would require a very high density map, with markers spaced at 1 cM apart or less, so that 3000 or more markers would be required to provide complete coverage. This would take several years using current technology, so not surprisingly this approach is yet to be tried, although it will undoubtedly become feasible in the future. In the meantime, it is worth noting that the marker data collected in the course of a linkage search can also be used for an allelic association study. For example, a linkage study based on 300 affected sibling pairs will also provide marker data on 600 affected individuals for a 'free' association study.

The feasibility of a genomic search based on linkage disequilibrium can be markedly improved by using populations with favourable structure. Theoretically, the best populations for such a study are those resulting from the recent admixture of two previously isolated populations. If the two founder populations have different frequencies of the disease alleles and marker alleles, linkage disequilibrium can be observed across distances of several centimorgans for several generations [67]. Such admixture has occurred, for example, in African American and Hispanic populations. Another potentially useful situation is where a large population has formed rapidly from a relatively small founder population; this can also lead to disequilibrium over larger distances. For example, the Finnish population has grown from a tiny founder population to about 5 million today over about 100 generations, in relative isolation, and linkage disequilibrium between loci separated by over 2 cM has been reported in this population [68].

One major difficulty which often arises in association studies is the choice of an appropriate control group. Allele frequencies for DNA polymorphisms often vary markedly between different populations and choosing suitable controls for a sample of cases drawn from, say, a hospital in a large ethnically diverse city can be problematic. Moreover, even if a perfectly matched control group is found, artefactual allelic associations can still arise through hidden population stratification, where for example a subset of the population with a distinct founder population has a high risk of the disease and different marker allele frequencies. However, it has been recognized fairly recently that this

difficulty can be avoided completely by the use of within-family controls. The ideal control group for this purpose is provided by the marker alleles in the parents of an affected individual which are not transmitted to their affected offspring [69, 70]. The statistical analysis of such data is extremely simple but elegant – one simply compares the proportion of alleles of a given type which are transmitted from a heterozygous parent with its expected proportion under independent Mendelian segregation, namely 1/2. This procedure has become known as the transmission disequilibrium test, or TDT [69]. One can also use this design to compute relative risks of disease due to a given allele, using the methodology of matched case-control analysis. The only difficulty with this approach is that for many common cancers a high proportion of parents will already be deceased. However, it is possible to construct a similar test, albeit with reduced power, using unaffected siblings as controls.

2.17 DISCUSSION

Linkage analysis has proved an extremely powerful tool for mapping and hence cloning of cancer susceptibility genes, and with the quantity and quality of DNA polymorphisms now available for typing, it is almost certain that a number of other cancer genes will be mapped over the next few years. Currently, the common familial cancers which appear to be most amenable to mapping by linkage analysis in large families include prostate cancer, breast cancer not due to *BRCA*1 or *BRCA*2 (although suitable families are rather rare, as *BRCA*1 and *BRCA*2 account for the majority of high risk families), and perhaps lung cancer. Linkage studies in colorectal cancer families may also still be worthwhile, if a substantial fraction of high-risk families prove not be due to the mismatch repair genes. It should also be feasible to map susceptibility genes for some of the rarer cancers by linkage in small families (such as relative pairs) where the familial relative risk is high, provided that one or two genes explain a high fraction of the familial effect; these include testis cancer, non-medullary thyroid cancer, laryngeal cancer, chronic lymphocytic leukaemia, non-Hodgkin's lymphoma and myeloma [44].

Identifying susceptibility genes for the other common cancers will be more problematic. The familial relative risks are generally less than three-fold, so affected relative pairs lack power to detect linkage unless one gene accounts for all the familial clustering; on the other hand, families with larger numbers of cases are rare, and there is no evidence from segregation analyses to indicate the existence of a gene with a major effect. Another difficult area is families involving several cancer types. For example, a large proportion of families with some features of the Li–Fraumeni syndrome (see Chapter 8) do not appear to be due to *TP*53 mutations. It seems likely that many of these families are genetic, but it is difficult to classify families into groups which might be due to a single gene. Elucidating the genetic basis of these weaker familial effects will require a broader range of strategies, including linkage analyses on a larger scale (probably involving collaborative analyses by several laboratories), direct analysis of candidate genes, use of associated phenotypic markers and linkage disequilibrium.

REFERENCES

1. Dausset, J., Colombani, J. and Hors, J. (1982) Major histocompatibility complex and cancer. *Cancer Surv.*, **1**, 120–47.
2. Simons, M.J., Wee, G.B., Chan, S.H., Shanmugaratnam, K., Day, N.E. and de Thé, G. (1975) Probable identification of an HLA second locus antigen associated with a high risk of nasopharyngeal carcinoma. *Lancet*, **i**, 142–3.
3. Hoskins, L.C., Loux, H.A., Britten, A. and Zamcheck, N. (1965) Distribution of ABO blood groups in patients with pernicious anemia, gastric carcinoma and gastric carcinoma associated with blood group A. *N. Engl. J. Med.*, **273**, 633–7.
4. Botstein, D., White, R., Skolnick, M.H. and Davis, R. (1980) Construction of a genetic linkage map in map using restriction fragment length polymorphisms. *Am. J. Hum. Genet.*, **32**, 314–31.
5. Bodmer, W.F., Bailey, C.J., Bodmer, J. *et al.* (1987) Localisation of the gene for familial adenomatous polyposis on chromosome 5. *Nature*, **328**, 614–16.
6. Mathew, C.G.P., Chin, K.S., Easton, D.F. *et al.* (1987) A linked genetic marker for multiple endocrine neoplasia type 2A on chromosome 10. *Nature*, **328**, 527–8.
7. Simpson, N.E., Kidd, K.K., Goodfellow, P.J. *et al.* (1987) Assignment of multiple endocrine neoplasia type 2A to chromosome 10 by linkage. *Nature*, **328**, 528–30.
8. Peltomaki, L., Aaltonen, L.A., Sistonen, P. *et al.* (1993) Genetic mapping of a locus predisposing to human colorectal cancer. *Science*, **260**, 810–12.
9. Lindblöm, A., Tannergard, P., Werelius, B. and Nordenskjord, M. (1993) Genetic mapping of a second locus predisposing to hereditary non-polyposis colon cancer. *Nature Genet.*, **5**, 279–82.
10. Cannon-Albright, L.A., Goldgar, D.E., Meyer, L.J. *et al.* (1992) Assignment of a locus for familial melanoma, MLM, to chromosome 9p13–p22. *Science*, **258**, 1148–52.
11. Hall, J.M., Lee, M.K., Morrow, J. *et al.* (1990) Linkage analysis of early onset familial breast cancer to chromosome 17q21. *Science*, **250**, 1684–9.
12. Wooster, R., Neuhausen, S., Mangion, J. *et al.* (1994) Localization of a breast cancer susceptibility gene to chromosome 13q12–q13. *Science*, **265**, 2088–90.
13. Easton, D.F., Bishop, D.T., Ford, D., Crockford, G.P. and the Breast Cancer Linkage Consortium (1993) Genetic linkage analysis in familial breast and ovarian cancer: results from 214 families. *Am. J. Hum. Genet.*, **52**, 678–701.

14. Narod, S.A., Ford, D., Devilee, P. *et al.* (1995) An evaluation of genetic heterogeneity in 145 breast-ovarian cancer families. *Am. J. Hum. Genet.*, **56**, 254–64.

15. Stratton, M.R., Ford, D., Neuhausen, S. *et al.* (1994) Familial male breast cancer is not linked to the BRCA1 locus on chromosome 17q. *Nature Genet*, **7**, 103–7.

16. Terwillinger, J.D. and Ott, J. (1994) *Handbook of Human Genetic Linkage*. Johns Hopkins University Press, Baltimore.

17. Morton, N.E. (1955) Sequential tests for the detection of linkage. *Am. J. Hum. Genet.*, **7**, 277–318.

18. Lander, E.S. and Schork, N.J. (1994) Genetic dissection of complex traits. *Science*, **265**, 2037–48.

19. Skolnick, M.H., Thompson, E.A., Bishop, D.T. and Cannon, L.A. (1984) Possible linkage of a breast cancer susceptibility locus to the ABO locus: sensitivity of LOD scores to a single new recombinant observation. *Genet. Epidemiol.*, **1**, 363–73.

20. Weeks, D.E., Lehner, T., Squires-Wheeler, E. *et al.* (1990) Measuring the inflation in the lod score due to its maximisation over model parameter values in human linkage analysis. *Genet. Epidemiol.*, **7**, 237–43.

21. Lathrop, G.M., Lalouel, J.M., Julier, C. and Ott, J. (1984) Strategies for multilocus linkage analysis in humans. *Proc. Natl Acad. Sci. USA*, **81**, 3443–6.

22. Lange, K., Weeks, D. and Boehnke, M. (1988) Programs for pedigree analysis: MENDEL, FISHER and dGENE. *Genet. Epidemiol.*, **5**, 471–2.

23. Cohen, B.B., Porter, D.E., Wallace, M.R., Carothers, A. and Steel, C.M. (1993) Linkage of a major breast cancer gene to chromosome 17q12–21: results from 15 Edinburgh families. *Am. J. Hum. Genet.*, **52**, 723–9.

24. Southern, E.M. (1975) Detection of specific sequences among DNA fragments separated by gel electrophoresis. *J. Mol. Biol.*, **98**, 503–17.

25. Jeffreys, A.J., Wilson, V. and Thein, S.L. (1985) Hypervariable 'minisatellite' regions in human DNA. *Nature*, **314**, 67–73.

26. Weber, J.L. and May, P.E. (1989) Abundant class of human DNA polymorphisms which can be typed using the polymerase chain reaction. *Am. J. Hum. Genet.*, **44**, 388–96.

27. Eeles, R.A. and Stamps, A.C. (1993) *Polymerase Chain Reaction (PCR): the Technique and its Applications*. R.G. Landes, Austin, Texas.

28. Lisitsyn, N., Lisitsyn, N. and Wigler, M. (1993) Cloning the differences between two complex genomes. *Science*, **259**, 946–51.

29. Nelson, S.F., McCusker, J.H., Sander, M.A. *et al.* (1993) Genomic mismatch scanning: a new approach to genetic linkage mapping. *Nature Genet.*, **4**, 11–18.

30. Ott, J. (1978) A simple scheme for the analysis of HLA linkages in pedigrees. *Ann. Hum. Genet.*, **42**, 255–7.

31. Kong, A., Cox, N., Frigge, M. and Irwin, M. (1993) Sequential imputation and multipoint linkage analysis. *Genet. Epidemiol.*, **10**, 483–8.

32. Guo, S.W. and Thompson, E.A. (1992) A monte carlo method for combined segregation and linkage analysis. *Am. J. Hum. Genet.*, **51**, 1111–26.

33. Claus, E.B., Risch, N.J. and Thompson, W.D. (1990) Age at onset as an indicator of familial risk of breast cancer. *Am. J. Epidemiol.*, **131**, 961–72.

34. Hastbacka, J., de la Chapelle, A., Mahtani, M.M. *et al.* (1994) The diastrophic dysplasia gene encodes a novel sulfate transporter – positional cloning by fine structure linkage disequilibrium mapping. *Cell*, **78**, 1073–87

35. Murray, J.C., Buetow, K.H., Weber, J.L. *et al.* (1994) A comprehensive human linkage map with centimorgan density. *Science*, **265**, 2049–54.

36. Smith, C.A.B. (1961) Homogeneity test for linkage data. *Proc. Sec. Int. Congr. Hum. Genet.*, **1**, 212–13.

37. Nyström-Lahti, M., Parsons, R., Sistonen, P. *et al.* (1994) Mismatch repair genes on chromosomes 2p and 3p account for a major share of hereditary nonpolyposis colorectal cancer families evaluable by linkage. *Am. J. Hum. Genet*, **55**, 659–65.

38. Leach, F.S., Nicolaides, N.C., Papadopoulos, N. *et al.* (1993) Mutations of a mutS homolog in hereditary nonpolyposis colorectal cancer. *Cell*, **75**, 1215–25.

39. Lander, E.S. and Botstein, D. (1986) Strategies for studying heterogeneous genetic traits in humans by using a linkage map of restriction

fragment length polymorphisms. *Proc. Natl Acad. Sci. USA*, **83**, 7353–7.

40. Holmans, P. (1993) Asymptotic properties of affected-sib-pair linkage analysis. *Am. J. Hum. Genet.*, **52** 362–74.

41. Risch, N.(1990) Linkage strategies for genetically complex traits. II. The power of affected relative pairs. *Am. J. Hum. Genet.* **46**, 226–41.

42. Bishop, D.T. and Williamson, J.A. (1990) The power of identity-by-state methods for linkage analysis. *Am. J. Hum. Genet.* **46**, 254–65.

43. Weeks, D.E. and Lange, K. (1988) The affected-pedigree-member method of linkage analysis. *Am. J. Hum. Genet.*, **42**, 315–26.

44. Clerget-Darpoux, F., Bonaiti-Pellie, C. and Hochez, J. (1986) Effects of misspecifying genetic parameters in lod score analysis. *Biometrics* **42**, 393–9.

45. Risch, N. and Giuffra, L. (1992) Model misspecification and multipoint linkage analysis. *Human Hered*, **42**, 77–92.

46. Green, P. (1990) Genetic linkage and complex diseases: a comment. *Genet. Epidemiol.*, **7**, 25–7.

47. MacClean, C.J., Bishop, D.T., Sherman, S.L. and Diehl, S.R. (1993) Distribution of lod scores under uncertain mode of inheritance. *Am. J. Hum. Genet.*, **52**, 54–61.

48. Weeks, D.E., Ott, J. and Lathrop, G.M. (1990) SLINK: a general simulation program for linkage analysis. *Am. J. Hum. Genet.* **47**, A204.

49. Ploughman, L.M. and Boehnke, M. (1989) Estimating the power of a proposed linkage study for a complex genetic trait. *Am. J. Hum. Genet.* **44**, 543–51.

50. Goldgar, D.E., Easton, D.F., Cannon-Albright, L. A. and Skolnick, M.H. (1994) A systematic population based assessment of cancer risk in first-degree relatives of cancer probands. *J. Natl Cancer Inst.*, **86**, 1600–8.

51. Easton, D.F. and Goldgar, D.E. (1994) Optimal sampling strategies for detecting linkage of a complex trait with known genetic heterogeneity. *Am. J. Hum. Genet.* **55**, A128.

52. Risch, N. (1984) Segregation analysis incorporating linkage markers. I. Single-locus models with an application to type 1 diabetes. *Am. J. Hum. Genet.*, **36**, 363–86.

53. Greenberg, D.A. (1989) Inferring mode of inheritance by comparison of lod scores. *Am. J. Med. Genet.*, **35**, 480–6.

54. Knudson, A. G. (1971) Mutation and cancer: a statistical study of retinoblastoma. *Proc. Natl Acad. Sci. USA*, **68**, 820–3.

55. Cavenee, W.K., Dryja, T.P., Phillips, R. A. *et al.* (1983) Expression of recessive alleles by chromosomal mechanisms in retinoblastoma. *Nature*, **305**, 779–89.

56. Smith, S.A., Easton, D.F., Evans, D.G.R. and Ponder, B.A.J. (1992) Allele losses in the region 17q12–q21 in familial breast and ovarian cancer involve the wild type chromosome. *Nature Genet.*, **2**, 128-31.

57. Rebbeck, T.R., Lustbader, E.D., and Buetow, K.H. (1994) Somatic allele loss in genetic linkage analysis of cancer. *Genet. Epidemiol.*, **11**, 419–29.

58. Easton, D.F. and Bishop, D.T. The power of linkage analysis to detect cancer susceptibility genes using affected relative pairs and loss of heterozygosity data in tumours. In preparation.

59. Burt, R.W., Cannon-Albright, L.A., Bishop, D.T. *et al.* (1993) Familial factors in sporadic adenomas and colorectal cancer. *Problems in General Surgery*, **10**, 688–94.

60. Green, A. and Swerdlow, A.J. (1989) Epidemiology of melanocytic naevi. *Epidemiol. Rev.*, **11**, 204–21.

61. Scott, D., Jones, L.A., Elyan, S.A.G. *et al.* (1992) Identification of A-T heterozygotes, in *Ataxia–Telangiectasia*, (eds R.A. Gatti and R.B. Painter), Springer-Verlag, pp. 101–16.

62. Barnes, D.M., Hanby, A.M., Gillett, C.E. *et al.* (1992) Abnormal expression of wild type p53 protein in normal cells of a cancer family patient. *Lancet*, **340**, 259–63.

63. Goldgar, D.E., Cannon-Albright, L.A., Meyer, L.J. *et al.* (1992) Inheritance of nevus number and size in melanoma/DNS kindreds. *Cytogenet. Cell Genet*, **59**, 200–2.

64. Risch, N. and Sherman, S. (1992) Genetic Analysis Workshop 7: summary of the melanoma workshop. *Cytogenet. Cell Genet.*, **59**, 148–58.

65. Krontiris, T.G., Devlin, B., Karp, D.D., Robert, N.J. and Risch, N. (1993) An association between the risk of cancer and mutations in the Hras1 minisatellite locus. *N. Engl. J. Med.*, **329**, 517–23.

66. Weir, B.S. (1990) *Genetic Data Analysis: Methods for Discrete Population Genetic Data*. Sinauer, Sunderland, MA.

67. Stephens, J.C., Briscoe, D. and O'Brien, S.J. (1994) Mapping by admixture linkage disequilibrium in human populations: limits and guidelines. *Am. J. Hum. Genet.*, **55**, 603–860.

68. Peterson, A., Slatkin, M., DiRienzo, A., Lehesjoki, A., de la Chapelle, A. and Freimer, N. (1994) A genomic survey of linkage disequilibrium. *Am. J. Hum. Genet.*, **55**, A124.

69. Spielman, R.S., McGinnis, R.E. and Ewens, W.J. (1993) Transmission disequilibrium test for linkage disequilibrium: the insulin gene region and insulin-dependent diabetes mellitus (IDDM). *Am. J. Hum. Genet.*, **52**, 506–16.

70. Self, S., Longton, G., Kopecky, K. and Liang, K.-Y. (1991) On estimating HLA/disease association with application to a study of aplastic anaemia. *Biometrics*, **47**, 53–61.

Chapter 3

From chromosomes to genes: how to isolate cancer-predisposition genes

HELEN PATTERSON and COLIN COOPER

3.1 INTRODUCTION

Linkage analysis in cancer families and the observation of rare cytogenetic abnormalities in the germline DNA of affected individuals can be used to identify the chromosomal location of the genetic defect associated with a familial cancer trait, as described in Chapter 2. The resolution of genetic mapping involving large consortium studies and multiple highly polymorphic marker probes is of the order of 1–2 cM, which corresponds to approximately 1–2 megabases (Mb). This compares to the size of whole chromosomes, which is of the order of 50 to 300 Mb.

A variety of techniques has been developed that allow candidate genes, typically spanning up to 100 kb of genomic DNA, to be isolated from the loci implicated in linkage and cytogenetic studies. Some techniques, such as conventional Southern analysis, cloning in phage and cosmid vectors and chromosome walking, allow cloning and mapping over short distances, whereas newer techniques such as pulse field gel electrophoresis,

the use of linking and jumping libraries, and cloning in yeast artificial chromosomes allow cloning and mapping over regions spanning several megabases (Figure 3.1). By combining these techniques it has been possible to devise flexible strategies for cloning cancer predisposition genes.

The aim of this chapter is to provide an understanding of these molecular strategies and the ways they have been employed to clone familial cancer genes such as the retinoblastoma gene (RB), a Wilms tumour gene (WT1), the gene for type I neurofibromatosis (NFI), and for familial adenomatous polyposis coli (APC). Terminology is defined in the Glossary.

3.2 PHYSICAL MAPPING TECHNIQUES

Once the chromosomal fragment implicated in a cancer predisposition syndrome has been identified by linkage or cytogenetic analyses, the next step in defining the gene locus, with sufficient accuracy to proceed with molecular

Genetic Predisposition to Cancer. Edited by R.A. Eeles, B.A.J. Ponder, D.F. Easton and A. Horwich. Published in 1996 by Chapman & Hall, London.
0 412 56580 3

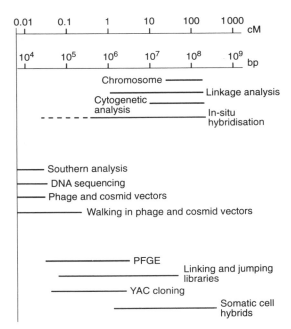

Fig. 3.1 Resolution of genetic and physical mapping techniques. The diagram illustrates the relative resolving capacities of the genetic and physical mapping and cloning techniques employed to clone cancer genes. Pulse field gel electrophoresis (PFGE), jumping and linking libraries and cloning in yeast using YAC vectors conveniently span the gap in resolution between conventional cloning and genetic mapping. The resolution of physical mapping and cloning techniques are given in base pairs (bp) and genetic mapping in centimorgans (cM). Although the relationship is not linear, 1 cM is approximately equivalent to 1×10^6 base pairs.

cloning, requires the availability of a large number of genetic probes from the region of interest and a means with which to map them.

3.2.1 SOMATIC CELL HYBRIDS

The development and use of somatic cell hybrids has been invaluable in promoting physical mapping projects. The basic methodology involves the rescue of human chromosomes or DNA fragments within rodent cells, thus allowing analysis of fragments of the human genome in isolation. Human–rodent hybrids are typically created by the fusion of human and rodent cells using Sendai virus, polyethylene glycol (PEG) or by the application of an electric field. Such hybrids, which may initially contain a complete set of parental chromosomes, are unstable in culture and typically a number of the human chromosomes are lost. Eventually, relatively stable hybrids retaining a reduced number of randomly selected human chromosomes are obtained. Hybrid clones retaining specific human chromosomes can be obtained by growth in selective media, or by screening for cell surface antigens encoded by genes on the chromosomes of interest. For example, addition of aminopterin to the culture media will inhibit cell division by blocking nucleotide synthesis. Salvage pathway enzymes such as thymidine kinase (chromosome 17), hypoxanthine–guanine phosphoribosyltransferase (chromosome X) and adenine phosphoribosyltransferase (chromosome 16) can overcome this inhibition provided that the culture medium is supplemented with thymidine and hypoxanthine or adenine. Rodent cells which lack these enzymes are chosen for hybrid preparation and in this way hybrids selectively retaining chromosomes X, 16 and 17 can be obtained.

Hybrids containing a more restricted quantity of human DNA can be obtained by microcell fusion, or by transfecting rodent cells with cell-free preparations of human chromosomes using calcium phosphate precipitation. In some cases fragments of human chromosomes of sufficient size to be characterized cytogenetically are taken up and stably incorporated in the rodent genome. In a further refinement, irradiation can be used to fragment chromosomal DNA which is again rescued by fusion with rodent cells. The initial cell is typically a hybrid containing a single human chromosome or fragment thereof. Irradiation-induced hybrids can be used to produce a panel of overlapping subchromosomal fragments which can be used to map the locus of a gene defect. The technique was successfully used to produce a complete physical map at the Wilms tumour locus (see p. 46).

Panels of hybrid clones each containing a different selection of human chromosomes or chromosomal fragments, can be used to ascribe chromosomal location to new genetic probes. Hybrids of particular importance in mapping projects are those carrying the deleted or translocated chromosomes from patients with familial cancer traits, in the absence of the normal homologue (Figure 3.2).

3.2.2 THE GENERATION OF MAPPING PROBES

Many of the probes used in physical mapping projects are cloned in a random and anonymous manner from genomic libraries generated from DNA which has been enriched for the chromosome or region of interest. This is typically a hybrid cell line containing that chromosome as its only human component, or chromosome-specific DNA obtained from a flow cytometer. Libraries generated from human–rodent hybrids will contain a majority of rodent clones and therefore human clones are first identified by hybridizing the library to a probe complementary to a human-specific repeat sequence such as *Alu*. *Alu*-positive clones are purified, characterized by means of a hybrid panel and clones of interest used in physical mapping projects.

DNA may also be microdissected from specific regions of metaphase chromosomes [1]. The chromosomes, carefully prepared to maintain their integrity for subsequent molecular analysis, are G-banded and individually microdissected for the region of interest using 2 μm glass rods. Approximately 40 copies from the same region are sufficient for

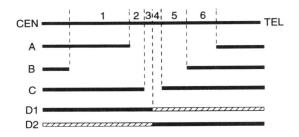

	P1	P2	P3	P4	P5	P6
A	+	-	-	-	-	-
B	-	-	-	-	-	+
C	+	+	-	-	+	+
D1	+	+	+	-	-	-
D2	-	-	-	+	+	+

Fig. 3.2 Physical mapping using hybrids from patients with constitutional deletions or translocations. In this example, hybrids carrying the mutated chromosome in the absence of the normal chromosome are available from three patients with overlapping deletions – A, B and C. Hybrids D1 and D2 carry the derivative chromosomes from a patient with a balanced translocation affecting the same gene. If sufficient appropriately spaced probes are available, this mapping panel will be able to divide the disease gene locus into six regions, 1 to 6, order the available probes within the region, and indicate which probes flank the disease gene most closely. The mapping panel is illustrated, and the results of hybridization of six probes P1→P6 to hybrid DNA are shown in the table below. The results show the order of the probes to be CEN—P1—P2—P3—DISEASE GENE—P4—P5—P6—TEL. CEN, centromeric; TEL, telomeric.

efficient amplification using the polymerase chain reaction (PCR). Two methods have typically been used to generate libraries of novel, region-specific probes using PCR. Sequences which lie between *Alu* repeat sequences can be amplified with *Alu*-specific primers [2]; alternatively the microdissected DNA is digested with a frequently cutting restriction enzyme, and short, synthetic DNA sequences called **linkers** are ligated to either end of the restriction fragments which are then amplified with linker specific primers. PCR products are cloned into plasmid vectors for subsequent analysis.

3.2.3 FLUORESCENT *IN SITU* HYBRIDIZATION (FISH)

In situ hybridization of metaphase or interphase chromosomes provides a visually direct way to map DNA probes. Appropriately prepared metaphase chromosomes are hybridized to biotinylated or digoxigenin-labelled DNA probes (typically cosmid inserts) and pre-annealed with repetitive DNA to avoid non-specific hybridization. Probe hybridization is detected using a fluorochrome bound to avidin or anti-digoxigenin antibodies. The limits of resolution of differentially labelled probes using metaphase chromosomes is of the order of 1–2 Mb, and with interphase nuclei is of the order of 50–100 kb. Recently, techniques using FISH to map stretched DNA released from interphase nuclei have been developed, and this allows the ordered mapping of probes separated by as little as 5–10 kb.

3.2.4 RESTRICTION ENZYMES: SITE-SPECIFIC DNA CLEAVAGE

Restriction enzymes are endonucleases derived from bacteria. They cleave double-stranded DNA at specific restriction sites determined by the exact nucleotide sequence. The restriction enzymes most frequently employed in the laboratory cleave DNA on average every 250–5000 bp. Much larger DNA fragments can be produced by carefully limiting the extent to which DNA is digested by these enzymes, or by digesting DNA with enzymes which will cut DNA only rarely.

Table 3.1 Examples of restriction enzymes useful in pulse field gel analysis of genomic DNA

Enzyme	Recognition site
*Not*I	GC/GGCCGC
*Sfi*I	GGCCNNNN/NGGCC
*Bss*HII	G/CGCGC
*Eag*I	C/GGCCG
*Nae*I	GCC/GGC
*Nru*I	TCG/CGA
*Sac*II	CCGC/GG
*Xho*I	C/TCGAG

N, any nucleotide, /, enzyme cleavage site.

Enzymes which cut DNA infrequently, such as *Not*I and *Sfi*I, have recognition sites requiring the occurrence of a specific 8-bp sequence, others have a 6-bp recognition sequence with a high C (cytosine) and G (guanine) content containing one or more CpG dinucleotides (Table 3.1). The CpG dinucleotide is significantly underrepresented in the mammalian genome, and is often methylated on cytosine, a modification which frequently blocks restriction enzyme cleavage. Clusters of rare cutter enzyme sites occur in what are known as HTF islands (Hpa II tiny fragments). These are small G- and C-rich regions of the genome with a high percentage of unmethylated CpG dinucleotides accessible to restriction enzyme cleavage. HTF islands are frequently associated with the 5' regions of actively transcribed genes, and therefore clusters of rare cutter sites can be used as pointers to the sites of these genes.

3.2.5 PULSE FIELD GEL ELECTROPHORESIS (PFGE): SIZE SEPARATION OF VERY LARGE DNA FRAGMENTS

Conventional agarose gel electrophoresis using a constant electrical field can be used to separate DNA fragments on the basis of molecular size up to a few tens of kilobases. This range of size separation can be extended to around 2–4 Mb by the application of pulsed, alternating orthogonal or inverted electrical fields to the gel [3]. Genomic DNA for pulse field gel analysis must be handled with great care, and conventional means of DNA preparation are inappropriate as they subject DNA to random shearing into fragments of around 100 kb or less which will interfere with subsequent analysis. High molecular weight DNA is typically prepared by embedding cultured cells in agarose blocks in which cell lysis, proteolysis and restriction enzyme digestion take place. The blocks are subsequently loaded into wells in the gel before electrophoresis. Subsequent Southern blotting produces a permanent record of these size-separated large DNA fragments. Sequential hybridization of multiple single copy probes to blots produced following the digestion of high molecular weight DNA with different combinations of rarely cutting restriction enzymes should allow all the DNA in a region of interest to be visualized and eventually ordered as a series of large restriction fragments. The location of a cancer gene within this physical map can be determined when hybridization of one of the mapping probes to a Southern blot of pulse field separated DNA demonstrates a deletion or rearrangement in the germline of a patient with the familial cancer trait. This probe provides an excellent starting point with which to clone the cancer gene.

3.3 CLONING STRATEGIES

3.3.1 LINKING AND JUMPING LIBRARIES

The development of a complete physical map, however, requires that sufficient numbers of appropriately spaced probes are available to identify and order all the restriction fragments in the region of interest. Frequently, sufficient numbers of probes are not available. Linking and jumping libraries are particularly useful in this respect as they are specifically designed to contain clones spaced at intervals of 100–1000 kb with deletion of the intervening DNA. Linking libraries [4] (Figure 3.3(a)) contain clones which consist of small regions of DNA on either side of a rare restriction enzyme site, for example *Not*I. A comprehensive *Not*I linking library will therefore contain clones which will identify all of the *Not*I fragments in a region of interest and will in addition identify adjacent restriction fragments. Jumping libraries are designed to contain clones which possess short sequences from either end of the same restriction fragment with selective deletion of all of the intervening DNA [5] (Figure 3.3(b)). Linking and jumping libraries can be used in a complementary fashion if they are constructed using the same rarely cutting restriction enzyme, as each jumping clone will identify two adjacent linking clones and likewise, each linking clone, will identify two jumping clones (Figure 3.3(c)). If clones from either library are used to screen the other library, it is possible, in principle, to walk and jump from clone to clone to generate an ordered map of the region. The concurrent use of these probes in PFGE analysis will provide the required information regarding the distance separating adjacent clones to generate a complete physical map of the region. It is of particular importance that clones from linking and jumping libraries constructed using rarely cutting enzymes will often contain HTF islands lying in the vicinity of actively transcribed genes. Such clones therefore provide a means with which to approach candidate genes in a region of interest.

3.3.2 CLONING LARGE REGIONS OF CONTIGUOUS DNA

Vectors based on bacteriophage lambda can be used to clone DNA fragments of up to 20–40 kb in a single step. This limitation on the size of clonable DNA fragments is caused by the limited capacity of the lambda phage head, used in both cosmid and phage cloning as a highly efficient means of introducing DNA into bacterial cells. Although this limitation can be overcome to a certain extent by chromosome walking (Figure 3.4), the technique is hindered by the fact that each step usually extends the region of contiguously cloned DNA by much less than the size of the insert accommodated by the vector, and the occurrence in human DNA of both highly repetitive and unclonable regions makes the method impractical for covering very extensive regions.

The development of a yeast artificial chromosome (YAC) by Olson and his colleagues in 1987 [6] allowing the propagation of large DNA molecules as linear, artificial chromosomes in the yeast *Saccharomyces cerevisiae* has been a major advance, allowing the cloning in a single step of up to 1 Mb of genomic DNA. The YAC vector is equivalent to a plasmid which supplies a cloning site within a gene whose interruption is phenotypically visible, an autonomously replicating region, a centromere flanked by selectable markers and two sequences which seed telomere formation *in vivo*. These features allow the YAC vector and its insert to be replicated alongside yeast chromosomal DNA, and for yeasts replicating YAC inserts to be selected. The cloning protocol is very similar to that employed in phage cloning systems. The YAC vector is cleaved to reveal two vector arms which are then ligated to large insert molecules generated by the partial or complete digestion of high molecular weight genomic DNA. The ligation products are then used to transform yeast spheroplasts. Typically, YACs carry inserts of 200–500 kb as single fragments, which is frequently sufficient to clone the entire region of interest in a single step. 'Walking' in YAC libraries can be used to generate more extensive regions of contiguously cloned DNA.

Although YACs frequently contain chimaeric inserts and have a tendency to develop internal deletions during their propagation, they are becoming increasingly invaluable in cloning projects. For example, they were used to clone 5.5 Mb of DNA from the *APC* locus on chromosome 5q, rapidly facilitating the cloning of the *APC* gene.

3.3.3   P1/BAC CLONING

Additional large insert DNA cloning systems have been developed in order to avoid the problems of insert instability and chimaerism associated with the YAC system. One of these uses a bacteriophage P1-based vector [7]. This vector will maintain stable inserts in the 70–100 kb size range and allows for the selection of recombinants over non-recombinants. A second system uses a BAC (bacterial artificial chromosome) vector based on the *E. coli* F factor [8]. This vector is capable of maintaining inserts up to 300 kb in size. An additional advantage of these two systems over YACs is the comparative ease with which the cloned DNA can be isolated and manipulated. This results from their circular plasmid structure as opposed to the linear structure of YACs. Both P1 and BAC clones were used in the recent isolation of the breast cancer susceptibility gene *BRCA*1 [9] (see Chapter 15).

3.4   ANALYSIS OF CLONED DNA FOR CANDIDATE GENES

As an alternative to sequencing long stretches of DNA and searching the sequence for open reading frames, a number of strategies have been developed to identify exons efficiently in genomic clones. One of the simplest, but also most time consuming, involves the hybridization of single-copy genomic subclones to Southern blots carrying

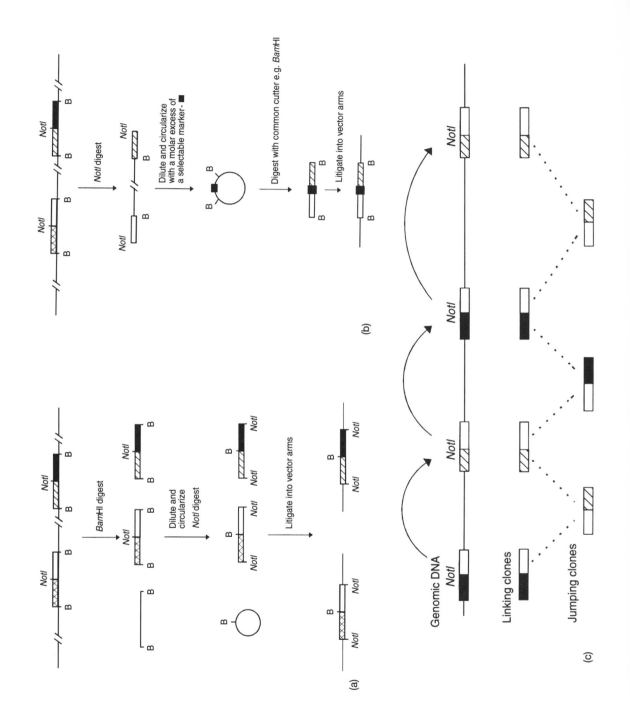

Digest with common cutter e.g. *Bam*HI

Dilute and circularize
with a molar excess of
a selectable marker - ■

*Not*I digest

Litigate into vector arms

(b)

*Bam*HI digest

Dilute and
circularize

*Not*I digest

Litigate into vector arms

(a)

Genomic DNA

Linking clones

Jumping clones

(c)

the DNA of several species (zoo blots). Clones which demonstrate cross-species hybridization carry sequences conserved between species, a feature of the coding region of genes. Such fragments can be used to probe Northern blots to assess tissue and tumour expression of the candidate gene, to confirm the size of the transcribed message and to identify cDNA clones corresponding to the gene. Alternatively, genomic fragments including whole cosmid and whole YAC inserts can be used to screen cDNA libraries directly, provided cross-hybridization of repetitive elements is adequately blocked by prehybridizing the library to total human DNA. In a third method, direct cDNA selection [10], genomic DNA usually in the form of overlapping cosmids or YAC DNA, is biotinylated and hybridized to a PCR-amplified cDNA library. Hybrid DNA is purified on streptavidin-coated magnetic beads, single-stranded PCR product eluted and then reamplified. After three rounds of hybridization–amplification the 'selected' cDNAs are cloned into plasmid vectors for analysis. A fourth method, 'exon trapping' [11], also allows the selective cloning of exonic sequences from genomic fragments. The technique makes use of a mammalian expression vector containing an intron flanked by 5' splice donor and 3' splice acceptor sequences. Genomic fragments of up to 10 kb are cloned within the intron and the vector transfected into appropriate mammalian cells. Gene expression requires that, following transcription, intronic sequences are spliced out to produce messenger RNA (mRNA) before translation. The splicing process depends upon the presence of specific splice donor and acceptor sequences at intron–exon boundaries. If the cloned genomic fragment contains exonic sequence, this will be spliced to vector sequence during mRNA production, which takes place following transfection, with the loss of the remaining genomic sequence. The 'trapped' exon is then amplified from mRNA by PCR (following cDNA synthesis), and the product cloned and sequenced. The identification of actively transcribed genes in the regions of HTF islands using linking and jumping libraries has already been discussed.

3.5 CLONING OF THE RETINOBLASTOMA GENE

Retinoblastoma is a childhood tumour of the developing retina which exists in sporadic

Fig. 3.3 (a) Construction of a *Not*I linking library. Genomic DNA, typically from a hybrid carrying the chromosome region of interest, or from flow-sorted chromosomes, is first digested with a frequently cutting enzyme such as *Bam*HI (B). The DNA is then diluted to a very low concentration to favour circularization during the ligation reaction. Subsequent cleavage with *Not*I will generate a subset of linear DNA fragments, representing the junction between adjacent *Not*I fragments. These are cloned into phage vector arms and propagated in bacteria. Human clones which map to the region of interest can be used in PFG analysis to create a physical map of the region. (b) Construction of a *Not*I jumping library requires the very careful preparation of high molecular weight DNA from an appropriate source. The DNA is then digested to completion with *Not*I, diluted and circularized in the presence of a molar excess of a selectable genetic marker. Subsequent digestion with a frequently cutting enzyme (B) will yield short junction fragments representing opposite ends of the same *Not*I restriction fragment. Junction fragments are recognized within the library by the presence of the selectable marker. (c) Complementation of linking and jumping libraries. Each *Not*I jumping clone will identify two adjacent linking clones when used to screen a *Not*I linking library. These linking clones when used in turn to screen the jumping library, will identify a novel jumping clone. In this way the region can be rapidly cloned in a series of jumps.

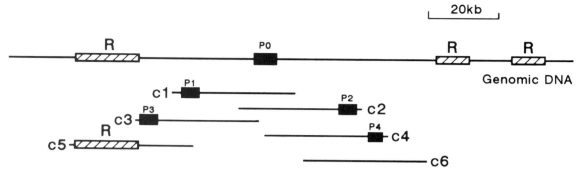

Fig. 3.4 Chromosome walking. An initial probe P0, in a region of interest is used to screen a partially digested genomic library and identify cosmid clones c1 and c2. Once orientated with respect to one another, single-copy probes are isolated from opposite ends of this cosmid contig and are used to rescreen the library, identifying cosmids c3 and c4, and extending the region of contiguously cloned DNA in both directions. Each round of walking is time consuming, requiring that the library is screened with the new probes, and positive clones purified, characterized and orientated within the contig, before being analysed for a distal single-copy fragment which will act as a probe for the next round of walking. The presence of regions of densely repetitive DNA (R) can completely block the progress in one or both directions. For example, cosmid c5 is unable to extend the contig further, as any probe from its distal end will identify multiple non-contiguous cosmid clones within the library.

and hereditary forms. It is discussed further in Chapter 4.

Cytogenetic observations of deletions of the long arm of chromosome 13 in the germline DNA of patients with hereditary retinoblastoma and in retinoblastoma tumours, gave rise to the hypothesis that retinoblastomas arose as a result of mutations in both alleles of a gene, possibly a tumour suppressor gene on the long arm of chromosome 13. Additional cytogenetic analyses demonstrated that the deletion centred on 13q14, and pedigree analysis demonstrated tight linkage of the retinoblastoma trait to the polymorphic enzyme esterase D [12].

Since nothing could be gleaned from the phenotype of patients with retinoblastoma of the structure or function of the retinoblastoma gene product, molecular cloning by reverse genetics was based on the chromosomal location of the retinoblastoma gene and the hypothesis that the gene would be expressed in normal retinoblasts, but not in retinoblastomas. The general strategy em-

ployed by several groups in the mid 1980s was to isolate DNA probes which localized to chromosome 13q14 and to 'walk' along chromosome 13 in both directions screening the contiguously cloned DNA periodically for features which indicated that it encoded a gene.

Tight linkage of esterase D to the retinoblastoma trait indicated that this gene would provide a useful starting point for such a chromosome walk. A partial amino acid sequence was deduced by analysis of the purified protein, and this sequence used to design a molecular probe with which to clone the esterase D gene. A bidirectional chromosome walk then isolated 120 kb of overlapping genomic clones at the esterase D locus and single-copy probes derived from these overlapping clones were used to screen cDNA libraries. Two cDNA clones were isolated but neither proved to represent a suitable candidate retinoblastoma gene.

At the same time a number of anonymous probes, cloned at random from a flow-sorted chromosome 13 genomic library [13] were available. Two probes, H2–42 and H3–8, were putatively assigned to 13q14 by the demonstration, using Southern analysis and densitometry, that they were hemizygously deleted in the germline DNA of an individual with a cytogenetic deletion of 13q14. Their location was confirmed by *in situ* hybridization. H3–8 was subsequently shown to be homozygously deleted in three out of 37 retinoblastomas examined [14], a feature which suggested it lay very close to the retinoblastoma gene. This probe was also used to initiate a second chromosome walk, and single copy probes were generated from 30 kb of contiguous genomic clones. One of these, p7H30.7R, demonstrated cross-species hybridization to mouse DNA and detected a 4.7 kb transcript in retinal RNA. The corresponding cDNA was subsequently cloned from a human retinal cDNA library. Expression of this gene was absent in retinoblastomas in which the gene was specifically mutated, consistent with the genetic criteria required of a candidate retinoblastoma gene [15, 16]. Confirmation that this cDNA did indeed represent the *RB* gene came from experiments in which the gene was expressed under the influence of a retroviral promoter in retinoblastoma cells lacking endogenous *RB* expression [17]. Expression of exogenous *RB* caused morphological changes and reduced the growth rate of these cells in culture. Most importantly, when transfected and previously tumourigenic cells were injected into nude mice, tumourigenicity was completely suppressed.

3.6 CLONING OF THE WILMS TUMOUR GENE

Wilms tumour is described in detail in Chapter 7.

Some patients with Wilms tumour (WT) suffer from a rare congenital dysplasia of the iris (aniridia, AN2), genitourinary abnormalities and mental retardation, the so-called WAGR syndrome. The 11p13 region was first implicated in the development of Wilms tumour by the observation of constitutional cytogenetic deletions in patients with WAGR.

As a first step towards the isolation of the Wilms tumour gene, lymphoblastoid cell lines were established from WAGR patients possessing cytogenetically visible constitutional deletions involving 11p13, and from aniridia patients with balanced translocations involving 11p13. These were then used to establish hybrid cell lines segregating the mutated chromosome 11 from the normal homologue. Cytogenetic analysis of constitutional deletions, and subsequent molecular analysis of hybrid DNA using probes for erythrocyte catalase (CAT) and the beta subunit of follicle-stimulating hormone (FSHB), both assigned to the WAGR locus at an early stage, and correlation of these findings with the phenotype exhibited by the corresponding patients, indicated that the order of genes in 11p13 was CEN–CAT–WT–AN2–FSHB–TEL [18, 19].

Subsequent analyses concentrated on further delineation of the *WT* locus using anonymous single-copy probes and extensive WAGR deletion panels. The anonymous probes, characterized by their differential hybridization patterns within the deletion panel, were used to establish physical maps of the WAGR locus using PFGE analysis. However, the shortage of probes within the WAGR locus meant that such maps were frequently incomplete.

Rose and colleagues [20] were able to produce a complete pulse field map and define the interval containing the *WT* gene using Goss–Harris irradiation-reduced hybrids. A hybrid cell line carrying 11p as its only human component was irradiated to fragment its DNA and the fragments rescued by fusion with hamster cells. Hybrid clones retaining the WAGR locus were selected by

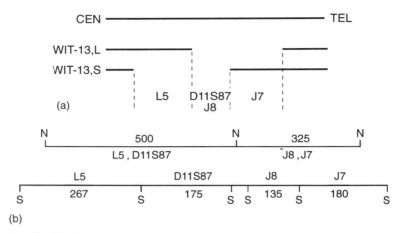

(a)

(b)

Fig. 3.5 Mapping the *WT* locus. (a) The position of the *WT* gene within the physical map was defined by analysis of a spontaneous Wilms tumour (WIT-13) possessing overlapping deletions involving the Wilms tumour locus. The chromosome carrying the distal deletion, WIT,L, defined the proximal boundary of the homozygously deleted region, and its homologue, WIT, S, which carries the proximal deletion, was used to define the distal boundary. Southern analysis of WIT,S and WIT,L hybrid DNA demonstrated that probes L5, D11S87 and J8 were deleted on the WIT,S chromosome with J7 retained, whereas J7, J8 and D11S87 were deleted on the WIT,L chromosome with L5 retained. Probes L5 and J8 therefore flanked the WT locus. (b) Subsequent pulse field gel electrophoresis demonstrated that probes L5 and D11S87 detected a 500 kb *Not*I fragment, whereas J7 and J8 detected a 325 kb fragment. The order of the probes defining the *WT* locus was therefore, CEN—L5—D11S87—J8—J7—TEL. The *WT* locus was more accurately defined using an *Sfi*I digest. L5, D11S87, J8 and J7 detected four *Sfi*I fragments of 267 kb, 175 kb, 135 kb and 180 kb respectively. (An additional 34 kb fragment mapping between the 175 kb and 135 kb fragments and carrying the *Not*I site was detected by concurrent examination of contiguous cosmids within the region.) As the 267 kb and 180 kb *Sfi*I fragments were shown to be unaffected by the deletions in WIT-13, the *WT* locus was limited to three *Sfi*I fragments spanning 345 kb genomic DNA. The genomic clone J8 was subsequently shown to contain exonic sequence of a gene whose narrow range of tissue expression included adult and fetal kidney.

screening for the cell surface antigen MICl, and the fragment of 11p retained, characterized using existing 11p13 probes. Because these hybrids contained so little human DNA, it could all be visualized as discrete pulse field restriction fragments using a human *Alu*-repeat probe. At the same time, genomic libraries constructed from the same hybrids provided a rich source of additional probes in and around the WAGR locus. The assignment of at least one single-copy probe to each of the pulse field restriction fragments identified by *Alu*-hybridization, and the use of single, double and partial digests to order

the restriction fragments, then allowed the production of a complete physical map of the WAGR locus. By examination of the end-points of small constitutional deletions (Figure 3.5) the *WT* gene was limited to a region within the map spanning 345 kb. A probe within this region demonstrating cross-species hyridization also detected a 3-kb transcript in fetal and adult kidney and in spleen. Several cDNAs corresponding to a transcription factor designated *WT1*, were subsequently cloned [21].

Gessler and colleagues [22] cloned the same gene using a different approach. They used a probe thought to be close to the *WT* gene, and containing a *Bss*HII cutting site, to screen a *Bss*HII jumping library. They identified four adjacent junction fragments, each representing a CpG island, by means of two consecutive bidirectional jumps. Conserved sequences identified in the flanking DNA of one of these junction fragments represented exonic sequence encoding a transcription factor highly expressed in fetal kidney – the same *WT*1 gene.

3.7 CLONING OF THE NEUROFIBROMATOSIS TYPE 1 GENE

Von Recklinghausen neurofibromatosis (NF1) is described in Chapter 5.

In 1987 the *NF*1 gene was linked by linkage analysis to a polymorphic probe, D17ZI, located near the centromere of chromosome 17. Subsequent analysis of nearly 200 *NF*1 families studied by over 30 groups worldwide, placed the *NF*1 gene in a 3 cM region flanked by the markers HHH202 and EW206. Additional evidence that the *NF*1 gene was flanked by these markers came from analyses of two balanced translocations t(1;17)(q34.3;q11.2) and t(17;22)(q11.2;q11.2) in two individuals with *NF*1 from separate pedigrees. These translocation breakpoints, flanked by HHH202 and EW206, provided crucial landmarks pinpointing the *NF*1 gene.

Physical mapping was carried out by two groups. Fountain and colleagues [23] used probes from a chromosome 17 linking library, which had been mapped to 17q11, to construct a 2.3-Mb pulse field map of the *NF*1 locus. One of their linking clones, 17L1, detected a rearrangement in the DNA of the individual with the t(1;17) translocation on pulsed field analysis. Reference to their physical map indicated that this probe lay within 240kb of the *NF*1 gene [23]. O'Connell and colleagues [24] used microcell hybrids, containing fragments of chromosome 17 spanning the *NF*1 locus, to construct cosmid libraries. Human cosmid clones from these libraries were mapped to 17q11.2 by means of a hybrid mapping panel, and were then used to produce a high-resolution physical map at the *NF*1 locus. One of these cosmids, c11-1F10, detected a 600-kb *Nru*I fragment rearranged in both the t(1;17) and t(17;22) translocations [24].

Fine mapping using cosmid walking, chromosome jumping and YAC cloning initiated from 17L1 and c11-1F10 demonstrated that the translocation breakpoints were approximately 60 kb apart. Subsequent analyses concentrated on the region between the breakpoints and identified three small genes, EV12, RC1 and OMGP. However, none of these genes was shown to be specifically mutated in *NF*1 patients. Finally, an additional fragment conserved between mouse and man was identified, and used to clone a large, ubiquitously expressed, and highly conserved gene interrupted by both translocation breakpoints [25, 26]. This gene contained the three genes EV12, RC1 and OMGP within a single large intron! Deletions and point mutations of this gene were demonstrated in additional *NF*1 patients, providing further evidence that this was the elusive *NF*1 gene.

3.8 FAMILIAL ADENOMATOUS POLYPOSIS COLI (APC)

APC, also known as FAP (familial polyposis coli), is a dominantly inherited cancer predisposition syndrome in which affected individuals develop numerous benign colorectal polyps by the second or third decade of life. There is an extremely high incidence of subsequent colorectal neoplasia (see Chapter 20).

Demonstration of a rare cytogenetic deletion of chromosome 5q21 in an APC patient provided the first clue as to the location of the gene. Subsequent pedigree analysis confirmed linkage of the trait to 5q21, and eventually limited the gene to an 8-cM region flanked by two cosmid markers tightly linked to the gene. Kinzler and colleagues [27] used numerous probes from 5q21 to screen a YAC library and cloned 5.5 Mb of genomic DNA from the *APC* locus in six separate contigs. These contigs were screened for exonic sequence using cross-species hybridization and cDNA library screening. Six genes, including the *APC* gene were identified and sequenced. Mutations of the *APC* gene were demonstrated in the germline of patients with *APC* and Gardner's syndrome, and in sporadic colorectal tumours. A second group narrowed the *APC* gene locus to a region of 100 kb, by analysis of small nested deletions in two *APC* patients [28]. cDNA screening using YACs spanning the deletion identified the same *APC* gene, and mutations in *APC* patients were confirmed.

3.9 CANDIDATE GENES

In contrast to the *RB*, *WT1*, *NF1* and *APC* genes, the genes responsible for the Li–Fraumeni syndrome, multiple endocrine neoplasia (MEN) types 2A and 2B, familial medullary thyroid carcinoma (FMTC) and hereditary non-polyposis coli (HNPCC) were first identified by alternative approaches and subsequently analysed as candidate genes for their respective cancer syndromes.

3.9.1 *TP53* AND THE LI–FRAUMENI SYNDROME

TP53 protein was first identified as a protein bound to the large T antigen in SV40 transformed cells. Although mutant *TP53* demonstrated the ability to transform primary cells when co-transfected with activated *ras*, wild-type *TP53* was shown conclusively in transfection experiments to be a tumour suppressor gene. Mutation of the *TP53* gene has been demonstrated in a significant proportion of every human tumour type examined, and its

contribution to human tumourigenesis is thought to be enormous. The *TP53* gene therefore represented a tumour suppressor gene looking for a syndrome, rather than a syndrome looking for a gene. The Li–Fraumeni syndrome, first described in 1969, is an autosomal dominant familial disorder in which childhood sarcomas are associated with a high risk of early-onset breast cancer and other tumours such as leukaemia, brain tumours and tumours of the adrenal cortex. The risk to affected family members of developing an invasive malignancy approaches 50% by the age of 30. Linkage and cytogenetic analyses failed to define the Li–Fraumeni locus, and germline mutations of the *RB* tumour suppressor gene were not thought to be involved because retinoblastomas were not seen in this syndrome. However, mutations of the *TP53* gene had been demonstrated in many of the tumour types seen in the Li–Fraumeni syndrome and transgenic mice, with germline mutations of the *TP53* gene, also developed a similar spectrum of tumours. Sequencing exonic sequence of the *TP53* gene identified germline mutations in the DNA of individuals from several Li–Fraumeni families [29] confirming the role of *TP53* in this familial cancer syndrome. This syndrome is discussed further in Chapter 8.

3.9.2 *RET* AND MULTIPLE ENDOCRINE NEOPLASIA

The *RET* gene was first identified as a dominantly transforming oncogene, activated by rearrangement in the DNA of papillary thyroid carcinomas, in the NIH3T3 DNA transfection–transformation assay. The gene was then localized to chromosome 10q11.2, the region implicated in the MEN 2A, MEN2B and FMTC syndromes by linkage analysis. Subsequent mutation analysis demonstrated mutations of *RET* in MEN 2A [30, 31], FMTC [31], MEN2B [32] and intriguingly in Hirschsprung's disease (congenital absence of parasympathetic innervation in the intestinal tract), not known to be associated with any form of cancer predisposition. Mutations in different domains of the gene appear to be responsible for the different phenotypes expressed. This is discussed in Chapter 6.

3.9.3 *MSH*2 AND HEREDITARY NON-POLYPOSIS COLON CANCER (HNPCC)

As recently as 1993 the HNPCC syndrome was linked to a telomeric locus on chromosome 2p. PCR amplification of polymorphic microsatellites such as di- and trinucleotide repeats is often used for linkage studies, and during these analyses HNPCC tumours frequently showed replication errors in these microsatellite sequences. A similar phenomenon had been seen in yeast cells possessing a defect in the *mutS* mismatch repair gene. Fishel and colleagues [33] then cloned the human homologue of the *mutS* gene, *MSH*2, and showed that it mapped to human chromosome 2p22. Mutations of the *MSH*2 gene were then demonstrated in affected individuals in HNPCC kindreds [33]. Since this time, further DNA mismatch repair genes have been examined as candidates for hereditary colon cancer genes (see Chapters 20 and 21).

3.10 CONCLUSION

Several approaches can be adopted in the search for familial cancer genes and the strategies which have been used to clone these genes reflect not only the techniques available at the time, but also the expertise and successes within an individual laboratory. Of crucial importance is the availability of cell lines carrying deletions or translocations, which can be identified cytogenetically or defined at the molecular level, as a means of pinpointing the gene. Where such a resource is not available, as with the familial

breast cancer gene on 17q, the only way forward is to clone all the genes in the region defined by multipoint linkage analysis and sequence these genes in affected individuals looking for mutations; a highly labour-intensive process.

The cloning of genes for the common cancers will be high priority over the next few years. Analysis of these genes will provide an understanding of the aetiology of not only the tumours occurring in their respective familial syndromes, but also of their sporadic counterparts.

REFERENCES

1. Ludecke, H.-J., Senger, G., Claussen, U. and Horsthemke, B. (1989) Cloning defined regions of the human genome by micro dissection of banded chromosomes and enzymatic amplification. *Nature*, **338**, 348–50.
2. Nelson, D.L., Ledbetter, S.A., Corbo, L. *et al.* (1989) *Alu* polymerase chain reaction: a method for rapid isolation of human-specific sequences from complex DNA sources. *Proc. Natl Acad. Sci. USA*, **86**, 6686–90.
3. Schwartz, D.C. and Cantor, C.R. (1984) Separation of yeast chromosome-sized DNA's by pulsed field gradient gel electrophoresis. *Cell*, **37**, 67–75.
4. Collins, F.S. and Weissman, S.M. (1984) Directional cloning of DNA fragments at a large distance from an initial probe: a circularization method. *Proc. Natl Acad. Sci. USA*, **81**, 6812–16.
5. Poustka, A. and Lehrach, H. (1986) Jumping libraries and linking libraries: the next generation of molecular tools in mammalian genetics. *Trends Genet*, **2**, 174–9.
6. Burke, D.T., Carle, G.F. and Olson, M.V. (1987) Cloning of large segments of exogenous DNA into yeast by means of artificial chromosome vectors. *Science*, **236**, 806–12.
7. Pierce, J.C., Sauer, B. and Sternberg, N. (1992) A positive selection vector for cloning high molecular weight DNA by the bacteriophage

P1 system: Improved cloning efficacy. *Proc. Natl Acad. Sci. USA*, **89**, 2056–60.

8. Shizuya, H., Birren, B., Kim, U. *et al.* (1992) Cloning and stable maintenance of 300-kilobase-pair fragments of human DNA in *Escherichia coli* using an F-factor-based vector. *Proc. Natl Acad. Sci. USA*, **89**, 8794–7

9. Miki, Y., Swenson, J., Shattuck-Eidens, D. *et al.* (1994) A strong candidate for the breast and ovarian cancer susceptibility gene *BRCA1*. *Science*, **266**, 66–71.

10. Lovett, M., Kere, J. and Hinton, L.M. (1991) Direct selection: a method for the isolation of cDNAs encoded by large genomic regions. *Proc. Natl Acad. Sci. USA*, **88**, 9628–32.

11. Auch, D. and Reth, M. (1990) Exon trap cloning: using PCR to rapidly detect and clone exons from genomic DNA fragments. *Nucleic Acids Res.*, **18**, 6743–4.

12. Sparkes, R.S., Murphree, A.L., Lingua, R.W. *et al.* (1983) Gene for hereditary retinoblastoma assigned to human chromosome 13 by linkage to esterase D. *Science*, **219**, 971–3.

13. Lalande, M., Dryja, T.P., Schreck, R.R. *et al* (1984) Isolation of human chromosome 13-specific DNA sequences cloned from flow sorted chromosomes and potentially linked to the retinoblastoma gene. *Cancer Genet. Cytogenet.*, **13**, 283–95.

14. Dryja, T.P., Rapaport, J.M., Joyce, J.M. and Petersen, R.A. (1986) Molecular detection of deletions involving band q14 of chromosome 13 in retinoblastomas. *Proc. Natl Acad. Sci. USA*, **83**, 7391–4.

15. Friend, S.H., Bernards, R., Rogelj, S. *et al.* (1986) A human DNA segment with properties of the gene that predisposes to retinoblastoma and osteosarcoma. *Nature*, **323**, 643–6.

16. Lee, W.-H., Bookstein, R., Hong, F. *et al.* (1987) Human retinoblastoma susceptibility gene: cloning, identification and sequence. *Science*, **235**, 1394–9.

17. Huang, H.-J.S., Yee, J.-K., Shew, J.-Y. *et al.* (1988) Suppression of the neoplastic phenotype by replacement of the RB gene in human cancer cells. *Science*, **242**, 1563–6.

18. van Heyningen, V., Boyd, P.A., Seawright, A. *et al.* (1985) Molecular analysis of chromosome 11 deletions in aniridia-Wilms' tumour syndrome. *Proc. Natl Acad. Sci. USA*, **82**, 8592–6.

19. Glaser, T., Lewis, W.H., Bruns, G.A.P. *et al.* (1986) The β-subunit of follicle-stimulating hormone is deleted in patients with aniridia and Wilms' tumour, allowing a further definition of the WAGR locus. *Nature*, **321**, 882–7.

20. Rose, E.A., Glaser, T., Jones, C. *et al.* (1990) Complete physical map of the WAGR region of 11p13 localizes a candidate Wilms' tumour gene. *Cell*, **60**, 495–508.

21. Call, K.M., Glaser, T., Ito, C.Y. *et al.* (1990) Isolation and characterization of a zinc finger polypeptide gene at the human chromosome 11 Wilms' tumour locus. *Cell*, **60**, 509–20.

22. Gessler, M., Poustka, A., Cavanee, W. *et al.* (1990) Homozygous deletion in Wilms' tumours of a zinc-finger gene identified by chromosome jumping. *Nature*, **343**, 774–8.

23. Fountain, J.W., Wallace, M.R., Bruce, M.A. *et al.* (1989) Physical mapping of a translocation breakpoint in neurofibromatosis. *Science*, **244**, 1085–7.

24. O'Connell, P., Leach, R., Cawthon, R.M. *et al.* (1989) Two NF1 translocations map within a 600-kilobase segment of 17q11.2. *Science*, **244**, 1087–8.

25. Wallace, M.R., Marchuk, D.A., Andersen, L.B. *et al.* (1990) Type 1 neurofibromatosis gene: identification of a large transcript disrupted in three NF1 patients. *Science*, **249**, 181–6.

26. Viskochil, D., Buchberg, A.M., Xu, G. *et al.* (1990) Deletions and a translocation interrupt a cloned gene at the neurofibromatosis type 1 locus. *Cell*, **62**, 187–92.

27. Kinzler, K.W., Nilbert, M.C., Su, L.–K. *et al.* (1991) Identifiction of FAP locus genes from chromosome 5q21. *Science*, **253**, 661–5.

28. Joslyn, G., Carlson, M., Thliveris, A. *et al.* (1991) Identification of deletion mutations and three new genes at the familial polyposis locus. *Cell*, **66**, 601–13.

29. Malkin, D., Li, F.P., Strong, L.C. *et al.* (1990) Germline p53 mutations in a familial syndrome of breast cancer, sarcomas, and other neoplasms. *Science*, **250**, 1223–8.

30. Mulligan, L.M., Kwok, J.B.J., Healey, C.S. *et al.* (1993) Germ-line mutations of the RET proto-oncogene in multiple endocrine neoplasia type 2A. *Nature*, **363**, 458–60.

31. Donis-Keller, H., Dou, S., Chi, D. *et al.* (1993) Mutations in the RET proto-oncogene are associated with MEN2A and FMTC. *Hum. Molec. Genet.*, **2**, 851–6.

32. Hofstra, R.M.W., Landsvater, R.M., Ceccherini, I. *et al.* (1994) A mutation in the RET proto-oncogene associated with multiple endocrine neoplasia type 2B and sporadic medullary thyroid carcinoma. *Nature*, **367**, 375–6.

33. Fishel, R., Lescoe, M.K., Rao, M.R.S. *et al.* (1993) The human mutator gene homologue MSH2 and its association with hereditary non-polyposis colon cancer. *Cell*, **75**, 1027–38.

Part Two

Inherited Cancer Syndromes

Chapter 4

Retinoblastoma: the paradigm for a genetically inherited cancer syndrome

JOHN K. COWELL

4.1 INTRODUCTION

Genetic analysis of human hereditary cancer has identified the chromosomal location of genes which predispose to tumourigenesis. In the majority of cases it has been shown that loss of function of both alleles of these genes is required for tumour initiation. Because at least one functional copy of the gene product is required to prevent tumour initiation these genes have collectively been called 'tumour suppressor genes'. Since their normal function is to ensure that differentiation and signal transduction occurs in the appropriate cell type, tumours cannot establish. The first tumour suppressor gene to be isolated was the retinoblastoma gene (*RB*), predisposing to the children's eye cancer, retinoblastoma (Rb). The study of this gene has established many of the precedents for the analysis and the cloning of other tumour suppressor genes.

4.2 RETINOBLASTOMA (Rb) GENETICS

As the name implies, Rb is a tumour of retinal cells. With only rare exceptions, it affects children under the age of 5 years, the majority of tumours occurring before 2 years or age. Individuals can present with Rb at birth, which demonstrates that the tumours have been growing since early fetal life. This view is supported by the histopathology of the tumour, which shows a relatively undifferentiated, embryonic-like organization, implying arrest in the development of a retinal precursor cell. Thus, clones of cells are frozen in a state in which further genetic changes can occur, giving rise to the full tumour phenotype. The exact identity of these precursor cells, however, remains unknown.

Approximately 10% of patients will have a prior family history, the remaining cases apparently sporadic. Since the new mutation rate is relatively high [1] many of these apparently sporadic cases will carry new germline mutations. In the familial form the

Genetic Predisposition to Cancer. Edited by R.A. Eeles, B.A.J. Ponder, D.F. Easton and A. Horwich. Published in 1996 by Chapman & Hall, London.
0 412 56580 3

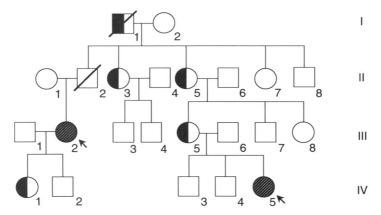

Fig. 4.1 Example of family pedigree segregating a 'mild' form of the disease. Individuals who have developed tumours are only unilaterally affected (◑) and two patients (arrows) have regressed tumours.

tumour phenotype segregates as an autosomal dominant trait. This implies that predisposition is due to inheritance of a single mutant. In fact, pedigree analysis shows that, in 10% of cases, individuals who inherit the mutant gene do not develop a tumour – so-called 'incomplete penetrance' – so it is clearly only a predisposition to tumourigenesis that is inherited and other genetic events must happen.

To estimate how many additional events are required, Knudson [2] analysed the incidence of tumours by age. This analysis led to the now classical 'two-hit hypothesis'. In hereditary cases the first mutation is present in all cells of the body. Only one additional mutation is required for tumour development. (Note that this event only affects the developing retina, suggesting a highly tissue-specific and developmental stage-specific role for this gene.) Since only one additional mutation is required for tumour formation and the chances of this are high, hereditary Rb is characterized by the presence of multiple tumours in both eyes. For this reason all bilaterally affected individuals must be considered carriers of a Rb gene mutation. This accounts for 40–50% of all patients. In truly sporadic cases, both mutations must occur,

one in each allele of the *RB* gene, in the same cell, during an early stage of development. The possibility of this occurring by chance is very small. Sporadic cases, therefore, are generally characterized by the presence of unilateral, unifocal tumours. However, we know empirically that approximately 10–15% of families have unilaterally affected individuals and, therefore some unilaterally affected sporadic cases will carry a predisposing mutation, although it is difficult to identify which ones. In our experience this group probably represents less than 5% of cases. In some families, apparently unaffected individuals have been seen to have retinal scars which resemble successfully treated tumours (Figure 4.1). These have been described as benign tumours – retinomas [3] – or as regressed tumours. Occasionally, several affected children can be born to unaffected parents with no prior family history. One possibility in these cases is that an unusual insertional translocation is segregating in the affected family and individuals should certainly be referred for cytogenetic analysis. It is also possible, however, that one of the parents is a mosaic carrying the mutation in the germline, but not in their own retinal cells.

If tumours are detected early they are usually more easily treated than those presenting later. The location of the tumour in the eye is also important. Treatment of small tumours usually involves cryosurgery, photocoagulation or radiation therapy, whereas larger tumours usually require enucleation. Tumours left to develop in the eye will eventually metastasize, often down the optic nerve, and prognosis in these cases is very poor indeed. Since early diagnosis offers a better prognosis, all 'at-risk' patients are screened regularly during the first years of life. In practice this involves all relatives of Rb patients since the possibility of incomplete penetrance means that lack of family history is not always an indication of the absence of heritable disease. Tumour formation is, for most patients, the only unequivocal clinical means of identifying mutant gene carriers. Clearly a system to identify those patients with germline mutations would make the clinical management of this disease more efficient (see later).

4.3 DEFINING THE *RB* LOCUS

The first clues to the location of the *RB*1 gene came from the cytogenetic analysis of rare Rb patients with mental retardation and other developmental abnormalities. These patients invariably had constitutional deletions of chromosome 13, the commonly deleted region being 13q14.3 [14]. Only 3% of Rb patients carry deletions but in most cases they also include the adjacent esterase-D gene (*ESD*). The gene responsible for the familial form of Rb was shown to be in 13q14 because of close linkage between the disease, Rb and *ESD* [5]. Sporadic tumours from individuals constitutionally heterozygous for polymorphic *ESD* alleles were shown to be homozygous at this locus [6]. This 'loss of heterozygosity' (LOH) was also demonstrated using polymorphic DNA probes [7]. The interpretation of these observations was

that the chromosome 13 homologue bearing the *RB*1 mutation in retinal precursor cells was duplicated at some stage and the normal chromosome 13 homologue was then lost. In this way the cell becomes homozygous for the initial *RB*1 mutation, which presumably results in failure to produce a functional protein. This prediction was confirmed by Cavenee *et al.* [8], who showed that, in a tumour from a patient with hereditary Rb, the allele which was retained was the one contributed by the affected parent. The mechanism by which LOH occurs was most frequently non-disjunction of chromosome 13 although it was also possible in some cases to demonstrate mitotic recombination – hitherto a mechanism which was considered very infrequent in mammalian cells. It appears that 70% of tumours arise as a result of LOH; presumably the other 30% are due to two independent mutations in the *RB*1 gene (see below). Similar molecular analyses allowed the parental origin of the *RB*1 mutation to be determined [9]. The heritable mutation arose on the paternally derived chromosome. However, in sporadic cases there was no differential susceptibility to somatic mutation between the homologous copies of the gene. These findings argue against genomic imprinting as an explanation for the parental origin and new mutations but point to new mutational events arising predominantly during spermatogenesis. There does not, however, seem to be a paternal age effect [10].

4.4 ISOLATION OF THE *RB*1 GENE

Following the random isolation of only 12 DNA probes from a flow-sorted chromosome 13-specific DNA library, one – H3–8 – was shown to be within the smallest of the constitutional deletions identified in Rb patients. A chromosome 'walk' from this locus generated adjacent probes which showed homozygous deletions in some tumours and which recognized a region of DNA highly conserved between species, suggesting it was within a gene. Using this probe Friend *et al.* [11] soon identified a cDNA, 4.7 kb long, which detected structurally abnormal mRNAs in Rb tumours with varying frequencies [11, 12]. Constitutional reciprocal translocations predisposing to Rb were shown to interrupt the *RB1* gene, confirming its authenticity [13]. The tissue distribution of expression of *RB1*, however, was slightly surprising, as expression was at high levels in all tissues examined [11]. This was unexpected, since the hypothesis was that this gene controls important aspects of the developing fetal retina. The *RB1* gene spans approximately 200 kb of genomic DNA and consists of 27 exons encoding 928 amino acids. There are no distinctive motifs in the gene structure or its promoter which clearly identify its function.

4.5 MUTATIONS IN THE *RB1* GENE

Only 20% of tumours showed structural abnormalities of *RB1*, so clearly the majority of mutations were more subtle. The nature of these mutations in tumours was demonstrated in a variety of ways. Dunn and colleagues [14] analysed RNA from tumour cells. Although this method is potentially very quick, since the majority of tumours are successfully treated *in situ*, mRNA from tumours is not always available. Of those which are removed, some do not produce *RB1* mRNA and from many others the samples are too small to analyse. Nonetheless, a variety of different mutations in tumours and cell lines were reported.

Formal proof of the role of *RB1* in predisposition to Rb could only be provided by demonstrating constitutional mutations in the *RB1* gene in Rb patients. Following the cloning of *RB1* the exon structure of the gene was established and sequence surrounding the 27 exons determined [15]. This allowed an exon-by-exon survey of the gene using PCR amplification of the individual exons and flanking intron regions followed by sequencing [16]. The efficiency of this procedure was improved using techniques to pre-screen the amplified exons before sequencing to identify those exons most likely to carry mutations [17]. In our own survey of tumours and constitutional cells from bilaterally affected patients, it is clear that mutations serve to produce a non-functional protein. It was also possible in many cases to show homozygous mutations in tumour cells confirming predictions suggested by LOH. In other tumours, two independent mutations were found in the two alleles of *RB1*, confirming the two-hit theory [18]. Mutations could be divided into three broad classes: those affecting correct splicing of the gene (presumably resulting in exon deletions), small deletions and insertions (which invariably generate premature stop codons downstream) and point mutations which generate stop codons directly [18]. The most common type of point mutation was a $C \rightarrow T$ transition, 70% of which converted CGA-arginine codons to TGA-stop codons.

Dryja *et al.* [9] presented evidence that the majority of new mutations arise in the male germline. Since these cells are rapidly dividing, and go through many generations, these mutations could be due to carcinogens or replication errors. In the majority of mutations in our survey there was evidence that replication errors were responsible [18]. Deletions and insertions occurred between direct repeat sequences, the intervening bases being lost, and point mutations occurred in the vicinity of quasi-repeats. If base pairing slipped during replication, the quasi-repeat sequence would be copied instead of the normal one (Figure 4.2).

Although there have still been too few mutations reported in Rb patients there do not appear to be any 'hot-spots' within *RB1*.

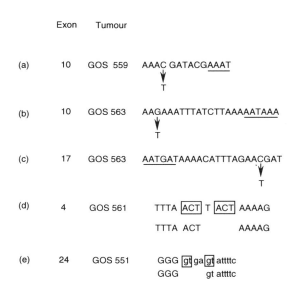

	Exon	Tumour
(a)	10	GOS 559
(b)	10	GOS 563
(c)	17	GOS 563
(d)	4	GOS 561
(e)	24	GOS 551

Fig. 4.2 Examples of mutations found in Rb tumours. Single base-pair mutations (a,b,c) induce stop codons directly but the mutated sequence is usually an identical copy of the same sequence (underlined) either upstream (c) or downstream (a,b) suggesting that they may arise as a result of replication errors. Small deletions (d,e) occur between perfect repeats (boxed). Again, slipped mispairing during replication results in one of the repeats, and the intervening sequence, being excised.

Missense mutations, simply substituting one amino acid for another, appear to be less common. In our own survey of hereditary Rb patients, a missense mutation was found in exon 20, which was associated with a 'low-penetrance' phenotype [19]. It was tempting to speculate that the substitution of a single amino acid only compromises the function of the protein and, unless the second mutation in the tumour precursor cell causes loss of *RB*1 function, duplication of the 'weak' mutation would allow sufficiently functional RB protein to be produced, so preventing tumourigenesis. This is consistent with our observa-tion in this particular family since many of the mutant gene carriers were either unaffec-ted or have regressed tumours. Sakai *et al.* [20] also investigated low-penetrance families and found mutations in recognition sequences for different transcription factors in the *RB*1 promoter region. Again the suggestion is that, as a result, a quantitative decrease in transcription occurs rather than complete inactivity. Sufficient RB protein is produced, however, and any phenotypic consequences are mild. Whether single amino acid changes will generally be found in patients with mild phenotypes remains to be determined.

4.6 CLINICAL APPLICATIONS IN THE IDENTIFICATION OF *RB*1

The autosomal dominant mode of inheritance of Rb predisposition makes genetic linkage analysis relatively straightforward, although there is some heterogeneity in the pheno-type. In the majority of families, affected individuals have bilateral, multifocal tumours with early-age onset and, since there is a family history of Rb, early detection is guar-anteed since newborns are screened regularly and tumours treated as they arise. Genetic linkage studies in these families have identi-fied, unequivocally, which individuals are at risk of tumour development and which are not [21]. In the majority of cases it is sufficient to use one or two very highly polymorphic probes, e.g. RS2.0 or RB 1.20 [21]. Using these tests, over 95% of families are informa-tive; this means that mutant gene carriers can be identified and, just as importantly, so too can those who do not carry the mutant allele, since they and their children will not have to undergo repeated ophthalmological examin-ation. This type of linkage analysis has also proved important in families where incom-plete penetrance is observed [19]. In these families unaffected mutant gene carriers can be identified and their children screened.

More recently it has been possible to offer prenatal screening using chorionic villus sampling [22] and, so far, this has proved to be a very successful screening programme. Only 10–12% of Rb cases, however, have a prior family history of the disease. Of the remaining 85%, approximately half will be bilaterally affected [23] and so, presumably, carry a germline mutation as a result of a new mutation. To offer these individuals screening for their firstborn it is necessary to identify the causative mutation and, since the majority of patients have their tumours successfully treated, this has to be carried out on constitutional cells where the mutation will be heterozygous. A number of techniques have been developed for this purpose, but perhaps the most commonly used is the single-strand conformation polymorphism (SSCP) method. This depends on the fact that a single base pair change in single-stranded DNA molecules alters their mobility in polyacrylamide gels (Figure 4.3). This procedure prescreens the RB1 exons quickly and likely mutations are identified which are then confirmed by sequencing (Figure 4.4). This approach has been successfully applied to the *RB*1 gene [18] and it is now theoretically possible that the mutations in all individuals could be identified. It is still not clear, however, whether in individuals where a mutation is not identified it has been missed or the gene is normal. The fact that several exons can be analysed simultaneously makes the procedure less labour intensive. PCR analysis can also be carried out on formalin-fixed, paraffin-embedded tissue sections [24], which means archival material can also be used to identify causative mutations.

4.7 THE FUNCTION OF THE *RB*1 GENE

The fact that Rb tumours are relatively undifferentiated, histopathologically, suggests an arrest in development of a retinal precursor cell at an early stage. By inference it

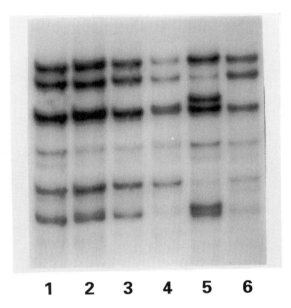

Fig. 4.3 Single-strand conformation polymorphism (SSCP) gel showing DNA samples from exon 18 from six different patients. The only aberrant banding pattern is seen in lane 5 where two novel bands appear which are not present in the other samples. For details of the technique used, see Chapter 26.

might appear, therefore, that *RB*1 controls the transition from this immature precursor cell to a photoreceptor cell. Either directly or indirectly, *RB*1 must, control the differentiation process, although analysis of the structure of the gene does not reveal any 'tell-tale' motifs implicating it as a regulator of transcription. The first clues to the function of the RB protein came from the demonstration that it could bind to proteins from certain DNA tumour viruses, which dominantly transform cells. After entry into a cell, DNA tumour viruses produce an 'early' set of proteins which trigger the normally quiescent cell into division. This is essential for successful virus propagation. The E1A protein from adenovirus, large-T-antigen (LT) from SV40 and E7 protein from human papilloma virus all form

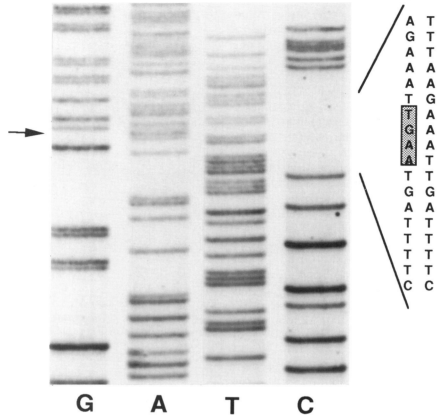

Fig. 4.4 Example of a DNA sequencing gel from exon 4 from an Rb patient showing a 4 base-pair deletion (boxed). Because this mutation is heterozygous the normal and the mutant sequence are superimposed from the point of the deletion (arrow), whereafter two bands are present at each position on the gel.

complexes with RB protein [25]. All of these viral transforming proteins share conserved regions which are necessary for their transforming function. Mutations in these conserved regions, which prevent cellular transformation, also prevent binding to RB protein. RB protein can be phosphorylated at many positions; in resting cells it is unphosphorylated but, as the cell moves into S-phase of the cell cycle, RB protein becomes phosphorylated until the end of mitosis where it is dephosphorylated again [26]. This led to the suggestion that the unphosphory-

lated form of RB protein promotes cell quiescence. LT binds specifically to the unphosphorylated form of the RB protein and LT – RB protein complexes are found only in G1 when the unphosphorylated form of the RB protein is present.

It appears, therefore, that, by sequestering RB protein from the cell during G1, the viral transforming proteins allow the cell to enter S-phase. The association of the viral early proteins with the RB protein is almost certainly an *in vitro* phenomenon, since it is unlikely that fetal retinal cells have been infected with these viruses. Rather, this model system points to associations of RB protein with other naturally occurring proteins. In fact, it has emerged that RB protein participates in the establishment of protein complexes which associate and dissociate during the cell cycle. The whole system is regulated by biochemical modifications of the participants which determine their availability to join the complex [27].

The E1A viral protein is thought to transform cells by altering the activity of cellular transcription factors. One such protein is E2F, which has been shown to be a transcriptional regulator of several cellular genes [28]. Ordinarily, E2F is complexed with specific cellular proteins which effectively suppress its function. E1A, however, can dissociate E2F from its protein complexes, releasing free E2F. To exert its transcriptional regulation E2F must form a stable complex with other proteins in order to bind to specific DNA sequences in the promotor regions of the genes it controls. The conserved regions of E1A facilitate E2F binding; the same regions are also responsible for binding RB. It was not surprising, therefore, to find that RB protein also forms complexes with E2F and that E1A can dissociate them. The E2F/RB protein complex ordinarily dissociates near the G1-S boundary, before S phase, releasing free E2F. It is thought that this process involves other cell-cycle specific proteins such as cyclins and kinases which alter the phosphorylation status of RB. The suggestion is that RB protein can control the transcriptional activities of E2F by binding to it. Dissociation of this complex allows free E2F to activate responsive cellular promotors which contribute to the release of cells from their proliferative suppression (Figure 4.5).

The *RB* gene is involved in a number of interactions in complex pathways leading to transcription regulation in the nucleus, the specifics of which have been described by Horowitz [27]. Several genes, such as *fos* and *myc*, the products of which appear soon after the decision for a cell to divide appear to be down-regulated by RB1. RB1 may also mediate the effects of transforming growth factor-β in down-regulating *myc*. Presumably, by blocking expression of these genes the cells are kept firmly in G0. Evidence is emerging to suggest that the effects of RB1 on transcription control may be cell-type dependent and that the function of RB1 in a given cell type may depend on the modulation of levels of other cell-specific transcription factors. If this is the case then this might also provide a mechanism for RB protein in the regulation of differentiation in fetal retinal cells.

To complete the E2F story, it is now known that another protein, p107, which is highly homologous to RB, recaptures E2F after it has exerted its effect on transcription, to inactivate it again (Figure 4.5). Once more these two proteins form joint protein complexes containing cyclins and kinases which influence their activity.

4.8 *RB*1 MUTATIONS IN OTHER TUMOURS

Patients carrying a constitutional RB gene mutation are also at significantly higher risk of developing second, non-ocular tumours later in life [23]. In childhood and early adulthood these are usually osteosarcomas and soft-tissue sarcomas. Both of these tumours have been shown to lose heterozygosity for markers on chromosome 13. The same classes of tumours also show frequent structural and transcriptional abnormalities of *RB*1, suggesting it plays a role in the development of the malignant phenotype in these cells. There is also evidence that *RB*1 mutation carries an increased risk of other cancers later in life, such as small cell lung cancer and bladder cancer.

Structural abnormalities in *RB*1 are also found in breast cancer [29] and small-cell

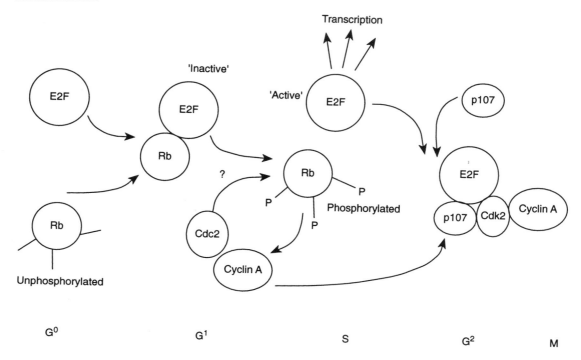

Fig. 4.5 Schematic representation of the function of the RB protein during different phases of the cell cycle. The unphosphorylated protein present in G0 binds a transcription factor E2F at the transition to G1, inactivating it. Possibly mediated by an association with cdc 2 kinase and cyclin A the RB protein is phosphorylated and E2F is released for a brief period to activate other genes presumably related to cell division. After this brief period of freedom E2F is again captured by the RB-related protein p107, which then forms a protein complex repressing E2F activity. Exactly what happens between G2 and G0 is unclear.

lung carcinoma tumour DNA [30]. A series of other tumours showing less frequent involvement of *RB*1 was presented by Horowitz *et al*. [31]. It is likely, however, that *RB*1 mutations in these other tissues only contribute to tumour progression since, in many cases, the frequency of tumours with mutations is still relatively low.

4.9 SUPPRESSION OF THE MALIGNANT PHENOTYPE

Loss of function of the *RB*1 gene is clearly vital for the development of tumours. It would be predicted, therefore, that the intro-

duction of a normal *RB*1 gene into cells with no RB function would reverse the malignant phenotype. Results from this type of experiment, however, have been difficult to interpret. Depending on the vector used, the nature of the recipient cell line, and the *in vivo* system being used to monitor the effects on tumourigenicity, different laboratories report different results [32]. In some cases transfected cells continued to grow in culture but did not produce tumours in nude mice. In other systems malignancy was apparently suppressed but, when the inoculation was intraocular, the same cells produced tumours, albeit at a slower rate. All of these experiments, however, used an *RB*1 gene which was not under the control of its own promoter, which was technically a more complicated procedure. However, it does appear that, when the *RB*1 gene is in its normal chromosomal environment, it can suppress the malignant phenotype, because introduction of an intact chromosome 13 into cell lines lacking a functional *RB*1 gene causes the cells to cease proliferation. It appears, therefore, that *RB*1 expression promotes arrest in G0. The same kinds of experiments have shown that reconstituting *RB*1 (deficient) cell lines derived from bladder, prostate and lung cancers with *RB*1 also suppresses malignancy in these cell types. This was slightly unexpected, since multiple genetic events appear to be responsible for the development of the malignant phenotype in these tumours. However, it has been shown in other tumours that, by correcting any of the defects in the multistep chain leading to malignancy with the introduction of the wild-type gene, malignancy can be suppressed [33].

4.10 TRANSGENIC MOUSE STUDIES

If the *RB*1 gene is responsible for tumour initiation in retinal precursor cells, it might be expected that disrupting this gene in mouse embryos would predispose them to Rb. Whether this would prove to be a realistic animal model was questionable since, for unknown reasons, mice do not naturally develop Rb. Using homologous recombination, one copy of the *RB*1 gene was 'knocked-out' in mouse embryonic stem cells which were then used to create chimaeric mice which eventually led to the production of mice heterozygous for the inactivated *RB*1 gene [34, 35]. None of these mice developed tumours, which was against Knudson's prediction, since a random mutational event in the homologous normal gene should initiate tumourigenesis. When the heterozygous

mice were interbred, fetuses which were *RB*1⁻/*RB*1⁻ developed apparently normally up to 11 days but then died *in utero* after 13–14 days of gestation. These mice did not have Rb or retinal defects but, instead, showed abnormal development of the mid-brain and haematopoietic system. Neuronal cell death was most obvious in the spinal cord and hind brain. Aberrant haematopoiesis was characterized by the deficiency of mature red cells which reflected an abnormal proliferation of immature erythrocytes in the liver. Clearly the *RB*1 gene is very important for normal development of mice, but loss of *RB*1 function does not appear to predispose to Rb. Remarkably, *RB*1 does not appear to be important for normal early development and is not crucial for normal cell division during this period in mice. When heterozygous mice were followed for longer periods they were shown to develop adenocarcinomas of the pituitary which is not one of the tumours often seen in hereditary cases of Rb in humans. These tumours showed loss of the normal *RB*1 allele and the development of tumours in homozygous *RB*1/*RB*1, mice could be prevented by introducing the normal *RB*1 gene [35]. The reason why *RB*1 mutation should predispose to pituitary tumours in mice and retinal tumours in humans is still not understood.

4.11 SUMMARY

The *RB*1 gene has proved to be the model tumour suppressor gene. Inactivation of this gene alone leads to the development of a highly specific type of cancer and its less frequent involvement in other tumours explains the increased risk that mutant gene carriers have to these malignancies. Reintroduction of a wild-type gene into cells deficient for its function apparently reverses the malignant phenotype. At present it seems that variations in phenotypic expression seen in different families are due to subtle differences in mutations in the *RB*1 gene. Hereditary cases carry inactivating mutations and their tumours either become homozygous for these initial mutations or sustain different inactivating mutation in the homologous gene. Molecular analysis of *RB*1 allows prenatal identification of mutant gene carriers and makes risk assessment for hereditary cases straightforward. It is still unexplained why mice do not develop retinal tumours when they carry an *RB*1 mutation, but it is entirely possible that the developmental pathways in the retina are subtly different between mice and humans although the basis for this is unknown. The way in which *RB*1 controls the developmental process in immature retinal cells appears to be through interaction with cell-specific, developmental stage-specific proteins which remain to be discovered. The way in which this tumour suppressor gene interacts with dominant transforming genes was unexpected and by fitting the RB protein into the puzzle, this has allowed a better understanding and development of many difficult, but related, areas of cancer research. It is likely that analysis of *RB*1 will continue to present more surprises for us in the future, a situation which will continue to make it an exciting gene with which to work.

REFERENCES

1. Vogel,F. (1979) Genetics of retinoblastoma. *Hum. Genet.*, **52**, 1–54.
2. Knudson,A.G. (1971) Mutation and cancer: statistical study of retinoblastoma. *Proc. Natl Acad. Sci. USA*, **68**, 820–23
3. Gallie, B.L., Ellsworth, R.M., Abramson, D.H. and Phillips, R.A. (1982) Retinoma: spontaneous regression of retinoblastoma or benign manifestation of the mutation? *Br.J.Cancer*, **45**, 513–21.
4. Cowell,J.K., Hungerford, J., Rutland, P. and Jay, M (1987) A chromosomal breakpoint which separates the esterase-D and retinoblas- toma predisposition loci in a patient with del(13) (q14-q31). *Cyto. Cell Genet.*, **27**, 27–31.
5. Sparkes, R.S., Murphree, A.L., Lingua, R.W. *et al*. (1983) Gene for hereditary retinoblastoma assigned to human chromosome 13 by linkage to esterase-D. *Science*, **219**, 971–3.
6. Godbout, R., Dryja, T.P., Squire, J., Gallie, B.L. and Phillips, R. A. (1983) Somatic inactiv- ation of genes on chromosome 13 is a common event in retinoblastoma. *Nature*, **304**, 451–3.
7. Cavenee,W.K., Dryja, T.P., Phillips, R.A. *et al* (1983) Expression of recessive alleles by chro- mosomal mechanisms in retinoblastoma. *Nature*, **305**, 779–84.
8. Cavenee,W.K., Hansen, M.F., Nordenskjold, M. *et al*. (1985) Genetic origin of mutations predisposing to retinoblastoma. *Science*, **228**, 501–3.
9. Dryja, T.P., Mukai, S., Petersen, R., Rapa- port, J.M., Walton, D. and Yandell, D.W. (1989) Parental origin of mutations of the retinoblastoma gene. *Nature*, **339**, 556–8.
10. Matsunaga, E., Minoda, K. and Sasaki, M.S. (1990) Parental age and seasonal variation in the births of children with sporadic retinoblas- toma: a mutation – epidemiologic study. *Hum. Genet.*, **84**, 155–8.
11. Friend, S.H., Bernards, R., Rogelj, S. *et al*. (1986) A human DNA segment with proper- ties of the gene that predisposes to retinoblas- toma and osteosarcoma. *Nature*, **323**, 643–6.
12. Goddard, A.D., Balakier, H., Canton, M. *et al*. (1988) Infrequent genomic rearrangement and normal expression of the putative RB1 gene in retinoblastoma tumours. *Mol. Cell. Biol.*, **8**, 2082–8.
13. Mitchell, C.D. and Cowell, J.K. (1989) Predis- position to retinoblastoma due to a transloca- tion within the 4.7R locus. *Oncogene*, **4**, 253–7.
14. Dunn, J.M., Phillips, R.A., Zhu, X., Becker, A. and Gallie, B.L. (1989) Mutations in the RB1 gene and their effects on transcription. *Mol. Cell. Biol.*, **9**, 4596–604.
15. McGee, T.L., Yandell, D.W. and Dryja, T.P. (1989) Structure and partial genomic sequence of the human retinoblastoma susceptibility gene. *Gene*, **80**, 119–28.
16. Yandell, D.W., Campbell, T.A., Dayton S.H. *et al*. (1989) Oncogenic point mutations in the human retinoblastoma gene: their application

to genetic counselling. *N. Engl. J. Med.*, **321**, 1689–95.

17. Hogg, A., Onadim, Z., Baird, P.N. and Cowell, J.K. (1992) Detection of heterozygous mutations in the RB1 gene in retinoblastoma patients using single-strand conformation polymorphism analysis and polymerase chain reaction sequencing. *Oncogene*, **7**, 1445–51.

18. Hogg, A., Bia, B., Onadim, Z. and Cowell, J.K. (1993) Molecular mechanisms of oncogenic mutations in tumours from patients with bilateral and unilateral retinoblastoma *Proc. Natl Acad. Sci. USA*, **90**, 7351–5.

19. Onadim, Z., Hogg, A., Baird, P.N. and Cowell, J.K. (1992) Oncogenic point mutations in exon 20 of the RB1 gene in families showing incomplete penetrance and mild expression of the retinoblastoma phenotype. *Proc. Natl Acad. Sci. USA*, **89**, 6177–81.

20. Sakai, T., Ohtani, N., McGee, T.L., Robbins, P.D. and Dryja, T.P. (1991) Oncogenic germline mutations in Sp1 and ATF sites in the human retinoblastoma gene. *Nature*, **353**, 83–6.

21. Onadim, Z.O., Mitchell, C.D., Rutland, P.C. *et al.* (1990) Application of intragenic DNA probes in prenatal screening for retinoblastoma gene carriers in the United Kingdom. *Arch. Dis. Child.*, **65**, 651–6.

22. Onadim, Z., Hungerford, J. and Cowell, J.K. (1992) Follow-up of retinoblastoma patients having prenatal and perinatal predictions for mutant gene carrier status using intragenic polymorphic probes from the RB1 gene. *Br. J. Cancer*, **65**, 711–6.

23. Draper, G.J., Sanders, B.M., Brownbill, P.A. and Hawkins, M.M. (1992) Patterns of risk of hereditary retinoblastoma and applications to genetic counselling. *Br. J. Cancer*, **66**, 211–9.

24. Onadin, Z. and Cowell, J.K. (1991) Application of PCR amplification from paraffin embedded tissue sections to linkage analysis in familial retinoblastoma. *J. Med. Genet.*, **28**, 312–6.

25. Weinberg, R.A. (1991) Tumour suppressor genes. *Science*, **254**, 1138–46.

26. Mihara, K., Cao, X.-R., Yen, A. *et al.* (1989) Cell cycle-dependent regulation of phosphorylation of the human retinoblastoma gene product. *Science*, **246**, 1300–3.

27. Horowitz, J.M. (1993) Regulation of transcription by the retinoblastoma protein. *Genes, Chromosomes Cancer*, **6**, 124–31.

28. Nevins, J.R. (1991) Transcriptional activation by viral regulatory proteins. *Trends Biochem. Sci.*, **16**, 435–9.

29. T'Ang, A., Varley, J.M., Chakraborty, S., Murphree, A.L. and Fung Y.-K.T. (1988) Structural rearrangement of the retinoblastoma gene in human breast carcinoma. *Science*, **242**, 263–6.

30. Harbour, W., Lai, S.-L., Whang-Peng, J., Gazdar, A.F., Minna, J.D. and Kaye F.J. (1988) Abnormalities in structure and expression of the human retinoblastoma gene in SCLC. *Science*, **241**, 353–7.

31. Horowitz, J.M., Park, S.-H., Bogenmann, E. *et al.* (1990) Frequent inactivation of the retinoblastoma anti-oncogene is restricted to a subset of human tumour cells. *Proc. Natl Acad. Sci. USA*, **87**, 2775–9.

32. Xu, H.-J., Sumegi, S.-X., Banerjee, A. *et al.* (1991) Intraocular tumour formation of RB reconstituted retinoblastoma cells. *Cancer Res.*, **51**, 4481–5

33. Stanbridge, E.J. (1992) Functional evidence for human tumour suppressor genes: chromosome and molecular genetic studies. *Cancer Surv.*, **12**, 5–24.

34. Jacks, T., Fazeli, A., Schmitt, E.M., Bronson, R.T., Goodell, M.A. and Weinberg R.A. (1992) Effects of an Rb mutation in the mouse. *Nature*, **359**, 295–300.

35. Lee, E.Y.-H.P., Chang, C.-Y., Hu, N. *et al.* (1992) Mice deficient for Rb are nonviable and show defects in neurogenesis and haematopoiesis. *Nature*, **359**, 288–94.

Chapter 5

Neurofibromatosis (NF) types 1 and 2

SUSAN M. HUSON

5.1 INTRODUCTION

In contrast to the majority of other genetic cancer syndromes reviewed in this book, neurofibromatosis 1 (NF1) and neurofibromatosis 2 (NF2) do not result in cancer development in the majority of affected individuals. In NF1, the tumours which develop in the majority of patients are benign cutaneous neurofibromas. People with *NF*1 have a small but significant risk of specific cancers which include peripheral nerve sarcomas, rhabdomyosarcomas, atypical forms of childhood leukaemia and astrocytomas. In *NF*2, the tumours are nearly always histologically benign and include vestibular schwannomas (also called acoustic neuromas), meningiomas, schwannomas and spinal ependymomas. Although the majority of these tumours are not malignant, curative surgery is often difficult and NF2 is associated with significant disease-related morbidity and mortality.

From a pathogenetic viewpoint, both the NF1 and NF2 genes have been cloned and appear to function as tumour suppressors. Clinically, NF2 fits well into the Knudson model [1]. In NF1 there are many non-tumourous manifestations, the cause of which remains to be elucidated. Loss of heterozygosity studies suggest that the *NF*1 and *NF*2 genes are also involved in the pathogenesis of some common cancers which do not occur with an increased risk in the neurofibromatoses.

5.1.1 HISTORICAL PERSPECTIVE

Although in the earliest reports, NF1 [2] and NF2 [3] appear to describe quite distinct diseases, following von Recklinghausen's report, patients with NF2 were recognized that had cutaneous features similar to those of NF1. In many reports in the first half of this century, NF1 and NF2 were not clearly distinguished, being described together under the umbrella term 'von Recklinghausen's disease'. As the inheritance of both NF1 and NF2 is autosomal dominant, this did not help to distinguish the different forms of NF. Gardiner and Frazier in reporting a large family in 1930 [4] did point out that the uniform expression of vestibular schwannomas in their family, with limited cutaneous involvement, was unusual for von Reck-

Genetic Predisposition to Cancer. Edited by R.A. Eeles, B.A.J. Ponder, D.F. Easton and A. Horwich. Published in 1996 by Chapman & Hall, London.
0 412 56580 3

linghausen's disease. Despite this, cases of NF1 and NF2 continued to be described together until the early 1970s. In 1970, Young *et al.* [5] reported a follow-up of the Gardiner and Frazier family. Their report resulted in NF2 becoming established as a distinct entity. They emphasized that the major disease feature in the family was bilateral vestibular schwannomas and that the cutaneous features, present in a few of the family, were much less prominent than in NF1. Other NF1 complications were notably absent.

Since the 1970s, there has been an escalation of activities specific to neurofibromatosis, stimulated in large part by the formation of lay organizations for patients and their families (e.g. the National Neurofibromatosis Foundation in the US, formed in 1978; the UK Neurofibromatosis Association formed in 1981). From a clinical perspective, work has concentrated on clearly delineating the different forms of NF and studying the natural history of NF1 and NF2. 'Splitting off' the various forms of the disease from the all-embracing umbrella of von Recklinghausen's disease may seem at first an academic exercise. The clinical importance however cannot be overstated, because the management and genetic advice for patients with different forms is quite different. The most significant advances in NF research in the past two decades have been in the molecular genetics. The gene for NF1 was cloned in 1990 [6–8] and for NF2 in 1993 [9, 10].

5.1.2 NOSOLOGY AND CLASSIFICATION

In many of the early reports, NF1 and NF2 are reported under the umbrella term of von Recklinghausen's disease. Later authors, aware of the different forms of the disease, used a number of terms which have now been superseded by the numerical classification recommended by the National Institutes of Health (NIH) Consensus Conference on

Neurofibromatosis [11]. Before this conference, NF1 was most commonly called von Recklinghausen's, multiple or peripheral NF and NF2 bilateral acoustic or central NF. These eponyms told us nothing about the nature of the underlying disease; the concept of peripheral and central disease seemed superficially sound, but confusion was created in those cases of NF1 with central nervous system (CNS) involvement. Bilateral acoustic neurofibromatosis now seems unsatisfactory since the acoustic neuromas actually arise from the vestibular and not the acoustic part of the eighth cranial nerve, and histologically are actually schwannomas. Throughout this chapter, acoustic neuromas are referred to as vestibular schwannomas, as recommended by the NIH Consensus Conference on Acoustic Neuroma in 1992 [12].

In addition to NF1 and NF2, there are other rarer forms of NF. In 1982, Riccardi [13] proposed a classification that included seven different types of NF and an eighth category for cases 'not otherwise specified'. Definition of the different forms depended on variations of the occurrence, number and distribution of the major defining features and associated complications, particularly tumours of the nervous system. Riccardi's classification has not come into widespread use, particularly because several of the forms are not defined sufficiently to permit their general use. At the 1988 NIH Consensus Conference, the panel concluded that although other forms did exist, they could not be precisely classified at that time. To review all the other forms of NF is beyond the scope of this chapter. Readers should, however, be aware that they do exist and that when they see patients that do not seem clearly to fit into either NF1 or NF2, an opinion from someone with a particular interest in neurofibromatosis may be of value. Viskochil and Carey [14] have recently proposed a new approach to classification, which has the attraction that it takes a combined molecular and clinical approach.

The best-defined of the other forms is segmental neurofibromatosis where patients present with the cutaneous features of NF1 limited to one or more body segments. Such patients are assumed to be mosaic for the NF1 gene (see pp. 82–83)

5.2 NEUROFIBROMATOSIS TYPE 1 (NF1)

NF1 is one of the most common single gene disorders in humans. It is by far the most frequent form of neurofibromatosis. It has an estimated birth incidence of 1 in 2500 to 1 in 3300 [15, 16]. Population-based studies have found the prevalence of NF1 to be between 1 in 4000 and 1 in 5000 [12].

Clinically, the disease features are divided into major defining features (café au lait spots, peripheral neurofibromas and Lisch nodules), minor disease features (short stature and macrocephaly), and disease complications. The morbidity and mortality caused by NF1 are largely dictated by the occurrence of complications; these are numerous and can involve any of the body systems. Their development is not predictable, even within families. The NIH Consensus Conference [11] recommended diagnostic criteria for NF1 which are shown in Table 5.1.

5.2.1 MAJOR DEFINING FEATURES

Café au lait spots are the first of these to appear, and may be present at birth. They are present in virtually all patients by the age of 2 years. In some patients they are associated with freckling in specific sites. The next disease features to develop during childhood are Lisch nodules. The peripheral neurofibromas develop from early adolescence onward in the majority of patients.

(a) Café au lait spots and freckling

Café au lait spots are not unique to NF1 sufferers. A number of studies have shown

Table 5.1 NIH Consensus statement, 1988(II): diagnostic criteria for neurofibromatosis type 1 (NF1)

The diagnostic criteria for NF1 are met in an individual if two or more of the following are found:

>   Six or more café au lait macules of over 5 mm in greater diameter in prepubertal individuals and over 15 mm in greatest diameter in postpubertal individuals
>
>   Two or more neurofibromas of any type or one plexiform neurofibroma
>
>   Freckling in the axillary or inguinal regions
>
>   Optic glioma
>
>   Two or more Lisch nodules (iris hamartomas)
>
>   A distinctive osseous lesion such as sphenoid dysplasia or thinning of the long bone cortex with or without pseudoarthrosis
>
>   A first-degree relative (parent, sibling, or offspring) with NF1 by the above criteria

that 10–25% of the general population have 1–3 of these lesions [17]. Clinically, there are no differences between the café au lait spots in NF1 patients and those in the general population; it is the increased number that is significant. The presence of six or more café au lait spots of a significant diameter (see Table 5.1) should lead to the presumptive diagnosis of NF1 in the absence of a family history. There are some patients with NF1 who only have four or five café au lait spots; these are usually older people with other disease features, the number of café au lait spots decreases with age [18].

Café au lait spots increase in number throughout childhood and appear to stop developing or even disappear in adulthood. Though varying in diameter from 0.5–50 cm or more, the majority are <10 cm. They usually have smooth contours, although some larger lesions may have irregular outlines. The intensity of their colour depends

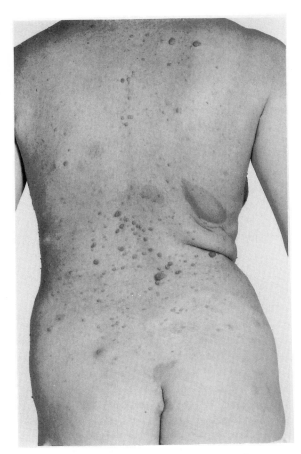

Fig. 5.1 Typical appearance of café au lait spots and cutaneous neurofibromas in an adult with neurofibromatosis type 1 (NF1). In childhood only the café au lait spots would have been present, making the skin appearance less obvious. The significance of multiple café au lait spots in childhood is often not appreciated unless other disease features are present.

on the background skin pigmentation. In some children with very pale complexions, the spots can be difficult to recognize by naked eye and are best assessed with an ultra violet lamp. Figure 5.1 shows the typical appearance of café au lait spots and dermal neurofibromas in an adult with NF1.

The other characteristic skin pigmentation unique to NF1 is freckling in the axilla, around the base of the neck, in the groins and in the submammary regions in women. In obese people with NF1, freckles can often be seen between skin folds. In some patients, there seems to be no demarcation in the zones of freckling and the patients have small freckles all over the trunk and proximal extremities. The freckles resemble café au lait spots and are 1–3 mm in diameter. Freckling tends to appear after the café au lait spots, the youngest patient in one study [18] with axillary freckling was 3 years of age. Some 67% of patients had freckling of the axilla, with 44% of the inguinal region; 29% of women aged more than 20 years had freckling in the submammary region.

The pigmentation in NF1 is asymptomatic and is not associated with a predisposition to malignant change.

(b)   Peripheral neurofibromas

Clinically, one can distinguish dermal and nodular peripheral neurofibromas. Dermal neurofibromas lie within the dermis and epidermis and move passively with the skin. Most adults with NF1 have dermal neurofibromas (Figure 5.1). The majority appear as discrete nodules with a violaceous colour and feel soft, almost gelatinous, on palpation; they vary from 0.1 cm to several cm in diameter. In older patients and in those with a lot of lesions, some of the dermal neurofibromas become papillomatous and grow larger. Dermal neurofibromas develop principally on the trunk. They are only present in large numbers on the face and other exposed areas of the body in more severe cases. They usually begin to appear around the onset of adolescence and the number of lesions is roughly proportional to age, but this is very variable even within families. There is no way to predict the number of neurofibromas that will develop. Although in a population-based study in South Wales [18], all the adults had dermal neurofibromas, with the increasing awareness of NF1, a small number of patients are being seen who just have pigmentary changes, even in adult life.

Although the majority of patients, once they understand the nature of the disease, come to accept the appearance of the dermal neurofibromas, some are continually distressed by their appearance and require the support of a sympathetic plastic surgeon. It is unrealistic to have all the neurofibromas that will develop removed, but patients often appreciate surgery for the largest legions, particularly in exposed areas. Dermal neurofibromas only occasionally cause symptoms. About 21% of cases in the Welsh study [18] complained of pruritus over the lesions, but these were rarely painful. Women with NF1 often comment that their neurofibromas increase in size and number during pregnancy, often with a partial regression after delivery. These lesions rarely, if at all, undergo sarcomatous change. However, haemorrhage into them may cause sudden painful enlargement.

The other form of peripheral neurofibroma is the nodular neurofibroma. These arise on the major peripheral nerve trunks, have a much firmer consistency and more defined margins than dermal neurofibromas. As they are on major nerve trunks, they often give rise to neurological symptoms which rarely occur with true dermal lesions. Removal of the nodular lesions is more difficult than for dermal neurofibromas because of major nerve trunk involvement, and requires the skill of a surgeon experienced in peripheral nerve surgery. No one has recorded systematically how many NF1 patients develop nodular neurofibromas; however, the proportion is estimated to be in the region of 5%.

(c) Lisch nodules

Lisch nodules are asymptomatic, harmless iris hamartomas. Although they can occasionally be seen by the naked eye, slit lamp examination is advisable to distinguish them from the more common iris nevus [19]. Using the slit lamp, they appear as smooth domed lesions, which are usually brown in colour but can be much paler, particularly on dark irides. As they develop in childhood after the café au lait spots but before peripheral neurofibromas, they are useful for confirming the diagnosis in children with no family history and only multiple café au lait spots. They are also useful in distinguishing NF1 and NF2 as they only occur in the former. Over 90% of adults with NF1 have Lisch nodules [17].

5.2.2 MINOR DISEASE FEATURES

These are features that occur in quite a high proportion of NF1 patients that are not specific to the disease. None of them is associated with significant morbidity. In the Welsh series [17, 18], after excluding patients with complications of the disease such as scoliosis and known unrelated causes of short stature, 31.5% of patients were at or below the third centile for height. When compared with the height of their normal siblings, the decrease in height in NF1 patients was highly significant. No endocrinological cause for this short stature has been found. However, very occasionally patients with pituitary/hypothalamic involvement from an optic chiasm tumour may have growth disturbance as a complication.

Macrocephaly (large head) is now a well-recognized feature of NF1 [17]. In the Welsh population study [18], 45% of patients had head circumferences at or above the 97 centile though again, the reason for this is unknown. In clinical practice, cranial neuro-imaging studies are reserved for children with other symptoms and signs or an increasing head circumference.

5.2.3 DIFFERENTIAL DIAGNOSIS

The clinical diagnosis of NF1 is usually straightforward. The most common misdiagnosis relates to other forms of neurofibromatosis not being distinguished. Patients with NF1 are rarely misdiagnosed as having another form, but patients with NF2 or one of the rarer forms have often been originally diagnosed as NF1. If a patient is being assessed who has some of the features of NF1 but who does not satisfy the diagnostic criteria given in Table 5.1, it is important to consider an alternative form of neurofibromatosis.

The other conditions that tend to be confused with NF1 either have abnormal skin pigmentation, which is confused with the café au lait spots, or some form of cutaneous tumour. In the former group, patients have been seen with McCune–Albright syndrome, Leopard syndrome, and urticaria pigmentosa, misdiagnosed as NF1. With regard to conditions with cutaneous/subcutaneous swellings, the most common condition misdiagnosed as NF1 is multiple lipomatosis. Other, much rarer conditions in this group are the Proteus syndrome and congenital generalized fibromatosis. One of the most famous patients originally diagnosed as having NF1 was Joseph Merrick, the 'Elephant Man'. It has now been realized that in fact, he had the much rarer Proteus syndrome; some of the swellings in this condition can be misdiagnosed initially as plexiform neurofibromas.

5.2.4 COMPLICATIONS

A complication of NF1 is defined as any condition that occurs at an increased frequency in patients with the disease compared with the general population. Many of the complications are also seen as isolated problems in the general population (e.g. scoliosis and the malignancies which occur). Others are relatively specific to NF1, such as sphenoid wing dysplasia. Table 5.2 shows the frequency of NF1 complications in the Welsh population study [18] along with the patients' age and presentation where this is known. Other problems which seem to be definitely associated with NF1, but were not seen in the study population are also listed; their presumed frequency is $\leq 1\%$. Some may argue that some of the things listed here as disease complications are actually disease associations (e.g. juvenile xanthogranulomas), but this further distinction seems unnecessary.

It is the complications which make NF1 a disease with significant morbidity and mortality. They only occur in a proportion of affected individuals and their occurrence cannot be predicted, even within families. This makes management of NF1 extremely difficult, achieving the balance between appropriate disease monitoring and creating unnecessary anxiety for the patient is difficult to achieve. For patients and their families, learning to deal with NF1 involves coming to terms with continuing uncertainty. Giving families detailed information about the frequency and age of presentation of the different NF1 complications is compounded by a lack of detailed knowledge about NF1's natural history. Many of the complications of NF1 were initially identified through case reports of one or more patients which gave little sense of a denominator to permit quantification of risk. A more complete picture comes from cross-sectional studies of large series of NF1 patients [15, 18, 20], and even then methods of case ascertainment tend to preferentially identify patients with more severe disease. The ideal study would be to follow a cohort of children with NF1 from birth in a defined geographical population, but this has not been done.

For discussion about presentation and management of the majority of complications of NF1, the interested reader is referred to one of the texts concentrating purely on

Table 5.2 Frequency of neurofibromatosis type 1 (NF1) complications in the Welsh study [18]. The age range at which these can present is also given unless it is obvious. (Data derived from Huson *et al.* [21].)

Complication	Frequency (%)	Age range at presentation (years)[1]
Plexiform neurofibromas		
All lesions	30.0	0–18
Large lesions of head and neck	1.2	0–1
Limbs/trunk lesions associated with significant skin/bone hypertrophy	5.8	0–5
Intellectual handicap		
Severe	0.8	
Moderate	2.4	
Minimal/learning difficulties	29.8	
Epilepsy		
No known cause	4.4	
Secondary to disease complications	2.2	Lifelong
Hypsarrhythmia	1.5	0–5
CNS tumours		
Optic glioma	1.5	0–20
Other CNS tumours	1.5	Lifelong
Spinal neurofibromas	1.5	Lifelong
Aqueduct stenosis	1.5	0–30
Malignancy		
Peripheral nerve sarcoma	1.5	Lifelong
Pelvic rhabdomyosarcoma	1.5	0–5
Orthopaedic complications		
Scoliosis – requiring surgery	4.4	0–18
Scoliosis – less severe	5.2	
Pseudoarthrosis of tibia and fibula	3.7	0–5
Gastrointestinal neurofibromas	2.2	Lifelong
Renal artery stenosis	1.5	Lifelong
Phaeochromocytoma	0.7	From 10 onwards
Duodenal carcinoid	1.5	From 10 onwards
Congenital glaucoma	0.7	0–1
Juvenile xanthogranuloma	0.7	0–5
Complications not seen in Welsh study but definitely associated with NF1		
Sphenoid wing dysplasia		Congenital
Lateral thoracic meningocoele	Presumed frequency ≤1%	Lifelong
Atypical forms of childhood leukaemia		0–18
Cerebrovascular disease		Usually in childhood

[1] Lifelong indicates cases have been reported presenting in all age groups.
CNS, central nervous system.

neurofibromatosis [20, 22, 23]. Before moving on to the specific malignancies associated with NF1, it is worth briefly mentioning the two most frequent complications: learning difficulties and plexiform neurofibromas. With regard to learning difficulties, the main thing to note is that they affect approximately one-third of children with NF1. They are usually not severe and may be associated with a tendency for the child to be generally clumsy. Because they are mild, in a classroom setting the child may appear to have good verbal skills and be labelled as being lazy when they fail to perform in their numerical or written work. For this reason, it is important that children with NF1 are assessed with a view to learning difficulties around the time they enter school.

Plexiform neurofibromas were found in 30% of the Welsh NF1 population. They are quite distinct both clinically and pathologically from dermal neurofibromas and can be divided into two types, the more common diffuse form and the nodular plexiform neurofibroma.

Diffuse plexiform neurofibromas present as large subcutaneous swellings, they have ill-defined margins, and vary from a few cm in diameter to those which involve a whole area of the body (Figure 5.2). They have a soft consistency, although sometimes hypertrophied nerve trunks can be palpated within the mass. The skin over the lesions is abnormal in about 50% of cases owing to a combination of hypertrophy, café au lait pigmentation or hypertrichosis. When these lesions occur on the trunk, they are often asymptomatic but those occurring on the face or on the limbs (particularly when associated with underlying bone hypertrophy) are a cause of significant cosmetic burden. Diffuse plexiform neurofibromas develop much earlier than other neurofibromas in NF1. The largest lesions are all probably obvious on careful clinical examination within the first 1–2 years of life.

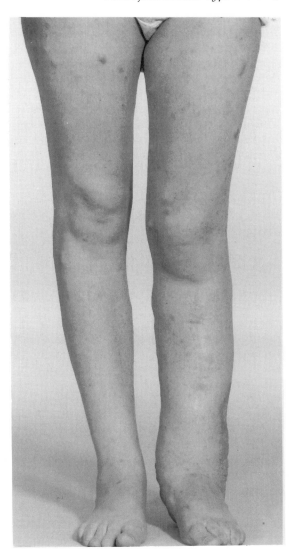

Fig. 5.2 Plexiform neurofibroma of the left leg in a 39-year-old patient with NF1. This resulted in overgrowth of the left leg in childhood. Several operations were performed to control this but the normal limb then outgrew the affected limb leaving the patient with the disproportion seen above.

A less common form of plexiform neurofibroma is the nodular form. The skin and other tissue surrounding the nerve trunks appears normal, but the nerve trunks themselves develop multiple nodular neurofibromas which seem to run into one another. The age of onset of these lesions is not known definitely; two patients have been seen who became symptomatic in their teens. They are much less frequent than the diffuse plexiform neurofibroma: in the Welsh study [18], none of the patients had a nodular lesion.

In terms of malignancy, plexiform neurofibromas harbour the potential for malignant change.

5.2.5 NF1 AND MALIGNANCY

Cancer is a frequently cited and much feared complication of NF1. The association of specific tumour types, often occurring at a younger age than usual, was first recognized through case reports. Reliable estimates for the frequencies of the different tumour types are limited because of the paucity of formal epidemiological studies. The frequency of particular malignancies in some published series of NF1 patients is vastly overestimated because of ascertainment bias. The other compounding factor in some earlier studies is that NF1 and NF2 are not clearly distinguished. In my opinion there is no clear evidence for stating that there is an increased frequency of meningiomas or Schwannomas in NF1. Overall cancer only occurs slightly more frequently in NF1 patients than in the general population. It is the relative risk of some specific tumour types which is high, the majority of these are so rare in the general population that the absolute risk of a patient with NF1 developing a particular tumour is still small. For the purpose of this section malignancy has been defined as a malignant neoplasm or benign CNS tumour; deep or cutaneous neurofibromas are excluded.

As discussed in the section on NF1 complications, the ideal epidemiological study would be to follow a cohort of NF1 children in a defined population from birth and look at the frequency of problems. Indeed, only one cohort has been retrospectively followed up, though this was identified 39 years previously [24]. Some 70 (33%) of the original cohort of 212 individuals had developed a malignancy (defined as a malignant neoplasm or benign CNS tumour). The numbers of expected cancers were calculated by applying the age-, year- and sex-specific incidence of total cancer to the corresponding numbers of years of risk in the cohort. For the total cohort, the point estimate of relative risk of malignancy was 2.5 (95% confidence interval [C.I.] 1.9–3.3) with 53 observed cases versus 20.8 expected. The excess was largely in the probands whose relative risk was 4 (C.I.2.8–5.6). The relative risk was higher in females and was statistically significant, even for female relatives (relative risk 1.9; C.I. 1.1–3.1). The cancers observed were very different from the general population; 47% of all malignant tumours in the cohort occurred in the nervous system, whereas in the general population lung, prostate and large bowel in men and breast, large bowel and uterus in women account for over 50% of all cancers. Finally, in the general population a second cancer develops in 4% of persons with a first cancer whereas 15/70 NF1 patients (21%) with a first malignancy developed a second malignancy.

The frequency of NF1 in cohorts of children with cancer has been studied [25], with 0.5% of childhood cancer estimated to be due to neurofibromatosis. Similar studies of adult cancer patients have not been performed, but would be valuable and would help to address the question as to whether NF1 has any effect on the frequency of the common adult cancers. The NF1 cross-sectional and Danish retrospective cohort studies do not suggest this, but the individual studies are probably too small to address the question adequately.

With regard to the prognosis and management of patients with NF1 who develop particular tumours, current treatment is generally similar to that in individuals with the same kind of tumour but who do not have NF1, an approach which seems appropriate. There is very little published data which review the natural history of the different kinds of tumours and when they occur in NF1 compared within the general population. Such a review would encourage studies looking at the natural history of specific tumours and response to standard therapies in NF1 patients compared with the general population.

(a) CNS tumours

When reviewing the literature about CNS tumours and NF1, the reader must be alert as to whether the particular paper groups NF1 and NF2 together or clearly distinguishes between the two conditions. As will be seen later in the chapter, CNS tumours are the hallmark of NF2 but occur relatively infrequently in NF1.

Optic nerve gliomas

Only two of 135 patients (1.5%) in the Welsh population study [18] had symptomatic optic gliomas. The proportion with NF1 in series of optic gliomas ranges from 10–65%, with an average of 25% [26]. This compares with 11/217 (5%) with NF1 who had symptomatic optic gliomas in one hospital-based series [27]. However, in the latter study all individuals underwent cranial imaging and a further 10% of patients were found to have asymptomatic optic gliomas on computed tomography (CT). Other studies have shown similar frequencies of asymptomatic optic gliomas when imaging is undertaken. The frequency is similar when magnetic resonance imaging (MRI) is used. MRI has the advantage of offering better delineation of the optic nerve lesion. MRI in patients with NF1 also identifies a number of other abnormalities, the significance of which at this point is uncertain. Increased intensity lesions are seen on T2-weighted images in approximately 60% of children with NF1. They are often referred to as UBOs (unidentified bright objects) and their significance is uncertain [28]. They occur predominantly in the basal ganglia, thalamus, brain stem and cerebellum. It was initially postulated that these may be slow-growing gliomas or hamartomas but they show a decrease in number with age, making this unlikely. Despite the apparent benign nature of UBOs their identification on MRI in so many children is a potential cause of parental anxiety.

The recognition of asymptomatic optic gliomas in a significant proportion of patients with NF1 on neuroimaging has led some authors to advocate routine screening [20] for children with NF1. I do not agree with this policy for reasons discussed in the section on management.

Other CNS tumours

These are principally astrocytomas which can occur anywhere in the nervous system, particularly in the cerebral and cerebellar hemispheres and brain stem. In a recent review of the literature Hughes [29] concluded that as neurological series of NF1 patients only identify 2–3% of patients with primary CNS tumours, the incidence of glioma in NF1 is at most four-fold greater than the general population, in which 0.7% of deaths are caused by primary malignant brain tumours. In the Welsh population [18], none of the living patients had CNS tumours other than optic gliomas, although one deceased affected family member had died from a frontal astrocytoma and another (where the diagnosis of NF1 was uncertain) died of a cerebellar astrocytoma, giving an overall frequency of 0.7–1.5% in the cohort used for this part of the study, depending on whether the case with an uncertain diagnosis is included.

(b) Malignant peripheral nerve sheath tumours

These are described as neurofibrosarcomas and malignant Schwannomas by different authors. The recently revised WHO classification of nervous system tumours [30] has introduced the diagnostic term 'malignant peripheral nerve sheath tumour' for both entities. The frequency of these tumours has been greatly overestimated in some series. Brasfield and Das Gupta [31] found a frequency of 29% (32/110), but this was a hospital-based series and one of the hospitals was a cancer centre. Subsequent hospital studies have shown a much lower frequency: based on his large experience, Riccardi [20] gives a lifetime risk of 5%. In the Welsh population-based study [18] the frequency was 1.5% (2/138). Despite this low absolute risk for NF1 patients, as the frequency of peripheral nerve sheath tumours in the general population is very low, the relative risk to patients with NF1 is much greater than for some of the other malignancies which occur. Patients with NF1 need to be aware of the importance of reporting growths which suddenly enlarge or become painful to their doctor. Peripheral nerve malignancies in NF1 either arise *de novo* or through malignant change in an existing plexiform neurofibroma. Cutaneous neurofibromas probably do not harbour the potential for malignant change.

(c) Rhabdomyosarcomas

Several series of rhabdomyosarcoma cases contain a higher than expected number of patients with NF1. In a US series [32] of 84 consecutive patients with rhabdomyosarcoma seen at the Children's Hospital of Philadelphia and the National Cancer Institute, five had NF1 (0.03 were expected by chance). Hartley *et al*. [33] found a similar excess in a UK series of childhood sarcomas. They drew attention to the fact that the tumours in their series all arose in the pelvis, and had presented between 7 and 13 months of age, compared with a median age at diagnosis for all cases in the series of 48 months. In retrospect, seven of the 10 children who presented at 5 years or under in the US series [32] had a rhabdomyosarcoma originating in the pelvis. In the Welsh population study [18] the estimated frequency of rhabdomyosarcoma was 1.5%, both of which arose in the pelvis, one presented at 6 months of age and the other at 2 years. There were no adults with rhabdomyosarcoma.

(d) Endocrine tumours

The association of phaeochromocytoma with NF1 is well established, but again despite a very large relative risk the absolute risk to an NF1 patient of developing a phaeochromocytoma is small. Seven of 72 patients (9.7%) in one series of patients with phaeochromocytoma had NF1 [34]. In the Welsh study [18], 1/135 (0.7%) of NF1 patients had a phaeochromocytoma.

More recently attention has been drawn to the association of duodenal carcinoid with NF1 [35]. In the Welsh study [18], 2/135 patients had a duodenal carcinoid, one of these being the patient who also had a phaeochromocytoma. The duodenal carcinoid was found as an incidental finding at operation, the surgeon being aware of the possible association. There is now a small but significant literature on the association of phaeochromocytoma and duodenal carcinoid occurring together in NF1. The practical outcome of this is that whenever a patient is diagnosed as having one of these tumours with NF1, a search must be made for the presence of the other.

(e) Haematological malignancy

The best-recognized association is of NF1 and the occurrence of atypical forms of childhood leukaemia. Again, the absolute risk to an NF1 patient of developing this complication is small, but the relative risk is quite large. Bader and Miller in a US series [36] found a probable increase in the number of cases and that the usual ratio of acute lymphocytic leukaemia to non-lymphocytic leukaemia in childhood, 4:1, was reversed among NF1 patients to 9:20, with the rare subtypes chronic myelogenous and acute myelomonocytic leukaemia comprising 13/18 cases. In a recent UK study Stiller *et al.* [37] found a marked increase in relative risk for chronic myelomonocytic leukaemia (CMML) with NF1 (relative risk 221; 95% C.I. 71–514) and a much lower increased risk for the development of acute lymphoblastic leukaemia (relative risk 54; 95% C.I. 2.8–9.4) and non-Hodgkin lymphoma (relative risk 10.0; 95% C.I. 3.3–23.4). However, as these are all rare in the general population, the chance of a child with NF1 developing a haematological malignancy is still <1%. None of the patients in the Welsh families had this form of malignancy.

The medical literature [38] draws our attention to the association of xanthogranuloma with NF1 and leukaemia. Xanthogranuloma are benign cutaneous lesions which develop in early childhood and resolve with age; they are usually multiple when seen in NF1.They are reported to occur at increased frequency in NF1 both with and without leukaemia, and to be associated with juvenile myeloid leukaemia. At this point I am convinced of an increased frequency of xanthogranuloma in NF1, but am uncertain whether the triple association of xanthogranuloma, leukaemia and NF1 is real or simply reflects reporting bias.

(f) Other malignancies

Hope and Mulvihill [39] and subsequently Mulvihill [40] have provided overviews of malignancy in NF1. Although the earlier review reported an association with neuroblastoma and Wilms tumour, this was later refuted. Given the abnormal pigmentation found in NF1 it is perhaps surprising that there is no clear evidence from the literature of an increased frequency of malignant melanoma.

5.2.6   NATURAL HISTORY

Because the morbidity and mortality of NF1 are largely dictated by the occurrence of its complications, all the limitations of our knowledge regarding frequency of those discussed above apply also to our understanding of the natural history of NF1. The only detailed follow-up information available at this time is that from the Danish NF1 cohort study [24]. Survival rates to June 1983 of patients alive on 1 January 1944 were lower than the year-, age- and sex-specific survival rate of the general population. Mortality was increased among probands, especially females, compared with affected relatives; affected female relatives had a survival rate just below that of the general population. The probands had been originally identified through hospital in-patient records and the authors concluded that patients requiring admission to hospital had a poor prognosis, whereas incidentally diagnosed relatives had a considerably better outcome. In the Welsh study [18], the contribution of NF1 to mortality was assessed in two ways. Firstly, by the association of disease prevalence with age, a decrease in prevalence was found from the second decade onwards which could not be accounted for by under-ascertainment.

Secondly, mortality attributable to NF1 was assessed by looking at the cause of death in 25 deceased affected relatives. Death was definitely attributable to NF1 in six cases (24%). Causes of death were rhabdomyosarcomas in two children; a frontal astrocytoma in a 32-year-old; neurofibrosarcoma in a 24-year-old; obstructive hydrocephalus following the removal of a neurofibroma at C1–2 in a 51-year-old; and acute left ventricular failure and haemorrhage into an undiagnosed phaeochromocytoma in a 54-year-old. Follow-up monitoring of the Welsh cohort is in progress (the author in collaboration with Dr J. Sampson and Dr I. Cordeiro).

5.2.7 THE GENETICS OF NF1

NF1 is an autosomal dominant disorder with virtually 100% penetrance [16]. The majority of affected individuals have developed multiple café au lait spots by the end of the second year of life. In practice, if at-risk children reach the end of the second year of life with no café au lait spots, parents can be reasonably reassured but one final check examination should be performed at the age of 5 years. Approximately 50% of cases represent new mutations and the mutation rate is one of the highest among humans. The Welsh study [18] found it to be between $3.1–10.5×10^{-5}$ per allele per generation. Evidence based on linkage analysis [41] has indicated that the majority of mutations arise from the paternal allele and that these occur during spermatogenesis. As NF1 does not show a definite paternal age effect [16], Jadayel *et al.* [41] argue that most NF1 mutations arise either at mitosis in cells that are not self-renewing stem cells, or independently of mitosis, for example in mature sperm. The molecular basis of the high new mutation rate is not understood at this time.

One of the most striking things about NF1 is its variable expressivity. In large families with multiple affected individuals a wide range of severity and complications is seen. Thus, the specific germline mutation at the NF1 locus does not predict accurately the phenotype in a particular individual, since all affected individuals in the same family carry the same mutation. In order to distinguish between genetic influences on the one hand, and environmental and/or chance influences on the other, Easton and colleagues [42] examined a series of monozygotic twins concordant for NF1 and compared them with relatives. There was a significant correlation between the number of café au lait spots and neurofibromas in identical twins, with a lower but significant correlation in first-degree relatives, but almost no correlation in more distant relatives. This suggests that these features are controlled by other influences than the *NF*1 mutation, and that the specific mutation in the *NF*1 gene itself plays a minor role. Several complications were also studied: in the twin pairs, optic glioma, scoliosis, epilepsy and learning disability were concordant but plexiform neurofibromas were not. All of these complications, with the exception of plexiform neurofibromas, showed a decreasing concordance with an increasing degree of relationship within the family. There was no evidence of any association between the different traits in affected individuals. The study concluded that the phenotypic expression of NF1 is to a large extent determined by the genotype at other modifying loci and that these modifying genes are trait-specific.

As 50% of patients represent new mutations, the most common question in clinical practice from the parents is 'what is the risk that a further child will be affected?' It is not possible to answer this without a careful examination of the skin and irides of the parents. This is because occasionally one finds a parent who is so mildly affected that they are not aware of having the disease. Also there are a few individuals with segmental neurofibromatosis that have been reported [17] who have children with full-blown NF1. It is presumed that these represent gonosomal mosaics for the *NF1* gene. In other words, a mutation in the *NF1* gene happened in early development in a progenitor cell of common origin to the affected segment involved with NF1 features and gonadal tissue. If the examination of the parents is entirely normal, then the chance of recurrence is barely increased above the background population risk of another new mutation. Certainly the large clinical studies of NF1 have not shown presumed gonadal mosaicism (observed clinically by finding two affected children with normal parents) to occur at a significant frequency and there are only a handful of families in the literature where two affected siblings are born to unaffected parents, some of which could have arisen by chance occurrence of two new mutations.

5.2.8 MANAGEMENT

Because of its extreme variability and large number of complications, NF1 is an extremely difficult disease to manage. As so many different specialties may be involved in the care of any one patient the coordination of medical care presents a significant challenge. Yet many NF1 patients will not develop major disease complications and so the health professional is continually performing a difficult 'balancing act' between providing adequate information and follow-up but not creating unnecessary anxiety. Until the last 10–15 years, the majority of NF1 patients did not receive any special form of health care and were independently managed by each specialty as complications arose. Although most patients were told the name of the disease, few received adequate information about NF1 and its genetic implications.

In the Welsh study [18], 94/135 cases had had at least one hospital consultation for NF1 before their assessment for the study. Only

30/135 were being regularly followed up in a hospital clinic, and in half of these it was to monitor a specific disease complication. Medical histories of many of the patients demonstrated that regular follow-up with more awareness of the disease would have avoided delay in diagnosis of complications and distress caused by uncertainty. Only nine individuals from seven families had received formal genetic counselling and in four cases this was after they had completed their families.

Fortunately, over the last two decades the approach to health care for NF1 patients has gradually changed, largely due to pressure from lay groups and the example of pioneering health professionals in the field such as Riccardi [13, 20]. It is now recommended that individuals with NF1 attend an annual clinical review, with a general physical examination geared to monitoring for complications. As shown in Table 5.2 the age at which particular complications may develop varies. For example, if a child reaches 2 years without obvious pseudoarthrosis or a large superficial plexiform neurofibroma, the parents can be reassured that these complications will not develop. Particular care over spinal examination needs to be taken during childhood, particularly through the adolescent growth spurt. The blood pressure needs to be monitored at all ages, as hypertension secondary to phaeochromocytoma or renal artery stenosis may not be symptomatic until a relatively advanced stage.

There are times when the NF1 patient and their family need more support. The time of diagnosis is particularly important and the author often offers a combination of two or three clinic and/or home visits with the clinic nurse to help families come to terms with the diagnosis and to learn about the natural history. As children enter full-time education it is important that they are assessed from the viewpoint of learning difficulties, so that if these are present they can receive appropriate help from an early age. Another important time is when adolescents and young adults begin to think about their own genetic risk, and referral for genetic counselling at an appropriate point is helpful. The risk of a child inheriting the gene is 50%. However, the risk of developing complications is more difficult to predict as these do not breed true, even within families. This is particularly important to mention if the affected parent has a disease complication, as they often think children will have the same presentation of NF1. Rather than go through the risks of each disease complication separately, the author finds it useful to group the complications together as to how they will affect the patient, using data derived from the Welsh population study [18]. The frequency of complications that fall into a particular group were totalled and then halved (and rounded to the nearest 0.5%) to give the risk to offspring of an affected parent. The groups are as follows:

1. Intellectual handicap, 16.5% (moderate/ severe retardation 1.5%, minimal retardation/learning difficulties 15%);
2. Complications developing in childhood and causing lifelong morbidity (severe plexiform neurofibromas of the head and neck, severe orthopaedic complications), 4.5%;
3. Treatable complications (aqueduct stenosis, epilepsy, internal neurofibromas, endocrine tumours, renal artery stenosis) that can develop at any age, 8%;
4. Malignant or CNS tumours, 2.3%

For some couples this approach is too complex, at which point it is important to try and identify those complications the couples would find a particular problem should they occur in the child, and talk about them. If it is assumed that these include moderate to severe retardation, the different complications that develop in childhood and cause

lifelong morbidity and the risk of developing a CNS or malignant tumour, then the combined risk to the offspring of an affected parent is 8%. Recent developments in molecular genetics (see pp. 85–87) mean that prenatal and pre-symptomatic diagnosis using linked DNA markers is available. The uptake of this has been relatively limited, as the clinical diagnosis of NF1 in a known family is usually straightforward, making the demand for pre-symptomatic diagnosis small. With regard to prenatal diagnosis many couples feel that they would only want such a test if it could predict disease severity and this is not possible at present.

The coordination of care of NF1 patients varies from country to country. In the US, Riccardi [20] and others have developed the concept of the multidisciplinary NF clinic. This involves one or two clinical coordinators, who are usually clinical geneticists, paediatricians or neurologists who liaise closely with identified colleagues in other specialties pertinent to NF1 complications, e.g. ophthalmologists, plastic surgeons, etc. It is not considered that all NF1 patients need to attend a specialist NF clinic on a regular basis. Although each country needs a number of specialist clinics to be available for diagnostic assessment of unusual cases, to assess cases with particular severe manifestations and to coordinate research programmes, most NF1 patients should be cared for in a 'local' setting, either by a hospital consultant or family physician. The question of which specialist should follow-up NF1 patients then arises. Because many NF1 complications present in childhood an annual follow-up by a consultant paediatrician is recommended during this period. In adults the family physician or any one of a number of specialists, (e.g. clinical geneticists, neurologists or dermatologists) are equally appropriate. In addition to medical care many families find it helpful to be in touch with a lay organization. The British Neurofibromatosis Patients' Association has a series of booklets covering all aspects of NF1 and NF2; however these detail many of the complication which can be quite rare. The Association also employs family support workers who can be in touch with families who contact it and helps them in coming to terms with the particular difficulties they are experiencing.

Some people feel that annual clinical examination of NF1 patients should be supplemented by screening investigations for particular disease complications. Riccardi [20] argues that because of the high frequency of asymptomatic optic gliomas NF1 patients should have cranial neuroimaging at least on their initial assessment. The author disagrees with this approach because so few of these lesions become symptomatic and treatment is only offered for progressive, symptomatic lesions.

There are no specific treatments for NF1, or any drug therapy which prevents growth or development of neurofibromas themselves. Patients with troublesome neurofibromas are helped by being in touch with sympathetic plastic surgeons for removal of particularly unsightly or troublesome lesions. The treatment of specific complications is beyond the scope of this chapter and is reviewed in detail elsewhere [20, 22, 23].

5.2.9 PATHOGENESIS

The cloning of the *NF*1 gene in 1990 [6–8] represented the first major step towards an eventual understanding of disease pathogenesis. Studies before those involving molecular genetics were relatively few and had not provided any major insights. Bolande [43] proposed that NF1 results from abnormal migration, growth or cytodifferentiation of primitive neural crest cells at various stages of development. The majority of NF1 manifestations arise in tissue of neural crest origin but others, such as the orthopaedic problems (scoliosis, pseudoarthrosis – mesodermal ori-

gin) and learning difficulties (neural tube origin) probably do not. Studies made possible by the cloning of the gene will now be able to address these issues. Given its role in the growth and maintenance of sympathetic and certain sensory neurones, nerve growth factor (NGF) has also been proposed to be important in the pathogenesis of neurofibromatosis. Molecular genetic studies have excluded NGF as being the primary gene involved in either NF1 or NF2 but NGF could still have a modifying effect on *NF*1 or *NF*2 gene expression.

Clinical studies have also given rise to a number of questions that may give clues to disease pathogenesis. The most important of these to date has been the identification of the different types of neurofibromatosis [13] which was essential to avoid problems with heterogeneity confounding the genetic linkage studies. The timing and rate of progression of different lesions in NF1 is striking. Why do café au lait spots appear during childhood, but then remain static or even disappear in adults? Why do dermal neurofibromas not appear until around the time of puberty? What hormonal influences cause neurofibromas to grow in pregnancy?

(a) The *NF*1 gene

As there was no information available on the structure and function of the *NF*1 gene before the late 1980s, the only feasible approach available to identify the gene was positional cloning. This and subsequent work has resulted in a large number of publications. It is beyond the scope and remit of this chapter to cite all the work that has contributed to these exciting developments, and therefore only an overview has been been provided and interested readers referred to recent reviews [44, 45].

The initial step in the isolation of the gene

was its localization to chromosome 17 in 1987 by linkage studies using DNA markers. Pooling of data from a number of groups excluded locus heterogeneity, and localized the *NF*1 gene to a 3 cM region on the proximal part of the long arm of chromosome 17. Shortly after this localization two patients with NF1 and balanced reciprocal translocations both involving 7q11.2 were identified – this was precisely where the *NF*1 gene had been mapped by linkage analysis. The identification of translocation breakpoints permitted analysis of this region by physical mapping techniques and this dramatically accelerated the gene cloning process.

Physical mapping narrowed the *NF*1 candidate region to an area of around 600 kb and within this region the translocation breakpoints were found to be about 60 kb part. Three potential candidate genes in the area (EVI2A, EVI2B and the oligodendrocyte myelin glycoprotein, OMGP) were identified. Even though EVI2A and EVI2B (through the role of their mouse equivalents in virally induced murine leukaemia) and OMGP (because of its almost exclusive expression in Schwann cells and oligodendrocytes) had some attraction as candidate genes, no mutations were found in these genes in NF1 patients.

The *NF*1 gene was the fourth candidate studied and was shown to be the disease gene in several ways [6–8]. The transcript was disrupted by both translocation breakpoints and more subtle mutations were identified in other NF1 patients. Subsequent analysis showed that the three previous candidate genes are embedded within one large intron of the true *NF*1 gene and transcribed from the opposite DNA strand. Whether or not they contribute in any way to the NF1 phenotype remains to be elucidated. The *NF*1 gene spans approximately 300 kb of genomic DNA and the messenger RNA has been estimated at 11–13 kb. There are approximately 51 exons, at least two of which are involved in alternative splice forms of the primary transcript [45].

(b) Mutation analysis

The large size of the gene has hampered mutation analysis, no particular hotspot for mutations having been identified. Those identified to date range from large deletions [46] to point mutations [47], all of which result in a loss of the functional protein. This fact is consistent with NF1 being a tumour suppressor gene. Analysis of some of the kinds of tumours that can occur in NF1 has given support to this in that loss of heterozygosity at the NF1 locus has been found in neurofibrosarcomas, phaeochromocytomas and myeloid leukaemia [48–50]. The molecular and pathogenetic basis of the major defining features and non-tumorous manifestations of NF1 remain to be elucidated.

(c) The *NF*1 gene product: neurofibromin

The protein product of the *NF*1 gene is a 250-kDa protein which has been named neurofibromin. Although messenger RNA appears to be present at some levels in all tissues, the highest level of protein is seen in the nervous system. Antibodies to neurofibromin label neurones, oligodendrocytes and non-myelinated Schwann cells but not astrocytomas or myelinated Schwann cells [51]. One region of the *NF*1 gene shows sequence homology with a family of GTPase activating proteins or GAP [52]. GAP proteins, both in mammals and yeast, accelerate the rate at which the p21 RAS protein hydrolyses GTP to become inactive ras–GDP and are therefore involved in mitogenic signal transduction. Neurofibromin has subsequently been shown to have GAP-like activity. It is therefore hypothesized that neurofibromin functions as a tumour suppressor gene by down-regulating *RAS* with inactivation of neurofibromin resulting in higher levels of active ras and therefore unlimited cell proliferation.

(d)   Mouse models of *NF*1

The cloning of the *NF*1 gene and identification of its highly related mouse homologue made construction and characterization of mice with *NF*1 mutations possible. Two groups have now created such mice both with targeted disruptions of exon 32 [53, 54]. Homozygosity for the *NF*1 mutation in mice leads to mid-gestational embryonic lethality with associated defects in cardiac development (double outlet right ventricle) which are postulated to result from failure of cardiac neural crest cells to migrate properly or function normally once in place. Heterozygote *NF*1 mice observed for more than 2 years have not developed any of the major defining features of NF1, but have shown an excess of both phaeochromocytoma and myeloid leukaemia, both of which are associated with the human disease. Furthermore, by crossing the mouse *NF*1 heterozygotes onto different murine genetic backgrounds, different disease phenotypes may be identified leading to the identification of *NF*1 modifying genes proposed to exist for the human *NF*1 gene by Easton *et al.* [42, 54].

(e)   Clinical applications

The immediate application to clinical practice of the above developments has been the availability of intragenic and closely linked DNA markers for prenatal and presymptomatic diagnosis. Diagnosis using linked markers is however limited to families with a suitable structure. In practice with regard to prenatal diagnosis, many families say they would only use a prenatal test if it could predict disease severity and this of course is not possible at this point: nor is the linkage approach applicable to the approximately 50% of patients who represent new gene mutations. Tests at the DNA level for these families must rely on mutation detection within the *NF*1 gene and as this has proven so difficult in the research setting, it is not applicable in the service laboratory at this time. Perhaps alternative diagnostic laboratory tests will be developed which are based on the protein, either by assaying neurofibromin levels or some measure of its biological activity.

Looking ahead, the cloning of the gene and the research subsequent to it in understanding neurofibromin function and distribution represent a major advance towards an eventual understanding of pathogenesis and development of disease treatments. With regard to disease treatment, the identification of the GAP activity of neurofibromin is important. Because of the involvement of *RAS* in a wide range of human cancers, several groups are working on drugs which interfere with the *RAS* pathway at various points. It could be that these drugs will also ultimately prove useful for therapy in NF1.

5.3   NEUROFIBROMATOSIS TYPE 2 (NF2)

NF2 is much less common than NF1, the only study of disease prevalence finding only 1 in 210 000 individuals to be affected [55]. The same study estimated the birth incidence to be between 1 in 33 000–40 000. The large difference between prevalence and incidence is explained by the late mean age of diagnosis of NF2 (usually in the late 20s) and the fact that many affected patients die from their disease at a relatively young age.

The diagnostic criteria for NF2 are given in Table 5.3. In contrast to NF1, cutaneous manifestations of the disease are relatively minor, if present at all. However nearly all affected individuals develop one or more schwannomas on the vestibular or other nerves, sometimes with other tumours such

Table 5.3 Diagnostic criteria for neurofibromatosis type 2 (NF2). (After Evans *et al.*[57].)

The criteria for NF2 are met by an individual with one of the following combinations of features

Bilateral vestibular schwannomas
A parent, sibling or child with NF2 plus:

(a) Unilateral vestibular schwannoma, or
(b) Any one of: meningioma, glioma, neurofibroma, schwannoma, posterior subcapsular lenticular opacities, cerebral calcification

Unilateral vestibular schwannoma plus one or more of the following: meningioma, glioma, neurofibroma, schwannoma, posterior subcapsular lenticular opacities, cerebral calcification

Multiple meningioma (two or more) plus any one or more of the following: glioma, neurofibroma, schwannoma, posterior subcapsular lenticular opacities, cerebral calcification.

Table 5.4 Neurofibromatosis type 2 (NF2): clinical features in 120 patients studied by Evans *et al.* [57]

Feature	*Frequency (percentage)*
Tumours of the nervous system	
Bilateral vestibular schwannoma	85
Unilateral vestibular schwannoma	6
Meningiomas	45
Spinal tumours (meningiomas, schwannomas)	26
Astrocytomas[1]	4
Ependymomas[1]	3
Café au lait spots ($n = 100$)	
1–4	42
6	1
Skin tumours	
Overall	68
>10 (maximum number: 27)	10
Cataracts and lens opacities ($n = 55$)[2]	60
Peripheral neuropathy	3

[1] All located in brain stem and/or upper cervical cord.
[2] Only 55 individuals had slit lamp examination.

as meningiomas during their lifetime (Figure 5.3). These tumours account for the morbidity and mortality seen in the disease. Disease features are summarized in Table 5.4.

5.3.1 NERVOUS SYSTEM TUMOURS OCCURRING IN NF2

(a) Vestibular schwannomas

These are the most consistent disease feature and were the cause of the initial symptom in the majority of cases in both of the large clinical studies [56, 57]. Early symptoms included hearing loss with tinnitus or vertigo resulting from pressure on the cochlear nerve. Compared with their unilateral counterparts, vestibular schwannomas in NF2 present at a younger age (median age of onset 27 years compared with over 50 years in non-NF2 cases usually). They also tend to have grown to a larger size before causing symptoms which presents difficulties in management [58]. (Figure 5.3.)

(b) Schwannomas

In addition to the eighth nerve, schwannomas can develop on any of the other cranial nerves (except 1 and 2), on the dorsal nerve roots of the spinal cord and on the major peripheral nerves. There may be multiple nerve involvement. The presenting features of the tumours are related to their anatomical localization.

The peripheral nerve schwannomas in NF2 appear clinically very like the nodular neurofibromas in NF1, and if they are the initial presentation of NF2 this often results in initial misdiagnosis as NF1 until other disease features develop.

(c) Meningiomas

Meningiomas were present in 45% of the patients in the large UK study [57]. There is

(d) Glial tumours

Glial tumours are much less common in NF2 than schwannomas or meningiomas. They include pilocytic astrocytomas of the brain and spinal cord, cerebral and spinal ependymomas. Optic nerve gliomas do not occur with increased frequency in NF2. In the UK study [57] 4% of patients had an astrocytoma and 2.5% ependymomas – they were low-grade tumours and affected the lower brain stem or upper cervical cord; syringomyelia can develop in association with intramedullary tumours.

(e) Cutaneous tumours

These occur less consistently and in much smaller numbers than in NF1. The most common kind, occurring in 48% of patients in the UK study [57], are sometimes referred to as NF2 plaques and have a distinctive appearance. They are discrete, well-circumscribed, slightly raised cutaneous lesions usually < 2 cm in diameter. Their surface may be slightly pigmented, roughened and often contain excess hair. Less commonly, NF2 patients have cutaneous tumours indistinguishable from the dermal lesions seen in NF1. They occurred in 27% of patients in the UK study, but were much fewer in number than would be normally seen in an adult with NF1. Histologically the cutaneous tumours in NF2 are usually schwannomas.

5.3.2 OTHER DISEASE FEATURES

(a) Café au lait spots

Some 43% of the patients in the UK study [57] had café au lait spots. Of these, 24 patients had one, 11 had two, four had three and three had four spots. Only one patient had six café au lait spots. Hence, although café au lait spots occur more frequently in

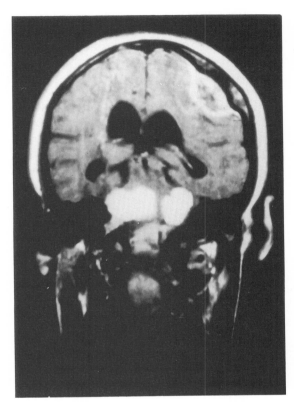

Fig. 5.3 An 18-year-old patient with severe neurofibromatosis type 2 (NF2). The cranial T1-weighted gadolinium-enhanced MR image demonstrates bilateral enhancing vestibular schwannomas dramatically compressing the brain stem. The brain stem and upper cervical cord are also expanded by an enhancing mass consistent with a brain stem glioma. There is also a left convexity meningioma. (Reproduced from [58] with permission.)

no site where they are particularly prone to occur; symptoms are related to location.

Meningioangiomatosis is a distinctive lesion with a meningiothelial and vascular component that can be associated with NF2. Although the lesions have been reported adjacent to meningiomas, it is thought that they present a dysplastic hamartomatous lesion rather than a neoplastic process.

NF2 than in the general population, they are much less frequent in number than in NF1. Axillary and groin freckling are not seen in NF2.

(b)   Ophthalmological features

Lisch nodules do not occur in NF2. Characteristic eye findings are posterior subcapsular lens opacities and sometimes cataracts. Kaiser-Kupfer *et al.* [59] found these changes in 18 of 22 affected individuals (82%). In the UK study opacities were found in 60% (33/55) of the patients who had slit lamp examination. Fifteen had been identified as having cataracts in childhood, of which four had minimal vision in the affected eye, probably from birth. Lens changes are therefore a valuable marker of NF2, and unless there are other obvious signs of NF2, individuals at risk should be screened for their presence in infancy.

The other eye findings in NF2 are retinal astrocytic hamartomas, found by Ragge *et al.* [60] in eight of 21 patients.

(c)   Other disease features

Mixed peripheral motor and sensory neuropathy is seen in some patients with NF2, occurring in 6% of patients in the UK study [57].

Intracranial calcifications on cranial neuroimaging not due to tumour and somewhat similar to those in tuberous sclerosis have been reported in a number of patients, but their frequency in a large series of patients has not been studied, nor is the pathological nature of the lesions known.

5.3.3   DIFFERENTIAL DIAGNOSIS

The most common misdiagnosis in the authors' experience is that patients with NF2 and marked cutaneous features are labelled as having NF1. The possibility of NF2 must be borne in mind when assessing young adults referred as having NF1 who subsequently have enough café au lait spots to satisfy the diagnostic criteria or who have atypical cutaneous tumours.

Another problem in misdiagnosis is that the possibility of NF2 is not considered when young people present with single vestibular schwannomas, meningiomas or spinal schwannomas. It is important that other signs of NF2 are sought in such patients and that they are offered long-term follow-up.

Bilateral vestibular schwannomas appear to be unique to NF2 but there do appear to be families in which multiple meningiomas segregate as an autosomal trait, and possibly others where spinal schwannomas with or without peripheral nerve schwannomas segregate without other NF2 features [58].

5.3.4   NATURAL HISTORY

In the UK study [57] the mean age at first symptom was 21.6 (range 2–52) years and at diagnosis 27.6 (range 5–66) years. Eleven patients (10%) presented before the age of 10 years. The mean age at onset of deafness was 24.3 (range 4–50) years in 87 patients. The natural history of NF2 is affected by the rate of growth of the vestibular schwannomas and the number of other tumours the individual may develop. The natural history is also affected by the surgical management. Inappropriate operations on large vestibular schwannomas can hasten the course of the disease [58]. In the large family followed up by Young *et al.* [5], the 20 deceased members who did not undergo surgery had a mean survival from onset of symptoms of 18.5 (range 4–44) years. The nine deceased members who had surgery had a mean survival of 9.2 (range 3–19) years. In the recent UK study [57] the mean age at death in 40 cases was 36.3 years. The mean actuarial survival from diagnosis was 15 years, which gave a mean age at death of 42–6 years if mean age at diagnosis was used. Overall the mean actuarial survival from birth for 150 cases was 62 years; however, over 40% would be expected to have died by 50 years and all cases by 70 years.

Some studies have suggested a deleterious effect of pregnancy on the natural history of NF2. The recent UK study did not find any evidence of this nor an effect of gender on the natural history of NF2 [57].

5.3.5 GENETICS

NF2 is an autosomal dominant condition with almost complete penetrance by the age of 60 years [55]. Approximately half the cases of NF2 are the first in their family and are presumed to be the result of new gene mutation. The mutation rate has been calculated to be 6.5×10^{-6} per allele per generation.

In contrast to NF1, all studies of NF2 have shown strong intrafamilial correlation in disease course but marked interfamilial variation. There is some suggestion that the families fall into two main groups (reviewed in [58]) as follows:

1. Mild (Gardner type) – characterized by relatively late onset (usually >25 years), bilateral vestibular schwannomas with only minimal skin manifestations and occasional other CNS tumours. Growth of the tumours is often very slow.
2. Severe (Wishart type) – with early onset (usually <25 years) and meningiomas and spinal tumours in large numbers (at least two of one type and usually multiple) in addition to bilateral vestibular schwannomas, which are the presenting feature in only 50% of cases. Disease course is often rapid, causing severe handicap or death before reproductive age.

In the recent UK study [55, 61] the families broadly fell into these two groups, but there was a significant number of cases that did not

fit exactly into this classification. The division of NF2 into two definite clinical types is therefore not clear-cut and studies of genotype/phenotype correlation are awaited to clarify the issue. Linkage studies in NF2 families at this point have shown no evidence of locus heterogeneity.

Two studies [55, 56] have shown an earlier age of onset in maternally inherited cases. Evans *et al.* [55] found an age of onset in maternal cases of 18.2 years compared with 24.5 years in paternal cases. This was very similar to the previous American study [56]. In addition, there was a general impression of a worse clinical course in maternally inherited cases. This may represent an imprinting effect in NF2, although there may be other explanations. The genetic fitness in NF2 is estimated to be 0.46–0.51 [55], the relative fitness in males being only 0.27 compared with 0.76 in females. The earlier onset of disease in maternally inherited cases could simply reflect that women with severe NF2 still go on to marry and have children, whereas only mildly affected males do the same – a later onset in their children would therefore be expected because of the more benign natural history of the disease.

5.3.6 MANAGEMENT

In contrast to NF1, the author recommends that all patients with NF2 and at-risk family members are followed in centres with experience of management of the condition. This is because the successful management of NF2 patients involves coordination between several different specialities, principally neurosurgeons, otolarygologists, ophthalmologists and geneticists. All patients with the condition, because of the high frequency of vestibular schwannomas and other serious nervous system tumours, need this multidisciplinary follow-up. Patients also need ongoing support from other health professionals such as teachers of communication to the deaf, and social workers. Several studies have shown improved surgical outcome when vestibular schwannoma surgery in NF2 is performed in centres specializing in this kind of surgery [12, 62]. The study of Evans *et al.* [57] also showed that very few families had any understanding of the natural history or genetic nature of their condition. Only 44 of 120 patients had received genetic counselling and many people were unaware that NF2 could be inherited [57].

(a) Management of affected individuals

Once an individual has been diagnosed as having NF2, they need life-long follow-up, since monitoring for the early diagnosis of developing tumours is essential. Even if patients only present with symptomatic vestibular schwannomas, they should always have a spinal MRI scan to exclude spinal tumours before any surgery is undertaken. The rate of growth of the tumours in NF2 is very variable, and with the advent of MRI imaging many asymptomatic tumours are being found in individuals with NF2 which, when followed for a number of years, either remain the same size or take several years before they enlarge enough to cause symptoms.

Surgery is geared toward the treatment of symptomatic lesions. For meningiomas and spinal tumours occurring in NF2, the surgical approach is the same as when these lesions arise in the general population. With regard to the bilateral vestibular schwannomas, surgery on small tumours in NF2 has been less successful than in unilateral cases [58, 63]. This has led to a relatively conservative approach in the management of patients. They should have regular careful evaluation with audiological examinations and neuro-imaging studies. In patients with no symptoms or mild stable symptoms, where MRI

shows no increase in tumour size, conservative observation is indicated. The detail of the different surgical approaches to vestibular schwannoma is beyond the scope of this chapter, and the interested reader is referred to other reference sources [58, 64].

(b) Genetic counselling and the management of at-risk individuals

Children of affected individuals have a 50% risk of inheriting the condition. In approximately half of those who present, there will be no obvious family history. Before concluding that they represent new mutations, it is important to draw up a very detailed family tree and, unless they are over 60 years of age, to screen the parents for NF2 with clinical examination, ophthalmological examination and cranial MRI.

It is recommended that at-risk individuals are followed annually from birth. The possibility of congenital or very early cataracts necessitates detailed early ophthalmological screening and slit lamp examination to exclude these and retinal hamartomas. Clinical review once a year will give the opportunity to check for other symptomatic lesions. Before the availability of molecular genetic diagnosis, the protocol for monitoring individuals [61] introduced specific screening for vestibular schwannomas with cranial MRI at around 10 years of age and annual brain stem-evoked responses after that point. Depending on the age of onset of disease in the family, these annual examinations were continued until around 30 years of age, when a further repeat MRI scan was recommended. In the majority of families, if individuals were negative at this point it would mean they had not inherited the gene; however, in families with very mild disease it was recommended that screening be continued.

The advent of molecular genetic diagnosis using linked DNA markers and direct mutation analysis means that these protocols have now been altered. The author's present practice is to offer DNA diagnosis, if this is possible, around the age of 9 or 10 years – at this point the children can understand to some degree the situation they are in, and a negative molecular genetic test would obviate the need to begin monitoring with MRI scans and brain stem-evoked responses. If a linkage approach has been used, those being shown to have a low risk of having inherited the gene can go on to less-frequent monitoring until a definitive molecular test becomes available in the family. Those shown to be negative for a gene mutation which has been shown to be present in the family can be reassured that they and their offspring are not at risk of the disease and screening can be discontinued. Molecular genetic testing should be accompanied by detailed genetic counselling. Those shown to be affected by molecular genetic techniques are followed with annual clinical examination, brain stem-evoked responses and MRI imaging. As stated earlier, the optimal management of these at-risk individuals requires close co-operation between the clinical geneticist and the teams involved in management of the affected individuals.

5.3.7 PATHOGENESIS

From a clinical viewpoint, NF2 fits well into the model of other familial cancers that have been shown to be caused by tumour suppressor genes. In the general population unilateral vestibular schwannomas develop in middle or old age. In NF2, vestibular schwannomas occur bilaterally and are often associated with other neoplasms, all of which develop at a relatively young age. Before the molecular genetic era, cytogenetic analysis of meningiomas had shown loss of the whole or part of chromosome 22 in 10–30% of tumours [65, 66]. With the development of molecular genetic techniques, this led Seizinger and

colleagues [67] to focus on chromosome 22 in their molecular genetic analysis of isolated vestibular schwannomas. Their hypothesis proved correct and preferential loss of chromosome 22 was found in unilateral vestibular schwannomas, in the general population. The studies were then extended to vestibular schwannomas from patients with NF2 who showed a similar loss of chromosome 22 [68]. This gave strong evidence that the most likely localization for the *NF2* gene was on chromosome 22, which was confirmed by study of the segregation of chromosome 22 markers in a large NF2 kindred [69]. Subsequent studies in other families has given no suggestion of genetic heterogeneity in NF2 [70].

(a) The *NF2* gene: Merlin/Schwannomin

Identification of flanking genetic markers enabled the application of physical mapping techniques to the intervening region in order to identify the *NF2* gene. In 1993, two groups reported the isolation of the *NF2* gene [9, 10]. This was achieved by identifying patients with molecular deletions within this region and studying the surrounding DNA. The *NF2* candidate gene was found to have deletions in some patients and more subtle forms of mutations at the single base level in others, all of which would have resulted in protein truncation compatible with the *NF2* being a tumour suppressor gene. Mutations were also identified in tumours, schwannomas and meningiomas from NF2-related patients.

The *NF2* gene has 16 exons, one of which is subject to alternative splicing. It encodes a protein consisting of 587 amino acids which shows homology to a growing family of proteins that have been proposed to act as links between the cell membrane and the cytoskeleton [9, 10, 71]. This group of proteins includes moesin, ezrin and radixin. This led Trofatter and colleagues [10] to name the

*NF*2 gene Merlin (*m*oesin-, *e*zrin-, *r*adixin-like gene). Rouleau *et al.* [9] suggested the name Schwannomin in view of the histology of most tumours in NF2.

The cloning of the gene now makes studies of tissue distribution, protein function and the creation of mice with the *NF*2 gene mutated possible.

5.3.8 CLINICAL APPLICATIONS

Once flanking markers had been identified [71] presymptomatic diagnosis using linkage analysis became possible in families with the correct structure. With linking markers, informative predictions are usually more than 99% accurate. The definitive test of course is for the presence of the mutation and, given the much smaller size of the *NF*2 gene compared with *NF*1, it is much easier to screen for mutations. These have been reported from a number of groups [72], and in the families of these individuals direct mutation testing is now clinically applicable with virtually 100% accuracy.

As we gain insight into the function of the normal and mutated *NF*2 gene, medical strategies for the prevention and control of growth of the tumours in NF2 may become possible.

REFERENCES

1. Knudson, A.G. Jr (1971) Mutation and cancer: statistical study of retinoblastoma. *Proc. Natl Acad. Sci. USA*, **68**, 820–3.
2. von Recklinghausen, F.D. (1882) *Ueber die multiplen Fibrome der Haut und ihre Beziehung zu den multiplen Neuromen*. Hirschwald, Berlin.
3. Wishart, J. (1822) Cases of tumors in the skull, dura mater and brain. *Edinb. Clin. Surg. J.*, **18**, 393–7.
4. Gardiner, W.T. and Frazier, C.H. (1930) Bilateral acoustic neurofibromas: a clinical study and field survey of a family of five generations with bilateral deafness in 38 members. *Arch. Neurol. Psychiatr.*, **23**, 266–300.
5. Young, D.F., Eldridge, R. and Gardner, W.J. (1970) Bilateral acoustic neuromas in a large kindred. *JAMA*, **214**, 347–53.
6. Cawthon, R.M., Weiss, R., Xu, G. *et al* (1990) A major segment of the neurofibromatosis type gene. CDNA sequence genomic structure and point mutations. *Cell*, **62**, 193–201.
7. Viskochil, D., Buchberg, A.M., Xu, G. *et al.* (1990) Deletions and a translocation interrupt a cloned gene at the neurofibromatosis type 1 locus. *Cell*, **62**, 187–92.
8. Wallace, M.R., Marchuk, D.A., Anderson, L.B. *et al.* (1990) Type 1 neurofibromatosis gene: identification of a large transcript disrupted in three NF1 patients. *Science*, **249**, 181–6
9. Rouleau, G.A., Merel, P., Lutchman, M. *et al.* (1993) Alteration in a new gene encoding a putative membrane organizing protein causes neurofibromatosis type 2. *Nature*, **363**, 515–21.
10. Trofatter, J.A., MacCollin, M.M., Rutter, J.L. *et al.* (1993) A novel moesin, ezrin, radixin-like gene is a candidate for the neurofibromatosis 2 tumour suppressor. *Cell*, **72**, 791–800.
11. NIH Consensus Development Conference (1988) Neurofibromatosis Conference Statement. *Arch. Neurol.*, **45**, 575–8.
12. NIH Consensus Development Conference (1992) Conference Statement: Acoustic Neuroma. *Neurofibromatosis Research Newsletter*, **8**, 1–7.
13. Riccardi, V.M. (1982) Neurofibromatosis: clinical heterogeneity. *Curr. Probl. Cancer*, **VII** (2), 1–34
14. Viskochil, D and Carey, J.C. (1994) Alternative and related forms of neurofibromatosis, in *The Neurofibromatoses: a Clinical and Pathogenetic Overview*, (eds S.M. Huson and R.A.C. Hughes), Chapman & Hall, London, pp. 445–74.
15. Crowe, F.W., Schull, W.J. and Neel, J.V. (1956) *A Clinical, Pathological and Genetic Study of Multiple Neurofibromatosis*, Charles C. Thomas, Springfield.
16. Huson, S.M., Clark, P., Compston, D.A.S. *et al.* (1989) A genetic study of von Recklinghausen's neurofibromatosis in South East Wales I: prevalence, fitness, mutation rate and effect of parental transmission on severity. *J. Clin. Genet.*, **26**, 704–11.
17. Huson, S.M. (1994) Neurofibromatosis I: a

clinical and genetic overview, in *The Neuro-fibromatoses: a Pathogenetic and Clinical Overview*, (eds S.M. Huson and R.A.C. Hughes), Chapman & Hall, London, pp. 160–203.

18. Huson, S.M., Harper, P.S. and Compston, D.A.S. (1988) von Recklinghausen neurofibromatosis: a clinical and population study in South East Wales. *Brain*, **III**, 1355–81.

19. Ragge, N.K., Falk, R.E., Cohen, W.E. and Murphree, A.L. (1993) Images of Lisch nodules across the spectrum. *Eye*, **7**, 95–101.

20. Riccardi, V.M. (1992) *Neurofibromatosis: Phenotype, Natural History and Pathogenesis*, 2nd edn, The Johns Hopkins University Press, Baltimore.

21. Huson, S.M., Compston, D.A.S. and Harper, P.S. (1989) A genetic study of von Recklinghausen neurofibromatosis in South East Wales II (guidelines for genetic counselling). *J. Clin. Genet.*, **26**, 712–21.

22. Huson, S.M. and Hughes, R.A.C. (eds) (1994) *The Neurofibromatoses: A Clinical and Pathogenetic Overview*, Chapman & Hall, London.

23. Rubenstein, A.E. and Korf, B.R. (eds) (1990) *Neurofibromatosis: A Handbook for Patients, Families and Healthcare Professionals*, Thieme Medical, New York.

24. Sorenson, S.A., Mulvihill, J.J. and Nielsen, A. (1986) Long-term follow up of von Recklinghausen neurofibromatosis: survival and malignant neoplasms. *N. Engl. J. Med.*, **314**, 1010–15.

25. Narod, S.A., Stiller, C. and Lenoir, G.M. (1991) An estimate of the heritable fraction of childhood cancer. *Br. J. Cancer*, **63**, 993–9.

26. Purvin, V.A. and Dunn, D.W. (1994) Ophthalmalogical manifestations of neurofibromatosis 1 and 2, in *The Neurofibromatoses: a Clinical and Pathogenetic Overview*, (eds S.M. Huson and R.A.C. Hughes), Chapman & Hall, London, pp. 253–74.

27. Lewis, R.A., Gerson, L.P., Axelson, K.A. *et al.* (1984) Von Reckinghausen neurofibromatosis II. Incidence of optic gliomata. *Ophthalmology*, **91**, 929–35.

28. Ferner, R.E., Chaudhuri, R, Bingham, J. *et al.* (1993) Magnetic resonance imaging in neurofibromatosis 1. The nature and evolution of increased intensity T2 weighted lesions and

their relationship to intellectual impairment. *J. Neurol. Neurosurg. Psychiatr.* **56**, 492–5.

29. Hughes, R.A.C. (1994) Neurological complications of neurofibromatosis 1, in *The Neurofibromatoses: a Clinical and Pathogenetic Overview*, (eds S.M. Huson and R.A.C. Hughes), Chapman & Hall, London, pp. 204–32.

30. Kleihues, P., Burger, P.C. and Scheithauer, B.W. (1993) *Histological typing of Tumours of the Central Nervous System*, 2nd ed, Springer Verlag, Berlin, Heidelberg.

31. Brasfield, R.D. and Das Gupta, T.K. (1972) Von Recklinghausen's disease: a clinicopathological study. *Ann. Surg.*, **175**, 86–104.

32. McKeen, E.A., Bodurtha, J., Meadows, A.T. *et al.* (1978) Rhabdomyosarcoma complicating multiple neurofibromatosis. *J. Pediatr.*, **93**, 992–3.

33. Hartley, A.L., Birch, J.M., Marsden, H.B. *et al.* (1988) Neurofibromatosis in children with soft tissue sarcoma. *Pediatr. Hematol Oncol.*, **5**, 7–16.

34. Modlin, I.M., Farndon, J.R., Shepherd, A. *et al.* (1979) Phaeochromocytoma in 72 patients: Clinical and diagnostic features, treatment and long-term results. *Br J. Surg.*, **66**, 456–65.

35. Griffiths, D.F.R., Williams, G.T. and Williams, E.D. (1987) Duodenal carcinoid, phaeochromocytoma and neurofibromatosis: islet cell tumor, phaeochromocytoma and the von Hippel Lindau complex: two distinctive neuroendocrine syndromes. *Q. J. Med.*, **64**, 69–82.

36. Bader, J.L. and Miller, R.W. (1978) Neurofibromatosis and childhood leukaemia. *J. Pediatr.*, **92**, 925–9.

37. Stiller, C.A., Chessells, J.M. and Fitchett, M. (1994) Neurofibromatosis and childhood leukaemia/lymphoma: a population-based UKCCSG study. *Br. J. Cancer*, **70**, 969–72.

38. Morier, P., Mérot, Y., Paccaud, D. *et al.* (1990) Juvenile chronic granulocytic leukaemia, juvenile xanthogranulomas and neurofibromatosis. Case report and review of the literature. *J. Am. Acad. Dermatol.*, **22**, 962–5.

39. Hope, D.G. and Mulvihill, J.J. (1981) Malignancy in neurofibromatosis. *Adv. Neurol.* **29**, 33–55.

40. Mulvihill, J.J. (1994) Malignancy: epidemiologically associated cancers, in *The Neurofibromatoses: a Clinical and Pathogenetic Overview*, (eds

S.M. Huson and R.A.C. Hughes), Chapman & Hall, London, pp. 305–15

41. Jadayel, D., Fain, P., Upadhyaya, M. *et al.* (1990) Paternal origin of new mutations in von Recklinghausens neurofibromatosis. *Nature*, **343**, 558–9.

42. Easton, D.F., Ponder, M.A., Huson, S.M. and Ponder, B.A.J. (1993) An analysis of variation in expression of NF 1: evidence for modifying genes. *Am. J. Hum. Genet.* **53**, 305–13.

43. Bolande, R.P. (1981) Neurofibromatosis – the quintessential neurocristopathy: pathogenetic concepts and relationships. *Adv. Neurol.*, **29**, 67–75.

44. Gutmann, D.H. *et al* (1993) The neurofibromatosis type 1 gene and its protein product, neurofibromin. *Neuron*, **10**, 335–43.

45. Viskochil, D., White, R. and Cawthorn, R. (1993) The neurofibromatosis type 1 gene. *Annu. Rev. Neurosci.*, **16**, 183–205

46. Kayes, L.M., Burke, W., Riccardi, V.M. *et al.* (1994) Deletions spanning the neurofibromatosis gene: Identification and phenotype of five patients. *Am J. Hum. Genet.*; **54**, 424–36.

47. Upadhyaya, M., Shen, M. and Cherryson, A. (1992) Analysis of mutations at the neurofibromatosis 1 (NF1) locus. *Hum. Mol. Genet.*, **1**, 735–40.

48. Legius, E., Marchuk, D.A., Collins, F.S. *et al.* (1993) Somatic deletion of the neurofibromatosis type 1 gene in a neurofibrosarcoma supports a tumour suppressor gene hypothesis. *Nat. Genet.*, **3**, 122–5.

49. Xu, W., Mulligan, L.M., Ponder, M.A. *et al.* (1992) Loss of NF1 alleles in phaeochromocytomas from patients with type 1 neurofibromatosis. *Genes Chromosomes and Cancer*, **4**, 337–42.

50. Shannon, K.M., O'Connell, P., Martin, G.A. *et al.* (1994) Loss of the normal NF1 allele from the bone marrow of children with type 1 neurofibromatosis and malignant myeloid disorders. *N. Engl. J. Med.*, **330**, 597–601.

51. Daston, M.M. Scrable, H., Nordlund, M. *et al.*, (1992) The protein product of the neurofibromatosis type 1 gene is expressed at highest abundance in neurons, Schwann cells and oligodendrocytes. *Neuron*, **8**, 415–28

52. Xu, G., O'Connell, P., Viskochil, D. *et al.* (1990) The neurofibromatosis type 1 gene

encodes a protein related to GAP. *Cell*, **62**, 599–608.

53. Brannan, C.I. Perkins, A.S., Vogel, K.S. *et al.* (1994) Targeted disruption of the neurofibromatosis type 1 gene leads to developmental abnormalities in heart and various neural crest-derived tissues. *Genes Dev.*, **8**, 1019–1029.

54. Jacks, T., Shane Shih, T., Schmitt, E.M. *et al.* (1994) Tumour predisposition in mice heterozygous for a targeted mutation in NF1. *Nature Genet.*, **7**, 353–61.

55. Evans, D.G.R., Huson, S.M., Donnai, D. *et al.* (1992) A genetic study of type 2 neurofibromatosis in the United Kingdom: I. prevalence, mutation rate, fitness and confirmation of maternal transmission effect on severity. *J. Med. Genet.*, **29**, 841–6.

56. Kanter, W.R., Eldridge, R., Fabricant, R. *et al.* (1980) Central neurofibromatosis with bilateral acoustic neuroma: genetic, clinical and biochemical distinctions from peripheral neurofibromatosis. *Neurology*, **30**, 851–9.

57. Evans, D.G.R., Huson, S.M., Neary, W. *et al.* (1992) A clinical study of type 2 neurofibromatosis. *Q. J. Med.*, **304**, 603–18.

58. Short, P.M. Martuza, R.L. and Huson, S.M. (1994) Neurofibromatosis 2: Clinical features, genetic counselling and management issues, in *The Neurofibromatoses: a Pathogenic and Clinical Overview*, (eds S.M. Huson and R.A.C. Hughes), Chapman & Hall, London, pp. 414–44.

59. Kaiser-Kupfer, M.I., Friedlin, V., Datiles, M.B. *et al.* (1989) The association of posterior capsular lens opacities with bilateral acoustic neuromas in patients with neurofibromatosis type 2. *Arch. Ophthalmol.*, **107**, 541–4.

60. Ragge, N.K., Baser, M., Falk, R.E. *et al.* (1992) Presymptomatic diagnosis of NF2: ocular expression. *Am. J. Hum. Genet.*, **51** (suppl.) A51, 113 (abstract).

61. Evans, D.G.R., Huson, S.M., Neary, W. *et al.* (1992) A genetic study of type 2 neurofibromatosis: II. Guidelines for genetic counselling. *J. Med. Genet.*, **29**, 847–52.

62. Evans, D.G.R., Ramsden, R., Huson, S.M. *et al.* (1993) Type 2 neurofibromatosis: The need for supraregional care? *J. Laryngol. Otolaryngol.*, **107**, 401–6.

63. Glasscock, M.E., Woods, C.I., Jackson, C.G.

et al. (1989) Management of bilateral acoustic tumors. *Laryngoscope*, **99**, 475–84.

64. Ojemann, R.G. and Martuza, R.L. (1990) Acoustic neuroma, in *Neurologic Surgery*, 3rd edn, (ed. J. Youmans), W.B. Saunders, Philadelphia, pp. 3316–50.

65. Zang, K.D. and Singer, H. (1967) Chromosomal constitution of meningiomas. *Nature*, **216**, 84–5.

66. Zang, K.D. (1982) Cytological and cytogenetical studies on human meningioma. *Cancer Genet. Cytogenet.*, **6**, 249–74.

67. Seizinger, B.R., Martuza, R.L. and Gusella, J.F. (1986) Loss of genes on chromosome 22 in tumorigenesis of human acoustic neuroma. *Nature*, **322**, 644–7.

68. Seizinger, B.R., Rouleau, G., Ozelius, L. *et al.* (1987) A common pathogenetic mechanism for three different tumour types in bilateral acoustic neurofibromatosis. *Science*, **236**, 317–19.

69. Rouleau, G., Wertelecki, W., Haings, J.L. *et al.* (1987) Genetic linkage analysis of bilateral acoustic neurofibromatosis to a DNA marker on chromosome 22. *Nature*, **329**, 246–8.

70. Narod, S.A., Parry, D.M., Parboosingh, J. *et al.* (1992) Neurofibromatosis type 2 appears to be a genetically homogeneous disease. *Am J. Hum. Genet.*, **51**, 486–96.

71. Bianchi, A.B., Hara, T., Ramesh, V. *et al.* (1994) Mutations in transcript isoforms of the neurofibromatosis 2 gene in multiple human tumour types. *Nature Genet.*, **6**, 185–92

72. Bourn, D., Carter, S.A., Mason, S. *et al.* (1994) Germline mutations in the neurofibromatosis type 2 tumour suppresser gene. *Hum. Mol. Genet.*, **3**, 811–16.

Chapter 6

Multiple endocrine neoplasia

BRUCE A.J. PONDER

6.1 INTRODUCTION

The multiple endocrine neoplasia (MEN) syndromes comprise dominantly inherited predisposition to tumours of specific endocrine glands. Two distinct syndromes are recognized:

- MEN 1, which most commonly affects the parathyroid, pancreatic islets and anterior pituitary.
- MEN 2, which is a constellation of three related but distinct syndromes of abnormal development and tumour formation, principally affecting the thyroid C cells, adrenal medulla, parathyroids, and the enteric ganglion cells of the autonomic nervous system.

Although families have been reported in which there have been tumours characteristic of both syndromes, there is no evidence that these are more than coincidence. Genetically, both MEN 1 and MEN 2 appear to be distinct and homogeneous, mapping respectively to genes on chromosome 11q13 and 10q11.2. Certain strains of rats do, however, appear to have a genuine susceptibility to a spectrum of

Table 6.1 Tumours in MEN 1

Tumour type/location	Cumulative risk (%)
Parathyroid	>90
Endocrine pancreatic tumours, gastrinoma, insulinoma, vipoma	~70
Anterior pituitary	~50
Carcinoid, adrenal cortex, lipomas	Uncommon

tumours which spans both MEN 1 and MEN 2, the genetic basis for which is unclear [1].

6.2 MULTIPLE ENDOCRINE NEOPLASIA TYPE 1 (MEN 1)

The prevalence of MEN 1 is unknown, but is probably between 1 in 5000 and 1 in 50 000 of the population [2]. The syndrome can be diagnosed when either two close relatives have one of the characteristic tumours (Table 6.1) or tumours at two or more sites occur in the same individual.

Formal studies of the probability of clinical presentation or detection by screening of

Genetic Predisposition to Cancer. Edited by R.A. Eeles, B.A.J. Ponder, D.F. Easton and A. Horwich. Published in 1996 by Chapman & Hall, London.
0 412 56580 3

Table 6.2   Guidelines for screening in MEN 1

---

1. Known MEN 1 family history; or individual with two MEN 1 syndrome tumours
    Affected individuals
    Every 1–2 years: clinical assessment
                      biochemical screening (serum calcium, prolactin, parathyroid hormone, growth
                      hormone, gastrin, pancreatic polypeptide, fasting serum insulin; blood glucose)
                      ?Stimulatory meal tests for early diagnosis of pancreatic tumours.

    Relatives at risk
        If you are not a specialist, contact clinical genetics department for advice about family tracing and
        possible DNA analysis
        Biochemical screening starting at age 5; 1–2-yearly serum calcium and prolactin. In the absence of
        DNA based data, the individual has a roughly 10% residual risk of being a carrier if testing is
        negative at age 40

2. Isolated case of MEN 1-type tumour: is this the family form?
        Clinical manifestations of other endocrine lesions in this patient
        Detailed family history – include peptic ulcer, renal stones, infertility, hypertension, acromegaly
        Histopathology: multicentric tumours suggest inherited syndrome
        Biochemical markers as above for other endocrine involvement
        If any suggestion of MEN 1, screen first-degree relatives (especially parents) by serum calcium
        level. Negative results are probably sufficient for exclusion of familial risk in most cases.

---

each of the components of MEN 1 by age have not been carried out in the same way as for MEN 2 [3]; nevertheless, experience of a large series of families suggests that elevated serum calcium is the first detectable manifestation in the vast majority of cases, preceded in a few cases by elevations of serum prolactin. A child of an MEN 1 parent has a 50% chance at birth of being an MEN 1 carrier; if he or she has a normal serum calcium and prolactin at the age of 40, this chance is reduced to about 10% [4]. These observations can be used to guide screening (see below).

6.2.1   MOLECULAR GENETICS

The MEN 1 gene has been mapped by genetic linkage to the region immediately distal to the *PYGM* locus on chromosome 11q13 [5]. Allele losses in this region in MEN 1-related tumours suggest that the MEN 1 gene probably acts as a tumour suppressor gene, and that the MEN 1 mutation results in loss of

activity [6]. At present, the gene has not been identified, and there are no clues as to the type of gene it might be.

6.2.2   CLINICAL IMPLICATIONS

Each of the component tumours of MEN 1 occurs more commonly in a truly sporadic (non-inherited) form. It is important to pick up those cases that are familial, so that biochemical or genetic screening and early diagnosis can be offered to family members at risk. The first step in the evaluation of any patient with an MEN 1 syndrome tumour must therefore be to take a careful and extensive family history. Screening can then follow the guidelines shown in Table 6.2. DNA-based screening is currently available only for extensive families, where the use of linked markers is possible. When the MEN 1 gene is identified, however, it should in principle be possible to extend DNA testing to all families to determine which individuals are at risk and require surveillance and which

Table 6.3 Tissue involvement in MEN 2 varieties

Syndrome	Thyroid cells (tumour)	Adrenal medulla (tumour)	Parathyroid (hyperplasia or adenoma)	Enteric ganglia (increased or absent)
MEN 2A	+	+	+	↓ ↓
MEN 2B	+	+	−	↑ ↑
F-MTC	+	−	−	−

are not. It should also be possible, provided that the majority of MEN 1 mutations are easily detected, to use DNA testing to distinguish sporadic cases of pituitary, pancreatic or parathyroid tumour from hereditary cases, and to focus biochemical screening accordingly.

6.3 MULTIPLE ENDOCRINE NEOPLASIA TYPE 2 (MEN 2)

MEN 2 is an autosomal dominant syndrome of disordered development and tumour formation which affects principally four tissues: thyroid C cells, adrenal medulla, the enteric autonomic nervous system, and the parathyroids. The first three of these share developmental origin from the neural ectoderm; the involvement of the parathyroids is explained by the expression, in the branchial arch endoderm which will give rise to the parathyroids, of the *RET* gene which is found to be mutated in MEN 2 (see below) [7].

There are three distinct clinical varieties of MEN 2, which differ in the pattern of tissues involved (Table 6.3). The most common form is MEN 2A, in which C cell tumours of the thyroid (medullary thyroid carcinoma; MTC) are associated with phaeochromocytoma in about 50% of individuals, and with parathyroid hyperplasia or adenoma in about 10–30% (depending on how energetically it is sought). The age at clinical diagnosis of tumours in MEN 2A ranges from early teens to 70 years or more; about 30% of gene carriers never manifest clinically significant

disease [3]. A few families have been described with variant forms of MEN 2A, including amyloid of the skin in the interscapular region, and aganglionosis of the colon resembling Hirschsprung disease [8].

Familial MTC (F-MTC) is a less common form of MEN 2, in which C cell tumours of the thyroid are the only abnormality. In these families, the disease tends to present later and to be less aggressive than in MEN 2A [9]. F-MTC is only clearly recognisable in the case of a very extensive family in which there is no evidence at all of phaeochromocytoma or parathyroid involvement: commonly, however, families are seen in which there are maybe two or three cases of MTC, and screening for phaeochromocytoma or parathyroid disease is incompletely documented. These families may be called 'F-MTC', when in fact it is equally or more probable that they should be classified as MEN 2A families in which by chance the adrenal or parathyroid involvement has not yet become manifest. This distinction is important in relation to the mutation data which will be presented below, and these families are better separated into an 'unclassified' group.

MEN 2B is also uncommon. It is distinguished by involvement of the thyroid C cells and the adrenal but not the parathyroids, and by a range of developmental abnormalities which include hyperplasia of the enteric ganglion cells and of nerve fibres in the oral mucosa and conjunctiva, skeletal abnormalities, and in a few cases, delayed puberty [10]. The onset of C cell and adrenal

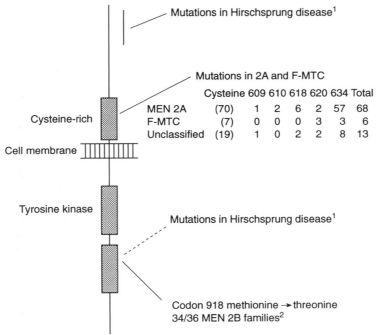

Fig. 6.1 Mutations in *RET* in MEN 2 and in Hirschsprung disease. The table of MEN 2A, F-MTC and Unclassified shows the numbers of mutations identified in these families in each of the five cysteine residues in the extracellular domain close to the cell membrane [14]. Cys634 is the closest to the membrane. Note that the mutation is yet to be identified in a few families. 1, refernces [19, 20]; 2, references [15, 16].

tumours tends to be earlier than in MEN 2A. Many cases of MEN 2B do not have a family history and are new mutations, appearing as sporadic cases with potentially heritable disease.

MTC and phaeochromocytomas also occur as truly sporadic tumours, with no inherited risk. However, as many as 10% of apparently isolated cases of MTC may in fact be of the heritable type: in these cases, the family history is not manifest for some reason, usually the failure of the gene to cause evident disease in the previous generation [11]. Recognition of these heritable cases with no family history can be a difficult clinical problem which may be resolved by DNA testing (see below).

6.3.1 THE MEN 2 GENE

The predisposing gene for the MEN 2 syndromes has been identified as *RET*, a member of the family of tyrosine kinase receptors [12] (Figure 6.1). These receptor molecules comprise an extracellular domain, a transmembrane region, and an intracellular tyrosine kinase domain. Binding of specific ligand to the extracellular domain activates the receptor (usually by causing dimerization, although this has not yet been demonstrated in the case of *RET* in MEN 2), causing the kinase domain to catalyse the phosphorylation of tyrosine residues on itself and possibly other interacting proteins, which initiates an onward signalling cascade [13].

In the majority of families with MEN 2A

and F-MTC, the mutations in *RET* affect one of several cysteine residues which lie in the extracellular domain of the protein, just outside the cell membrane (Figure 6.1). Most commonly, in MEN 2A, the mutations affect 634Cys, the cysteine closest to the membrane. Each of the possible amino-acid changes from cysteine has been seen. Interestingly, there seems to be a correlation between the precise mutation and the spectrum of tissues involved. In F-MTC families, the mutations are more likely to affect one of the cysteines further out from the cell membrane, whereas in MEN 2A families 634Cys is most often affected; and 634Cys mutations which lead to substitution of cysteine by arginine are the most likely to be associated with parathyroid disease [14]. In about 5% of MEN 2A families (defined as MTC with either phaeochromocytoma or parathyroid disease) and in about 30% of families in which MTC is the only tumour, *RET* mutations have still not been found.

In MEN 2B, the mutations are quite distinct. Almost all are identical, a point mutation leading to replacement of methionine to threonine at codon 918, in the catalytic core of the tyrosine kinase domain [15, 16]. Two apparently typical MEN 2B cases have been reported so far in which this mutation is not present.

Hirschsprung disease is associated with absence of the enteric autonomic ganglion plexus, in contrast to MEN 2B where there is hyperplasia of the plexus. The finding that predisposition in some families with Hirschsprung mapped by linkage to the MEN 2 region of chromosome 10 [17], and that transgenic mice in which *RET* had been inactivated developed a gut pathology resembling Hirschsprung disease [18], suggested *RET* as a candidate gene for human Hirschsprung as well. This has been confirmed by the finding of germline mutations in both the extracellular [19] and tyrosine kinase [20] domains of *RET* in Hirschsprung families.

The functional consequences of these different *RET* mutations are beginning to become clear [19–22]. The deletion of one allele of *RET* in some cases of Hirschsprung disease suggests that loss of activity of one copy of the gene causes this phenotype, and consistent with this, point mutations in the *RET* gene in Hirschsprung disease are predicted to result in an inactive protein [19, 20]. The contrasting hyperplasia of the enteric nervous system in MEN 2B, and the apparent lack of mutations in the wild-type *RET* allele in MEN 2-related tumours, suggested that the mutations in F-MTC, MEN 2A and MEN 2B might result in inappropriate activation of the *RET* gene. This has recently been confirmed by studies in which transfection of *RET* constructs bearing an MEN 2A mutation into 3T3 cells resulted in transformation [21]. The activation of MEN2A *RET* probably results from the formation of covalently linked dimers between adjacent *RET* protein molecules, through the cysteines which have lost their normal partners on the same molecule as a result of the MEN 2A mutation [21]. By contrast, it is still unclear whether the MEN 2B mutation is activating, in the sense that the activity of the receptor is independent of ligand. The methionine residue at codon 918 which is critical in MEN 2B lies at the bottom of the substrate-binding pocket in the catalytic domain of the *RET* tyrosine kinase. The mutation is produced to alter the substrate specificity of *RET*, and hence the pathway of downstream signalling from the receptor. This has now been confirmed in two ways: by demonstrating different substrate affinity of the wild-type and MEN 2B tyrosine kinase [22], or by showing that a different pattern of phosphorylated intracellular peptides is produced upon activation of the wild-type or MEN 2B mutant receptor [21].

102

Preliminary results from analysis of sporadic MTC tumour DNA and phaeochromocytomas suggest that mutations similar to that seen in MEN 2B are not uncommon, but that there are few, if any, mutations of the MEN 2A type. This suggests that the functional consequences of the MEN 2B tyrosine kinase mutation are more effective than are mutations of the type seen in MEN 2A, in driving tumour formation in somatic cells.

6.3.2 CLINICAL IMPLICATIONS

(a) Predictive genetic testing in families

Prediction of the inheritance of the predisposing gene is now possible in the majority of families with classical MEN 2A or MEN 2B, and in many families with MTC only, by direct mutation analysis without the need for typing several family members to establish the inheritance of a linked genetic marker. Because the number of different mutations is quite small, mutation screening should be rapid; for several of the mutations, a simple restriction enzyme recognition site assay can be used instead of DNA sequencing [23]. It is not yet possible to predict with enough accuracy to be of clinical value the risk of either phaeochromocytoma or parathyroid disease within a given family, nor the likely age at development or aggressiveness of the disease. Requests for DNA testing should be made through a clinical genetics laboratory.

(b) The apparently sporadic case of MTC

The recognition of the potentially familial cases among those presenting with apparently sporadic disease is an important clinical problem. Screening of DNA from the blood of such cases is now recommended, as the finding of a typical MEN 2 mutation will provide strong evidence that this is a familial case, and indicate the possibility of screening the rest of the family for the same mutation. Failure to find a mutation in the original case cannot, however, completely rule out inherited disease (though it can reduce the chances), because the mutations have still not been identified in some 30% of familial cases.

REFERENCES

1. Boorman, G.A. and Hollander, C.F. (1976) Animal model of human disease: medullary carcinoma of the thyroid. *Am. J. Pathol.*, **83**, 237–40.
2. Lips, C.J., Vasen, H.F. and Lamens, C.B. (1984) Multiple endocrine neoplasia syndromes. *Crit. Rev. Oncol. Haematol.*, **2**, 117–84.
3. Easton, D.F., Ponder, M.A., Cummings. T. *et al.* (1989) The clinical and screening age-at-onset distribution for the MEN 2 syndrome. *Am. J. Hum. Genet.*, **44**, 208–15.
4. Thakker, R.V. (1993) The molecular genetics of the multiple endocrine neoplasia syndromes. *Clin. Endocrinol.*, **38**, 1–14.
5. Thakker, R.V., Wooding, C., Pang, J.T. *et al.* (1993) Linkage analysis of 7 polymorphic markers at chromosome 11p11.2-11q13 in 27 multiple endocrine neoplasia type I families. *Ann. Hum. Genet.* **57**, 17–25.
6. Larsson, C., Skogseid, B., Oberg, K. *et al.* (1988) Multiple endocrine neoplasia type I gene maps to chromosome 11 and is lost in insulinoma. *Nature*, **332**, 85–7.
7. Pachnis, V., Mankoo, B. and Constantini, F. (1993) Expression of the c-ret proto-oncogene during mouse embryogenesis. *Development*, **119**, 1005–17.
8. Verdy, M., Weber, A.M., Roy, C.C. *et al.* (1982) Hirschsprung's disease in a family with MEN type 2. *Paediatr. Gastroenterol. Nutr.*, **1**, 603–7.
9. Farndon, J.R., Dilley, W.G., Baylin, S.B. *et al.* (1986). Familial medullary thyroid carcinoma without associated endocrinopathies: a distinct clinical entity. *Br. J. Surg.*, **73**, 278–81.
10. Dyck, P.J., Carney, A., Sizemore, G.W. *et al.* (1979). Multiple endocrine neoplasia type 2B: phenotype recognition. *Ann. Neurol.*, **6**, 302–14.

11. Ponder, B.A.J., Ponder, M.A., Coffey, R. *et al.* (1988) Risk estimation and screening of families of patients with medullary thyroid carcinoma. *Lancet*, **i**, 397–400.

12. Mulligan, L.M., Kwok, J.B.J., Healey, C.S. *et al.* (1993) Germ-line mutations of the RET proto-oncogene in multiple endocrine neoplasia type 2A. *Nature*, **363**, 458–60.

13. Ullrich, A. and Schlessinger, J. (1990) Signal transduction by receptors with tyrosine kinase activity. *Cell*, **61**, 203–12.

14. Mulligan, L.M., Eng, C., Healey, C.S. *et al.* (1994) Specific mutations of the ret proto-oncogene are related to disease phenotype in MEN 2A and FMTC. *Nature Genet.*, **6**, 70–4.

15. Hofstra, R.M.W., Landsvater, R.M., Ceccherini, I. *et al.* (1994) A mutation in the ret protooncogene associated with multiple endocrine neoplasia type 2B and sporadic medullary thyroid carcinoma. *Nature*, **367**, 375–6.

16. Eng, C., Smith, D.P., Mulligan, L.M. *et al.* (1994) Point mutation within the tyrosine kinase domain of the RET proto-oncogene in multiple endocrine neoplasia type 2B and related sporadic tumours. *Hum. Mol. Genet.*, **3**, 237–41.

17. Lyonnet, S., Bolina, A., Pelet, A. *et al.* (1993) A gene for Hirschsprungs disease maps to the proximal long arm of chromosome 10. *Nature Genet.*, **4**, 346–50.

18. Schuchardt, A., D'Agati, V., Larsson-Blomberg, L. *et al.* (1994) Defects in the kidney and enteric nervous system of mice lacking the tyrosine kinase receptor ret. *Nature*, **367**, 380–2.

19. Edery, P., Lyonnet, S., Mulligan, L.M. *et al.* (1994) Mutations of the RET proto-oncogene in Hirschsprung's disease. *Nature*, **367**, 378–80.

20. Romeo, G., Ronchetto, P., Luo, Y. *et al.* (1994) Point mutations affecting the tyrosine kinase domain of the ret protooncogene in Hirschsprungs disease, *Nature*, **367**, 377–8.

21. Santoro, M., Carlomango, F., Romano, A. *et al.* (1995) Activation of *RET* as a dominant transforming gene by germline mutations of MEN 2A and MEN 2B. *Science*, **267**, 381–3.

22. Songyang, Z., Carraway, K.L., Eck, M.J. *et al.* (1995) Catalytic specificity of protein tyrosine kinases is critical for selective signalling. *Nature*, **373**, 536–8.

23. McMahon, R., Mulligan, L.M., Healey, C.S. *et al.* (1994) Direct, non-radioactive detection of mutations in multiple endocrine neoplasia type 2A families. *Hum. Mol. Genet.*, **3**, 643–6.

Chapter 7

Wilms tumour and other genetic causes of renal cancer

KATHRYN PRITCHARD-JONES

7.1 INTRODUCTION

Primary cancers of the kidney are rare at any age. Although only a small proportion of cases are clearly inherited, genetic predisposition is the most important aetiological factor thus far identified in this group of tumours. The histological type of tumour depends very much on the age at tumour diagnosis; congenital mesoblastic nephroma is most common in the first 3 months of life, followed by a predominance of Wilms tumour (nephroblastoma) in early childhood which is overtaken by renal cell carcinoma in adult life. Kidney cancer is extremely rare between the ages of 7 and 40 years (see Figure 7.1).

By mid-1994, three genes predisposing to kidney cancer have been cloned, the Wilms tumour (WT1) gene at chromosome 11p13, the Von Hippel–Lindau gene at 3p25 and the tuberous sclerosis gene at 16p13. The chro-mosomal loci of several other such genes are known and they are close to being isolated.

7.2 RENAL TUMOURS IN CHILDHOOD

The majority of kidney cancers in childhood occur before the age of 7 years. Such an early onset implies either that genetic factors are predominant or that early, perhaps intrauterine, exposure to strong enviromental carcinogens results in the development of these tumours. Such an intrauterine effect has been shown in the ethylnitrosourea-induced rat model of nephroblastoma [1]. However, in humans, case-control studies have failed to identify consistent environmental risk factors, the strongest association being paternal occupation as a welder or mechanic, which has been shown to confer up to an eight-fold increased risk of Wilms tumour in their offspring [2]. Wilms tumour accounts for about 90% of childhood renal cancers and is the only such tumour for which genetic

Genetic Predisposition to Cancer. Edited by R.A. Eeles, B.A.J. Ponder, D.F. Easton and A. Horwich. Published in 1996 by Chapman & Hall, London.
0 412 56580 3

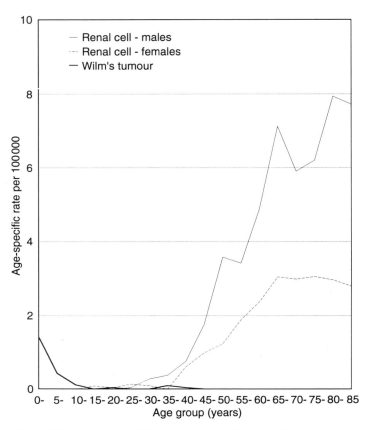

Fig. 7.1 Age-specific incidence rates for Wilms tumour and renal cell carcinoma in south-east England; average annual rates 1980–89. (Data from the Thames Cancer Registry.)

predisposition has been proven. Despite the very early onset of congenital mesoblastic nephroma, no predisposing genetic factors have yet been identified. A similar situation holds for the rare malignant rhabdoid tumour of kidney, which accounts for about 2% of all childhood renal cancers. This tumour presents at a median age of only 13 months and is associated with a high risk of independent primary brain tumours, both observations suggesting a genetic predisposition, which remains to be elucidated. Clear cell sarcoma of kidney, which accounts for about 4% of all childhood renal cancers, has no

special features suggestive of genetic predisposition.

7.2.1 WILMS TUMOUR

Wilms tumour, otherwise known as nephroblastoma, is one of the embryonal tumours of childhood, so-called because the growth pattern of the tumour shows a remarkable mimicry of structures seen during normal embryonic kidney development. At least 90% of Wilms tumours occur as a sporadic event in an otherwise normal child. Less than 1% of cases are clearly inherited and approxi-

Table 7.1 Genetics of Wilms tumour-associated syndromes

	Wilms tumour – aniridia	*Denys–Drash syndrome*	*Beckwith– Wiedemann syndrome*	*Perlman syndrome*
Prevalence among Wilms tumour cases	~1%	<1%	~0.5%[1]	Extremely rare[2]
Risk of Wilms tumour	30–50%	High (>50%)	3–5%	High (>50%)[2]
Genetics and mode of inheritance	Sporadic *de novo* germline mutation	Sporadic *de novo* germline mutation	Sporadic *de novo* germline mutation 85%	Familial (AR)
	Rarely familial (AD)		Familial 15% (AD variable expressively)	
Chromosomal locus	11p13	11p13	11p15.5	Unknown
Disease gene(s)	WT1 (and aniridia gene)	WT1	Unknown	Unknown
Types of mutation	Contiguous gene syndrome Complete deletion of one allele of WT1 and aniridia genes	Point mutation (mainly missense) Frameshift Aberrant mRNA splicing	–	–

[1] A further 2.5% of all cases have hemihypertrophy, which may represent a 'forme fruste' of BWS.
[2] Only 14 cases reported in world literature [62–67]. Risk of Wilms tumour (WT) probably very high if they survive beyond 1 year of age (6/14 had WT, 7/8 without WT died in neonatal period).

mately 1–2% occur in children with congenital malformation syndromes which carry a greatly increased risk of Wilms tumour – the WAGR (Wilms tumour-aniridia), Denys–Drash, Beckwith–Wiedemann and Perlman syndromes (Table 7.1). Wilms tumour is associated with presumed precursor lesions in the kidney, known as nephrogenic rests, which have been classified into two major types (perilobar and intralobar) according to position and morphology [3]. Intralobar nephrogenic rests (ILNRs) are thought to result from a very early, probably germline, mutation whereas perilobar nephrogenic rests (PLNRs) are thought to represent a slightly later insult to the embryonic kidney. Overall, nephrogenic rests are found in adjacent normal kidney in 40% of unilateral and almost 100% of bilateral Wilms tumours.

(a) Genetics of Wilms tumour and Knudson's two-hit hypothesis

In 1972, Knudson proposed that his two-hit mutational model, which had been formulated originally for retinoblastoma, could also serve as a model for Wilms tumour [4,5] (see Chapter 4). Briefly, the hypothesis states that as few as two mutations are sufficient to allow tumour development and that the first of these mutations can be in the germline, in which case tumours tend to occur earlier and be bilateral. The assumption was made that all familial and bilateral cases were carriers of a germline mutation.

107

Although the initial statistical analysis of small numbers of familial and bilateral cases of Wilms tumour suggested that the two-hit hypothesis should apply, the situation is now clearly more complex than for retinoblastoma. Allele loss and genetic linkage studies have provided evidence for the existence of up to four Wilms tumour genes, the *WT1* gene at chromosome 11p13, the Beckwith–Wiedemann gene at 11p15, a familial *WT* gene which does not map to chromosomes 11 or 16 and a gene within chromosome 16q, based on a 20% allele loss rate in sporadic Wilms tumours [6]. Furthermore, in those Wilms tumours which do involve mutations in the *WT1* gene, while the majority do carry mutations in both *WT1* alleles, several cases have been described where only one *WT1* allele is mutated [7, 8]. Until the promoter region of the *WT1* gene has been fully examined in these tumours, one cannot be confident that they do not conform to the two-hit model, but it seems likely, especially since several have allele loss confined to chromosome 11p15, that other genes are interacting.

A further prediction of the two-hit model is the proportion of unilateral sporadic cases which represent carriers of germline predisposing mutations. For retinoblastoma, the predicted 10–12% was borne out by the observed 5.5% tumour rate among offspring of survivors of unilateral retinoblastoma. Originally, Knudson and Strong [4] calculated that 30% of unilateral Wilms tumour might be prezygotically determined, based on an 8% incidence of bilateral tumours and the assumption that all bilateral cases indicated a heritable mutation [9]. Subsequently, Knudson revised this estimate downwards to 10–15% when much larger studies of thousands of cases showed a lower incidence of bilaterality (4–5%). However, even this figure must be too high, as using a penetrance of 0.67, the predicted 3–5% of offspring of survivors of unilateral Wilms tumour who

should develop the tumour has not been observed; only one case has been seen among 270 such children [10–12]. The figure for penetrance seems a reasonable approximate based on the observed risk in the albeit small numbers of known gene carriers (familial and *WT1*-associated cases), although the risk of Wilms tumour in BWS is only 3–5% [13, 14]. However, it now seems that the bilateral cases are a heterogeneous group, not all of whom carry germline mutations. First, their age at diagnosis shows a bimodal distribution [2]. Second, the type of associated nephrogenic rest differs for synchronous (PLNR) and metachronous (ILNR) presentation [3]. A further group likely to be of similarly heterogeneous aetiology is the unilateral multifocal Wilms tumours. The two-hit hypothesis assumes that these should all indicate a germline mutation and should occur less frequently than bilateral tumours. In fact, two large epidemiological studies have shown an excess of multifocal unilateral cases and one has proven mathematically that these data do not fit the two-hit model [2, 15]. This, together with the observation that their median age of onset is intermediate between the bilateral and unilateral unifocal cases, with a clearly bimodal curve, is strong evidence that only a subset of children with unilateral multifocal tumours are carriers of germline mutations [2].

(b)   Wilms tumour-aniridia syndrome and the *WT1* gene

The association of aniridia (lack of iris formation) with Wilms tumour has been recognized since the 1960s. Approximately 1% of children with Wilms tumour also have congenital aniridia, which is far in excess of the 1 in 50 000 prevalence of aniridia in the general population. Geneticists recognize two forms of aniridia: familial and sporadic. Only the latter group have this greatly increased risk of

Wilms tumour, which affects 30–50%. The explanation for this discrepancy is that in the familial form, the mutation is confined to the aniridia gene, whereas the sporadic form is the result of an interstitial deletion on the short arm of chromosome 11, which causes constitutional hemizygosity for both the aniridia and Wilms tumour genes as well as many other neighbouring genes. Such individuals frequently have other phenotypic abnormalities, hence the name WAGR (Wilms tumour, Aniridia, Genitourinary malformation and mental Retardation) syndrome. Aniridia is dominant and a marker for the syndrome whereas development of Wilms tumour is recessive at a cellular level, requiring at least a second mutation. There is a high incidence of genitourinary malformation in this syndrome, particularly among XY individuals.

High-resolution molecular mapping of the smallest region of common overlap of chromosomal deletions from several WAGR patients has established that the aniridia gene lies about 1 Mb telomeric to the Wilms tumour gene within 11p13 and has led to the cloning of both genes – human *PAX6* and *WT1* respectively [16–18]. Molecular analysis of individuals with submicroscopic deletions suggests that at least some of the genitourinary abnormalities in the WAGR syndrome are due to dominant effects of mutation in the *WT1* gene rather than to deletion of neighbouring genes [19]. This has been confirmed by mutational analysis in the Denys–Drash syndrome and in a case of familial Wilms tumour (see later).

Six out of eight WAGR patients whose Wilms tumours have been subjected to molecular analysis have a mutation in their remaining *WT1* allele, in accord with the two-hit hypothesis [20–24]. The two negative cases could still harbour *WT1* promoter mutations, as this region of the *WT1* gene was not examined. The nature of the second hit in the Wilms tumours developing in WAGR patients is nearly always a small deletion/ insertion or point mutation, in contrast to the more usual mechanism of mitotic recombination to duplicate the mutant allele. This presumably signifies that homozygous deletion of genes adjacent to *WT1* is cell-lethal.

(c) Characterization of the *WT1* gene

The *WT1* gene encodes a 3-kb mRNA which shows tissue-specific expression in the developing embryo, mainly in the genitourinary tract and mesothelium [25, 26]. Expression continues at lower levels in the adult kidney and gonad. The predicted protein contains four zinc finger motifs and an N-terminal effector domain (Figure 7.2). *In vitro* studies have shown that the protein binds to DNA, the target sequence depending on the presence or absence of an alternative three amino acid splice (KTS) between zinc fingers 3 and 4. The effector domain appears to contain two regions, one a repressor and the other an activator of transcription. The functional balance is usually in favour of repression, though the ratio of +/− KTS isoforms or mutations in either the target promoter or the effector domain of *WT1* can reverse this in *in vitro* assays [45, 46]. The genes regulated by the *WT1* protein *in vivo* have not yet been established, but several proliferative genes (insulin-like growth factor II, platelet-derived growth factor A chain) have been implicated in *in vitro* assays. The *WT1* gene is known to be essential for formation of the metanephric kidney and gonad, as shown by the complete absence of these two organs in homozygous *WT1* null mice [47]. About 10–20% of sporadic Wilms tumours have been found to have *WT1* gene mutations, most of which result in premature termination codons and presumed loss of protein function [7, 8, 40–43, 48–51]. In the majority of cases, the two-hit model is followed but three tumours have been described where only one *WT1* allele can be shown to be mutated.

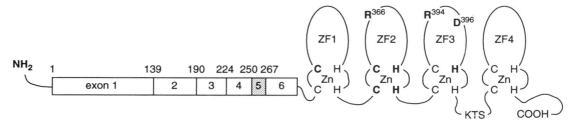

Fig. 7.2 Schematic representation of the *WT1* protein, numbered from the initiator methionine, showing the position of exon boundaries. Exon 5 (shaded) and the three extra amino acids (KTS) between zinc fingers (ZF) 3 and 4 are subjected to alternative splicing. Amino acids indicated in bold are sites of missense mutations in the Denys–Drash syndrome – R[394] is by far the most common mutation, occurring in 24/51 cases, with missense mutations in zinc fingers 2 or 3 accounting for a total of 41/51 cases [27–39]. This is in contrast to other germline intragenic *WT1* mutations, where 6/7 introduce premature stop codons [40–44].

(d) Other syndromes predisposing to Wilms tumour

Denys–Drash syndrome

Denys–Drash syndrome (DDS) is a very rare, sporadic syndrome which was described originally as a triad of male pseudohermaphroditism, early onset protein-losing nephropathy and Wilms tumour [52, 53]. The nephropathy appears to be due to a distinctive glomerular lesion which involves the podocyte layer. It has been suggested that the syndrome should be expanded to include patients with any two of these three features and normal females with the characteristic nephropathy [54]. The risk of Wilms tumour and other gonadal tumours is high but difficult to quantify exactly as, until recently, tumour occurrence was almost a prerequisite for defining the syndrome. Certainly, any child with a congenital gonadal abnormality and nephropathy should be considered at greatly increased risk of Wilms and gonadal tumours.

The observation that the *WT1* gene was expressed in the three cell types showing abnormalities in DDS (i.e. metanephric blastema, podocytes, developing gonad) made it an ideal candidate gene for this syndrome

[26]. This prediction was borne out when 10 children with a clinical diagnosis of DDS were found to have constitutional *WT1* missense mutations in the zinc finger region [27]. Initially, it appeared that missense mutations affecting amino acids critical for the stability of DNA binding of zinc fingers 2 and 3 were responsible for the syndrome, with the genital malformation being dominant but tumour development requiring a second hit. Subsequently, although missense mutations of Arg[394] remain the most common group, several cases with nonsense mutations causing truncated proteins have been described (see Figure 7.2). As a unifying hypothesis, it has been suggested that the constitutionally mutant *WT1* protein may behave as a dominant-negative or antimorph, somehow interfering with the function of the remaining wild-type allele [28, 55]. It is also now apparent that a normal ratio of the second alternative splice in zinc finger 3 is essential for both gonadal development and podocyte function as four DDS patients with intronic mutations preventing formation of the +KTS splice have been described [29–31]. It is an interesting paradox that complete deletion of the *WT1* gene, as in the WAGR syndrome, gives a less severe genitourinary phenotype

than the presence of a mutant *WT*1 protein, which must therefore be somehow interfering with the function of other cellular proteins. However, the final phenotypic expression of *WT*1 mutations must depend on the host genetic make-up, as two children with DDS phenotype but constitutional *WT*1 deletions have been described [54, 56]. Conversely, the most common DDS mutation (Arg^{394}→Trp) has been found in the germline of a normal female with unilateral Wilms tumour who has no evidence of nephropathy at the age of 7 years, making it unlikely that it will develop [40]. There is also a case of germline transmission of the same mutation from an unaffected father to a son with DDS [32]. Furthermore, a review of the genital phenotype of 20 children with identical Arg^{394}→Trp mutations shows a wide range, from normal female to complete ambiguity [30]. This paradox should be clarified once transgenic mice bearing the Arg^{394} mutation become available.

Beckwith–Wiedemann syndrome

The Beckwith–Wiedemann syndrome (BWS) is characterized by pre- and postnatal gigantism, which may be asymmetric leading to hemihypertrophy, as well as malformation, particularly of the heart and genitourinary system [57]. There is hyperplasia of many organs including the tongue and intra-abdominal organs with defects of closure of the abdominal wall (omphalocoele). The kidneys often show persistent fetal characteristics and medullary dysplasia. These children have a 7.5–10% overall risk of developing a childhood tumour, half of which are Wilms tumour, the remainder comprising rhabdomyosarcoma, hepatoblastoma or adrenocortical carcinoma [13, 14]. Of interest, while hemihypertropy is found in 12.5% of all children with BWS, it is found in 40% of those who develop tumours. Most cases are sporadic but familial cases have been described. The familial cases show genetic link-

age to chromosome 11p15.5 and there is an excess of maternal inheritance [58]. Apparently balanced 11p15 translocations occurring in BWS patients also involve the maternal allele. Several sporadic cases have been shown to have uniparental disomy or trisomy for 11p15.5, with the extra copy being of paternal origin. These findings have been interpreted to signify the involvement of genomic imprinting and it is not clear whether BWS is due to a single gene or disruption of contiguous genes, which may be imprinted in opposite directions. A potential candidate gene within 11p15 is the fetal mitogen, insulin-like growth factor II (IGF-II), which is normally imprinted (i.e. inactive) on the maternal allele [59]. However, in some sporadic Wilms tumours, imprinting is relaxed in the tumour cells so that both alleles are expressed [60]. This relaxation has also been documented in the germline of a child with Wilms tumour and gigantism, whereas in a single case of BWS, constitutional imprinting of the *IGF*-II gene was maintained [59, 61]. Children with isolated hemihypertrophy, which may be of a single limb or digit, but without other stigmata of BWS, are also considered at increased risk of Wilms tumour. Hemihypertrophy is found in 2.5–3.3% of Wilms tumour patients, which is about 500-fold greater than the prevalence in the general population. It is possible that all these children represent 'forme fruste' of the BWS but confirmation of this will have to await the cloning of the BWS gene(s) and its analysis in this group of patients. The BWS locus is also implicated in the development of sporadic Wilms tumours as approximately one-third show allele loss on chromosome 11p, which is restricted to 11p15 in a third of such cases.

Perlman syndrome

Perlman syndrome is a rare congenital malformation syndrome which includes fetal gigantism, nephroblastomatosis and cryptorchidism and which has so far been reported in only seven separate families [62–67]. It shows some phenotypic overlap with BWS but appears to be a distinct entity, with autosomal recessive inheritance, high neonatal mortality and an extremely high risk of Wilms tumour: of 14 cases reported, eight were neonatal deaths, one with a congenital Wilms tumour, and five of the six survivors developed Wilms tumour at an early age, three being bilateral. A single case subjected to molecular analysis did not show allele loss for chromosome 11p [63].

Other phenotypes associated with Wilms tumour

A retrospective study found three cases of neurofibromatosis type I among 342 children with Wilms tumour and suggested that this condition conferred a 29-fold increased risk of Wilms tumour [68]. Subsequent larger studies have failed to confirm this level of risk [69], though anecdotal reports suggest a link does exist [70]. Indeed, it is interesting that in the rat, transplacental carcinogenic insults can give rise to either plexiform neurofibromas or Wilms tumour [1]. A retrospective study of a population-based series of 176 Wilms tumour patients in Manchester suggested that up to 3% of cases may occur within Li–Fraumeni syndrome families [71]. Molecular analysis of the p53 gene in these cases is awaited. Several other syndromes have been reported in association with Wilms tumour, e.g. trisomy 18 and other overgrowth syndromes such as Sotos and Klippel–Trelaunay syndromes, but their small numbers make the causality of these associations uncertain [72].

7.2.2 FAMILIAL WILMS TUMOUR

Familial Wilms tumour has been documented in 0.5–1.2% of cases in two large series [2, 73]. The rare pedigrees reported fall into two main categories: small families with an affec-

ted parent and child(ren) or large pedigrees with several cases among cousins and uncles or aunts. These have been interpreted to show autosomal dominant inheritance of the predisposition to Wilms tumour but with variable penetrance. The median age at diagnosis of familial cases is intermediate between that of bilateral and unilateral cases, with a bimodal distribution, and the incidence of bilateral tumours and congenital abnormalities is no higher than for sporadic cases [2]. This suggests that only a proportion of familial Wilms tumour follows a simple two mutation model. The three largest pedigrees subjected to linkage analysis have excluded chromosomes 11 or 16 as the site of the Wilms tumour gene in these families [74–76]. However, two cases of direct parent – child transmission have been shown to be due to *WT1* gene mutation. In one family, both father and son had a constitutional single base-pair deletion in exon 6 which would result in a premature termination codon; of interest, the father had a normal genital phenotype whereas his son had cryptorchidism and hypospadias [44]. In the second, an apparent example of familial aniridia transmitted from mother to son, the son developed a Wilms tumour at the age of 18 months [77]. Molecular analysis revealed a submicroscopic chromosome 11p13 deletion in both mother and child and therefore this represents a case of familial WAGR syndrome with very limited phenotypic abnormalities. In another case of direct parent – child transmission from the mother to two children, the *WT1* gene has been excluded by sequence analysis [78]. An attempt to estimate the heritability rate of Wilms tumour was made by analysing disease concordance rates in monozygotic (MZ) and dizygotic (DZ) twins [79]. Of 31 MZ pairs, none was concordant for Wilms tumour, leading to a heritability estimate of zero. One of 35 DZ pairs was concordant for Wilms tumour. Of interest, in one pair, the co-twin, who is still at risk for Wilms tumour, also had hypospadias, suggesting that a shared genetic defect could manifest as either tumour or malformation. The co-twins of two MZ twins with bilateral tumours have not developed Wilms tumour, reinforcing the previously stated view that not all bilateral tumours represent carriers of germline mutations. Four twin pairs had a family history of Wilms tumour in an aunt or cousin, three were MZ pairs who remain discordant for tumour development well beyond the normal risk period. This suggests that at least some of the Wilms tumour genes have a low penetrance or very variable expressivity.

7.2.3 IDENTIFICATION AND SCREENING OF WILMS TUMOUR PATIENTS WITH GENETIC PREDISPOSITION

The possibility of genetic predisposition should be considered in any child with an early onset (before age 2 years) Wilms tumour or an additional congenital abnormality, particularly of the genitourinary tract. All patients should be examined repeatedly for evidence of hemihypertrophy or neurofibromatosis, which may only become evident sometime after the diagnosis of Wilms tumour. Full-blown Beckwith – Wiedemann syndrome or aniridia will usually have been diagnosed previously and the child should be under follow-up. Children with bilateral and multifocal Wilms tumour should be considered to carry a germline mutation until proved otherwise. Currently, there are no documented survivors of bilateral disease who have gone on to reproduce, so their genetic burden is not established. Children in whom nephrogenic rests are found, particularly of the intralobar variety, should be considered at increased risk of developing a Wilms tumour in their remaining kidney.

Currently, all such children can only be examined for *WT*1 gene mutations and then only in a research setting, although this could be set up as a diagnostic service. Failure to identify a *WT*1 mutation will not exclude a genetic predisposition, as there are at least two other Wilms tumour genes as yet uncloned. Screening of children at known or presumed increased risk of Wilms tumour remains problematic. It is controversial as to whether planned regular abdominal ultrasound examinations are successful in reducing the overall stage of the tumour at diagnosis [80]. It has been suggested that teaching the parents to perform regular abdominal palpation on their child would be a more fruitful strategy. The period of maximum risk is up to about 7 years of age, as 90% of Wilms tumour have presented by then. The risk to a sibling of an otherwise normal child with unilateral Wilms tumour seems to be extremely low and does not justify instituting a regular screening policy.

7.2.4 DOES GENETIC PREDISPOSITION CONTRIBUTE TO SECOND PRIMARY TUMOURS IN WILMS TUMOUR SURVIVORS?

Wilms tumour survivors do not have a particularly high risk of developing a second primary tumour (SPT) and there is no clear-cut pattern of SPTs. This is in contrast to the paradigm of retinoblastoma, where the heritable group have a greatly increased risk of SPT, particularly osteosarcoma, whose aetiology probably involves homozygous *RB*1 gene mutations, as these are found in many sporadic osteosarcomas [5]. Most of the SPTs after Wilms tumour have occurred in previously irradiated tissues and radiation has been suggested as the most likely aetiological factor [81]. However, some SPTs in Wilms tumour patients have arisen in tissues that normally express the *WT*1 gene (mesotheliomas and leukaemias), raising the possibility that they are the result of genetic predisposition. Certainly, it is known that germline

113

WT1 mutations can predispose to tumours of non-renal tissues, as a child with the Denys – Drash syndrome had not only Wilms tumour but also bilateral gonadoblastoma and juvenile granulosa cell tumour of the ovary and the latter tumour was shown to have lost the remaining normal *WT1* allele [27]. Mesothelioma is an unusual SPT following childhood cancer and has occurred in four Wilms tumour survivors [82]. A single case of sporadic mesothelioma has been shown to carry a homozygous *WT1* gene mutation, making it more likely that these four cases involved genetic predisposition [83]. We have found a second mutation in the remaining *WT1* allele in a case of acute myeloid leukaemia developing in a survivor of Wilms tumour with the WAGR syndrome [84]. Thus, it seems likely that a small proportion of Wilms tumour survivors have a genetic predisposition to second primary tumours. It is difficult to quantify the magnitude of such a risk as the number of survivors who carry germline mutations is not established.

7.3 KIDNEY TUMOURS IN ADULTS

The majority (85%) of primary kidney tumours in adults are renal cell carcinoma (RCC). Most of the remainder are tumours of the renal pelvis, which share a common pathology with the transitional cell carcinomas of the lower urinary tract.

7.3.1 RENAL CELL CARCINOMA

Renal cell carcinoma (RCC) is a relatively rare tumour, comprising about 2% of all adult cancers in the UK. Incidence rates show a 10-fold variation around the world, with the Scandinavians having the highest rates (11.8 per 100 000 males) and Asian countries amongst the lowest, the UK figures being intermediate (5.1–6.6 per 100 000 males) [85]. It is not clear how much of this ethnic variation is due to genetic predisposition or

enviromental factors but the commonly observed 2:1 male excess is thought partly to reflect smoking habits and about one-third of RCC is attributable to tobacco exposure. Furthermore, the overall incidence of RCC has slowly increased in many countries, by 0.5–2 % per annum, again thought to reflect enviromental influences. This increase in risk seems to be slowing down for those born after 1940 [86]. Around 1% of cases are familial and two distinct groups can be distinguished: those forming part of the von Hippel–Lindau syndrome (VHL) and isolated familial RCC. In both, inheritance is autosomal dominant with high, age-dependent penetrance. These heritable cases have a higher incidence of bilateral and/or multifocal tumours and an earlier age of onset than sporadic cases, suggesting that Knudson's two-hit model might be operating [87].

(a) Familial renal cell carcinoma

Clues to the location of the RCC gene(s) came from the finding of a consistent chromosomal translocation involving the short arm of chromosome 3 segregating with the disease in a family with 10 cases of RCC in three generations [88]. An unrelated pedigree with a t(3;6) in three generations is also likely to represent hereditary RCC as two of the three translocation carriers are below the usual age for developing RCC and the affected older member has multiple bilateral tumours [89]. In both these families, the breakpoints have been localized to 3p13-14.2 [90]. This translocation breakpoint has been shown to lie close to a fragile site and flanking markers have been cloned, which should soon lead to the identification of candidate genes [91]. Tumour cells from another unrelated familial case also showed chromosome 3p abnormalities [t(3;11)(p13 or 14;p15)] though in this individual the constitutional karyotype was normal [92]. Of interest, in three families where it could be studied, the tumour cells have lost the derivative 3p and retained an apparently normal chromosome 3 [89, 93, 94]. This unexpected finding might be explained if disruption or deregulation of a gene on chromosome 3p predisposed to RCC, which only developed if a second event, such as a point mutation or small deletion occurred on the normal allele. Once tumorigenesis was initiated, the derivative chromosome might be inherently unstable and prone to loss, leaving the tumour cells hemizygous for the somatically mutated 3p allele(s). This mechanism has been substantiated in one of these familial cases by the finding of mutation of a more distal gene (*VHL* gene) on the normal chromosome 3, with loss of the derivative 8 chromosome carrying the translocated 3p sequences in the tumour (see page 117) [95]. Further evidence that loss of a tumour suppressor gene(s) on chromosome 3 is important in RCC comes from the observation that reintroduction of a normal chromosome 3p into an RCC cell line suppresses tumorigenicity [96]. It should be emphasized that the majority of cases of hereditary RCC (based on family history, early age of onset before 45 years or bilateral disease) do not have constitutional karyotypic abnormalities [97].

A high frequency of chromosome 3p abnormalities has been found subsequently in sporadic RCC by both conventional cytogenetics and allele loss studies [98]. The latter show an 80–90% incidence of chromosome 3p allele loss in sporadic RCC [99, 100]. As with Wilms tumour, more detailed molecular studies have shown that RCC is not as simple as the retinoblastoma paradigm. High-resolution allele loss studies have defined at least two distinct regions on chromosome 3p, at 3p13-14.3 and 3p21.3 [90]. Both are distinct from the Von Hippel–Lindau locus (see below) at 3p25-6. Many other sites of allele loss in sporadic RCC have been described, including 5q, 6q and 10q [100]. 17p allele loss has been found in two studies and may be

inversely related to 3p allele loss [101]. None occurs with the high frequency seen for chromosome 3p but their levels are probably significant and suggest either that RCC is a heterogeneous disease or they represent further genetic events occurring with tumour progression. Indeed, Morita *et al.* [100] have provided evidence for the accumulation of genetic events signalled by allele loss being associated with tumour progression.

RCC has been subdivided according to growth pattern (papillary or non-papillary) and cell type. The non-papillary subtype is the most common (80%) and is the type found in both familial and VHL-associated cases. Recently, a classification based on molecular changes has been proposed, where 3p changes characterize the non-papillary subtype [99]. Further subdivisions into clear cell and granular subtypes are debatable, as these morphological appearances may reflect only differences in tumour blood supply rather than underlying biology, although Ogawa *et al.* [101] have shown that the granular subtype is more likely to have 17p rather than 3p allele loss. Papillary RCC is also distinct at a molecular level, not having 3p or 5q loss but showing a high incidence of trisomy 7, 16 and 17 and loss of the Y chromosome [101]. But is even non-papillary RCC a single disease? At a molecular level the answer is probably so, as there is evidence for at least three loci on chromosome 3p within the non-papillary group (see Figure 7.3).

(b) Von Hippel–Lindau

Von Hippel–Lindau (VHL) syndrome is a dominantly inherited familial cancer syndrome characterized by the development of haemangioblastomas, mainly of the retina and cerebellum, RCC, phaeochromocytomas and renal, epididymal and pancreatic cysts [103]. The risk of RCC is lower than in 'pure' familial RCC but again the tumours present earlier and are more likely to be bilateral and/

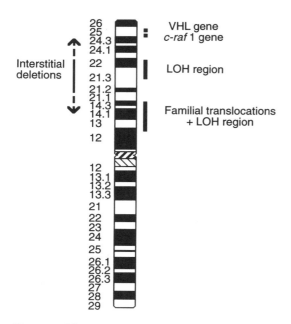

Fig. 7.3 Idiogram of chromosome 3, showing the three non-overlapping loci implicated in RCC: the *VHL* gene at 3p25, loss of heterozygosity (LOH) at 3p22 and 3p13-14.3, the latter also being the site of translocations in familial RCC. All three loci are included in the 3p interstitial deletions described by Teyssier, where the *c-raf* 1 gene at 3p25 is brought adjacent to 3p14 [102].

or multifocal than sporadic cases. There is some interfamily phenotypic variation with some pedigrees showing a very high frequency of phaeochromocytoma, but there is no evidence to suggest that this represents two separate genes. The *VHL* locus was mapped to chromosome 3p25-26 by genetic linkage and allele loss studies. An intensive collaborative mapping effort led to the identification of three unrelated VHL patients with nested constitutional deletions, the smallest of which was only about 100 kb [104]. By using evolutionarily conserved DNA sequences from within the region, two cDNAs were isolated from a teratocarcinoma cDNA library. One of these cDNAs detected partial deletions by Southern analysis in 28 of

221 (12%) of VHL patients. The deletions were non-overlapping into the 5′ and 3′ termini of the gene, suggesting that this was indeed the *VHL* gene. This was strengthened by the finding of constitutional small intragenic deletions/insertions introducing premature stop codons into the predicted open reading frame in three further VHL patients. This newly cloned *VHL* gene maps within 3p25 and seems to be expressed in all adult tissues examined, where there are 6 kb and 6.5 kb transcripts. In the fetus, there is presumed tissue-specific splicing in kidney and brain, the two most frequently affected tissues in VHL, which express only the 6.5 kb or 6 kb transcripts respectively. The predicted protein is short, only 284 amino acids, and has no significant homology to any proteins in the current database. The type of *VHL* gene mutation seems to correlate with disease phenotype, those patients with missense mutations being more likely to develop phaeochromocytoma than those with mutations causing loss of VHL protein expression [95].

In a study of 40 RCCs from six VHL patients, Kovacs *et al.* [105] found that nearly all had lost 3p13-pter sequences and that this was a very early change, found even in tumours <1 cm diameter. They also noted that 50% of tumours had gained 5q22-qter sequences, a similar percentage to that found in sporadic RCC. What does this tell us about the molecular events necessary for the development of RCC? At a histological level, the RCCs of VHL and familial cases are indistinguishable from the sporadic form of non-papillary RCC. At least some cases of familial RCC involve translocations in 3p13-14 but are these disrupting an RCC gene? The answer is possibly no, since it may be that the critical event is the loss of distal 3p sequences occurring secondary to the translocation. Such an argument would be strengthened by the familial case where the translocation is in 3q but the 3pter sequences are lost in the tumour [93]. The only argument against this is that a few cases of sporadic RCC show allele loss confined to 3p13-14 [90]. Certainly, one case of familial RCC has developed a *VHL* gene mutation in the tumour with loss of the remaining normal *VHL* allele [95]. This implies that the constitutional 3;8 translocation is a predisposing mutation with the development of full-blown RCC requiring 'two hits' at the *VHL* gene. It will be important to examine other cases of familial RCC for *VHL* mutations as these could be 'forme fruste' of VHL, manifesting only RCC (i.e. phenotype would be mutation-dependent) or *VHL* gene mutations may be associated with tumour progression, with initiation being due to another 3p gene mutation. This would be analogous to the situation seen in Wilms tumour, where a presumed tumour initiating mutation in the *WT1* gene at 11p13 is followed by allele loss confined to 11p15, presumed to indicate mutation of the Beckwith–Wiedemann gene.

The *VHL* gene is also involved in sporadic RCC. In a study of 110 tumours, 56 of 98 cases of non-papillary RCC contained *VHL* mutations whereas none of 12 cases of papillary RCC had mutations, again confirming the different pathogenesis of these two subtypes [95]. The majority of the *VHL* gene mutations were homozygous, producing either a truncated protein or an altered amino acid. Of interest, the spectrum of *VHL* mutation in RCC differs between germline and sporadic cases, with the latter being mainly in exon 2.

(c) Tuberous sclerosis – renal hamartomas

Individuals with tuberous sclerosis (TSC), an autosomal dominant syndrome, commonly develop benign renal hamartomas or angiomyolipomas, but also have a small increased risk of developing renal cell carcinoma [106]. The type of RCC is usually renal oncocytoma,

which is considered to be relatively benign. Most of these tumours do not appear to have any specific chromosomal changes other than in mitochondrial DNA [99]. Approximately 60% of TSC cases are thought to be new mutations, though the great variation in phenotypic expression of the trait makes this estimate uncertain. TSC has been mapped to two separate chromosomal loci, at chromosome 9q34 and 16p13. Following a tremendous international collaboration, the tuberous sclerosis gene at chromosome 16p13 (designated *TSC*2) has now been cloned [107]. Five of 255 unrelated cases were found to have small non-overlapping interstitial 16p13 deletions by pulse-field gel electrophoresis. A candidate gene spanning both deleted areas was isolated and shown to encode a 5.5-kb mRNA which was expressed in all tissues examined. The predicted protein product, termed tuberin, shows homology to a GTPase-activating protein, GAP3 as well as containing possible membrane-spanning hydrophobic domains. Five further TSC patients were shown to have intragenic deletions, thus confirming its identity as the *TSC*2 gene. The presence of 16p allele loss in hamartomas from TSC patients suggested that the *TSC*2 gene would function as a tumour suppressor, with loss of gene function being responsible for tumour development [108]. In accordance with this, reduced expression of *TSC*2 is seen in fibroblasts from affected individuals, with one expressing a truncated mRNA. Of interest, the *TSC*2 gene shows linkage to a marker for adult polycystic kidney disease (APKD) and it had been suggested that they could be allelic variants. However, the *APKD* gene has now been isolated and shown to be a separate gene lying adjacent to the *TSC*2 gene [109]. Currently, the slightly increased risk of RCC in APKD is thought to be secondary to dialysis treatment rather than genetic predisposition. Analysis of the *APKD* gene in these rare tumours should resolve this issue.

In conclusion the molecular basis for cancers of the kidney in both adults and children is beginning to be unravelled. Three predisposing gene have now been cloned and studies of the *WT1* gene in particular have emphasized the intimate relationship of cancer predisposition and developmental abnormalities. A greater understanding of the biology of these genes should lead to novel therapeutic and preventative strategies. In the future, it should be possible to define, at a molecular level, individuals at increased risk of kidney cancers, which should lead to a rational approach to screening and therapy.

REFERENCES

1. Cardesa, A., Ribalta, T., Von, S.B. *et al.* (1989) Experimental model of tumors associated with neurofibromatosis. *Cancer.* **63** (9) 1737–49.

2. Breslow, N., Olshan, A., Beckwith, J.B. *et al.* (1993) Epidemiology of Wilms Tumor. *Med. Pediatr. Oncol.*, **21** (3) 172–81.

3. Beckwith, J.B., Kiviat, N.B. and Bonadio, J.F. (1990) Nephrogenic rests, nephroblastomatosis and the pathogenesis of Wilms tumour. *Pediatr. Pathol.*, **10**, 1–36.

4. Knudson, A.G. and Strong, L.C. (1972) Mutation and cancer: a model for Wilms tumor of the kidney. *J. Natl Cancer Inst.*, **48**, 313–24.

5. Goodrich, D.W. and Lee, W.-H. (1990) The molecular genetics of retinoblastoma. *Cancer Surv.*, **9**, 529–54.

6. Maw, M., Grundy, P., Millow, L. *et al.* (1992) A third Wilms tumor locus on chromosome 16q. *Cancer Res.*, **52**, 3094–8.

7. Haber, D.A., Buckler, A.J., Glaser, T. *et al.* (1990) An internal deletion within a 11p13 zinc finger gene contributes to the development of Wilms tumor. *Cell*, **61**, (7) 1257–69.

8. Little, M.H., Prosser, J., Condie, A. *et al.* (1992) Zinc finger point mutations within the WT1 gene in Wilms tumor patients. *Proc. Natl Acad. Sci. USA*, **89** (11) 4791–5.

9. Knudson, A. (1980) Genetics and the child cured of cancer, In *Status of the Curability of Childhood Cancers* (eds J. van Eys and M.P. Sullivan), Raven Press, New York, p. 296.

10. Li F., Williams, W. Gimbere, K. *et al.* (1988) Heritable fraction of unilateral Wilms tumour. *Pediatrics*, **81**, 147–9.

11. Hawkins, M., Draper, G. and Smith, R.A. (1989) Cancer among 1,348 offspring of survivors of childhood cancer. *Int. J. Cancer*, **43**, 975–8.

12. Byrne, J., Mulvihill, J., Connelly, R. *et al.* (1988) Reproductive problems and birth defects in survivors of Wilms tumour and their relatives. *Med. Pediatr. Oncol.*, **16**, 233–40.

13. Wiedemann, H.R. (1983) Tumours and hemihypetrophy associated with Wiedemann–Beckwith syndrome. *Eur. J. Pediatr.*, **141**, 129–36.

14. Sotelo-Avila, C., Gonzalez-Crussi, F. and Fowler, J. (1980) Complete and incomplete forms of Beckwith – Wiedemann syndrome: their oncogenic potential. *J. Pediatr.*, **96**, 47–50.

15. Bonaïti-Pellié, C., Chompret, A., Tournade, M.-F. *et al.* (1993) Excess of multifocal tumours in nephroblastoma: implications for mechanisms of tumour development and genetic counselling. *Hum. Genet.*, **91**, 373–6.

16. Ton, C., Hirvonen, H., Miwa, H. *et al.* (1991) Positional cloning and characterisation of a paired box- and homeobox-containing gene from the aniridia region. *Cell*, **67**, 1059–74.

17. Gessler, M., Poustka, A. Cavenee, W. *et al.* (1990) Homozygous deletion in Wilms tumours of a zinc-finger gene identified by chromosome jumping. *Nature*, **343**, 774–8.

18. Call, K.M., Glaser, T., Ito, C.Y. *et al.* (1990) Isolation and characterization of a zinc finger polypeptide gene at the human chromosome 11 Wilms tumor locus. *Cell*, **60** (3), 509–20.

19. Van Heyningen, V., Bickmore, W.A., Seawright, A. *et al.* (1990) Role for the Wilms tumor gene in genital development? *Proc. Natl Acad. Sci. USA*, **87** (14), 5383–6.

20. Baird, P.N., Groves, N., Haber, D.A. *et al* (1992) Identification of mutations in the WT1 gene in tumours from patients with the WAGR syndrome. *Oncogene*, **7** (11), 2141–9.

21. Brown, K.W., Watson, J.E., Poirier, V. *et al.* (1992) Inactivation of the remaining allele of the WT1 gene in a Wilms tumour from a WAGR patient. *Oncogene*, **7**, 763–8.

22. Gessler, M., Konig, A., Moore, J. *et al.* (1993) Homozygous inactivation of WT1 in a Wilms

tumor associated with the WAGR syndrome. *Genes Chromosom. Cancer*, **7** (3) 131–6.

23. Park, S., Tomlinson, G., Nisen, P. *et al.* (1993) Altered trans-activational properties of a mutated WT1 gene product in a WAGR-associated Wilms tumour. *Cancer Res.*, **53**, 4757–60.

24. Santos, A., Osorio, A.L., Baird, P.N., *et al.* (1993) Insertional inactivation of the WT1 gene in tumour cells from a patient with WAGR syndrome. *Hum. Genet.*, **92** (1), 83–6.

25. Armstrong, J.F., Pritchard J.K., Bickmore, W.A. *et al.* (1993) The expression of the Wilms tumour gene, WT1, in the developing mammalian embryo. *Mech. Dev.*, **40** (1–2), 85–97.

26. Pritchard-Jones, K., Fleming S., Davidson, D. *et al.* (1990) The candidate Wilms tumour gene is involved in genitourinary development. *Nature*, **346**, 194–7.

27. Pelletier, J., Bruening W., Kashtan, C.E., *et al.* (1991) Germline mutations in the Wilms tumor suppressor gene are associated with abnormal urogenital development in Denys–Drash syndrome. *Cell*, **67** (2), 437–47.

28. Little, M., Williamson, K., Mannens M., *et al.* (1993) Evidence that WT1 mutations in Denys–Drash syndrome patients may act in a dominant-negative fashion. *Hum. Mol. Genet.*, **2** (3), 259–64.

29. Bruening, W., Bardeesy, N., Silverman, B. *et al.* (1992) Germline intronic and exonic mutations in the Wilms tumour gene (WT1) affecting urogenital development. *Nature Genet.*, **1**, 144–8.

30. Coppes, M.J., Campbell, C.E. and Williams, B.R. (1993) The role of WT1 in Wilms tumorigenesis. *FASEB J.*, **7** (10), 886–95.

31. König, A., Jakubiczka, S., Wieacker P. *et al.* (1993) Further evidence that imbalance of WT1 isoforms may be involved in Denys–Drash syndrome. *Hum. Mol. Genet.*, **2**, 1967–8.

32. Coppes, M., Liefers, G., Higuchi, M. *et al.* (1992) Inherited WT1 mutation in DDS. *Cancer Res.*, **52**, 6125–8.

33. Baird, P.N., Santos, A., Groves, N. *et al.* (1992) Constitutional mutations in the WT1 gene in patients with Denys–Drash syndrome. *Hum. Mol. Genet.*, **1** (5), 301–5.

34. Baird, P. and Cowell, J. (1993) A novel zinc finger mutation in a patient with Denys–Drash syndrome. *Hum. Mol. Genet.*, **2**, 2193–4.

35. Schneider, S., Wildhardt, G., Ludwig, R. *et al.* (1993) Exon skipping due to a mutation in a donor splice site in the WT-1 gene is associated with Wilms tumor and severe genital malformations. *Hum. Genet.*, **91** (6), 599–604.

36. Sakai, A., Tadokoro, K., Yanagisawa, H. *et al.* (1993) A novel insertional mutation of the WT1 gene in a patient with Denys–Drash syndrome. *Hum. Mol. Genet.*, **2**, 1969–70.

37. Ogawa, O., Eccles, M., Yun, K. *et al.* (1993) A novel insertional mutation at the third zinc finger coding region of the WT1 gene in Denys–Drash syndrome. *Hum. Mol. Genet.*, **2**, 203–4.

38. Nordenskjöld, A., Friedman, E. and Anvret, M. (1994) WT1 mutations in patients with Denys–Drash syndrome: a novel mutation in exon 8 and paternal allele origin. *Hum Genet.*, **93**, 115–20.

39. Clarkson, P., Davies, H., Williams, D. *et al.* (1993) Mutational screening of the Wilms tumour gene. WT1, in males with genital abnormalities. *J.Med. Genet.*, **30**, 767–72.

40. Akasaka, Y., Kikuchi, H., Nagai, T. *et al.* (1993) A point mutation found in the WT1 gene in a sporadic Wilms tumor without genitourinary abnormalities is identical with the most frequent point mutation in Denys–Drash syndrome. *FEBS Lett.*, **317**, 39–43.

41. Coppes, M.J., Liefers G.J., Paul, P. *et al.* (1993) Homozygous somatic WT1 point mutations in sporadic unilateral Wilms tumor. *Proc. Natl Acad. Sci. USA*, **90** (4), 1416–19.

42. Huff, V., Miwa, H., Haber, D.A. *et al.* (1991) Evidence for WT1 point Wilms tumor (WT) gene: intragenic germinal deletion in bilateral WT. *Am. J. Hum. Genet.*, **48** (5), 997–1003.

43. Tadokoro, K., Fujii, H., Ohshima, A. *et al.* (1992) Intragenic homozygous deletion of the WT1 gene in Wilms tumor. *Oncogene*, **7** (6), 1215–21.

44. Pelletier, J., Bruening, W., Li, F.P. *et al.* (1991) WT1 mutations contribute to abnormal genital system development and hereditary Wilms tumour. *Nature*, **353**, 431–4.

45. Wang, Z.Y., Qiu, Q.Q., Enger, K.T. *et al.* (1993) A second transcriptionally active DNA-binding site for the Wilms tumor gene product, WT1. *Proc. Natl Acad. Sci. USA*, **90**, 8896–900.

46. Wang, Z.Y., Qiu, Q.Q. and Deuel, T.F. (1993) The Wilms tumor gene product WT1 activates or suppresses transcription through separate functional domains. *J. Biol. Chem.*, **268** (13), 9172–5.

47. Kreidberg, J.A., Sariola, H., Loring, J.M. *et al.* (1993) WT-1 is required for early kidney development. *Cell*, **74** (4), 679–91.

48. Cowell, J.K., Wadey, R.B., Haber, D.A. *et al.* (1991) Structural rearrangements of the WT1 gene in Wilms tumour cells. *Oncogene*, **6** (4), 595–9.

49. Kikuchi, H., Akasaka, Y., Nagai, T. *et al.* (1992) Genomic changes in the WT-gene (WT1) in Wilms tumors and their correlation with histology. *Am. J. Pathol.*, **140** (4), 781–6.

50. Radice, P., Pilotti, S., De, B.V. *et al.* (1993) Homozygous intragenic loss of the WT1 locus in a sporadic intralobar Wilms tumor [letter]. *Int. J. Cancer*, **55** (1), 174–6.

51. Ton, C.C., Huff, V., Call, K.M. *et al.* (1991) Smallest region of overlap in Wilms tumor deletions uniquely implicates an 11 p13 zinc finger gene as the disease locus. *Genomics*, **10** (1), 293–7.

52. Drash, A., Sherman, F., Hartman, W. *et al.* (1970) A syndrome of pseudohermaphroditism. Wilms tumour, hypertension and degenerative renal disease. *J. Pediatr*, **76**, 585–93.

53. Denys, P., Malvaux, P., Van den Berghe, H. *et al.* (1967) Association d'un syndrome anatomo-pathologique de pseudohermaphrodisme masculin, d'une tumeur de Wilms, d'une nephropathie parenchymateuse et d'un mosaicisms XX/XY. *Arch. Fr. Pediatr.*, **24**, 729–39.

54. Jadresic, L., Bleake, J., Gordon, I. *et al.* (1990) Clinico-pathological review of 13 children with nephropathy, Wilms tumour and genital abnormalities (DRASH syndrome). *J. Pediatr.*, **117**, 717–25.

55. Hastie, N.D. (1992) Dominant negative mutations in the Wilms tumour (WT1) gene cause Denys–Drash syndrome – proof that a tumour-suppressor gene plays a crucial role in normal genitourinary development. *Hum. Mol. Genet.*, **1** (5), 293–5.

56. Henry, I., Hoovers, J., Barichard, F. *et al.* (1993) Pericentric intrachromosomal insertion responsible for recurrence of del(11)(p13p14) in a family. *Genes Chromosom. Cancer*, **7** (1), 57–62.

57. Pettenati, M.J., Haynes, J.L., Wappmer, R. *et al.* (1986) Wiedemann–Beckwith syndrome: presentation of clinical and psychogenetic data on 22 new cases and review of the literature. *Hum. Genet.*, **74**, 143–54.

58. Moutou, C., Junien, C., Henry, I. *et al.* (1992) Beckwith–Wiedmann syndrome: a demonstration of the mechanisms responsible for the excess of transmitting females. *J. Med. Genet.*, **29**, 217–20.

59. Ohlsson, R., Nyström, A., Pfeifer-Ohlsson, S. *et al.* (1993) IGF2 is parentally imprinted during human embryogenesis and in the Beckwith–Wiedmann syndrome. *Nature Genet.* **4**, 94–7.

60. Ogawa, O., Eccles, M.R., Szeto, J. *et al.* (1993) Relaxation of insulin-like growth factor II gene imprinting implicated in Wilms tumour. *Nature*, **362**, 749–51.

61. Ogawa, O., Becroft, D., Morison, I. *et al.* (1993) Constitutional relaxation of insulin-like growth factor II gene imprinting associated with Wilms tumour and gigantism. *Nature Genet.*, **5**, 408–12.

62. Dao, D., Schroeder, W.T., Chao, L. *et al.* (1987) Genetic mechanisms of tumor-specific loss of 11p DNA sequences in Wilms tumor. *Am. J. Hum. Genet.*, **41**, 202–17.

63. Hamel, B., Mannens, M. and Bökkerink, J. (1990) Perlman syndrome: a report of a case and results of molecular studies. *Am. J. Hum. Genet.*, **45** (4), *A*48.

64. Neri, G., Martini-Neri, M., Katz, B. *et al.* (1984) The Perlman syndrome: familial renal dysplasia with Wilms tumor, fetal gigantism and multiple congenital anomalies. *Am. J. Med. Genet.*, **19**, 195–207.

65. Greenberg, F., Copeland, K. and Gresik, M. (1988) Expanding the spectrum of Perlman syndrome. *Am. J. Med. Genet.*, **29**, 773–6.

66. Perlman, M., Levin, M. and Wittels, B. (1975) Syndrome of fetal gigantism, renal hamartomas and nephroblastomatosis with Wilms tumour. *Cancer*, **35**, 1212–17.

67. Grundy, R.G., Pritchard, J., Baraitser, M. *et al.* (1992) Perlman and Wiedemann–Beckwith syndromes: two distinct conditions associated with Wilms tumour. *Eur. J. Pediatr.*, **151**(12), 895–8.

68. Stay, E. and Vawter, G. (1977) The relation-

ship between nephroblastomata and neuro-fibromatosis. *Cancer*, **39**, 2550–5.

69. Blatt, J., Jaffe, R., Deutsch, M. *et al.* (1986) Neurofibromatosis and childhood tumours. *Cancer*, **57**, 1225–9.

70. Perilongo, G., Felix, C.A., Meadows, A.T. *et al.* (1993) Sequential development of Wilms tumor, T-cell acute lymphoblastic leukemia, medulloblastoma and myeloid leukemia in a child with type 1 neurofibromatosis: a clinical and cytogenetic case report. *Leukemia*, **7** (6), 912–15.

71. Hartley, A.L., Birch, J.M., Tricker, K. *et al.* (1993) Wilms tumor in the Li–Fraumeni cancer family syndrome. *Cancer Genet. Cytogenet.*, **67** (2), 133–5.

72. Clericuzio, C.L. (1993) Clinical phenotypes and Wilms tumor. *Med. Pediatr. Oncol.*, **21**, 182–7.

73. Pastore, G., Carli, M., Lemerle, J. *et al.* (1988) Epidemiological features of Wilms tumour: results of studies by the International Society of Paediatric Oncology (SIOP). *Med. Pediatr. Oncol.*, **16**, 7–11.

74. Huff, V., Compton, D.A., Chao, L.Y. *et al.* (1988) Lack of linkage of familial Wilms' tumour to chromosomal band 11p13. *Nature*, **336**, 377–8.

75. Schwartz, C.E., Haber, D.A., Stanton, V.P. *et al.* (1991) Familial predisposition to Wilms tumor does not segregate with the WT1 gene. *Genomics*, **10** (4), 927–30.

76. Huff, V., Reeve, A.E., Leppert, M. *et al.* (1992) Nonlinkage of 16q markers to familial predisposition to Wilms tumor. *Cancer Res.*, **52** (21), 6117–20.

77. Fantes, J., Bickmore, W., Fletcher, J. *et al.* (1992) Submicroscopic deletions at the WAGR locus, revealed by nonradioactive *in situ* hybridisation. *Am. J. Hum. Genet.*, **51**, 1286–94.

78. Baird, P., Pritchard, J. and Cowell, J. (1994) Molecular genetic analysis of chromosome 11p in familial Wilms tumour. *Br. J. Cancer*, **69**, 1072–7.

79. Olson, J., Breslow, N. and Barce, J. (1993) Cancer in twins of Wilms tumour patients. *Am. J. Med. Genet.*, **47**, 91–4.

80. Green, D., Breslow, N., Beckwith, J.B. *et al.* (1993) Screening of children with hemihypertrophy, aniridia and Beckwith–Wiedemann syndrome in patients with Wilms tumour: a report from the National Wilms Tumor Study. *Med. Paediatr. Oncol.*, **21**, 188–92.

81. Hawkins, M., Draper, G. and Kingston, J. (1987) Incidence of second primary tumours among childhood cancer survivors. *Br. J. Cancer*, **56**, 339–47.

82. Austin, M.B., Fechner, R.E. and Roggli, V.L. (1986) Pleural malignant mesothelioma following Wilms tumour. *Am. J. Clin. Pathol.*, **86**, 227–30.

83. Park, S., Schalling, M., Bernard, A. *et al.* (1993) The Wilms tumour gene WT1 is expressed in murine mesoderm-derived tissues and mutated in a human mesothelioma. *Nature Genet.*, **4** (4), 415–20.

84. Pritchard–Jones, K., Renshaw, J. and King–Underwood, L. (1994) The Wilms tumour (WT1) gene is mutated in a secondary leukaemia in a WAGR patient. *Hum. Molec. Genet.*, **3**, 1633–7.

85. Whelan, S.L., Parkin, D.M. and Masuyer, E. (eds) (1990) *Patterns of Cancer in Five Continents*, vol. 102, International Agency for Research on Cancer, Lyon.

86. Coleman, M.P., Esteve, J., Damiecki, P. *et al.* (eds) (1993) *Trends in Cancer Incidence and Mortality*, vol. 121, IARC, Lyon.

87. Erlandsson, R., Boldog, F., Sumegi, J. *et al.* (1988) Do human renal cell carcinomas arise by a double-loss mechanism? *Cancer Genet. Cytogenet.*, **36**, 197–202.

88. Cohen, A.J., Li, F.P., Berg, S. *et al.* (1979) Hereditary renal cell carcinoma associated with a chromosomal translocation. *N. Engl. J. Med.*, **301**, 592–5.

89. Kovacs, G., Brusa, P. and De Riese, W. (1989) Tissue-specific expression of a constitutional 3;6 translocation: development of multiple bilateral renal cell carcinomas. *Int. J. Cancer*, **43**, 422–7.

90. Yamakawa, K., Morita, R., Takahashi, E. *et al.* (1991) A detailed deletion mapping of the short arm of chromosome 3 in sporadic renal cell carcinoma. *Cancer Res.*, **51**, 4707–11.

91. Yamakawa, K., Takahashi, E., Murata, M. *et al.* (1992) Detailed mapping around the breakpoint of the (3;8) translocation in familial renal cell carcinoma and FRA3B. *Genomics*, **14**, 412–16.

92. Pathak, S., Strong, L.C., Ferrell, R.E. *et al.* (1982) Familial renal cell carcinoma with a 3;11 chromosome translocation limited to tumour cells. *Science*, **217**, 939–41.

93. Kovacs, G. and Hoene, E. (1988) Loss of der (3) in renal carcinoma cells of a patient with constitutional t(3;12). *Human Genet.*, **78**, 148–50.

94. Li, F.P., Decker, H.-J.H., Zbar, B. *et al.* (1993) Clinical and genetic studies of renal cell carcinomas in a family with a constitutional chromosome 3;8 translocation. *Ann. Intern. Med.*, **118**, 106–11.

95. Gnarra, J.R, Tory, K., Weng, Y. *et al.* (1994) Mutations of the VHL tumour suppressor gene in renal carcinoma. *Nature Genet.*, **7**, 85–9.

96. Shimizu, M., Yokota, J., Mori, N. *et al.* (1990) Introduction of a normal chromosome 3p modulates the tumorigenicity of a human renal cell carcinoma cell line YCR. *Oncogene*, **5**, 185–94.

97. Kantor, A.F. (1982) Hereditary renal carcinoma and chromosomal defects. *N. Engl. J. Med.*, **307** (22), 1403–4.

98. Walter, T.A., Berger, C.S. and Sandberg, A.A. (1989) The cytogenetics of renal tumours. *Cancer Genet. Cytogenet.*, **43**, 15–34.

99. Kovacs, G. (1993) Molecular differential pathology of renal cell tumours. *Histopathology*, **22**, 1–8.

100. Morita, R., Saito, S., Ishikawa, J. *et al.* (1991) Common regions of deletion on chromosomes 5q, 6q and 10q in renal cell carcinoma. *Cancer Res.*, **51**, 5817–20.

101. Ogawa, O., Habuchi, T., Kakehi, Y. *et al.* (1992) Allelic losses at chromosome 17p in human renal cell carcinoma are inversely related to allelic losses at chromosome 3p. *Cancer Res.*, **52**, 1881–5.

102. Teyssier, J., Henry, I., Dozier, C. *et al.* (1986) Recurrent deletion of the short arm of chromosome 3 in human renal cell carcinoma: shift of the c-raf 1 locus. *J. Natl Cancer Inst.*, **77**, 1187–94.

103. Maher, E.R. and Yates, J.R.W. (1991) Familial renal cell carcinoma: clinical and molecular genetic aspects. *Br. J. Cancer*, **63**, 176–9.

104. Latif, F., Tory, K., Gnarra J. *et al.* (1993) Identification of the von Hippel–Lindau disease tumor suppressor gene. *Science*, **260**, 1317–20.

105. Kovacs, G., Emanuel, A., Neumann, H. *et al.* (1993) Cytogenetics of renal cell carcinoma associated with von Hippel–Lindau disease. *Genes Chromosom., Cancer*, **3**, 256–62.

106. Gomez, M.R. (1988) *Tuberous Sclerosis.* 2nd edn, Raven Press, New York.

107. Consortium ECITS. (1993) Identification and characterisation of the tuberous sclerosis gene on chromosome 16. *Cell* **75**, 1305–15.

108. Green, A. Smith, M. and Yates, J. (1994) Loss of heterozygosity on chromosome 16p13.3 in hamartomas from tuberous sclerosis patients. *Nature Genet.*, **6**, 193–6.

Chapter 8

The Li–Fraumeni syndrome and the role of *TP*53 mutations in predisposition to cancer

JILLIAN M. BIRCH

8.1 INTRODUCTION AND DEFINITIONS

The familial cancer syndrome which is now known as the Li–Fraumeni syndrome (LFS) was first described by Dr F.P.Li and Dr J.F. Fraumeni in 1969. As part of a survey of nearly 650 children with rhabdomyosarcoma in the United States, Li and Fraumeni identified three pairs of affected siblings when less than one would have been expected by chance. In addition one pair of affected cousins was identified. Li and Fraumeni obtained information by interview with the families and from medical records about the occurrence of cancer in these four families, and found an unusually high incidence of premenopausal breast cancer, sarcomas occurring at an early age, and other unusually early-onset cancers in the close relatives of the index cases. It is notable that three of the mothers of the index children had developed breast cancer under the age of

30. Li and Fraumeni proposed that these observations were due to inherited predisposition to the observed cancers [1]. In a more detailed report, a second pair of cousins with childhood soft tissue sarcoma were identified, and the finding of adrenocortical carcinoma and brain tumours in first-degree relatives of children with soft tissue sarcoma suggested that these cancers may also be components of the syndrome [2].

A report of one family showing a similar pattern of cancers had previously been published [3], and following Li and Fraumeni's report, descriptions of a number of other families which were also consistent with their findings, appeared in the literature [4–6].

At this time, however, it was uncertain as to whether these observations were due to inherited predisposition to a diverse but specific number of neoplasms, whether these familial aggregations might be due to exposure to a common environmental agent, or

Genetic Predisposition to Cancer. Edited by R.A. Eeles, B.A.J. Ponder, D.F. Easton and A. Horwich. Published in 1996 by Chapman & Hall, London.
0 412 56580 3

whether the reported families simply represented rare chance aggregations of cancers within the families. One problem in accepting the notion of genetic predisposition was the diverse nature of the component cancers. Given the then prevailing concept that inherited predisposition to cancer could only occur in a site-specific fashion, there was difficulty in accepting that a single gene trait could confer susceptibility to such a diverse collection of tumours. Subsequently systematic studies of families and patient populations provided a number of pieces of evidence which strongly supported the notion of inherited susceptibility.

Firstly, Li and Fraumeni carried out a follow-up study of their original four families, and found that over a 12-year period, 10 of 31 surviving members of the families had between them developed 16 additional cancers, compared with an expected number of less than 1. The cancers occurring during this follow-up period showed the same pattern as had been observed originally, and included five breast cancers, four soft tissue sarcomas and two brain tumours. The excess was particularly marked for breast cancers, with five observed and only 0.08 expected. The soft tissue sarcomas all occurred within previous radiotherapy fields, but when these were excluded, there was still a highly significant excess above expectation (12 observed, 0.5 expected). The idea of genetic susceptibility was further supported in this follow-up study by the observation that 12 of the cancers occurred as second or subsequent primaries. These 12 cancers, which were predominantly sarcomas and carcinoma of the breast, had occurred in eight patients. This remarkable tendency to the development of second and subsequent cancers of types consistent with the initial description of the syndrome added further weight to the idea of genetic susceptibility in these individuals [7].

Definitive evidence came from two groups who studied the cancer incidence in the families of a population-based series of children with soft tissue sarcoma, and a hospital-based series of survivors of childhood soft tissue sarcoma respectively [8–11]. The first report was based on an analysis of cancer incidence in the mothers of children who were registered with the Manchester Children's Tumour Registry with a diagnosis of soft tissue sarcoma. There was an increased incidence of cancer among these mothers, particularly premenopausal breast cancer, where the observed to expected ratio was 3 [8, 9].

This group went on to study the cancer experience among all first-degree relatives of children with soft tissue sarcoma who were included in the Manchester Children's Tumour Registry. The results of this study showed a statistically significant excess of cancers among all first-degree relatives (relative risk 1.6), which was accounted for by cancers in mothers and siblings, there being no excess in the fathers. The cancer excess was mainly due to carcinoma of the breast and paediatric tumours. The risk was highest for cancers diagnosed at younger ages. Multivariate analysis of clinical characteristics in the index patient identified young age at diagnosis, histological subtype of embryonal rhabdomyosarcoma, and male sex, as independent indicators of increased cancer risk in first-degree relatives [10].

Among first-degree relatives of a hospital-based series of survivors of childhood soft tissue sarcoma, a similar excess of cancers was also found, with 34 observed compared with 20.7 expected, the excess again being predominantly due to breast cancers and cancers of bone and soft tissue, diagnosed at young ages. In this series, the relatives of children with multiple primary cancers, soft tissue sarcoma diagnosed at younger ages, and with histologic type of embryonal rhabdomyosarcoma were at highest risk [11]. Thus the results of these two series were highly consistent, although the index patients were selected according to different criteria, and were from different countries.

Segregation analysis demonstrated that the cancer distribution in the families of children included in the hospital-based series was compatible with a rare autosomal dominant gene (gene frequency 0.00002), with a penetrance of almost 50% by age 30 years and 90% by age 60. In children who are gene carriers, the estimated relative risk of developing cancer was 100 times the background rate. Although age-specific penetrance was slightly higher in females, maternal and paternal lineages contributed equally to the evidence favouring a dominant gene [12, 13].

In order to study the characteristic components of the syndrome, Li assembled 24 kindreds conforming to standard criteria, as follows: bone or soft tissue sarcoma, diagnosed under the age of 45 years, in an individual designated the proband, one first-degree relative with cancer under 45 years of age, and one first - or second-degree relative in the same lineage, with cancer under 45 or sarcoma diagnosed at any age. These criteria have been widely accepted as a clinical definition of the syndrome, and families conforming to these criteria are hereafter referred to as having classic LFS. An example of a family with classic LFS is shown in Figure 8.1.

Among the 24 kindreds, in addition to bone and soft tissue sarcoma and breast cancer, brain tumours, adrenocortical carcinoma and leukaemia were found to excess compared with US population-based cancer incidence data. Among the 151 blood relatives developing cancer, 119 (79%) were affected under the age of 45 years, compared with 10% of all cancers occurring below this age in the general population. Fifteen patients had multiple primary cancers, and the types of cancer which emerged as the principal components of the syndrome on the basis of first primary cancers, also predomi-

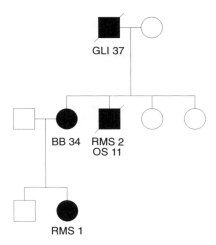

Fig. 8.1 Family conforming to the syndrome criteria of Li *et al.* [14], 'classic LFS'. BB, bilateral breast carcinoma; GLI, glioma; RMS, rhabdomyosarcoma. Numbers indicate age at diagnosis.

nated as second and subsequent primaries [14].

The population-based and hospital-based series of families of children with soft tissue sarcoma, in addition to confirming bone and soft tissue sarcomas, breast cancer, brain tumours, adrenocortical carcinoma and leukaemia as the principal components of LFS also suggest that melanoma, germ cell tumours and Wilms tumour may represent further components of the syndrome [10, 11, 13, 15–17]. The syndrome had therefore been well characterized, both statistically and in terms of cancer phenotype.

These systematic studies provided compelling evidence that in certain families there did appear to be an inherited predisposition to a diverse but specific range of cancers. Furthermore, studies of survivors of retinoblastoma and their families had demonstrated that what had originally been assumed to be an inherited site-specific genetic trait was in fact associated with predisposition to a number of other diverse types of cancer, notably bone and soft tissue sarcoma and melanoma, but probably also to a variety of other cancers including brain tumours and early onset carcinomas [18–20].

8.2 IDENTIFICATION OF *TP*53 AS A CAUSE OF LFS

The probable location of the gene responsible for retinoblastoma was indicated by the association of a congenital malformation syndrome, characterized by constitutional deletion in the long arm of chromosome 13, which included retinoblastoma as one of the component features. The retinoblastoma gene was mapped to chromosome 13q14 and was subsequently isolated and characterized in 1986 [21].

Identification of the gene(s) responsible for the high cancer incidence in families with LFS, however, was more problematical. No characteristic constitutional chromosomal aberrations had been found in any of the families with the syndrome, and classic genetic linkage analysis was difficult because of the lethal nature of the component tumours. Collection of biological samples for genetic marker typing from sufficient numbers of affected family members was therefore extremely difficult. Furthermore, because some of the component cancers are frequent in the general population, for example, breast cancer, the problem of phenocopies also arose. For these reasons, Malkin *et al.* [22] adopted an alternative approach, in choosing to analyse candidate genes. They reasoned that the LFS gene was most likely to be a tumour suppressor gene. The retinoblastoma gene (*RB*), which was the first tumour suppressor gene to be cloned, is associated with a number of the cancers characteristic of LFS, including bone and soft tissue sarcoma. However, the *RB* gene did not seem a likely candidate, since retinoblastoma had not been observed in LFS families.

The *TP*53 gene, located on chromosome 17p13, was the second tumour suppressor gene to be recognized and deletions and/or mutations in the *TP*53 gene had been found in tumour tissue from sporadic osteosarcomas, soft tissue sarcomas, brain tumours, leukaemias and carcinoma of the breast. In addition, mice with a constitutional *TP*53 mutation had been shown to develop bone and soft tissue sarcomas, adrenal and lymphoid tumours as well as other tumours at an increased level [23]. The *TP*53 gene therefore appeared to be a plausible candidate gene in families with LFS.

Constitutional samples from affected members of five families with LFS and unaffected members from one of these families were therefore analysed for the presence of germline mutations in the *TP*53 gene. Germline *TP*53 mutations were found in all affected individuals tested. In the family where multiple members were tested, each of the three affected members carried the same germline *TP*53 mutation, and two of the three unaffected individuals tested also carried this mutation. These two individuals were respectively the grandfather of the proband who, at the time of the study was 57 and alive and well, and the first cousin of the proband, who was aged five and whose mother had developed bilateral breast cancer at the age of 28. These two individuals were regarded as being at high risk of developing malignancies.

The *TP*53 gene has been conserved through evolution, and more specifically contains five domains within the coding region of the gene which are evolutionarily highly conserved. In sporadic tumours, *TP*53 mutations have been found throughout the coding sequence, but tend to cluster in four of the highly conserved domains in exon 5, encompassing two of these domains, exon 7 and exon 8. Certain codons have emerged as mutational hot spots. The three most commonly affected codons are 175, 248 and 273, with 245, 249 and 282 also frequently affected [24]. The germline mutations detected in LFS families by Malkin *et al.* [22] affected codons 245, 248 (two families) 252 and 258. Shortly after this report a sixth LFS family with a germline mutation in codon 245 was published [25]. These germline mutations had therefore all occurred in a stretch of 14 codons within the fourth evolutionarily conserved domain of *TP53*, which resides in exon 7 of the gene. Following these two reports, there was much speculation about the possible significance of this positional clustering, and it was suggested that there may be restriction on the types of *TP53* mutations which could occur in the germline with other mutations being lethal [26].

Subsequently, a number of groups throughout the world have analysed LFS families, families with cancer clusters suggestive of LFS (LFS-like families), and series of patients with LFS-associated cancers. Because of the frequency of premenopausal breast cancer in LFS families, examples of site-specific early-onset familial breast cancer were also studied. A number of reports of single LFS or LFS-like families with germline mutations in *TP53* have been published [27–30]. In these families germline mutations were observed in exons 5 and 8 as well as in exon 7. Other groups analysed series of families with features of LFS. Sameshima *et al.* [31] found germline *TP53* mutations in one classic LFS and one LFS-like family, which were both in exon 8. Both families were identified through a young child with adrenocortical carcinoma.

Brugières *et al.* [32] analysed 10 families of children with solid tumours, including eight with sarcomas and two with neural tumours, where at least one first- or second-degree relative of the index cases had been diagnosed with cancer before 45 years of age. The series comprised five families with classic LFS, three families in which the index child had an affected first-degree relative (incomplete LFS), one LFS-like family (three affected relatives, but not fulfilling the definition for classic LFS), and one family in which a second-degree relative of the proband had developed childhood cancer. Two of the families with classic LFS had germline *TP53* mutations in exon 8, and one family with incomplete LFS had a germline mutation in exon 7 of TP53. In this study, however, only exons 5 through to 8 were analysed. It is therefore possible that germline mutations outside these regions may have been present in one or more of the remaining families.

Birch *et al.* [33] analysed the entire coding sequence of the *TP53* gene for the presence of germline mutations in 12 families with classic LFS and nine LFS-like families. The families were ascertained systematically through patient registers of children with cancer and adults with bone or soft tissue sarcoma. Among the 12 families with classic LFS, nine probands were children, and among the LFS-like families, seven were children. Germline *TP53* mutations were detected in seven of the families, six with classic LFS and one LFS-like family. The mutations occurred in exons 4, 5, 6 and 7. Families which included young children with rhabdomyosarcoma and/or adrenocortical carcinoma were more likely to be associated with germline *TP53* mutations.

8.3 GERMLINE *TP53* MUTATIONS AND SARCOMAS AND LEUKAEMIAS

A series of 196 patients with bone or soft tissue sarcoma were analysed for the presence of germline mutations in exons 2 through to 11 of the *TP53* gene by Toguchida *et al.* [34]. Fifteen of these patients were selected because of an unusual family history of cancer, or the presence of multiple primary cancers. Among the remaining sporadic group, three patients all with osteosarcoma, were found to have *TP53* mutations in the germline. Although these patients were from the unselected series, two of them had multiple primary cancers, and one of these

127

also had a young daughter with soft tissue sarcoma. The third patient had a sibling with osteosarcoma. Among the patients who were selected as having an unusual personal or family history of cancer, germline *TP*53 mutations were detected in five. These eight examples of germline *TP*53 mutations involved exons 4, 5, 6, 7 and 8. The family histories of these patients included classic LFS, incomplete LFS, and LFS-like aggregations of cancer.

Felix *et al.* [35] analysed the coding sequence of *TP*53 in samples from 25 children with acute lymphoblastic leukaemia. A germline *TP*53 mutation in exon 8 was detected in one of these. On investigation, the family history was found to be consistent with classic LFS.

8.4 GERMLINE *TP*53 MUTATIONS AND MULTIPLE TUMOURS

Because of the high incidence of multiple primary tumours in members of LFS families, Malkin *et al.* [36] investigated a series of 59 children and young adults with second malignant neoplasms for the presence of germline *TP*53 mutations. The analysis included the four conserved domains of the *TP*53 gene, encompassing all the mutational hot spot regions. Germline mutations were detected in four of the patients in exons 7, 8 (two cases) and 9. Investigation of the family history in these four patients showed that one family could be classified as LFS-like, one family demonstrated incomplete LFS, and the remaining two had close relatives with breast cancer diagnosed at 57, and colon cancer diagnosed at 63 years respectively [36]. Among four cases of multifocal osteosarcoma, Iavarone *et al.* [37] found one case with a germline mutation in exon 8. There was no significant family history of cancer in this latter patient.

8.5 GERMLINE *TP*53 MUTATIONS AND BREAST CANCER

Three groups have analysed series of breast cancer patients for the presence of germline *TP*53 mutations. One of these series was completely unselected, and the remaining two included patients selected for early age at onset. Børresen *et al.* [38] studied an unselected series of 167 breast cancer patients, including 30 who had a family history of breast cancer and 40 who had developed breast cancer under the age of 35. Exons 5 through to 8 of the *TP*53 gene were analysed in constitutional samples from each of these patients. Two patients were found to carry germline mutations in *TP*53. The first of these, in codon 181, occurred in one of the patients from the unselected series, and the second mutation in codon 245 occurred in one of the patients with early-onset breast cancer. Both these patients had a family history of cancers, including breast cancer, which were suggestive of the Li–Fraumeni syndrome.

Sidransky *et al.* [39] analysed samples from 126 consecutively diagnosed patients with breast cancer diagnosed under the age of 41 for the presence of germline mutations in exons 5 through 8 of *TP*53. One patient was found to have a constitutional mutation in codon 181. On examination of her family history, her mother was found to have been diagnosed with bilateral premenopausal breast cancer and her grandmother had breast cancer at age 72, having previously developed carcinoma of the colon. The index patient, whose breast cancer was diagnosed at age 33, was subsequently diagnosed with a melanotic spindle-cell carcinoma of the mediastinum at age 35 [39].

Among a series of 136 breast cancer patients unselected with respect to age and family history, Prosser *et al.* [40] found one patient with a germline mutation in codon 267. The index patient had developed breast cancer at age 49, and family history showed that her mother had developed lung cancer at age 53 and cervix cancer at age 62; her maternal grandmother had had breast cancer at age 42, and her sister had died of breast cancer at age 67. The daughter of this latter patient had ovarian cancer at age 62. Thus, in this family the ages at onset of cancer were somewhat later than in other reported families with germline *TP*53 mutations. No samples were available for analysis from affected family members other than the index patient, but analysis of a number of unaffected relatives revealed two individuals who were carriers of this mutation and alive and well at the ages of 37 and 74 respectively. The mutation occurs outside of the conserved regions of the *TP*53 gene, and had been observed only once before in a sporadic cancer [24]. It would seem therefore that this particular mutation is either of low penetrance or may not be associated with cancer predisposition in this family, but rather may represent a polymorphic variation with no biological significance.

From these studies it would appear that germline *TP*53 mutations are uncommon among breast cancer patients in general, but a low frequency is observed in patients diagnosed at young ages and with family histories of early-onset cancers including carcinoma of the breast.

8.6 DISTRIBUTION OF GERMLINE MUTATIONS IN *TP*53

Details of 41 germline mutations in the coding region of *TP*53 have been published. Sixteen of these have occurred in exon 7, including eight affecting codon 248 and four affecting codon 245. Exon 8 was the next most frequently affected region, with 12 mutations including four affecting codon 273 and four affecting codon 282. Seven muta-

tions occurred in exon 5, two in exon 6, and only four mutations occurred outside of exons 5 through 8. However, these latter may be underrepresented, since most investigators have analysed only the conserved regions. The distribution of these germline mutations, in contrast to the marked positional clustering within part of exon 7 with respect to the initial six reported *TP*53 germline mutations, now much more closely resembles the distribution of *TP*53 mutations found in sporadic tumours.

Considering the nature of these 40 documented germline mutations in the coding region of the *TP*53 gene, it can be seen that 29 were transitions, and of these, 22 occurred at CpG dinucleotides. Only six transversions were seen and five examples of deletion and/ or insertion mutations were found.

Although carcinoma of the breast is the most common cancer occurring in adult members of LFS families, it is of interest that in tissue from sporadic breast cancers, transversions are as common as transitions, with mutations at CpG sites occurring relatively infrequently. The distribution of types of *TP*53 mutations occurring constitutionally most closely resembles that found among sporadic colon cancers. Although carcinoma of the colon has occurred in families with germline *TP*53 mutations, it is not among the most frequent types of cancer found in these families.

The hypermutability of CpG dinucleotides resulting from the spontaneous deamination of 5-methylcytosine has previously been described [24]. The frequency of this type of mutation among the documented examples of germline *TP*53 mutations suggests that the majority of these may arise as a result of spontaneous events. Exogenous mutagenic agents may play only a minor role in the generation of such mutations. The aetiology of germline *TP*53 mutations will be an important subject for future research.

8.7 MUTATIONS OUTSIDE THE CODING REGIONS OF THE *TP*53 GENE

In the majority of studies described above, only the conserved exons of the *TP*53 gene have been analysed, with the whole of the coding region being analysed in the remaining studies. This leaves open the possibility of mutations occurring in other regions of the gene, and two examples of intronic mutations have thus far been reported. One of these was found in a patient with osteosarcoma diagnosed during childhood, and a second primary abdominal malignancy as a young adult. The mutation was detected in intron 5 and consisted of the deletion of an 11-basepair sequence involving a region of splicing recognition [41].

The second example occurred in a family with hereditary breast and ovarian cancer. The proband in this family developed choroid plexus carcinoma at the age of 2 years. Three maternal aunts and the maternal grandmother had developed bilateral breast cancer, ovarian and colon cancer, all below the age of 40. The proband was found to carry a germline mutation affecting the splice acceptor site of exon 6, resulting in deletion of exon 6 and creating a frameshift leading to a premature stop codon. The mutation was found in each of the three cancer-affected maternal aunts and was also present in the unaffected mother of the index patient, who was alive and well at age 38, and in two first cousins unaffected at the ages of 18 and 16 respectively [42]. These findings suggest that intronic mutations may account for cancer predisposition in at least a proportion of those families with classic LFS who were negative for the presence of germline *TP*53 coding mutations.

8.8 PENETRANCE AND PHENOTYPIC EXPRESSION OF *TP*53

It will be seen from the above review that germline mutations in the *TP*53 gene have been found in association with familial clusters of cancers other than classic LFS, and in individual patients prone to the development of multiple primary cancers, Although breast cancers and sarcomas are common findings in patients and families with such mutations, a very wide spectrum of cancers has been observed, including most of the common carcinomas, as well as rare paediatric tumours. The phenotype associated with germline *TP*53 mutations thus appears to be broad. The penetrance is very variable, with malignancies occurring in the first year of life, and several cancers occurring in sequence in some individuals. In contrast, carriers of such mutations who have remained cancer-free into old age, have also been observed, even in families manifesting classic LFS.

Table 8.1 shows the age-distribution of the principal cancers which have occurred in known carriers of germline *TP*53 mutations and their first-degree relatives. It will be seen that the most common cancers in probands are childhood bone and soft tissue sarcoma. This is partly accounted for by the way individuals and families were selected for analysis. However, even though the definition of classic LFS allows for probands with sarcomas up to 44 years of age, all the sarcomas in probands with germline *TP*53 mutations were diagnosed under 30 years of age. Similarly, in the relatives nearly half the cancers occurred below 30 years of age. It is particularly striking that among the 42 breast cancers in probands and their relatives 12 (29%) occurred under 30 years of age. Only 0.6% of breast cancers in general occur within this age range.

The issue of whether penetrance and phenotypic expression is influenced by the type of germline mutation has not yet been resolved. The number of families so far reported are too few to attempt studies of possible correlations between specific mutations and cancer phenotype. Although *TP*53 behaves as a tumour suppressor gene, certain

Table 8.1 Cancers in carriers of germline *TP53* mutations and their first-degree relatives

Type of cancer	Age at diagnosis in probands (years)				Age at diagnosis in relatives (years)			
	0–14	15–29	30–49	50+	0–14	15–29	30–49	50+
Soft tissue sarcoma	14	2	–	–	8	2	4	1
Osteo/chondrosarcoma	12	10	–	–	1	8	–	–
Breast cancer	0	3	4	–	0	9	25	1
Brain tumour	4	1	–	–	4	1	2	2
Leukaemia	–	1	–	–	2	2	1	–
Adrenocortical carcinoma	3	–	–	–	3	–	–	–
Other	2	5	2	0	0	7	12	4
Totals	35	22	6	0	18	29	44	8
All tumours in probands or relatives (%)	55.6	34.9	9.5	0	18.2	29.3	44.4	8.1

mutant protein products show a gain of function or transdominant effect on the wild-type *TP53* product which influences phenotype at the cellular level [43, 44]. It is possible that such gain of function mutations, if they occur in the germline, may result in a more highly penetrant cancer phenotype in terms of lifetime risk of malignancy, age at onset and probability of developing multiple primary cancers, than mutations which result in a simple loss of function of properties associated with the wild-type protein.

The influence of exogenous factors on cancer development in carriers of germline *TP53* mutations is also unknown, but factors such as exposure to environmental carcinogens, lifestyle and social habits, may in part determine the type of cancer that develops and the age at onset. Such lifetime experiences, together with the genetic background in an individual, may explain the apparent wide variations in types of cancer and ages at onset in carriers of identical mutations which have been observed even within the same family. Such issues will only be resolved when detailed information on many more families accumulates, especially planned prospective follow-up of carriers of germline TP53 mutations, together with a deeper understanding of the function of wild-type TP53 and its partners in comparison with the spectrum of mutant protein products.

8.9 LFS AND LFS-LIKE FAMILIES NOT DUE TO *TP*53

It appears that approximately half of the families with classic LFS do not have germline mutations in the coding region of *TP53*. Some of these families may have intronic or promoter region mutations. A second possibility is that a constitutional mutation in another gene, which interacts with TP53 such that the normal function of TP53 wild-type protein is compromised, may be present. This is suggested by two families with a Li–Fraumeni-like pattern of cancers, in whom no *TP53* germline mutation could be detected. In both families increased expression of apparently wild-type TP53 protein was detected by immunohistochemistry in normal tissue as well as tumour tissue in affected family members [45, 46]. In one of these families direct involvement of *TP53* by linkage analysis has been excluded [46]. This latter family is shown in Figure 8.2. The basis of cancer predisposition in LFS families in whom germline mutations in the *TP53* gene have not been detected is at present an area of intense research activity.

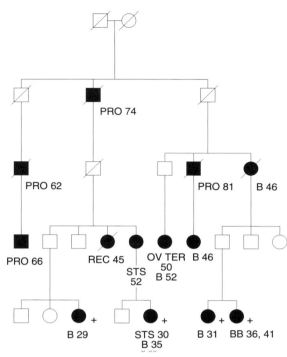

Fig. 8.2 Family with LFS in whom direct involvement of *TP*53 has been excluded by linkage analysis. Individuals marked + show increased expression of TP53 protein by immunohistochemical analysis in their normal tissue and tumour tissue. B, breast carcinoma; BB, bi-lateral breast carcinoma; OVTER, ovarian teratoma; PRO, carcinoma of the prostate; REC, rectal carcinoma; STS, soft tissue sarcoma. Numbers indicate age at diagnosis.

8.10 PREDICTIVE GENETIC TESTING

The finding of germline mutations in the *TP*53 gene in LFS and LFS-like families means that it is now possible to test asymptomatic members of these families for the presence of such mutations. Predictive testing in this way, however, presents a number of ethical, technical and clinical difficulties which need to be addressed. Present data suggest that the prevalence of germline *TP*53 mutations among cancer patients in general is very low.

Even among patients with LFS-associated cancers, for example bone and soft tissue sarcoma and premenopausal breast cancer, the incidence of germline *TP*53 mutations appears to be of the order of 1% [34, 38–40]. It would therefore be inappropriate to screen the generality of patients with these cancers for the presence of germline *TP*53 mutations. Testing would only be appropriate in the close relatives of individuals shown to carry a germline *TP*53 mutation. These individuals would be likely to be members of LFS families or patients with multiple primary LFS-associated cancers. Counselling families on cancer risks associated with germline *TP*53 mutations is difficult, since the morphology, site-, age- and sex-specific incidence of cancers in carriers of such mutations are unknown. Furthermore, as discussed above, it is possible that there may be mutation-specific variations in cancer risks and risks may be modified according to an individual's life experiences. Childhood cancers are a common feature of families with classic LFS, and a further difficulty therefore arises as to whether it would be ethical to test healthy children for the presence of a germline *TP*53 mutation. This would only be justified if it could be demonstrated that screening for early detection of cancers in such children conferred a survival benefit or reduction in morbidity. At present there is no evidence to suggest that this is the case. In adult carriers of these mutations, it is equally difficult to envisage a programme of screening procedures which would be effective in early detection of associated cancers. For example, even mammography aimed at early detection of breast cancer, the most common adult-onset cancer in LFS families, is of unproven benefit in premenopausal women. There is also concern about the use of X-irradiation in carriers of *TP*53 mutations because mice heterozygous for *TP*53 mutation tolerate radiation-induced DNA damage. If this can be extrapolated to humans there may be a risk of radiation-induced tumour from such screening.

The psychological impact of imparting to individuals the knowledge that they are at increased risk of developing cancer and that they may have passed this risk on to their children is poorly understood, and represents a further area which should be addressed in any predictive testing programme. It has therefore been recommended that any such genetic predictive testing should be carried out according to a standard protocol within the context of a multicentre collaborative study aimed at evaluating the benefits and disadvantages of such testing. It is mandatory that predictive testing for genetic susceptibility to cancer should be carried out in centres with the appropriate expertise in clinical genetics and molecular biology, and that psychological assessment should be built in to a standard protocol. Such coordinated programmes are being implemented in North America and the UK, and it is hoped these will provide a model for predictive testing for carriers of other cancer susceptibility genes in the future [47–49].

8.11 CONCLUSIONS

In conclusion, the study of the Li–Fraumeni syndrome and the discovery of germline *TP*53 mutations in families with LFS is a good example of how basic cancer research involving clinical observations in patients with rare paediatric cancers, painstaking epidemiological research, together with biochemical and molecular biological research, initially in a purely experimental system, have come together and progressed in little over 10 years to yield results of profound scientific and clinical importance.

REFERENCES

1. Li, F.P. and Fraumeni, J.F., Jr (1969) Soft-tissue sarcomas, breast cancer, and other neoplasms. A familial syndrome? *Ann. Intern. Med.*, **71**, 747–52.
2. Li, F.P. and Fraumeni, J.F., Jr (1969) Rhabdomyosarcoma in children: epidemiologic study and identification of a familial cancer syndrome. *J. Natl Cancer Inst.*, **43**, 1365–73.
3. Bottomley, R.H., Trainer, A.L. and Condit, P.T. (1971) Chromosome studies in a 'cancer family'. *Cancer*, **28**, 519–28.
4. Lynch, H.T., Krush, A.J., Harlan, W.L. and Sharp, E.A. (1973) Association of soft tissue sarcoma, leukemia, and brain tumors in families affected with breast cancer. *Am. Surg.*, **39**, 199–206.
5. Blattner, W.A., McGuire, D.B., Mulvihill, J.J. *et al.* (1979) Genealogy of cancer in a family. *JAMA*, **241**, 259–61.
6. Pearson, A.D.J., Craft, A.W., Ratcliffe, J.M. *et al.* (1982) Two families with the Li–Fraumeni cancer family syndrome. *J. Med. Genet.*, **19**, 362–5.
7. Li, F.P. and Fraumeni, J.F., Jr (1982) Prospective study of a family cancer syndrome. *JAMA*, **247**, 2692–4.
8. Birch, J.M., Hartley, A.L., Marsden, H.B. *et al.* (1984) Excess risk of breast cancer in the mothers of children with soft tissue sarcomas. *Br. J. Cancer*, **49**, 325–31.
9. Birch, J.M., Hartley, A.L., Blair, V. *et al.* (1990) Cancer in the families of children with soft tissue sarcoma. *Cancer*, **66**, 2239–48.
10. Birch, J.M., Hartley, A.L., Blair, V. *et al.* (1990) Identification of factors associated with high breast cancer risk in the mothers of children with soft tissue sarcoma. *J. Clin. Oncol.*, **8**, 583–90.
11. Strong, L.C., Stine, M. and Norsted, T.L. (1987) Cancer in survivors of childhood soft tissue sarcoma and their relatives. *J. Natl Cancer Inst.*, **79**, 1213–20
12. Williams, W.R. and Strong, L.C. (1985) Genetic epidemiology of soft tissue sarcomas in children, in *Familial Cancer. First International Research Conference on Familial Cancer, Basel, 1985*, (eds H. Muller and W. Weber), Karger, Basel, pp. 151–3.
13. Lustbader, E.D., Williams, W.R., Bondy, M.L. *et al.*, (1992) Segregation analysis of cancer in families of childhood soft-tissue-sarcoma patients. *Am. J. Hum. Genet.*, **51**, 344–56.

14. Li, F.P., Fraumeni, J.F., Jr., Mulvihill, J.J. *et al.* (1988) A cancer family syndrome in twenty-four kindreds. *Cancer Res.*, **48**, 5358–62.

15. Hartley, A.L., Birch, J.M., Marsden, H.B. and Harris, M. (1987) Malignant melanoma in families of children with osteosarcoma, chondrosarcoma and adrenal cortical carcinoma. *J. Med. Genet.*, **24**, 664–8.

16. Hartley, A.L., Birch, J.M., Kelsey, A.M. *et al.* (1989) Are germ cell tumors part of the Li–Fraumeni Cancer Family Syndrome? *Cancer Genet. Cytogenet.*, **42**. 221–6.

17. Hartley, A.L., Birch, J.M., Tricker, K. *et al.* (1993) Wilms' tumour in the Li Fraumeni cancer family syndrome. *Cancer Genet. Cytogenet.*, **67**, 133–5.

18. Draper, G.J., Sanders, B.M. and Kingston, J.E. (1986) Second primary neoplasms in patients with retinoblastoma. *Br. J. Cancer*, **53**, 661–71.

19. Strong, L.C., Herson, J., Haas, C. *et al.*, (1984) Cancer mortality in relatives of retinoblastoma patients. *J. Natl Cancer Inst.*, **73**, 303–11.

20. DerKinderen, D.J., Koten, J.W., Nagelkerke, N.J.D. *et al.* (1988) Non-ocular cancer in patients with hereditary retinoblastoma and their relatives. *Int. J. Cancer*, **41**, 499–504.

21. Friend, S.H., Bernards, R., Rogelj, S. *et al.* (1986) A human DNA segment with properties of the gene that predisposes to retinoblastoma and osteosarcoma. *Nature*, **323**, 643–6.

22. Malkin, D., Li, F.P., Strong, L.C. *et al.* (1990) Germ line p53 mutations in a familial syndrome of breast cancer, sarcomas, and other neoplasms. *Science*, **250**, 1233–8.

23. Lavigueur, A., Maltby, V., Mock, D. *et al.* (1989) High incidence of lung, bone, and lymphoid tumors in transgenic mice over-expressing mutant alleles of the p53 oncogene. *Mol. Cell. Biol.*, **9**, 3982–91.

24. Caron de Fromental, C. and Soussi, T. (1992) The *TP53* tumor suppressor gene: a model for investigating human mutagenesis. *Genes Chromosom. Cancer*, **4**, 1–15.

25. Srivastava, S., Zou, Z., Pirollo, K. *et al.* (1990) Germ-line transmission of a mutated *p53* gene in a cancer-prone family with Li–Fraumeni syndrome. *Nature*, **348**, 747–9.

26. Vogelstein, B. (1990) A deadly inheritance. *Nature*, **348**, 681–2.

27. Law, J.C., Strong, L.C., Chidambaram, A. and Ferrell, R.E. (1991) A germ line mutation in exon 5 of the *p53* gene in an extended cancer family. *Cancer Res.*, **51**, 6385–7.

28. Kovar, H., Auinger, A., Jug, G. *et al.* (1992) p53 mosaicism with an exon 8 germline mutation in the founder of a cancer-prone pedigree. *Oncogene*, **7**, 2169–73.

29. Metzger, A.K., Sheffield, V.C., Duyk, G. *et al.* (1991) Identification of a germ-line mutation in the p53 gene in a patient with an intracranial ependymoma. *Proc. Natl Acad. Sci. USA*, **88**, 7825–9.

30. Eeles, R.A., Warren, W., Knee, G. *et al.* (1993) Constitutional mutation in exon 8 of the p53 gene in a patient with multiple primary tumours: molecular and immunohistochemical findings. *Oncogene*, **8**, 1269–76.

31. Sameshima, Y., Tsunematsu, Y., Watanabe, S. *et al.* (1992) Detection of novel germ-line p53 mutations in diverse-cancer-prone families identified by selecting patients with childhood adrenocortical carcinoma. *J. Natl Cancer Inst.*, **84**, 703–7.

32. Brugières, L., Gardes, M., Moutou, C. *et al.* (1993) Screening for germ line *p53* mutations in children with malignant tumors and a family history of cancer. *Cancer Res.*, **53**, 452–5.

33. Birch, J.M., Hartley, A.L., Tricker, K.J. *et al.* (1994) Prevalence and diversity of constitutional mutations in the p53 gene among 21 Li–Fraumeni families. *Cancer Res.*, **54**, 1298–304.

34. Toguchida, J., Yamaguchi, T., Dayton, S.H. *et al.* (1992) Prevalence and spectrum of germline mutations of the p53 gene among patients with sarcoma. *N. Engl. J. Med.*, **326**, 1301–8.

35. Felix, C.A., Nau, M.M., Takahashi, T. *et al.* (1992) Hereditary and acquired p53 gene mutations in childhood acute lymphoblastic leukemia. *J. Clin. Invest.*, **89**, 640–7.

36. Malkin, D., Jolly, K.W., Barbier, N. *et al.* (1992) Germline mutations of the p53 tumor-suppressor gene in children and young adults with second malignant neoplasms. *N. Engl. J. Med.*, **326**, 1309–15.

37. Iavarone, A., Matthay, K.K., Steinkirchner, T.M. and Israel, M.A. (1992) Germ-line and somatic p53 gene mutations in multifocal

osteogenic sarcoma. *Proc. Nat. Acad. Sci. USA*, **89**, 4207–9.

38. Børresen, A.-L., Andersen, T.I., Garber, J. *et al.* (1992) Screening for germ line TP53 mutations in breast cancer patients. *Cancer Res.*, **52**, 3234–6.

39. Sidransky, D., Tokino, T., Helzlsouer, K. *et al.* (1992) Inherited *p53* gene mutations in breast cancer. *Cancer Res.*, **52**, 2984–6.

40. Prosser, J., Porter, D., Coles, C. *et al.* (1992) Constitutional p53 mutation in a non-Li–Fraumeni cancer family. *Br. J. Cancer*, **65**, 527–8.

41. Felix, C.A., Strauss, E.A., D'Amico, D. *et al.* (1993) A novel germline p53 splicing mutation in a pediatric patient with a second malignant neoplasm. *Oncogene*, **8**, 1203–10.

42. Jolly, K.W., Malkin, D., Douglass, E.C. *et al.* (1994) Splice-site mutation of the p53 gene in a family with hereditary breast-ovarian cancer. *Oncogene* **9**, 97–102.

43. Dittmer, D., Pati, S., Zambetti, G. *et al.* (1993) Gain of function mutations in p53. *Nature Genet.*, **4**, 42–5.

44. Srivastava, S., Wang, S., Tong, Y.A. *et al.* (1993) Several mutant p53 proteins detected in cancer-prone families with Li–Fraumeni syndrome exhibit transdominant effects on the biochemical properties of the wild-type p53. *Oncogene*, **8**, 2449–56.

45. Barnes, D.M., Hanby, A.M., Gillett, C.E. *et al.* (1992) Abnormal expression of wild type p53 protein in normal cells of a cancer family patient. *Lancet*, **340**, 259–63.

46. Birch, J.M., Heighway, J., Teare, M.D. *et al.* (1994) Linkage studies in a Li–Fraumeni family with increased expression of p53 protein but no germline mutation in p53. *Br. J. Cancer*, **70**, 1176–81.

47. Li, F.P., Garber, J.E., Friend, S.H. *et al.* (1992) Recommendations on predictive testing for germ line p53 mutations among cancer-prone individuals. *J. Natl Cancer Inst.*, **84**, 1156–60.

48. Birch, J.M. (1992) Germline mutations in the p53 tumour suppressor gene: scientific, clinical and ethical challenges. *Br. J. Cancer*, **66**, 424–6.

49. Eeles, R.A. (1993) Predictive testing for germline mutations in the p53 gene: are all the questions answered? *Eur. J. Cancer*, **29A**, 1361–5.

Chromosome Fragility Syndromes and the Gorlin Syndrome

Chapter 9

Malignant disease and variations in radiosensitivity in ataxia telangiectasia patients

A.M.R. TAYLOR, D. HERNANDEZ, C.M. MCCONVILLE, C.G. WOODS, M. STACEY, P. BIGGS, P.J. BYRD, C.F. ARLETT and D. SCOTT

9.1 INTRODUCTION

Ataxia telangiectasia (A-T) is a progressive neurological disorder with a birth incidence of about 1 in 300 000 [1, 2]. Although generally believed to be a Mendelian recessive disorder there is some evidence that this may not always be the case [2]. The major neurological features include progressive cerebellar ataxia presenting in infancy, oculomotor dyspraxia and dysarthria. Immunodeficiency is an important feature of this disorder although it is not usually severe. A majority of patients, if not all, have a deficiency of cell-mediated immunity, with deficiencies in humoral immunity being more variable. The resulting predisposition to infection is very variable between patients with some not noticably affected and others showing several episodes of severe infection. In addition, patients show thymic hypo-plasia, hypogonadism, a high level of serum alphafetoprotein, growth retardation and an abnormality of blood vessels (telangiectasia) [3]. The *A-T* gene also confers an increased radiosensitivity which can be observed both in patients and in cultured cells from patients [4, 5].

9.2 MALIGNANT DISEASE IN ATAXIA TELANGIECTASIA

Approximately 10% of all A-T homozygotes develop a malignancy in childhood or early adulthood. A minority of tumours are epithelial cell cancers with an unusually high predisposition to stomach carcinoma and smaller excesses of liver, uterus and ovarian cancers [6]. The majority of tumours are, however, either lymphoid leukaemias or lymphomas [6, 7]. A greater proportion of

Genetic Predisposition to Cancer. Edited by R.A. Eeles, B.A.J. Ponder, D.F. Easton and A. Horwich. Published in 1996 by Chapman & Hall, London.
0 412 56580 3

A-T patients with leukaemia, compared with patients in the non-A-T population, have markers for T cell leukaemia [6, 8]. Cases of T cell lymphoma, T cell acute lymphoblastic leukaemia (T-ALL) and T cell prolymphocytic leukaemia (T-PLL) have been reported [8].

Our limited number of observations suggest that A-T patients with T cell tumours can clearly be grouped into either an older or a younger category. Older patients (with a mean age of about 33 years) develop T-PLL. Two of our patients in this category showed proliferation of a t(X;14) (q28;q11)-containing lymphocyte clone to 100% of T cells and a further patient showed a large inv(14) (q11;q32) clone. In all cases the tumour arose from the clone following the appearance of additional chromosome translocations [9, 10]. There are several other examples in the literature showing the association between T-PLL (sometimes referred to as T-CLL) and translocation clone proliferation in A-T patients in early adulthood [8]. In some patients with leukaemia of mature post-thymic lymphocytes, progress of the disease in the later stages may be as rapid as in T-ALL. Younger patients (2–12 years in our group) developed T cell acute leukaemia or T cell lymphoma. There are far fewer observations on the chromosomal changes associated with these tumour types in A-T patients, but inv(14) and t(14;14) translocations are seen [8]. It seems that the constitutional gene defect in A-T patients allows the formation of a much higher level of chromosome translocations involving interlocus recombination of T cell receptor (TCR) genes in T lymphocytes than occurs in non A-T patients. The wide range of translocations associated with T-ALL in non-A-T patients [11] presumably also occurs in A-T patients and, because of a likely defect in recombination in A-T cells [12], may even be present at an increased frequency. The presence of this variety of initial chromosome translocations explains the potential for the development of any of the several forms of T cell tumour in a population of A-T patients. In some A-T patients a translocation which affects a gene at the top of the regulatory cascade will be associated with the development of T-ALL; in other patients the translocation may activate a gene which allows a steady proliferation of lymphocytes in which further mutational events accumulate to give the eventual transformation to, say T-PLL, which we observe in older patients. There is a curious complication seen in some families. Although one might expect that, within families, the development of different forms of T cell tumour might occur at random there are reports of concordance within families for the development of either T-PLL (T-CLL) or ALL [8]. While the numbers of families are small perhaps this is an indication of the effect of different *A-T* mutations and therefore heterogeneity.

9.3 THE *A-T* GENE IN THE HETEROZYGOUS STATE

Although the *A-T* gene in the homozygous state clearly predisposes patients to lymphoid leukaemia/lymphoma the gene may be numerically more important in the heterozygous state. About 1% of the population carry the gene [1] and carriers have been reported to have a risk of cancer which is 2–6 times higher than for the normal population. In a prospective study Swift *et al.* [13] estimated that women heterozygous for the *A-T* gene were 5.1 [95% C.l. 1.5–16.9] times more likely to have breast cancer than non-carriers of the gene. If this is correct it follows that individuals heterozygous for the *A-T* gene may comprise 9–18% of patients with breast cancer (in the US) [13]. Two other studies have reported an excess of breast cancer (but low patient numbers) in patients heterozygous for the *A-T* gene [14, 15]. In neither of these latter two studies was an excess of tumours observed in the grandparents of A-T patients where half would be expected to be A-T heterozygotes. Separate estimates for the parental and grandparental generations of excess cancer risk were not given by Swift *et al.* [13]. A recent study found no evidence for linkage between breast cancer and chromosome 11q markers and the authors concluded that the contribution of the *A-T* gene to familial clustering of breast cancer was likely to be familial [16]. *A-T* could still be important, however, in contributing to single cases by conferring a moderate breast cancer risk. It is not known why there is apparently no obvious increase in the heterozygotes of leukaemia/lymphomas, which are the tumours most frequent in homozygotes. The increased numbers of other tumour types seen in A-T heterozygotes are not statistically significant. It may not be possible to test whether a clear association exists between the *A-T* gene in the heterozygous state and other tumour types because of the paucity of tumours. It has also been reported that diagnostic or occupational exposure to ionizing radiation might increase the risk of breast cancer in women heterozygous for the *A-T* gene [13], although this suggestion has met some criticism [17].

9.4 LOCALIZATION AND ISOLATION OF THE *A-T* GENE

The gene for ataxia telangiectasia was first mapped to chromosome 11q22–23 by Gatti *et al.* [18] by linkage to the gene *THY* 1 and the DNA marker D11S144. This localization was confirmed [19] and subsequently linkage and recombination evidence pointed to the existence of a single *A-T* locus between the markers A4 (DS11S1819) and A2 (DS11S1818) at this position [20]. The *A-T* gene was recently partially cloned from the region between D11S384 and D11S535 [21]. It codes for a major 12kb transcript present in all tissues and cell types examined but there may be several additional transcripts result-

ing from alternative splicing. The coding region has now been completely sequenced and extends over more than 9kb and mutations have been shown to be scattered throughout its whole length [21, 22] with most leading to premature truncation of the protein product and the remainder, small in-frame deletions. There is significant homology of the *A-T* gene product with several yeast and mammalian phosphatidylinositol 3-kinases that are involved in signal transduction, meiotic recombination and cell cycle control [21]. These homologies are consistent with the known pleiotropic effects of the *A-T* mutation that lead to defects in signal transduction, cellular differentiation, cell cycle control and an abnormal response to DNA damage.

Genetic complementation indicating the presence of four complementation groups in A-T has previously been reported [27] although the finding of a single *A-T* gene makes the existence of these groups more difficult to interpret especially as patients apparently in different complementation groups have been reported to be homozygous for the same mutation [21]. There is little evidence for locus heterogeneity, although one family with two affected cousins that we have studied showed no clear evidence that the *A-T* gene in this family was on chromosome 11q22–23 [23].

9.5 CLINICAL HETEROGENEITY IN ATAXIA TELANGIECTASIA

Although generally regarded as a homogeneous entity some clinical heterogeneity in A-T cases has been observed [3, 24, 25]. The progressive cerebellar degeneration is usually first noted in infancy or early childhood [3] but the rate of progress of the cerebellar ataxia may be variable. Some patients may show a much slower course [3, 23] and the degree of bulbar telangiectasia and levels of serum AFP are also very variable [3, 26].

Table 9.1 Induced chromosome damage in lymphocytes from classical A-T patients following exposure to 1 Gy X-rays at G_2

Family no.	Patient identifi-cation	Sex	No. of cells	Ring chromo-somes	Dicentric chromo-somes	Chromo-some fragments	Chroma-tid gaps	Chroma-tid breaks	Chromo-some gaps	Triradial chromo-somes	Quadri-radial chromo-somes
45	II-1	M	50	0	0	3	93	20	0	1	1
47	II-1	F	50	0	0	2	104	46	0	1	0
48	II-3	F	35	0	0	7	66	25	0	1	0
51	II-4	M	50	0	0	0	78	26	0	8	5
54	II-2	F	50	0	0	4	86	9	0	2	4
55	II-3	M	22	0	0	0	28	25	0	1	4
56	II-1	F	50	0	0	0	85	16	0	4	4
57	II-1	M	50	0	0	0	43	6	1	2	1
58	II-1	M	50	0	1	1	81	11	0	2	0
	II-2	F	50	0	0	3	74	7	0	7	0
60	II-1	F	16	0	0	0	41	5	0	1	1
	II-3	M	50	0	0	5	93	11	0	5	1
61	II-1	F	50	0	0	2	67	16	0	3	1

9.6 LOW RADIOSENSITIVITY VARIANTS OF ATAXIA TELANGIECTASIA

The classical group of ataxia telangiectasia patients show the characteristically high level of radiosensitivity, measured either chromo-somally in lymphocytes or by the survival of skin fibroblasts. Within this group of patients there appears to be some variation in the level of induced chromosome damage in response to exposure of lymphocytes to X-rays (Table 9.1). When the colony-forming ability of fibroblasts from these patients is analysed, no difference in survival is observed in cells from different patients [26–28]. There also appears to be another group of A-T patients showing a much lower level of chromosomal radiosensitivity [29]. We present here a comparison (Tables 9.1 and 9.2) between a classical group and a group of low-radiosensitivity A-T patients. All the patients described here were diagnosed clin-ically as having A-T. The criteria for diagnosis were the presence of progressive cerebellar ataxia and horizontal and vertical saccades,

together with at least two of the following: choreoathetosis, impassive face, dysarthria and bulbar telangiectasia (Table 9.1).

9.6.1 RADIOSENSITIVITY OF CHROMOSOMES IN LOW-RADIOSENSITIVITY VARIANTS

In a study of 60 A-T families, chromosomal radiosensitivity, following exposure of lym-phocytes to 1 Gy X-rays at G_2, was measured as a matter of course. During the study it became apparent that a few A-T patients had a much lower level of chromosomal radio-sensitivity measured in terms of chromatid type damage compared with the majority of patients. This was so marked in some instances as to be no different from normal. There were no hard criteria for judging low radiosensitivity. Rather, an assessment of the low radiosensitivity of a patient's lympho-cytes was based on our experience of the levels of radiosensitivity in about 100 families over many years. In most cases the level of radiosensitivity in the initial blood sample

Table 9.2 Chromatid type aberrations induced in lymphocytes from low-radiosensitivity variants following exposure to 1 Gy X-rays at G_2

Family no.	Patient identification	Sample no.	Sex	Ring chromosomes	Dicentric chromosomes	Chromosome fragments	Chromatid gaps	Chromatid breaks	Chromosome gaps	Chromosome breaks	Interchanges[1]
1	II-1	i	F	0	0	0	31	10	0	0	1
		ii		0	0	0	15	10	0	0	3
		iii		0	0	2	39	11	0	0	0
14	II-1	i	F	0	0	0	20	9	1	0	0
		ii		0	0	0	48	8	0	0	1
38	II-1		M	0	0	1	10	1	0	0	0
	II-2		M	0	0	0	10	1	0	0	0
40	II-1		M	0	0	3	17	1	2	0	1
	II-2		M	0	0	0	9	2	0	0	0
44	II-1	i	F	0	0	0	13	0	0	0	0
		ii		0	0	0	1	0	1	0	1
46	II-1	i	M	0	0	4	16	4	0	0	0
		ii		0	0	1	23	6	0	0	0
	II-2		M	0	0	0	24	1	0	0	1
52	II-3		F	0	0	0	26	2	1	0	1
53	II-1		M	0	0	2	41	9	0	0	6
	II-2		M	0	0	2	26	4	1	0	2
59	II-1	i	F	0	1	0	12	0	1	0	0
		ii		0	0	0	11	1	0	0	1
62	II-2		F	0	0	0	18	3	0	0	0
90	II-1	i	F	0	0	1	14	2	0	0	2
		ii		0	0	0	5	7	0	0	0
91	II-1	i	M	0	0	1	19	1	0	0	1
		ii		0	0	3	36	6	0	0	0

[1] Sum of triradial and quadriradial chromosomes.

from a patient designated as a low-radiosensitivity patient was very close to the mean level seen in controls. During the time required to accumulate the 60 families, patients with low levels of radiosensitivity were identified in 10 families (14 patients), giving a frequency for low-radiosensitivity variants of about 16% of all A-T families. The levels of induced chromatid type damage ranged from 11–57 gaps/breaks with a mean of 25 in the 10 families (Table 9.2). This compared with a mean of 9 for the controls (Table 9.3). In addition to this group from the cohort of 60 families we have also identified two other families (90 and 91) showing low

radiosensitivity. In all 12 families the levels of chromatid-type damage ranged from 1–57 chromatid gaps/breaks in 50 cells, with a mean of 25. The radiosensitivity of this group can be compared with that of the last eleven consecutively ascertained families of the total of 60 in our linkage study (Table 9.1). In this group the mean level of chromatid gaps/breaks in 50 cells was 107 compared with normals at 9 (Table 9.3). The ratio of X-ray-induced damage in normal, A-T variants and classical A-T patients is therefore approximately 1:3:12. The mean level of induced damage in these variants is at least two standard deviations less than the mean levels

Table 9.3 Induced chromosome damage in lymphocytes from normal individuals following exposure to 1 Gy X-rays at G_2

Control subject	No. of cells	Ring chromo-somes	Dicentric chromosome	Chromo-some fragments	Chromatid gaps	Chromatid breaks	Chromo-some gaps	Triradial chromo-somes	Quadri-radials
1	50	0	0	1	10	0	0	0	0
2	50	0	0	0	14	1	0	0	0
3	50	0	0	0	2	0	0	0	0
4	50	0	0	0	9	0	0	0	0
5	50	0	0	0	8	0	0	0	1
6	50	0	0	0	8	1	1	0	0
7	22	0	0	0	4	1	0	0	0

in classical patients. Two additional observations are important in confirming the unusually low chromosomal radiosensitivity in these patients. First, in the four families with two affected siblings the level of induced damage is the same in both siblings (families 38, 40, 46 and 53) with family 38 showing the lowest level. Second, when patients have been sampled at different times, the level of induced chromosome damage was seen to be the same at each sampling time (families 1, 14, 44, 46, 59, 90 and 91).

9.6.2 RADIOSENSITIVITY OF LYMPHOCYTES AT DIFFERENT FIXATION TIMES

Only a single fixation time of 4h following X-irradiation was used for measuring the level of radiosensitivity. This may not represent an identical stage in G_2 in all the cultures examined. Abnormally low levels of chromosomal radiosensitivity therefore might have been due to failure to fix cells at equivalent points in the cell cycle following irradiation. This is unlikely for two reasons. First, repeated blood samples from the same individual, at different sampling times, showed the same level of aberrations. Second, lymphocytes, from low-radiosensitivity patients, fixed over a range of sampling times showed

no large differential between the A-T patients and controls.

9.6.3 COLONY-FORMING ASSAYS IN FIBROBLASTS FROM LOW-RADIOSENSITIVITY A-T PATIENTS

Fibroblast cultures were only available from eight patients in six low-radiosensitivity families (1, 14, 38, 44, 46 and 52). Cell strains from all eight of these patients showed an intermediate level of survival compared with normal controls and classical A-T strains (Figure 9.1). These results show that it is possible that our population of low-radiosensitivity variants falls into different groups. The more radiosensitive group indicated by ● and ■ have six individuals from five families. The less radiosensitive pair (▲) are two brothers from family 46.

9.6.4 LOW RADIOSENSITIVITY, CHROMOSOME TRANSLOCATION FREQUENCY AND CLINICAL VARIATION IN A-T

The cellular radiosensitivity measurements and clinical assessment of patients were made independently. In four low-radiosensitivity families the sibship consisted of only two affected males. The significance of this is not known. The clinical details of the

143

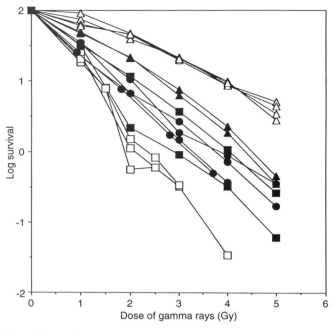

Fig. 9.1 Colony-forming ability of primary skin fibroblast strains following exposure to gamma rays. △, fibroblast strains from four normal individuals; □, fibroblast strains from typical highly radiosensitive A-T patients. Closed symbols are all fibroblast strains from low-radiosensitivity variant A-T patients. ●, patients 1, II-1; 14, II-1; 44, II-1 and 52, II-2. ▲ represent brothers 46, II-1 and 46 II-2; ■ represent brothers 38, II-1 and 38, II-2.

low-radiosensitivity patients are summarized in Table 9.4. In five of the 16 patients (1, II–1; 14, II–1; 38, II–1; 38, II–2 and 52, II–3, group 1) the clinical progress of the cerebellar ataxia could definitely be described as being slow. The age of onset of symptoms in these patients may have been only a little later than usual (2–3 years) with the exception of patient 1, II–1 (6 years). Three further patients (44, II–2; 59, II–1 and 62, II–2, group 2) showed no problem of gait until the ages of 13, 8 and 11 years respectively and at the ages now of 16, 12 and 19 years are still walking, even if some aid is required.

These three patients therefore appear to be different insofar as they showed a late onset form of A-T. Of the two brothers (46, II-1 and 46, II–2, group 3) whose fibroblasts showed

the highest survival, one was still ambulatory at age 22 years and did not use a wheelchair, while his younger brother (46, II–2) at 13 years of age had only minimal physical signs including clumsiness and jerky eye movements. Six patients (in families 40, 53, 90 and 91, group 4) appeared to have onset at the usual age and a normal rate of progress, although it should be stressed that two of these patients are still very young.

Even allowing for some loss of objectivity in judging similarities and differences there is clearly evidence of clinical heterogeneity in this group of radiosensitivity variants and the 12 families may fall into four different groups. The low chromosomal radiosensitivity is matched by higher survival for at least one patient in each of the groups 1–3 but

144

Table 9.4 Clinical features of A-T low-radiosensitivity variants

Patient	Age (years)	Sex	Facies[1]	Conjunctival telangiectasia[2]	Speech[3]	Eye movement[4]	Choreoathetosis[5]	Presenting feature to parents	Infections[6]	Progress[7]
1-1	23	F	imp	1	1	2	1	Gait at 6 years	0	S
14-1	17	F	imp	2	2	2	2	Gait at 3 years	1	S
38-1	26	M	imp	1	1	2	2	Gait at 2 years	0	S
38-2	23	M	imp	1	1	3	1	Gait at 2 years	1	S
40-1	26	M	imp	1	2	2	1	Gait at 2 years	2	N
40-2	22	M	imm	2	2	2	1	Gait at 2 years	0	?N
44-2	16	F	imp	1	1	2	?	Drooling at 3 years	0	L/S[8]
46-1	24	M	–	1	2	1	?	Clumsy at ?		S[9]
46-2	13	M	–	0	0	1	1	Clumsy at 11 years	?	S[10]
52-3	32	F	imp	1	1	?	?	Gait at 1 year	1	S
53-1	17	M	imp	1	2	2	2	Gait at 14 months	0	?N
53-2	15	M	imp	1	2	2	2	Gait at 17 months	0	?N
59-2	12	F	–	1	1	1	1	Gait at 8 years	0	L/S
62-2	19	F	imm	2	1	1	2	Gait at 11 years	0	L/S
90-1	2	F	?	?	2	0	?	Gait at 13 months	0	?
91-1	5	M	imp	?	2	?	?	?		?

[1] Facies: imp, impassive; imm, immobile.
[2] Conjunctival telangiectasia: 0, none; 1, mild or fine vessels; 2, moderate; 3, prominent.
[3] Speech: 0, normal; 1, mild slurring; 2, dysarthria; 3, difficult to comprehend without time and effort.
[4] Eye movement: 0, normal; 1, full movement but difficult; 2, saccades deficient; 3, forward vision only.
[5] Choreoathetosis: 0, none; 1, occasional; 2, easily noticeable.
[6] Infections: 0, none; 1, possible; 2, definite increased number or one severe infection; 3, severe infection.
[7] Progress: N, normal; R, rapid; S, slow; L, late onset.
[8] No gait problem until age 13 years.
[9] Ambulatory at age 24 years.
[10] No gait problem at 11 years.

survival data is not available for any of the group 4 patients.

In addition to the clinical criteria of A-T, all the low-radiosensitivity patients showed the presence of translocations involving chromosomes 7 and 14 in their lymphocytes, as did the group of classical patients (Table 9.5). The translocations mostly involved inv(7) (p14;q35), t(7;14)(p14;q11) and t(7;14) (q35;q11). Overall the levels of translocations in the two groups is approximately the same and with the same variation between patients in the two groups. In the variant group, one individual (44,II–2) showed no translocations in 50 cells analysed at one sampling time but 3/50 at a subsequent time. Patient 52, II–3 showed only two in 100 cells with an inv(7) at one sampling time. Spontaneous translocation levels were 0.0325, 0.035, 0.13 and 0.0625 translocations per cell in groups 1–4 respectively and 0.067 in the classical patients. The levels of radiation-induced chromatid type damage at G_2 were 0.647, 0.252, 0.533 and 0.565 chromatid gaps/chromatid breaks/ interchanges per cell in groups 1–4 respectively and 2.11 in classical patients shown in Table 9.1. The later onset patients are interesting in showing both a lower level of spontaneously occurring translocations and a lower level of radiation-induced chromosome aberrations.

9.7 DISCUSSION

We address three main questions. First, is there truly a group of A-T patients in which the level of radiosensitivity is so low as to approach normal levels in some individuals; second, are there any clinical features in these patients which can be associated with the low radiosensitivity phenotype; third, is there any association between the level of radiosensitivity in A-T patients and their likelihood of developing malignant disease?

In answer to the first question, the evidence presented here suggests that there is indeed a low-radiosensitivity group of A-T patients and this evidence can be summarized as follows: (i) Measurements of low levels of chromosomal radiosensitivity at a single fixation time are repeatable between sample times from the same A-T individual; (ii) the reduced level of radiosensitivity is the same in both siblings of an affected pair; (iii) the reduced chromosomal radiosensitivity is seen across different fixation times, suggesting that the lower level is not an artefact of differential cell cycle times; and (iv) this reduced radiosensitivity can also be observed as an increased survival in fibroblasts from these patients, compared with classical patients, in colony-forming assays. The reverse correlation is however stronger; that is, in patients whose fibroblasts show increased survival, chromosomal radiosensitivity is less. This is because there appear to be some patients with fairly low chromosomal radiosensitivity but with typical low colony- forming ability following exposure of cells to gamma rays [29]. The approximate correlation of survival levels in fibroblasts with chromosomal radiosensitivity of lymphocytes seen in A-T patients is not likely to be universally applicable. In the case of A-T it is a reflection of the increased radiosensitivity of all the tissues in these patients. In other syndromes there may be evidence for a tissue-specific increased radiosensitivity as is seen in the mouse mutant 'wasted' [30]. Following these observations on low radiosensitivity the criteria now for describing a patient as a low-radiosensitivity variant include: the clinical features of A-T, a small increase in chromosomal radiosensitivity (with the mean being more than 2 SD lower than the mean for classical patients); an intermediate level of colony-forming ability of skin fibroblasts from the patient; and the presence of typical A-T chromosome translocations in lymphocytes

In answer to the second question there are no clinical features associated only with the

Table 9.5 Spontaneous chromosome rearrangements observed in cells from both classical A-T patients and low-radiosensitivity variants. Figures in columns refer to the numbers of cells in 50 analysed with the translocations indicated at the head of the column

Patient	inv(7)	7p;7q	7p;14q	7q;14q	14q;14q	inv(14)	Other
Classical patients							
45,II-1	2		3				comp[1]
47,II-1			1				
50,II-1	1[2]						
51,II-4	2	1	2	2			
54,II-2	4			1			
55,II-3	1[3]						
57,II-1			1				7p−comp
58,II-1				1			
58,II-2				1			7p−t(3;14)
60,II-3	2		2	1			
61,II-1	1			2			comp
Low-radiosensitivity variants							
1,II-1	1	1				1	t(6;15)
14,II-1	(i) 2						14q+
	(ii) 1					1	
	(iii) 1						
38,II-1	2						
38,II-2	1						del13q
40,II-1		1	1				
40,II-2	1		1				
44,II-2	(i)						
	(ii) 2		1				
46,II-1	4	1	2	1			
46,II-2	2		2			1	t(7;9)
52,II-3	2						
53,II-1							
53,II-2				1			
59,II-1	2			1			
62,II-2		1					
90,II-1	(i) 1		1	1			
	(ii) 3		1				t(3;14)
91,II-1	(i) 4	2		2			comp[4]
	(ii) 5		1				

Inv(7), inv(7) (p14;q35); 7;7, t(7;7) (p14;q35); 7p;14q, t(7;14) (p14;q11); 7q;14q, t(7;14) (q35;q11); 14;14, t(14;14) (q11;q32); inv(14), inv(14) (q11q32).
[1] Complex rearrangement, −7, −9, dic(7;9) (qter;p13), 17q−, +frag(17q)?
[2] 1/16 cells analysed with inv(7).
[3] 1/24 cells analysed with inv(7).
[4] Complex rearrangement, −5, −17, −19, +3 markers, +22 like.

147

low-radiosensitivity cellular phenotype. The low-radiosensitivity cellular phenotype in A-T patients can be associated with either a slow rate of progression of the condition (group 1) or a late onset of the features (group 2). These clinical phenotypes might result from less severe cellular defects caused by particular mutations. This being the case, the patients showing the least severe clinical features might also be the least radiosensitive and show the fewest spontaneous chromosome translocations. This appears to be the case, particularly for the late-onset (group 2) A-T patients. An advantage to this group also might be that they might be less likely to develop leukaemia/lymphoma.

It seems clear, however, that at both the clinical and the cellular level the group of A-T low-radiosensitivity variants may not be very homogeneous. It is intriguing that fibroblasts from the two brothers in family 46 showed a higher survival than the remainder of the low-radiosensitivity variants, possibly indicating heterogeneity in this group. These two brothers (together with patient 91,II-1) also showed the highest levels of spontaneously occurring chromosome translocations. It cannot always be the case, therefore, that a milder clinical phenotype is accompanied by both a smaller increase in radiosensitivity and fewer translocations. Indeed, in rare families there is evidence of a milder clinical presentation but with a high level of radiosensitivity [23].

Our more recent results show that a majority of patients (1, II-1; 14, II-1; 38, II-1; 38, II-2; 40, II-1; 40, II-2; 44, II-2; 52, II-3; 59, II-1 and 62, II-1), but not all, in the intermediate radiosensitivity group share a haplotype (designated the '418' haplotype) on one chromosome, inferring the presence of a common mutation [31]. The second chromosome does not show the presence of the same haplotype and in fact the haplotype of the second chromosome is different for each patient. This suggests a different mutation on the second chromosome in each of these patients. It is interesting that the brothers in families 46 and 53 and together with patients 90, II-1 and 91, II-1 do not share the '418' haplotype found in the majority of our low radiosensitivity patients, bearing in mind their different clinical and chromosomal features.

Some of the low-radiosensitivity patients described here may actually be at the low end of a normal distribution of radiosensitivity seen in classical patients, but this probably only applies to patients described as being in group 4. Patient 91, II-1 is such an example. Although showing a smaller increase in radiosensitivity, compared with classical patients, he has a higher level of spontaneously occurring translocations and has also developed T cell lymphoma.

Despite the low level of radiosensitivity of variants the clinical end-point appears to be the same in both low-radiosensitivity and classical A-T patients (an exception may be family 46). Insufficient comparative data are, however, available on clinical variation, in age of onset and rate of progress of the disease.

Thus, what is the relationship of the variable radiosensitivity in A-T to the basic gene defect and to tumour development? Some patients described here with lower radiosensitivity clearly show a slower rate of cerebellar degeneration. As has already been stated, classically high levels of radiosensitivity may also be associated with a less severe cerebellar ataxia in some instances [23]. Similarly, patients with severe, early-onset ataxia but intermediate levels of radiosensitivity have also been reported [32–33]. An important conclusion is that in different patients there are real variations in clinical presentation and in cellular radiosensitivity which are concordant within families.

All A-T patients described so far have some degree of increased radiosensitivity which can be measured at least by colony survival, suggesting that the mutation producing the clinical features of A-T is always associated with some increase in radiosensitivity, even though it is variable. Other features including telangiectasia, the degree of immunodeficiency and susceptibility to infections can be more variable between siblings. It seems likely therefore that the *A-T* mutation(s) has a more direct effect on cerebellar function, on cellular radiosensitivity and translocation production (recombination defect?) and that other clinical features may be more readily influenced by additional genes. The presence of this variety of phenotypes might suggest that there are many mutant alleles and/or many genes capable of modifying the phenotype.

The clinical and cellular variation may be explained in one of several ways: (i) there is more than one mutant allele at the same locus and each allele has a slightly different effect on the function of the gene. The phenotype of the individual may be different depending on whether the patient is a true homozygote or a compound heterozygote; (ii) the effect of a single gene mutation on the phenotype may be variable depending on the presence of modifying genes; and (iii) a combination of (i) and (ii). A phenotype resulting from the effects of compound heterozygosity and modifying genes seems quite plausible. The clinical and cellular variation in A-T is consistent with the existence of several or even many *A-T* mutations at a single locus.

There is no evidence that the lymphoid tumours in A-T patients are caused by an increased sensitivity of patients to the effects of ionizing radiation. Rather, the evidence points to the importance of particular chromosome translocations in the development of leukaemia/lymphoma as outlined above. The basic defect in A-T cells has the effect of producing both the abnormal chromosomal response to ionizing radiation and producing a high level of specific chromosome translocations. From the observations of levels of these

chromosome changes in different patients (? different mutations) these responses appear to be independently regulated, i.e. a low chromosomal radiosensitivity is not always associated with a low spontaneous level of translocations. The presence of a T cell lymphoma in patient 91, II-1, who showed a relatively low level of radiosensitivity but normal or higher levels of translocations, emphasizes both the independent regulation of these responses and possibly the importance of translocations in leukaemia/lymphoma development.

In patients with the Nijmegen breakage syndrome (NBS) [35–37] an increased radiosensitivity, measured chromosomally or by survival, is present in the absence of any cerebellar defect. These NBS patients have essentially the same cellular defects as A-T patients, including the spontaneous translocations seen in lymphocytes. A-T and NBS are, however, genetically distinct, as shown by the ability of cells to complement each other, in terms of radio-resistant DNA synthesis, and show quite distinct clinical phenotypes. There is evidence, however, strongly suggesting that the NBS locus is not linked to the *A-T* gene region on 11q22–23 [38, 39]. Cloning the gene for ataxia telangiectasia is an important step towards our understanding of the mechanism of radiosensitivity and the fundamental defect leading to the development of some forms of leukaemia. It will also answer the controversy about whether the *A-T* gene confers a moderate breast cancer risk in A-T heterozygotes which may account for a proportion of sporadic cases.

ACKNOWLEDGEMENTS

We thank the Cancer Research Campaign, the Medical Research Council, the Ataxia Telangiectasia Society of the U.K., the A-T Medical Research Trust (U.K.) and the Ataxia Telangiectasia Research and Support Trust for continued support.

REFERENCES

1. Swift, M., Morell, D., Cromartie, E., Chamberlin, A.R., Skolnick, M.H. and Bishop, D.H. (1986) The incidence and gene frequency of ataxia telangiectasia in the United States. *Am. J. Hum. Genet.*, **39**, 573–83.
2. Woods, C.G. Bundey, S.E. and Taylor, A.M.R. (1990) Unusual features in the inheritance of ataxia telangiectasia. *Hum. Genet.*, **84**, 555–62.
3. Sedgwick, R.P. and Boder, E. (1991) Ataxia telangiectasia, in *Handbook of Clinical Neurology. Hereditary Neuropathies and Spinocerebellar Atrophies*, vol 16, (ed. J.M.B.V. de Jong), Elsevier Science Publishers BV, Amsterdam, pp.347–423.
4. Cunliffe, P.N., Mann, J.R., Cameron, A.H., Roberts, K.D. and Ward, H.W.C. (1975) Radiosensitivity in ataxia telangiectasia. *Br. J. Radiol.*, **48**, 374–6.
5. Taylor, A.M.R., Harnden, D.G., Arlett, C.F. *et al.* (1975) Ataxia telangiectasia: a human mutation with abnormal radiation sensitivity. *Nature*, **258**, 427–9.
6. Spector, B.D., Filipovich, A.H., Perry, G.S. and Kersey, J.H. (1982) Epidemiology of cancer in ataxia telangiectasia, in *Ataxia Telangiectasia – a Cellular and Molecular Link between Cancer, Neuropathology and Immunodeficiency*, (eds B.A. Bridges and D.G. Harnden), John Wiley, Chichester, pp. 103–38.
7. Morrell, D., Cromartie, E. and Swift, M. (1986) Mortality and cancer incidence in 263 patients with ataxia telangiectasia. *J. Natl Cancer Inst.*, **77**, 89–92.
8. Taylor, A.M.R. (1992) Ataxia telangiectasia genes and predisposition to leukaemia, lymphoma and breast cancer. *Br. J. Cancer*, **66**, 5–9.
9. Taylor, A.M.R. and Butterworth, S.V. (1986) Clonal evolution of T cell chronic lymphocytic leukaemia in a patient with ataxia telangiectasia. *Int. J. Cancer*, **37**, 511–16.
10. Taylor, A.M.R., Lowe, P.A., Stacey, M. *et al.* (1992) Development of T cell leukaemia in an ataxia telangiectasia patient following clonal selection in t (X;14) containing cells. *Leukaemia*, **6**, 961–6.
11. Rabbitts, T.H.(1991) Translocations, master genes and differences between the origins of acute and chronic leukaemias. *Cell*, **67**, 641–4.
12. Meyn, M.S. (1993) High spontaneous intrachromosomal recombination rates in ataxia telangiectasia. *Science*, **260**, 1327–30.
13. Swift, M., Morell, D., Massey, R.B. and Chase, C.L. (1991) Incidence of cancer in 161 families affected by ataxia telangiectasia. *N. Engl. J. Med.*, **325**, 1831–5.
14. Pippard, E.C., Hall, A.J., Barker, D.J. P. and Bridges, B.A. (1988) Cancer in homozygotes and heterozygotes of ataxia telangiectasia and xeroderma pigmentosum in Britain. *Cancer Res.*, **48**, 2929–32.
15. Borresen, A.L., Andersen, T.I., Tretli, S., Heiberg, A. and Moller, P. (1990) Breast cancer and other cancers in Norwegian families with ataxia telangiectasia. *Genes, Chromosomes Cancer*, **2**, 339–40.
16. Wooster, R., Ford, D., Mangion, J. *et al.* (1993) Absence of linkage to the ataxia telangiectasia locus in familial breast cancer. *Hum. Genet.*, **92**, 91–4.
17. Boice, J.D. and Miller, R.W. (1992) Risk of breast cancer in ataxia telangiectasia. *N. Engl. J. Med.*, **326**, 1357–8
18. Gatti, R.A., Berkel, I., Boder, E., *et al.* (1988) Localisation of an ataxia telangiectasia gene to chromosome 11q22–23. *Nature*, **336**, 577–80.
19. McConville, C.M., Formstone, C.J., Hernandez, D., Thick, J. and Taylor, A.M.R. (1990) Fine mapping of the chromosome 11q22–23 region using PFGE, linkage and haplotype analysis; localisation of the gene for ataxia telangiectasia to a 5cM region flanked by NCAM/DRD2 and STMY/CJ52.75/ f2.22. *Nucleic Acids Res.*, **11**, 4335–43.
20. Lange, E., Borresen, A-L., Chen, X. *et al.* (1995) Localisation of an ataxia telangiectasia gene to a 500kb interval on chromosome 11q23.1: linkage analysis of 176 families by an international consortium. *Am. J. Hum. Genet.*, **57**, 112–19.
21. Savitsky, K., Bar-Shira, A., Gilad, S. *et al.* (1995) A single ataxia telangiectasia gene with a product similar to PI-3 kinase. *Science*, **268**, 1749–53.
22. Byrd, P.J., McConville, C.M., Cooper, P. *et al.* (1996) Mutations revealed by sequencing the

150

5' half of the gene for ataxia telangiectasia. *Hum. Mol. Genet.*, (in press).

23. Hernandez, D., McConville, C.M., Stacey, M. *et al.* (1993) A family showing no evidence of linkage between the ataxia telangiectasia gene and chromosome 11q22–23. *J. Med. Genet.*, **30**, 145–50.

24. Cox, R, Hosking, P. and Wilson J. (1978) Ataxia telangiectasia, evaluation of radiosensitivity in cultured skin fibroblasts as a diagnostic test. *Arch. Dis. Child.*, **53**, 386–90.

25. Ying, K.L. and Decoteau, W.E. (1981) Cytogenetic anomalies in a patient with ataxia, immune deficiency and high alpha-fetoprotein in the absence of telangiectasia. *Cancer Genet. Cytogenet.*, **4**, 311–17.

26. Woods, C.G. and Taylor, A.M.R. (1992) Ataxia telangiectasia in the British Isles. The clinical and laboratory features of 70 affected individuals. *Q. J. Med. (New Series)*, **82**, 169–79.

27. Jaspers, N.G.J., Gatti, R.A., Baan, C., Linssen, P.C.M.L. and Bootsma, D. (1988) Genetic complementation analysis of ataxia telangiectasia and Nijmegen Breakage Syndrome: a survey of 50 patients. *Cytogenet. Cell. Genet.*, **49**, 259–63.

28. Murnane, J.P. and Painter, R.B. (1982) Complementation of the defects in DNA synthesis in irradiated and unirradiated ataxia telangiectasia cells. *Proc. Natl Acad. Sci. USA*, **79**, 1960–3.

29. Taylor, A.M.R., Flude, E., Laher, B. *et al.* (1987) Variant forms of ataxia telangiectasia. *J. Med. Genet.*, **24**, 669–77.

30. Inoue, T., Aikawa, K., Tezuka, H., Kada, T. and Schulz, L.D. (1986) Effect of DNA damaging agents on isolated spleen cell and lung fibroblasts from the mouse mutant 'wasted', a putative model for ataxia telangiectasia. *Cancer Res.*, **46**, 3979–82.

31. Taylor, A.M.R., McConville, C.M., Rotman, G., Shiloh, Y. and Byrd, P.J. (1994) A haplotype common to intermediate radiosensitivity variants of ataxia telangiectasia in the U.K. *Int. J. Radiat. Biol.*, **66**, S35–S41.

32. Fiorilli, M., Antonelli, A., Russo, G., Crescendi, M., Carbonari, M. and Petrinelli, P. (1985) Variants of ataxia telangiectasia with low level radiosensitivity. *Hum. Genet.*, **70**, 274–7.

33. Chessa, L., Petrinelli, P., Antonelli, A. *et al.* (1992) Heterogeneity in ataxia telangiectasia: classical phenotype associated with intermediate cellular radiosensitivity. *Am. J. Med. Genet.*, **42**, 741–6.

34. Ziv, Y., Amiel, A., Jaspers, N.G.J., Berkel, A. I. and Shiloh, Y. (1989) Ataxia telangiectasia: a variant with altered *in vitro* phenotype of fibroblast cells. *Mutation Res.*, **210**, 211–19.

35. Weemaes, C.M.R., Hustinx, J.W.J., Scheres, J.M.J.G., van Munster, P.J.J., Bakkeren, J.A.J.M. and Taalman, R.D.F.M. (1981) A new chromosomal instability disorder. The Nijmegen breakage syndrome. *Acta Paed. Scand.*, **70**, 557–64.

36. Jaspers, N.G.J., Taalman, R.D.F.M. and Baan, C. (1988) Patients with an inherited syndrome characterised by immunodeficiency, microcephaly and chromosomal instability: genetic relationship to ataxia telangiectasia. *Am. J. Hum. Genet.*, **42**, 66–73.

37. Taalman, R.D.F.M., Hustinx, T.W.J., Weemaes, C.M.R. *et al.* (1989) Further delineation of the Nijmegen Breakage Syndrome. *Am. J. Med. Genet.*, **32**, 425–31.

38. Green, A.J., Yates, J.R.W., Taylor, A.M.R. *et al.* (1995) Severe microcephaly with normal intellectual development: the Nijmegen Breakage Syndrome. *Arch. Dis. Childh.*, **73**, 431–4.

39. Stumm, M., Gatti, R.A., Reis, A. *et al.* (1995) The ataxia telangiectasia variant genes 1 and 2 are distinct from the ataxia telangiectasia gene on chromosome 11q22–23. *Am. J. Hum. Genet.*, **57**, 960–2.

151

Chapter 10

Fanconi's anaemia

CHRISTOPHER G. MATHEW

Fanconi's anaemia (FA) is an inherited disorder which is associated with a variety of congenital abnormalities, bone marrow failure, and a predisposition to leukaemia. A comprehensive review of clinical and scientific aspects of FA has been published [1], and several shorter and more recent reviews on clinical and molecular findings are available [2–5]. This review will focus on cancer predisposition in FA, and on progress in identifying the Fanconi anaemia genes, but we begin with a summary of clinical and genetic aspects of FA.

10.1 CLINICAL AND LABORATORY DIAGNOSIS OF FANCONI'S ANAEMIA

10.1.1 CLINICAL FEATURES

The most common congenital abnormalities seen include low birth weight and growth retardation, café au lait patches of skin hyperpigmentation, absent or hypoplastic thumbs, and renal abnormalities such as horseshoe kidney. However, a diverse spectrum of anomalies may exist in the same patient [6]. Bone marrow failure in FA is progressive, usually presenting clinically as a pancytopenia between the ages of 5 and 10 years. A subset of families with the haemato-

logical manifestations of FA but without developmental abnormalities were originally classified as having the Estren–Dameshek syndrome [7]. However, classical FA with congenital abnormalities was later detected in relatives of the original kindreds, so this is unlikely to be a separate syndrome [8].

The median survival of FA patients after the occurrence of haematological symptoms is 5 years, but a minority survive to their third decade. Conventional therapy for FA includes regular transfusion support and the administration of androgens and steroids to stimulate haematopoeisis. The response rate for reversal of the pancytopenia by androgen therapy is about 50% [1]. However, patients finally become resistant to this treatment, and there are side effects such as virilization and the development of hepatic tumours. Many patients eventually die from acute non-lymphoblastic leukaemia. Bone marrow transplantation (BMT) currently provides the most realistic prospect for a cure, especially if an HLA-matched donor can be found. Success rates for this have improved substantially with the introduction of a modified conditioning regimen which takes account of the increased sensitivity of FA patients to alkylating agents and irradiation [9].

Genetic Predisposition to Cancer. Edited by R.A. Eeles, B.A.J. Ponder, D.F. Easton and A. Horwich. Published in 1996 by Chapman & Hall, London.
0 412 56580 3

10.1.2 LABORATORY DIAGNOSIS

The wide spectrum of congenital anomalies seen in FA patients, often initially in the absence of haematological changes, complicates the clinical diagnosis of this condition. The observation that cells from many FA patients displayed an increase in spontaneous chromosomal instability [10] led to the classification of FA as a chromosome breakage disorder. Further work showed that FA cells were hypersensitive to the bifunctional alkylating agents mitomycin C (MMC) [11] and diepoxybutane (DEB) [12], and these agents are now used to provide a sensitive and specific laboratory test for both prenatal and postnatal diagnosis [13]. However, it is noteworthy that FA patients have been described whose lymphocytes are completely resistant to MMC but whose fibroblasts were clearly MMC-sensitive [14], and there are FA patients in whom only a proportion of lymphocytes show cross-link sensitivity [13, 14]. These findings imply that if a negative chromosome breakage result is obtained with one or other of these cross-linking agents in peripheral blood lymphocytes in the face of a highly suggestive clinical diagnosis, the test should be repeated with both MMC and DEB in a fibroblast culture from a skin biopsy. Positive and negative controls should also be analysed in the same experiment as the test sample to check the cross-linking activity of these chemicals.

10.2 GENETICS OF FANCONI'S ANAEMIA

FA is a rare disorder, and little information on its incidence and prevalence are available. The exception to this is the Afrikaner population of South Africa, in whom the birth incidence of FA is 1 in 26 000 [15]. This unusually high frequency has been attributed to a founder effect [15] in this population. Swift has estimated the minimum incidence of FA in New York State as 1 in 348 000 [16],

and the minimum prevalence of FA in South African Black children was estimated to be 1 in 476 000 [17]. Formal segregation analysis of FA has demonstrated simple autosomal recessive inheritance for this disorder [18, 19]. Genetic heterogeneity in FA has been investigated by complementation analysis. Lymphoblastoid cell-lines from different FA patients were fused together to create a panel of somatic cell hybrids which were then tested for sensitivity to MMC [20]. This, together with more recent work from Buchwald's laboratory [21] has identified at least four different complementation groups, called A,B,C and D. Since these four groups were identified from only seven FA cell-lines, genetic heterogeneity may be even more extensive.

In view of the uncertain estimates of incidence and prevalence of FA homozygotes, and of the extensive genetic heterogeneity, the heterozygote frequency of *FA* genes is unknown. As has been pointed out by Heim *et al.* [22], the heterozygote frequency for a heterogeneous disorder will be higher than that calculated from the incidence of homozygotes, since matings between heterozygotes for different complementation groups will not produce affected offspring. Thus, from a FA homozygote incidence of 1 in 348 000 we calculate a heterozygote frequency of 1 in 300, but if we assume four complementation groups of equal frequency, then the total heterozygote frequency is 1 in 148. The true frequency cannot be determined at present, since no accurate assay for FA heterozygotes is available [23].

10.3 CANCER PREDISPOSITION IN FANCONI'S ANAEMIA

10.3.1 CANCER IN HOMOZYGOTES

Acute leukaemia is reported as the cause of death in 5–20% of FA patients (reviewed in

[24]). In most cases the leukaemia is of the acute non-lymphocytic type (ANLL), but some cases of lymphoblastic leukaemia do occur. The mean time between the onset of pancytopenia and the development of leukaemia is 5 years. In a study of 222 FA cases in the International Fanconi anaemia registry, 19 patients (9%) had acute leukaemia or myelodysplastic disease [25]. The mean age at diagnosis was 14.8 years, and mean age at death 15.5 years, indicative of the very poor prognosis for leukaemic FA patients. The high incidence of ANLL in FA, and the potentially disastrous consequences of standard pre-BMT conditioning for FA patients, has led Gyger *et al.* [26] to suggest that chromosome breakage studies should be performed routinely as part of the BMT work-up for ANLL cases.

The causes of predisposition to leukaemia in FA are not well understood. The chromosomal instability in FA might lead to an increased frequency of the chromosomal translocations associated with the development of leukaemia. The hypersensitivity of FA cells to alkylating agents may also contribute. Auerbach and Allen [25], in noting the increased incidence of ANLL in cancer patients who have received chemotherapy with alkylating agents, have suggested that FA patients might be at increased risk of ANLL from exposure to low levels of such chemicals in their environment.

There is also some evidence for an increased incidence of squamous cell carcinoma and hepatic tumours in FA [24, 27]. The hepatic tumours may be a consequence of prolonged androgen therapy, but no published comparison of the incidence of these tumours in androgen-treated versus untreated FA cases is available.

10.3.2 CANCER IN HETEROZYGOTES

Since FA is a very rare disorder, its overall contribution to cancer incidence is small.

Swift *et al.* [28], however, suggested that FA heterozygotes had an increased susceptibility to malignancies. If this were so, then as many as 1% of all cancer deaths could occur in FA heterozygotes [16]. A further study of 25 families by the same group [28, 29] did not confirm the original findings, but indicated an excess of bladder, stomach and breast cancer in blood relatives of FA patients which was not statistically significant. The theoretical basis for such a predisposition is that heterozygotes may have a marginal increase in chromosomal instability and hypersensitivity to carcinogens, which increases their probability of acquiring oncogenic somatic mutations. This hypothesis is supported by some experimental evidence for increased chromosomal instability in heterozygotes in response to agents such as MMC, DEB and nitrogen mustard (reviewed in [22]). These differences are not, however, sufficiently pronounced to form the basis for a reliable diagnostic test of heterozygote status.

It is unlikely that this question will be resolved satisfactorily until much larger data sets of cancer incidence in obligate heterozygotes are analysed. This would only be possible by means of an international collaborative effort. It could also be addressed more effectively if a facile and reliable test for heterozygotes were available, but this will depend on the cloning of the genes for the major FA complementation groups (see pages 155–7).

10.4 WHAT IS THE BASIC DEFECT?

Research relating to the identification of the basic defect in FA has been thoroughly reviewed recently by Gordon-Smith and Rutherford [2] and Strathdee and Buchwald [5]. Despite the existence of a substantial literature, limited consensus and even less understanding of the primary causes of the phenotype are evident. What is clear is that FA cells are very sensitive to chemicals that cause cross-linking of DNA, but relatively insensitive to closely related chemicals that do not [11]. Thus, it is likely that FA cells are deficient in some part of the process by which the cell repairs DNA cross-links, but there is disagreement about their capability for incision of cross-links [2, 5]. Some of the variability in experimental findings may relate to the genetic heterogeneity in FA. The use of cell-lines from different complementation groups (which may have different defects) by the various investigators certainly has the potential for confusion [30], and there is also evidence that capacity for cross-link repair is passage-dependent [31].

Further clues to the nature of the FA defect stem from the work of Nordenson [32] who showed that addition of superoxide dismutase (SOD) or catalase to FA cells in culture reduced the frequency of chromosomal aberrations. The protective effect on FA cells of a variety of antioxidants has since been demonstrated by many investigators. The FA defect is unlikely to be in SOD itself, since SOD levels are normal in FA fibroblasts [33], and purified SOD from FA cells appears to be normal [34]. Joenje *et al.* [35] then found that chromosome breakage in FA cells increased with increasing oxygen tension, and proposed that the primary defect in FA was a failure to tolerate oxidative stress. The prolonged G_2 phase and frequent G_2 arrest seen in FA cell cultures is also reduced at low oxygen tension. These findings could be explained either by a reduced capacity to inactivate mutagenic oxygen derivatives such as free radicals, or by a failure to repair the genetic damage which they induce.

In summary, the underlying defect in FA has not been clearly defined in the way that it has been for some other chromosome fragility syndromes such as xeroderma pigmentosum or Bloom's syndrome.

10.5 IDENTIFICATION OF THE FA GENES

The key to a deeper understanding of the basic defect in FA is the cloning of the genes which are mutated in this condition, and a detailed study of the properties of the proteins which are made from them. There are two general methods by which this might be achieved. One is the positional cloning approach [36] in which the gene is first mapped by genetic linkage analysis using polymorphic DNA markers, and then cloned by a systematic search of the appropriate region for candidate genes. The other is functional complementation, in which DNA or RNA sequences from normal cells are inserted into FA cell-lines, and the gene is then isolated from cells which have become resistant to MMC or DEB.

10.5.1 POSITIONAL CLONING

There are several problems associated with this approach in FA. The rarity of the disorder, and the fact that many of the affected children die at a young age make it difficult to collect sufficient informative families with multiple affected siblings for a linkage study. Family members need to be tested for chromosome breakage not only to support the clinical diagnosis, but also to identify siblings who have FA but have not yet manifested any of the clinical symptoms. The major problem, however, is the genetic heterogeneity of FA, reflected in the existence of at least four different complementation groups [21]. If these different groups are specified by genes with different functions in the DNA repair pathway, it is very likely that they will be located in different regions of the genome. Thus if linkage analysis is carried out on families from a mixture of unknown complementation groups, it is unlikely to be successful.

Linkage studies in FA were initiated before

the extent of the heterogeneity was known. Mann *et al.* [37] obtained a LOD score of +3.04 at $\theta = 0.12$ at the locus D20S20 on chromosome 20q, but other markers from the region showed either no or only weak evidence of linkage. An admixture test produced significant evidence for genetic heterogeneity, and it was estimated that about 10% of the 34 FA families in the study were linked. One of the two kindreds in which a LOD score of over 2 was obtained was from complementation group A. We typed 14 FA families with nine markers from chromosome 20q, and found positive LOD scores for all markers tested, but no significant evidence for linkage [38; R.A. Gibson and C.G. Mathew, unpublished data]. We obtained a LOD score of +2.4 at $\theta = 0.0$ in a single family with a marker from the ADA locus at chromosome 20q12–q13.1, but this locus is more than 50 cM proximal to D20S20.

It is unlikely that the provisional assignment of a FA gene to chromosome 20q [37] will be confirmed or rejected until the linkage is tested on a panel of FA families of known complementation group. The starting point for this study should be group A families, since one family with a LOD score of over 2 is from group A. If sufficient families of a particular group can be sampled, it will be possible to map the FA gene for that group by linkage analysis using the extensive set of highly polymorphic markers which are now available from all regions of the genome.

10.5.2 FUNCTIONAL COMPLEMENTATION

In this method, nucleic acid sequences from normal cells are introduced into FA cell-lines either as genomic DNA, mRNA or as a complementary DNA (cDNA) library cloned into an expression vector. The major difficulties associated with this approach are ensuring that the full coding sequence of the relevant gene is likely to be inserted, the fact that human cells are refractory to stable transfer of DNA, and the significant frequency of reversion in the transfectants.

The method most commonly used has been transfection of FA cell-lines with genomic DNA from normal rodent cells [39, 40]. Although these experiments showed that at least partial complementation of the FA defect could be achieved, they have yet to result in the isolation of a FA gene. Since human cells incorporate DNA of 50 kb or less [41], this procedure will only work if the target FA gene is of average size. A variant of this method is transfection of the Chinese hamster mutant cell-line V-H4, which is homologous to FA complementation group A [42] with human DNA. This has the advantage that rodent cells can incorporate larger DNA fragments than human cells, and take up more DNA [5].

Digweed *et al.* [43] have isolated an mRNA fraction that partially restores DNA synthesis in FA(A) cells by microinjection. Construction of cDNA libraries from a mRNA fraction enriched for the FA gene followed by transfection with the enriched library would have a greater chance of success, but only if the fraction fully corrected the FA phenotype.

The only successful approach to functional complementation of the FA defect to date has been that developed by Buchwald's laboratory, which led to the cloning of the Fanconi anaemia group C gene [44]. A cDNA library from normal cells was constructed in an Epstein–Barr virus-based expression shuttle vector, and transfected into the FA(C) cell-line. After antibiotic selection of cells that had taken up plasmid, cells were then exposed to MMC and finally DEB. Resistant clones of cells were shown to contain cDNAs that fully corrected the defect in FA(C) cells, but not in cells from the other complementation groups. The FA(C) cell-line was also found to have a mutation in the coding sequence of the cDNA, which was later shown to abolish its complementing activity [45]. This powerful approach enhances the efficiency with which sequences are transfected into the FA cells, and removes the need to reclone the complementing cDNA since the plasmid conferring resistance can be recovered by shuttling it back into *Escherichia coli*. However, it must be said that the cloning of the FA group C gene (*FAC*) was announced over 2 years ago, and at the time of writing no further FA genes have been identified. It may be that further technical developments will be required in order to clone the other FA genes by functional complementation.

Finally, a promising approach involving the *Drosophila* mutant *mus308* has been pursued by the late Dr Jim Boyd. The phenotype of this mutant includes hypersensitivity to cross-linking agents such as nitrogen mustard, but not to monofunctional agents, increased chromosomal breakage in larval neuroblasts, and an altered wing position with reduced flight capacity [46]. The similarity of the *mus308* phenotype with Fanconi anaemia suggests that it may provide a genetic model for FA, and possibly a further means of cloning at least one of the human FA genes. The *mus308* locus has been genetically mapped [46], and cloning of the gene is in progress.

10.6 THE FA GROUP C (*FAC*) GENE

10.6.1 THE *FAC* cDNA AND PROTEIN

The *FAC* cDNA has been cloned in its entirety, and its nucleotide sequence determined [44] (see also [47, 48] for corrections). The cDNA is 4569 base pairs (bp) in length, and has an open reading frame of 1677 bp. This encodes a predicted protein of 558 amino acid residues, with a molecular weight of 63 kDa. Alternatively spliced forms of the cDNA have been identified. Two different 5′ untranslated regions were detected which converge 77 bp upstream of the initiation codon [44]. There is also heterogeneity in the

end-point of the cDNA in the 3′ untranslated region, which generates cDNAs with lengths of 2.3, 3.2 and 4.6 kb [44]. An alternatively spliced cDNA which lacked exon 13 (see below) was also observed upon amplification of FAC cDNA from lymphocytes [49]. The functional significance of these alternative cDNAs remains to be established. The gene is ubiquitously expressed in both regenerating and non-replicating tissues [44].

When a new gene is isolated, a comparison of its predicted protein sequence with other sequences in the database often reveals homologies of amino acid sequence which provide clues to the function of the new gene. No such homologies were detected with the *FAC* gene product [44]. Its only notable feature is a preponderance of hydrophobic amino acid residues. *FAC* is therefore a completely novel gene, and an understanding of its function will only emerge from a detailed study of the properties of its encoded protein.

10.6.2 *FAC* GENOMIC STRUCTURE

Since the coding sequence of most eukaryotic genes is divided into a number of exons, it is generally not possible to investigate all classes of mutations in the gene without knowledge of its genomic structure. In particular, exon boundaries and the sequences of part of the adjacent introns need to be defined in order to characterize mutations which involve aberrant splicing. This information is also needed in order to amplify the exons of the gene from genomic DNA samples by polymerase chain reaction (PCR) [50]. The genomic structure of genes can now be determined using an efficient PCR-based method known as vectorette PCR [51]. This method was used to show that the coding region of the *FAC* gene was composed of 14 exons, ranging in size from 53–204 bp [48]. Sequencing of the introns at the exon boundaries revealed that all donor and acceptor splice sites fitted well with consensus sequences for these regions in other eukaryotic genes, and these sequences were used to design PCR reactions to amplify all 14 exons from genomic DNA [48]. This is particularly important in the context of FA, since genomic DNA is often the only sample available from the index patient. Further interruptions of the cDNA which occur in the 5′ untranslated region of the gene are being characterized (A. Savoia and M. Buchwald, unpublished data).

10.6.3 PHYSICAL AND GENETIC MAPPING OF *FAC*

The *FAC* gene has been localized to chromosome 9q22.3 by *in situ* hybridization [5]. Thus, if the FA locus detected on chromosome 20q by linkage analysis [37] is confirmed, it must contain a FA gene or genes from other complementation groups.

The location of *FAC* on the human genetic linkage map was made possible by the detection of a restriction fragment length polymorphism (RFLP) within *FAC* [52]. Typing of this RFLP in the international set of reference families in the CEPH collaboration [53], allowed us to localize *FAC* within a 7 cM interval on chromosome 9q between the loci D9S134 and D9S176 (R.A. Gibson *et al.* submitted for publication). The most likely order of markers in this region is D9S134–D9S196/D9S197–FAC–D9S176. This region of the genome seems to be particularly well endowed with genes involved in DNA repair and cancer, since it also contains the genes for xeroderma pigmentosum group A, Gorlin's syndrome, and multiple self-healing squamous epitheliomata.

The location of *FAC* between three highly informative microsatellite polymorphisms [54] allowed us to address the question of the proportion of FA families that might be linked to *FAC*. Typing of these markers in a panel of 36 FA families showed that only about 8% of families were likely to be linked

to this locus (R.A. Gibson *et al.* submitted for publication). This figure agrees well with our estimates based on mutation analysis (see below).

10.6.4 MUTATION ANALYSIS OF *FAC*

The original report of the cloning of the *FAC* gene [44] described two mutations in FA cell-lines. The FA(C) cell-line was heterozygous for a missense mutation which changed a leucine to a proline at amino acid residue 554 (L554P). Since no other mutation was detected in the cDNA, it was suggested that the mutation in the other allele resulted in a lack of detectable *FAC* mRNA. Subsequently, site-directed mutagenesis of the *FAC* cDNA confirmed that the L554P mutation abolished the function of the FAC protein [45]. The other mutation, which removed a single nucleotide at cDNA position 322 and which would produce a truncated peptide of 44 residues, was observed in two FA cell-lines of unknown complementation group.

A Scottish FA patient was found to be homozygous for a nonsense mutation in exon 6 (R185X) which would result in premature termination of translation of the FAC protein [49]. An interesting feature of this mutation is that it was associated with skipping of exon 6 from a proportion of *FAC* transcripts [48]. Loss of exon 6 generates an in-frame transcript [48], which might produce a partially functional FAC protein. This hypothesis is testable using the functional complementation assay of Strathdee *et al.* [21]. A mutation in the *FAC* gene was detected by Whitney *et al.* [55] in Ashkenazi Jewish FA patients. This altered a splice site in intron 4, leading to transcripts which lacked exon 4. Subsequent analysis of further Jewish FA patients revealed that this is the most common mutation in this population group [55, 56].

The *FAC* mutations detected thus far are summarized in Table 10.1. It is important to

Table 10.1 Sequence changes in the *FAC* gene

Change	Exon	No. of families	Status[1]	Reference
Q13X	1	3	M	[56, 58]
ΔG322	1	10	M	[44]
S26F	1	4	P	[56], Gibson et al.[2]
G139E	4	5	P	[55]
IVS4+4A>T	14	13	M	[55]
R185X	6	3	M	[49]
L190F	6	1	P	Gibson et al.[2]
D195V	6	1	?	[56]
R548X	14	1	M	[58]
L554P	14	1	M	[44]

[1] M, disease-causing mutation; P, polymorphism; ?, status unknown.

[2] R.A. Gibson et al., manuscript in preparation.

note that not all missense mutations would give rise to the FA phenotype. Thus Whitney et al. [55] reported a G139E mutation in a patient from complementation group A, and this mutation was subsequently shown not to segregate with the FA phenotype in a family with multiply affected siblings [56]. This is also true for the S26F mutation [56] (see also R.A. Gibson et al. in preparation), which is conserved in the mouse *Fac* gene [57]. Thus missense mutations which cause non-conservative amino acid substitutions and which are evolutionarily conserved may have nothing to do with the FA phenotype in affected families. The consequences of mis-classification of a FA family as group C are potentially severe, since the mutations might be used to provide the family with prenatal diagnosis, and they might be encouraged to believe that they are future candidates for gene therapy (see pages 160–1).

What proportion of FA patients are from group C? Mutation analysis of the *FAC* gene is beginning to provide an answer which the very labour-intensive method of comple-mentation analysis could not. Whitney et al.

[55] and our group [49] (also R.A. Gibson et al., in preparation) have screened the full coding sequence of the *FAC* gene by chemical cleavage analysis, and detected disease-causing mutations in three of 17 and two of 26 FA patients respectively, giving a total of 5/43 or 11.6% group C patients. Verlander et al. [56] have screened genomic DNA from 174 patients by single-stranded conformational polymorphism analysis, and observed muta-tions in 25 families (14.4%). The detection rate in the current North American samples may turn out to be relatively high because of a substantial number of Jewish patients with the common splice site mutation in intron 4. A group C frequency of 10% in an unselected FA patient population is a reasonable esti-mate at this stage.

The number of FA patients with specific *FAC* mutations identified thus far is too limited to allow correlations of genotype with clinical phenotype, except for the common IVS4+4A>T mutation, which appears to be associated with a severe form of the disease [56]. In cases where the *FAC* mutation is clearly sufficient to cause FA, the information can be used to provide prenatal diagnosis for subsequent pregnancies in the family. DNA analysis provides a rapid and qualitative alternative to prenatal diagnosis based on the analysis of chromosome breakage. We have confirmed a cytogenetic prenatal diagnosis of FA by detection of two nonsense mutations in fetal tissue [58], and recently performed a rapid DNA-based prenatal diagnosis which was subsequently confirmed by cytogenetic analysis [R.A. Gibson and C.G. Mathew, unpublished data].

10.6.5 THE MURINE FA GROUP C GENE, *Fac*

An important research goal is to develop a mouse model of FA. This would enable a variety of strategies for treatment to be evaluated, including gene replacement therapy. It would also permit a detailed study of the development of the FA phenotype in an experimental system. As a first step towards this goal, Wevrick *et al.* [57] have cloned the mouse homologue of the human *FAC* gene, termed *Fac*. The credentials of this gene as the mouse homologue were demonstrated convincingly by the fact that insertion of Fac into the human FA(C) cell-line restored cellular sensitivity to cross-linking agents to normal levels. Sequence analysis of *Fac* revealed a surprisingly modest degree of homology between the mouse and human genes. Although the mouse gene also encodes a protein of 558 amino acid residues, it is only 67% identical to the human amino acid sequence, with 79% similarity if conservative changes are disregarded. It is remarkable that the Fac protein fully complements the function of the human gene at this degree of homology, and this underscores the point that non-conservative missense mutations may not inactivate the human gene.

An interesting feature of the *Fac* gene is that one of the cloned cDNAs contained an additional 99 bp of coding sequence, and would therefore produce a protein of 591 amino acids [57]. This insertion is at the position of the exon 13/14 boundary in the human gene, and probably represents an alternatively spliced exon. This location is interesting in view of the alternative splicing of exon 13 in the human *FAC* gene [49], and suggests that this region of the gene may have tissue or developmental-specific functions. The *Fac* gene has been mapped to mouse chromosome 13, and its rat homologue to rat chromosome 17 [59]. An anaemic mouse mutant, known as flexed-tail, maps to the same chromosomal region, but no differences in size or quantity of *Fac* mRNA have been detected in its RNA [59].

RNA–PCR analysis of the tissue distribution of the murine *Fac* gene showed that it was widely expressed, and *in situ* hybridiza-

tion revealed a uniform pattern of expression in both adult and early embryonic tissue [57]. Higher levels of expression were noted in the bones of 14 to 16-day-old embryos, but the significance of this finding is not yet clear.

10.7 THE FUTURE

It is clear that all FA patients should be screened for group C mutations wherever the resources for this work exist. The screening may reveal functionally important domains in the FAC protein which will shed light on its function. The information could also be used to provide a rapid and accurate molecular prenatal diagnostic test for group C families. It will also identify a group of patients for whom gene replacement therapy might become a therapeutic option. FA is an obvious candidate for gene therapy, given the fact that the primary effect of the disorder is on the bone marrow, and that FA cells which have taken up the normal gene will be at a growth advantage over those which have not. Work is in progress to identify suitable vectors to deliver the normal *FAC* gene to FA cells at a workable efficiency. The development of a mouse model for FA by targeted disruption of the *Fac* gene would be an important breakthrough. This would allow treatment protocols to be tested, and would further our understanding of the function of the FAC protein.

The FA group A gene has recently been localized to chromosome 16q24.3 by genetic linkage analysis [60]. Interestingly, strong evidence of allelic association was found with the marker D16S303 in Afrikaner families, indicating that a founder *FACA* mutation is responsible for the high incidence of the disease in this population. The FA group D gene has also now been localized to chromosome 3p by microcell mediated chromosome transfer. The identification of these FA genes and the others which remain to be mapped is clearly a major research priority at this time.

ACKNOWLEDGEMENTS

Fanconi Anaemia Research in the author's laboratory is supported by the Medical Research Council (United Kingdom) and The Generation Trust. We are also grateful to members of Fanconi Anaemia Breakthrough, UK, for their support and cooperation.

REFERENCES

1. Schroeder-Kurth, T.M., Auerbach, A.D. and Obe, G. (eds) (1989) *Fanconi Anaemia. Clinical, Cytogenetic and Experimental Aspects*, Springer-Verlag, Berlin.
2. Gordon-Smith, E.C. and Rutherford, T.R. (1991) Fanconi anemia: constitutional aplastic anemia. *Semin. Hematol.*, **28** (2), 104–12.
3. Alter, B.P. (1992) Fanconi anemia: current concepts. *Am. J. Pediatr. Hematol. Oncol.*, **14** (2), 170–6.
4. Chaganti, R.S.K. and Houldsworth, J. (1991) Fanconi anemia: a pleotropic mutation with multiple cellular and developmental abnormalities. *Ann. Genet.*, **34** (3–4), 206–11.
5. Strathdee, C.A. and Buchwald, M. (1992) Molecular and cellular biology of Fanconi anemia. *Am. J. Pediatr. Hematol. Oncol.*, **14** (2), 177–85.
6. Porteous, M.E.M., Cross, I. and Burn, J. (1992) VACTERL with hydrocephalus: one end of the Fanconi anemia spectrum of anomalies? *Am. J. Med. Genet.*, **43**, 1032–4.
7. Estren, S. and Dameshek, W. (1947) Familial hypoplastic anemia of childhood: report of eight cases in two families with beneficial effects of splenectomy in one case. *Am. J. Dis. Child.*, **73**, 671–87.
8. Glanz, A. and Fraser, F.C. (1982) Spectrum of anomalies in Fanconi's anaemia. *J. Med. Genet.*, **19**, 412–16.
9. Gluckman, E., Devergie, A. and Dutreix, J. (1989) Bone marrow transplantation for Fanconi anemia, in *Fanconi Anemia. Clinical, Cytogenetic and Experimental Aspects*, (eds T.M. Schroeder-Kurth, A.D. Auerbach and G. Obe), Springer-Verlag, Berlin, pp. 60–8.
10. Schroeder, T.M., Anschutz, F. and Knopp, A. (1964) Spontane chromosomenabberrationen bei familiarer panmyelopathie. *Hum. Genet.*, **1**, 194–6.
11. Sasaki, M.S. and Tonomura, A. (1973) A high susceptibility of Fanconi's anemia to chromosome breakage by DNA cross-linking agents. *Cancer Res.*, **33**, 1829–33.
12. Auerbach, A.D. and Wolman, S.R. (1976) Susceptibility of Fanconi anaemia fibroblasts to chromosome damage by carcinogens. *Nature*, **261**, 494–6.
13. Auerbach, A.D., Ghosh, R., Pollio, P.C. and Zhang, M. (1989) Diepoxybutane test for prenatal and postnatal diagnosis of Fanconi anemia, in *Fanconi Anemia. Clinical, Cytogenetic and Experimental Aspects*, (eds T.M. Schroeder-Kurth, A.D. Auerbach and G. Obe), Springer-Verlag, Berlin, pp. 71–82.
14. Arwert, F. and Klee, M.L. (1989) Chromosomal breakage in response to cross-linking agents in the diagnosis of Fanconi anemia, in *Fanconi Anemia. Clinical, Cytogenetic and Experimental Aspects* (eds T.M. Schroeder-Kurth, A.D. Auerbach and G. Obe), Springer-Verlag, Berlin, pp. 83–92.
15. Rosendorff, J., Bernstein, R., Macdougall, L. and Jenkins, T. (1987) Fanconi anemia: another disease of unusually high prevalence in the Afrikaans population of South Africa. *Am. J. Med. Genet.*, **27**, 793–7.
16. Swift, M. (1971) Fanconi's anaemia in the genetics of neoplasia. *Nature*, **230**, 370–3.
17. Macdougall, L.G., Greeff, M.C., Rosendorff, J. and Bernstein, R. (1990) Fanconi anemia in Black African children. *Am. J. Med. Genet.*, **36**, 408–13.
18. Schroeder, T.M., Tilgen, D., Kruger, J. and Vogel, F. (1976) Formal genetics of Fanconi's anemia. *Hum. Genet.*, **32**, 257–88.
19. Rogatko, A. and Auerbach, A.D. (1988) Segregation analysis with uncertain ascertainment: application to Fanconi anemia. *Am. J. Hum. Genet.*, **42**, 889–97.
20. Duckworth-Rysiecki, G., Cornish, K., Clarke, C.A. and Buchwald, M. (1985) Identification of two complementation groups in Fanconi anemia. *Somatic Cell. Mol. Genet.*, **11**(1), 35–41.
21. Strathdee, C.A., Duncan, A.M.V. and Buchwald, M. (1992) Evidence for at least four Fanconi anaemia genes including *FACC* on chromosome 9. *Nature Genet.*, **1**, 196–8.

22. Heim, R.A., Lench, N.J. and Swift, M. (1992) Heterozygous manifestations in four autosomal recessive human cancer-prone syndromes: ataxia telangiectasia, xeroderma pigmentosum, Fanconi anemia, and Bloom Syndrome. *Mutat. Res.*, **284**, 25–36.

23. Dallapiccola, B. and Porfirio, B. (1989) Chromosomal studies in Fanconi anemia heterozygotes, in *Fanconi Anemia. Clinical, Cytogenetic and Experimental Aspects*, (eds T.M. Schroeder-Kurth, A.D. Auerbach and G. Obe), Springer-Verlag, Berlin, pp. 145–58.

24. Ebell, W., Friedrick, W. and Kohne, E. (1989) Therapeutic Aspects of Fanconi anemia, in *Fanconi Anaemia. Clinical. Cytogenetic and Experimental Aspects*, (eds T.M. Schroeder-Kurth, A.D. Auerbach, and G. Obe), Springer-Verlag, Berlin, pp. 47–59.

25. Auerbach, A.D. and Allen, R.G. (1991) Leukemia and preleukemia in Fanconi anemia patients. A review of the literature and report of the International Fanconi Anemia Registry. *Cancer Genet. Cytogenet.*, **51**, 1–12.

26. Gyger, M., Perreault, C., Belanger, R. *et al.* (1989) Unsuspected Fanconi's anemia and bone marrow transplantation in cases of acute myelomonocytic leukaemia. *N. Engl. J. Med.*, **321**(2), 120–1.

27. Okuyama, S. and Mishina, H. (1987) Fanconi's anaemia as Nature's evolutionary experiment on carcinogenesis. *Exp. Med.*, **153**, 87–102.

28. Swift, M., Caldwell, R.J. and Chase, C. (1980) Reassessment of cancer predisposition of Fanconi anemia heterozygotes. *J. Natl Cancer Inst.*, **65**(5), 863–7.

29. Swift, M., Kupper, L.L. and Chase C.L. (1990) Effective testing of gene-disease associations. *Am. J. Hum. Genet.*, **47**, 266–74.

30. Moustacchi, E., Papadopoulo, D., Diatloff-Zito, C. *et al.* (1987) Two complementation groups of Fanconi's anemia differ in their phenotypic response to DNA-crosslinking treatment. *Hum. Genet.*, **75**, 45–7.

31. Sognier, M.A. and Hittelman, W.D. (1983) Loss of repairability of DNA interstrand crosslinks in Fanconi's anemia cells with culture age. *Mutat. Res.*, **108**, 383–93.

32. Nordenson, I. (1977) Effect of superoxide dismutase and catalase on spontaneously occurring chromosome breaks in patient with Fanconi's anaemia. *Hereditas*, **86**, 147–50.

33. Abeliovich, D. and Cohen, M.M. (1978) Normal activity of nucleoside phosphorylase, superoxide dismutase and catalase in skin fibroblast cultures from Fanconi anaemia patients. *Isr. J. Med. Sci.*, **14**, 284–7.

34. Joenje, H. and Gille, J.J.P. (1989) Oxygen metabolism and chromosomal breakage in Fanconi anemia, in *Fanconi Anaemia. Clinical, Cytogenetic and Experimental Aspects*, (eds T.M. Schroeder-Kurth, A.D. Auerbach and G. Obe), Springer-Verlag, Berlin, pp. 174–82.

35. Joenje, H., Arwert, F., Eriksson, A.W. *et al.* (1981) Oxygen-dependence of chromosomal aberrations in Fanconi's anaemia. *Nature*, **290**, 142–3.

36. Wicking, C. and Williamson, R. (1991) From linked marker to gene. *Trends Genet.*, **7**, (9), 288–93.

37. Mann, W.R., Venkatraj, V.S., Allen, R.G. *et al.* (1991) Fanconi anemia: evidence for linkage heterogeneity on chromosome 20q. *Genomics*, **9**, 329–37.

38 Lee, R., Jansen, S., Milner, R. *et al.* (1991) Genetic heterogeneity in Fanconi anaemia? *J. Med. Genet.*, **29** (4), 273.

39. Diatloff-Zito, C., Rosselli, F., Heddle, J. and Moustacchi, E. (1990) Partial complementation of the Fanconi anaemia defect upon transfection by heterologous DNA. *Hum. Genet.*, **86**, 151–61.

40. Shaham, M., Adler, B., Ganguly, S. and Chaganti, R.S.K. (1987) Transfection of normal human and Chinese hamster DNA corrects diepoxybutane-induced chromosomal hypersensitivity of Fanconi anemia fibroblasts. *Proc. Natl Acad. Sci. USA*, **84**, 5853–7.

41. Buchwald, M., Clarke, C., Ng, J. *et al.* (1989) Complementation and gene transfer studies in Fanconi anemia, in *Fanconi Anemia. Clinical. Cytogenetic and Experimental Aspects*, (eds T.M. Schroeder-Kurth, A.D. Auerbach and G. Obe), Springer-Verlag, Berlin, pp. 226–35.

42. Arwert, F., Rooimans, M.A., Westerveld, A. *et al.* (1991) The Chinese hamster cell mutant V-H4 is homologous to Fanconi anemia (complementation group A). *Cytogenet. Cell. Genet.*, **56**, 23–26.

43. Digweed, M., Zakrzewski-Lüdcke, S. and

Sperling, K. (1989) Complementation studies in Fanconi anemia using cell fusion and microinjection of mRNA, in *Fanconi Anemia. Clinical, Cytogenetic and Experimental Aspects*, (eds T.M. Schroeder-Kurth, A.D. Auerbach and G. Obe), Springer-Verlag, Berlin, pp. 236–54.

44. Strathdee, C.A., Gavish, H., Shannon, W.R. and Buchwald, M. (1992) Cloning of cDNAs for Fanconi's anaemia by functional complementation. *Nature*, **356**, 763–7.

45. Gavish, H., Dos Santos, C.C. and Buchwald, M. (1993) A Leu$_{554}$-to-Pro substitution completely abolishes the functional complementing activity of the Fanconi anemia (FACC) protein. *Hum. Molec. Genet.*, **2** (2), 123–6.

46. Leonhardt, E.A., Henderson, D.S., Rinehart, J.E. and Boyd, J.B. (1993) Characterization of the *mus308* gene in *Drosophila melanogaster*. *Genetics*, **133**, 87–96.

47. Strathdee, C.A., Gavish, H., Shannon, W.R. and Buchwald, M. (1992) Correction: cloning of cDNAs for Fanconi's anaemia by functional complementation. *Nature*, **358**, 434.

48. Gibson, R.A., Buchwald, M., Roberts, R.G. and Mathew, C.G. (1993) Characterisation of the exon structure of the Fanconi anaemia group C gene by vectorette PCR. *Hum. Molec. Genet.*, **2** (1), 35–8.

49. Gibson, R.A., Hajianpour, A.K., Murer-Orlando, M., Buchwald, M. and Mathew, C.G. (1993). A nonsense mutation and exon skipping in the Fanconi anaemia group C gene. *Hum. Molec. Genet.*, **2** (6), 797–9.

50. Saiki, R.K., Gelfand, D.H., Stoffel, S. *et al.* (1988) Primer-directed enzymatic amplification of DNA with a thermostable DNA polymerase. *Science*, **239**, 487–91.

51. Riley, J., Butler, R., Ogilvie, D. *et al.* (1990) A novel, rapid method for the isolation of terminal sequences from yeast artificial chromosome (YAC) clones. *Nucleic Acids Res.*, **18** (10), 2887–90.

52. Gibson, R.A., Savoia, A., Buchwald, M. and Mathew, C.G. (1993). EcoRI-RFLP in the Fanconi anaemia complementation group C gene (FACC). *Hum. Molec. Genet.*, **2** (9), 1509.

53. Dausset, J. (1990) The CEPH collaboration. *Genomics*, **6**, 575–7.

54. Weissenbach, J., Gyapay, G., Dib, C. *et al.* (1992) A second-generation linkage map of the human genome. *Nature*, **359**, 794–801.

55. Whitney, M.A., Saito, H., Jakobs, P.M. *et al.* (1993) A common mutation in the FACC gene causes Fanconi anaemia in Ashkenazi Jews. *Nature Genet.*, **4**, 202–5.

56. Verlander, P.C., Lin, J.D., Udono, M.U. *et al.* (1994) Mutation analysis of the Fanconi anemia gene FACC. *Am. J. Hum. Genet.*, **54**, 595–601.

57. Wevrick, R., Clarke, C.A. and Buchwald, M. (1993) Cloning and analysis of the murine Fanconi anemia group C cDNA. *Hum. Molec. Genet.*, **2**, 655–62.

58. Murer-Orlando, M., Llerena J.C., Jr, Birjandi, F., Gibson, R.A. and Mathew, C.G. (1993) FACC gene mutations and early prenatal diagnosis of Fanconi's anaemia. *Lancet*, **342**, 686.

59. Wevrick, R., Barker, J.E. and Nadeau, J.H. (1993) Mapping of the murine and rat FACC genes and assessment of flexed-tail as a candidate mouse homolog of Fanconi anemia group C. *Mammalian Genome*, **4** (8), 440–4.

60. Pronk, J.C., Gibson, R.A., Savoia, A. *et al.* (1995) Localisation of the Fanconi anaemia complementation group A gene to chromosome 16q24.3. *Nature Genetics*, **11**, 338–40.

61. Whitney, M., Thayer, M., Reifsteck, C. *et al.* (1995) Microcell mediated chromosome transfer maps the Fanconi anaemia group D gene to chromosome 3p. *Nature Genetics*, **11**, 341–3.

Chapter 11

The Gorlin (nevoid basal cell carcinoma) syndrome

PETER A. FARNDON

11.1 THE GORLIN SYNDROME

11.1.1 INTRODUCTION

Patients with the Gorlin syndrome (McKusick number 109400, gene symbol NBCCS) may present to any medical or surgical speciality as there are over 100 recognized features. The most frequent and important components of the syndrome are nevoid basal cell carcinomas and odontogenic keratocysts. Nonprogressive skeletal anomalies are present in a high proportion of cases and are helpful diagnostically, as is the presence of ectopic calcification. Congenital malformations occur at an increased frequency.

The first reported cases appear to be those of Jarisch and White in 1894, but mummies from early Egyptian times have been found with skeletal signs of the syndrome. The syndrome was delineated by Gorlin and Goltz in 1960 [1] when they reported two patients and reviewed cases in the literature. Gorlin presented an extensive review of the syndrome in 1987 [2], combining information from a personal series of patients and a review of 216 papers.

The information in this chapter is taken from a review of the literature and the author's own observations in a series of over 100 patients.

11.1.2 NOMENCLATURE

The syndrome has been given many different names, reflecting the multiplicity of presenting signs and symptoms. The names include basal cell naevus syndrome, nevoid basal cell carcinoma syndrome, epitheliomatose multiple generalisee, fifth phakomatosis, hereditary cutaneomandibular polyoncosis, multiple basalioma syndrome and Gorlin syndrome.

The term basal cell naevus syndrome is inappropriate because histologically the naevi are basal cell carcinomas (BCCs), although not all behave aggressively. Throughout Europe the condition is known as Gorlin syndrome, reflecting Professor Robert Gorlin's contributions to the understanding of the condition. He has suggested that it be known as the nevoid basal cell carcinoma syndrome, although this too may not be the most appropriate name because 10% of adults do not develop BCCs. In addition, patients seem to prefer an eponymous title

Genetic Predisposition to Cancer. Edited by R.A. Eeles, B.A.J. Ponder, D.F. Easton and A. Horwich. Published in 1996 by Chapman & Hall, London.
0 412 56580 3

rather than one which contains the word 'carcinoma'.

11.1.3 PREVALENCE

The prevalence in a population-based study in North-West England was 1 in 55 600 [3]; this, however, is likely to be the minimum prevalence.

(a) Frequency among patients with one or more BCCs

Rahbari and Mehregan [4] reported a group of 59 children under the age of 19 with a histologically proven BCC. Ten had a BCC which had developed in a pre-existing naevus sebaceous. Of the others, 13 (26%) had features of the Gorlin syndrome. Two other children were developing a second BCC but they had no signs of the syndrome on X-ray or examination.

In 1904 cases with one or more BCCs, Summerly [5] found that 198 (10.4%) were under 45 years. Two unequivocal cases of the syndrome were found in 125 of these patients available for study – 1.9% of patients under 45. However, this may be an underestimate, because an additional 21 patients in this group had facial milia, two had cervical ribs and two had jaw cysts. A Russian study [6] found five cases among 122 patients with multiple and/or early-onset basal cell carcinomas.

(b) Frequency among patients with odontogenic keratocysts

In a series of 122 patients [7], 113 had single cysts, and nine (7%) had multiple cysts. Gorlin syndrome was diagnosed in three of nine patients who had more than one odontogenic keratocyst. The minimum estimate is therefore 2.5% of patients with one or more cysts.

It has been suggested that an isolated odontogenic keratocyst may represent the 'least complete' form of the syndrome. No family member at risk of the syndrome in the North-West England longitudinal study [3] is known to have an odontogenic keratocyst in the absence of other signs or symptoms. In addition, there appears to be no evidence that there is a familial tendency to develop odontogenic keratocysts in the absence of other features of the syndrome.

11.1.4 INHERITANCE, PENETRANCE AND VARIABILITY IN EXPRESSION

The syndrome is inherited as an autosomal dominant, with a one in two chance that a child of an affected parent will inherit the condition. Penetrance appears to be complete, but there is wide variability in expression both between and within families. The variability manifests itself not only in the presence or absence of a particular feature, but also in its severity.

11.1.5 NEW MUTATION RATE

Gorlin *et al.* [8] suggested a new mutation rate of 40% from a review of the literature. In the author's personal series, several patients were referred as isolated cases, but physical and X-ray examinations revealed that one of the parents also had the syndrome. Parents of apparently isolated cases should therefore be examined and investigated carefully, being mindful of the variation in expression. The condition appeared to be the result of a new mutation in 17% of the fully investigated families in the author's series.

As in some other dominant conditions, a paternal age effect was shown in a study of 12 sporadic cases [9] – the mean paternal age was 36.9 years (control population 29.9 years) and maternal age 31.7 (control 26.5).

11.2 FEATURES OF THE SYNDROME

The major features of the syndrome are shown in Table 11.1. The frequencies are

Table 11.1 Features of Gorlin syndrome

Feature	Frequency (%)
Multiple basal cell carcinomas	90
Odontogenic keratocysts of jaws	90
Calcified falx cerebri	>85
Characteristic face	70
Palmar and/or plantar pits	65
Rib anomalies (splayed, fused, partially missing, bifid, etc.)	60
Spina bifida occulta of cervical or thoracic vertebrae	60
Calcified diaphragma sellae (bridged sella, fused clinoids)	60–80
Hyperpneumatization of paranasal sinuses	60
Epidermoid cysts of skin	>50
Enlarged occipitofrontal circumference	>50
Mild ocular hypertelorism	>50
Calcification of tentorium cerebelli	40
Lumbarization of sacrum	40
Kyphoscoliosis or other vertebral anomalies	30–40
Pseudocystic lytic lesion of bones (hamartomas)	35
Facial milia	30
Calcified ovarian fibromas	24
Calcification of petroclinoid ligament	20
Short fourth metacarpals	20
Pectus excavatum or carinatum	15–49
Strabismus (exotropia)	14
Cataract, glaucoma, coloboma of iris, retina, optic nerve, medullated retinal nerve fibres	7
Grand mal seizures	6
Sprengel deformity of scapula	5–25
Cleft lip and/or palate	5.7
Medulloblastoma	5
Cardiac fibroma	2.5
Meningioma	1

Features with less than 5% frequency
  Lymphomesenteric cysts
  Inguinal hernia
  Fetal rhabdomyoma
  Marfanoid build
  Agenesis of corpus callosum
  Cyst of septum pellucidum
  Postaxial polydactyly – hands or feet
  Subcutaneous calcifications of skin
  Minor kidney malformations
  Hypogonadism in males
  Undescended testes
  Mental retardation

Features are arranged in descending order of approximate frequency, with figures given when available. Features where a more precise figure is unavailable are listed at the end of the table. In addition many other features have been reported, but it is unclear whether these are truly related to the syndrome, or have occurred in an affected patient by chance.

adapted from 53 patients reported by Professor Gorlin in his review, over 100 patients known to the author and information from the literature.

11.2.1 SKIN

(a) Milia

Small keratin-filled cysts (milia) are found on the face in 30%, most commonly in the infraorbital areas, but they can also occur on the forehead. Larger epidermoid cysts occur on the limbs and trunk in over 50% of cases. They are usually 1–2 cm in diameter, and are particularly common around the knee.

(b) Palmar/plantar pits

Some 65% of patients have small (1–2 mm) asymmetric pits, found more commonly on the palms than on the soles. In one case known to the author the pits have been found on the neck. The pits are shallow depressions, with the colour of the base being white, flesh-coloured or pale pink (Figure 11.1). Some patients report that they notice a small mound appearing on the skin which, when squeezed, results in the centre falling away leaving a typical pit. The pits are easier to see in patients who undertake manual labour, and may be better visualized if the patient's hands are soaked in warm water for about 10 minutes. Occasionally, pits are found on the sides of the fingers or toes, where they appear as bright red pinpricks. They appear to increase in number with age, being relatively uncommon in children (although when present in childhood are a strong diagnostic indicator). They may vary in number from only a few to greater than 100. Basal cell carcinomas have rarely arisen in the base of the pits.

The pits appear to be caused by premature desquamation of horny cells along the inter-cellular spaces, but they are not due to degeneration of the horny cells themselves. Light microscopy reveals a lack of keratinization of pit tissue and a proliferation of basaloid cells in irregular rete ridges [10].

(c) Café au lait patches

A few café au lait patches are commonly present, usually on the trunk, which may lead to consideration of a diagnosis of neurofibromatosis, especially in those patients with a large head circumference. Axillary freckling, however, is not found.

(d) Naevi and basal cell carcinomas

A patient may develop no naevi, a few, or many thousands. Histologically, the naevi are basal cell carcinomas (BCCs) from the time they first appear, but their behaviour differs from isolated BCCs.

The nevoid basal cell carcinomas (NBCCs) appear most commonly between puberty and about 40 years of age, although they can also occur in infancy and childhood. Some 10% of patients over the age of 40 do not develop a BCC.

NBCCs may arise in any area of the skin, affecting the face, neck and upper trunk in preference to the abdomen, lower trunk and extremities. The areas around the eyes, the nose, the malar regions and the upper lip are the most frequently affected sites on the face, leading to a widespread view in the literature that sun exposure is an important factor.

Patients report that NBCCs tend to appear multiply in clusters, often following a feeling of intense itching in a particular area of skin. NBCCs can also appear as isolated lesions. They can be flesh-coloured, reddish-brown or pearly, and the groups may resemble moles, skin tags, ordinary naevus cell naevi or haemangiomas. They may grow rapidly for a few days to a few weeks, but then most

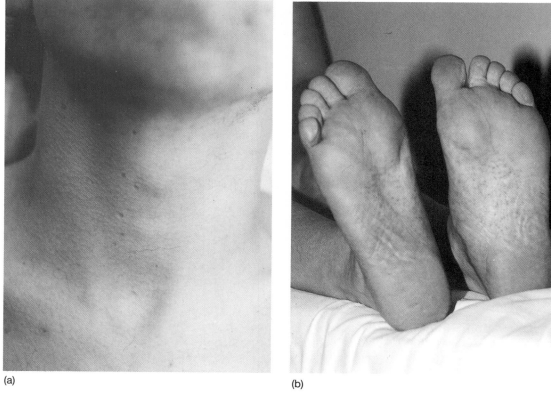

(a)

(b)

Fig. 11.1 Palmar/plantar pits. (a) The typical 'white' pits associated with the syndrome, most commonly found on the palms. As palmar pits can be difficult to photograph, shown here are typical pits on the neck of a 21-year-old man, although it is very unusual to develop the pits elsewhere than the palms and soles. (b) A large number of small pink pits of pin-prick size on the soles. These are found more often on the soles than the larger 'white' pits as shown in (a). The pink pits are also often found on the sides of fingers.

remain static. Usually only a few become aggressive, when they may be locally invasive and behave like ordinary BCCs. Evidence of aggressive transformation of an individual lesion includes, as expected, an increase in size, ulceration, bleeding, or crusting. It is rare for metastasis to occur. It is unusual to develop aggressive BCCs before puberty.

About one-third of patients have two or more types of BCCs, including superficial, multi-centric, solid, cystic, adenoid and lattice-like. NBCCs are more commonly asso-ciated with melanin pigmentation and foci of calcification than ordinary BCCs.

11.2.2 JAW CYSTS

Cysts of the jaws are a major feature of the syndrome. They are termed odontogenic keratocysts because a great deal of evidence suggests that their origin is the primordial odontogenic epithelium, and their linings keratinize.

Some odontogenic keratocysts appear on X-rays to be dentigerous cysts, that is, a cyst

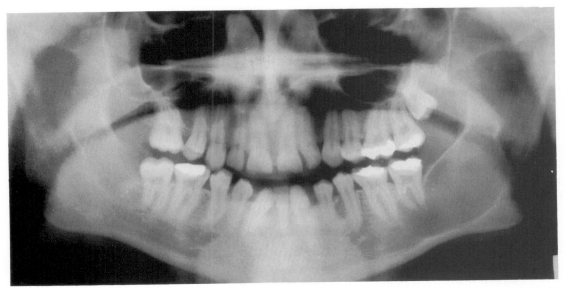

Fig. 11.2 Orthopantomogram of the jaws of a 16-year-old male showing a large cyst beginning in the posterior body of the left mandible, extending into the ramus.

which encloses the crown of an unerupted tooth, and is attached at its neck. However, the majority of these are not true dentigerous cysts when examined histologically – a layer of fibrous tissue separates the crown from the adjacent cyst cavity. A cyst may impede the eruption of a related tooth, or envelop an unerupted tooth to produce a dentigerous appearance.

The cysts may develop during the first decade of life, usually after about the seventh year, with a peak incidence in the second or third decade. This peak is about 10 years earlier than that associated with isolated odontogenic keratocysts. In one series [3], 82% of patients had developed a cyst by the age of 20, and only 10% of patients over the age of 40 had not developed a cyst.

(a) Site

The mandible is involved far more frequently (75%) than the maxilla (Figure 11.2). About one-half of odontogenic keratocysts occur at the angle of the mandible. The cysts also occur mainly in the canine to premolar area, in the mandibular retromolar–ramus area and in the region of the maxillary second molar. They may form in the mid-line of the mandible and maxilla, and may cross the mid-line. They may be relatively small, single, or multiple, but at diagnosis are more often large, bilateral, unilocular or multilocular, involving both jaws.

(b) Clinical presentation

Most cysts are diagnosed on X-ray examination in the absence of symptoms. Occasionally they become infected and cause pain or discharge, or cause swelling by expansion of the jaws. Patients are usually remarkably free of symptoms until the cysts have reached a large size, especially when the ascending ramus is involved because the cyst extends into the medullary cavity. The enlarging cyst may cause displacement or loosening of teeth. It is rare for a cyst to cause a patholog-

169

ical fracture but they can cause swelling by extending into the soft tissues after perforating the cortex.

(c)   Recurrences

The odontogenic keratocyst has a tendency to recur after surgical treatment, with reported rates as high as 62%. New cysts may form from satellite cysts associated with the original, or from the dental lamina. True recurrences may be the result of incomplete surgical eradication.

(d)   Pathology

The histological features are characteristic. The cysts are lined by a parakeratotic stratified squamous epithelium which is usually about 5–8 cell layers thick and without rete ridges. Rarely the form of keratinization is orthokeratotic. The basal layer is well-defined with regularly orientated palisaded cells. Satellite cysts, epithelial rests and proliferating dental lamina are sometimes seen in the cyst capsules.

Histological evidence has been presented [11] to suggest that cysts in the ascending ramus which have no relationship to a tooth follicle or dental lamina may arise from proliferation of the basal cells of the oral epithelium.

11.2.3   MUSCULOSKELETAL SYSTEM

Musculoskeletal features may be readily apparent on clinical examination, but X-ray investigation should always be undertaken when the syndrome is suspected.

(a)   Height

Patients tend to be very tall. Their heights are usually over the 97th centile, often in marked

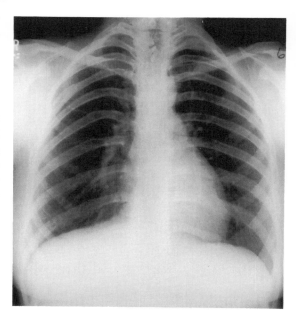

Fig. 11.3 Chest X-ray of a 25-year-old female, showing spina bifida occulta of T1 and T2, bifid right fourth and fifth ribs, and variation in thickness of the anterior ends of the ribs, particularly the right second rib.

contrast to unaffected siblings. Some patients exhibit a marfanoid build.

(b)   Shape and size of cranium

The calvarium is usually large, with frontal and biparietal bossing. The occiput is low and the interorbital distance increased (usually in proportion to the head circumference). Platybasia is frequent.

(c)   Spine and chest

Bifid, anteriorly splayed, fused, partially missing or hypoplastic ribs are found in 60% (Figure 11.3) and may give an unusual shape to the chest, including a characteristic downward sloping of the shoulders. The rib anomalies, together with kyphoscoliosis may cause pectus excavatum or carinatum in about 30–40% of patients.

Abnormalities of the cervical or thoracic vertebrae are helpful diagnostic signs, being found in about 60% of cases. Spina bifida occulta of the cervical vertebrae, or malformations at the occipitovertebral junction are common. In addition to lack of fusion of the cervical or upper thoracic vertebrae, fusion or lack of segmentation has been documented in about 40%. Sprengel deformity has been found in some surveys to be as common as 25%.

Bifid ribs, cervical ribs and synostosis of ribs occur in 6.25, 1.7 and 2.6 per 1000 respectively of the normal population [12].

(d) Other bone anomalies

Pre- or post-axial polydactyly of hands or feet, hallux valgus, syndactyly of second and third fingers, and a defective medial portion of the scapula have all been reported occasionally. The fourth metacarpal is short in 15–45% of patients, but as this occurs in about 10% of the normal population, it is not a good diagnostic sign.

At least 35% of patients have small pseudocystic lytic bone lesions, most often in the phalanges, metapodial and carpal and tarsal bones. These may vary from just one or two lesions to their involving almost the entire bone. The long bones, pelvis and calvarium may also be affected. Histologically these bone radiolucencies are hamartomas composed of fibrous connective tissue, nerves and vessels. Calcification may occur subcutaneously in apparently otherwise normal skin of the fingers and scalp.

11.2.4 ECTOPIC CALCIFICATION

Calcification of the falx cerebri occurs in at least 85% of cases. It can appear very early in

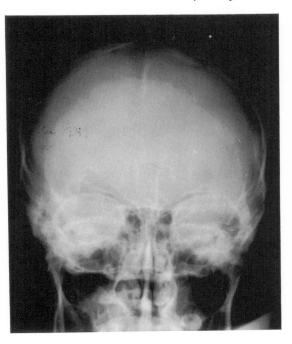

Fig. 11.4 Skull X-ray of a 17-year-old male showing calcification of the upper falx, with the typical lamellar appearance.

life, and is often strikingly apparent from late childhood. It has a characteristic lamellar appearance (Figure 11.4), in comparison with the single sheet of calcification found in 7% of the normal older population. Calcification of the falx cerebri in a child should strongly raise Gorlin syndrome as a diagnosis. A normal variant of the skull, a prominent frontal crest, can simulate falx calcification on the AP skull film, and should be considered if the calcification appears to be a single line beginning inferiorly.

Ectopic calcification also occurs in other membranes – the tentorium cerebelli (40%), petroclinoid ligaments (20%) the dura, pia, and choroid plexus. Calcification of the diaphragma sellae causing the appearance of bridging of the sella turcica is found in 80% and is an early sign; this is found in 4% of the normal population in later life.

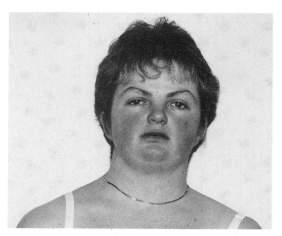

Fig. 11.5 A patient showing many of the facial features associated with the syndrome – arched eyebrows, down-slanting palpebral fissures, prominent jaw, naevi on the neck and chest, sloping shoulders. The frontal bossing is disguised by the cut of the hair.

11.2.5 CRANIOFACIAL FEATURES

(a) Facies

About 70% of patients have a characteristic facies (Figure 11.5), but there is intrafamilial variation. Some members of a sibship may have the typical shape to the skull, for instance, while others do not. One of the most striking features is the increased head size (in all adults in our series the head circumference was over 60 cm and above the corresponding centile line for height). The head gives the appearance of being long in the anterior–posterior plane, with a prominent and low occiput. Frontal, temporal and biparietal bossing give a prominent appearance to the upper part of the face, and patients often adopt hairstyles which disguise the bossing. There is often facial asymmetry. Some patients have well developed supraorbital ridges, giving the eyes a sunken appearance. The eyebrows are often heavy, fused and arched. There is a broad nasal root and hypertelorism. The inner canthal, inter-

pupillary and outer canthal distances are all generally above the 97th centile, but appear to be in proportion with the head circumference. The mandible is long and often prominent with the lower lip protruding in front of the upper.

(b) Ophthalmic problems

In a personally examined series, 26% of cases had ophthalmic problems. Of these 18 patients, 10 had a convergent strabismus, and three members of a family had rotatory nystagmus. Cataracts were present in four cases and microphthalmia in one. Between 10–15% of patients reported in the literature have ophthalmic abnormalities including congenital blindness due to corneal opacity, congenital glaucoma, coloboma of the iris, choroid or optic nerve, convergent or divergent strabismus and nystagmus. Medullated nerve fibres and retinal hamartomas have also been noted.

(c) Cleft lip and palate

There is a well-established association with cleft lip/palate which occurs in 5–6%.

11.2.6 CENTRAL NERVOUS SYSTEM

Medulloblastoma is a well-recognized complication of the syndrome, with an incidence of about 5%. Gorlin syndrome is found in 1–2% of children with medulloblastoma [13], presenting at an average age of about 2 years. This is about 5 years before the average age of presentation in children with isolated medulloblastoma. Meningioma, glioblastoma multiforme and craniopharyngioma have also been described.

In the literature, 'mental retardation' has been reported in about 3%. In the population study in North-West England [3] (apart from treated cases of medulloblastoma) there were no cases of moderate or severe mental retardation in 84 cases. About 6% of patients in that study required prolonged anticonvulsant therapy for grand mal seizures.

11.2.7 DEVELOPMENTAL HISTORY

Some 62% of children in a personal series had an operative delivery. The average birth weight was 4.1 kg and head circumference 38 cm, both greatly increased when compared with siblings. Walking was delayed until an average of 18 months; sibs walked at 12–13 months. Several children had investigations for hydrocephalus because of macrocephaly – the head circumference was above the 97th centile, but growth continued parallel with the centile lines. Many children initially have a mild motor delay, but appear to catch up. All children known to the author have attended mainstream school, a few needing additional help.

11.2.8 GENITOURINARY SYSTEM

(a) Ovarian fibroma

Calcified ovarian fibromas have been reported to occur in over 50% women with the syndrome. In a recent study [3], 25 asymptomatic women with the syndrome underwent abdominal ultrasound and pelvic X-ray examination; 24% had evidence of an ovarian fibroma. Fibromas were found at caesarean section in a woman in whom no abnormality had been detected with imaging.

Ovarian fibromas do not seem to reduce fertility; the main concern is that they may undergo torsion. The fibromas may be mistaken for calcified uterine fibroids, especially if they overlap medially. However, there is no evidence to suggest that they should be removed prophylactically.

Ovarian fibromas which are bilateral, calcified and multinodular should suggest a search for other features of Gorlin syndrome. Ovarian fibromas in general usually form a single mass replacing one ovary and less than 10% are bilateral or demonstrate calcification.

Ovarian fibrosarcoma and other ovarian tumours have been reported but these are rare.

(b) Hypogonadotrophic hypogonadism in males

Scanty mention is made in a few case reports that males may have cryptorchism, hypogonadotrophic hypogonadism, female pubic escutcheon, and scanty facial or body hair. The incidence is unknown, but no cases were found in the North-West England population study [3].

(c) Renal malformations

Kidney malformations (horseshoe kidney, unilateral renal agenesis, renal cysts) have been described in isolated case reports but detailed information is not available.

11.2.9 OTHER FINDINGS

(a) Mesentery

Just as cysts of the skin and jaws are integral parts of the syndrome, so are chylous or lymphatic cysts of the mesentery, though these are rare. They may present, if large, as painless movable masses in the upper abdomen, or rarely may cause symptoms of obstruction. In most cases, however, they are discovered at laparotomy or on X-ray if calcified.

(b) Cardiovascular system

In the North-West England population study [3], cardiac fibroma was found to have a frequency of 2.5%. One child died at 3 months of age from multiple cardiac fibromas, while another case has been followed for over 20 years with a single 2-cm cardiac fibroma in the interventricular septum, and this has remained unchanged. Long-term prognosis is generally good, but resection may be necessary. The incidence in childhood of an isolated cardiac fibroma is between 0.027–0.08%, affecting most frequently the interventricular septum.

(c) Neoplasia in other organs

Tumours in many other organs have been reported in patients with the syndrome. They include renal fibroma, melanoma, leiomyoma, rhabdomyosarcoma, adenoid cystic carcinoma, adrenal cortical adenoma, seminoma, fibroadenoma of the breast, thyroid adenoma, carcinoma of the bladder, Hodgkin's disease, and chronic leukaemia. In a personal series, affected people died from Hodgkin's disease, myeloma, renal cell carcinoma, seminoma and lung cancer. There does not appear to be a particular neoplasm occurring at a frequency which would warrant selective screening.

(d) Response to therapeutic radiation

Patients treated for eczema by irradiation to the hands have developed multiple BCCs on the palms. Children who received craniospinal irradiation as part of the treatment for a medulloblastoma have developed thousands of BCCs in the irradiated area as have some patients whose BCCs were treated with therapeutic radiation [15, 16] (Figure 11.6).

11.3 DIAGNOSIS AND DIFFERENTIAL DIAGNOSIS

11.3.1 DIAGNOSIS

Confirming or refuting the diagnosis of Gorlin syndrome in a patient with some of the condition's features is vital in determining subsequent surveillance and treatment.

There are implications for other family members, who may be completely asymptomatic at the time of diagnosis. They can then be offered surveillance for complications such as BCCs and jaw cysts, and given genetic information. Diagnosis depends on a detailed family history, and physical and X-ray examinations.

(a) Family history

While taking the family history the physician should be mindful of the different presentations of the syndrome, especially the variability in severity between family members. A detailed physical examination and X-ray investigations of the parents of an apparently isolated case should be obligatory before reaching the conclusion that the patient's condition is the result of a new mutation.

(b) Physical examination

The physical features outlined above should be specifically sought and documented; measurements should include height, head circumference, and inner and outer canthal and interpupillary distances. The head circumference should be plotted on a chart which takes height into account [17]. Examination should include a search for palmar/plantar pits.

(c) X-ray investigations

X-ray signs may aid diagnosis in family members who have equivocal physical signs. X-rays recommended include:

- Panoramic views of the jaws (plain films may miss lesions)
- Skull – antero-posterior
- Skull – lateral
- Chest X-ray
- Cervical and thoracic spine
- Hands (for pseudocysts)

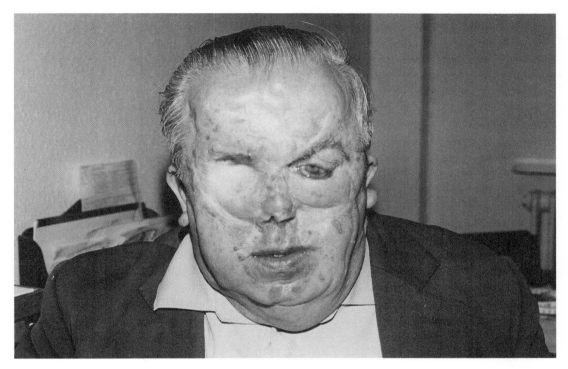

Fig. 11.6 A patient aged 63 showing the effects of multiple facial basal cell carcinomas and treatment. Facial BCCs appeared when he was 28; at the age of 40, multiple BCCs involving the whole of his right and left lower eyelids, and extending onto the upper eyelids were treated with excision and radiotherapy. Although new lesions continued to appear in areas not previously irradiated, at the age of 46 he developed multiple recurrences in the area previously treated by DXT. These BCCs behaved extremely aggressively so that at the age of 47 his right eye had to be enucleated because of carcinomatous invasion of the cornea. The BCCs in the irradiated area were multifocal and cicatricial with diffuse dermal infiltration.

(d) Ultrasound examination

Ultrasound examinations for ovarian and cardiac fibromas may be helpful.

(e) Diagnostic criteria

Diagnostic criteria are given in Table 11.2 based on the most frequent and/or specific features of the syndrome. These criteria were based on examination of family cases in England, a country not noted for excessive sunlight. The numbers of BCCs acceptable as a major criterion will vary according to the climate, and will need adaptation for countries such as Australia.

(f) Diagnosis by gene tracking

Following the demonstration that loss of heterozygosity on chromosome 9 occurred frequently in sporadic BCCs [18], Gorlin syndrome was mapped to 9q22.3–q31 in families from central Europe [19], the UK [20] and the USA [21]. The syndrome also maps to the same area in 15 Australasian families [22]. Locus heterogeneity had not been reported by

Table 11.2 Diagnostic criteria for nevoid basal cell carcinoma syndrome. A diagnosis can be made when two major *or* one major and two minor criteria are fulfilled.

Major criteria
1. Multiple (>2)[1] basal cell carcinomas or one under the age of 30 years or >10 basal cell naevi
2. Odontogenic keratocyst (proven on histology) or polyostotic bone cyst
3. Palmar or plantar pits (three or more)
4. Ectopic calcification: lamellar or early (<20 years) falx calcification
5. First-degree relative with NBCCs

Minor criteria
1. Congenital skeletal anomaly: bifid, fused, splayed or missing rib or fused vertebrae
2. OFC (occipitofrontal circumference) >97th centile with bossing
3. Cardiac or ovarian fibroma
4. Medulloblastoma
5. Lymphomesenteric cysts
6. Congenital malformation: cleft lip and/or palate, polydactyly, eye anomaly (cataract, coloboma, microphthalmia)

[1]Note that the numbers of BCC given were based on a study carried out in England; the numbers of BCC for diagnosis will be inappropriate for sunnier climes!

December 1994, despite the wide range of features of the syndrome both between and within families.

There are useful flanking DNA markers, such as D9S196/D9S197 and D9S180[23]. These have an intermarker distance of about 3.6 cM, and where DNA is available from several family members, allow gene tracking. No common ancestral haplotype has been found, in keeping with the relatively high new mutation rate.

Male chiasmata studies [23] and linkage analysis [24, 25] suggest that there is apparently complete positive genetic interference over 9q22.3–31: only one chiasma would be expected to occur in this region. The error due to double recombinants when using flanking DNA markers for diagnosis will therefore be extremely low.

11.3.2 DIFFERENTIAL DIAGNOSIS

Unilateral linear nevoid basal cell carcinomas with comedones [26] is probably the result of a somatic mutation of the Gorlin syndrome gene. There are multiple basal cell carcinomas, comedones, and epidermoid cysts in a unilateral distribution.

Rasmussen [27] reported a family with trichoepitheliomas, milia and cylindromas presenting in the second and third decades. Inheritance was autosomal dominant. The milia were miniature trichoepitheliomas and appeared only in sun-exposed areas. In some cases cylindromatosis [28] (Turban tumour syndrome) may be the same condition; it shows considerable variation within families in the size and extent of distribution, and age of onset.

Bazex syndrome [29] is characterized by multiple basal cell carcinomas, follicular atrophoderma on the dorsum of hands and feet, decreased sweating and hypotrichosis. The pitting on the backs of the hands is reported to be reminiscent of orange peel and quite unlike the pits of Gorlin syndrome. The inheritance pattern is uncertain – either autosomal or X-linked dominant.

Rombo syndrome [30] is a dominantly inherited condition characterized by vermiculate atrophoderma, milia, hypotrichosis, trichoepitheliomas, basal cell carcinomas and peripheral vasodilation with cyanosis, reported in one family. The features are very similiar to Bazex syndrome, except that the skin is normal until later childhood, BCCs develop later and there is no reduction in sweating.

A single family with another syndrome of hypotrichosis (coarse sparse scalp hair), basal cell carcinomas and milia was reported by Oley *et al.* [31]. The family pedigree was consistent with either an autosomal or X-linked dominant mode of transmission. Affected members of the family showed excessive sweating. Pseudohypoparathyroidism may be considered because of ectopic calcification and short fourth metacarpals.

In Cowden syndrome (multiple hamartoma syndrome) [32] mucocutaneous changes develop in the second decade. Multiple facial papules, both smooth and keratotic, are associated with hair follicles and concentrated around the orifices. Small hyperkeratotic and verrucous growths are numerous on the dorsal aspect of the hands and feet, and round translucent palmoplantar keratoses are also common. Similar lesions, including verrucous papules, occur on the oral mucosa. Multiple skin tags are also frequent. Most patients have a broad forehead and a large head circumference. Neoplasms occur in the gastrointestinal system, thyroid, and breast.

Arsenic exposure may cause multiple basal cell carcinomas.

Cardiac fibromas are also found in tuberous sclerosis and Beckwith–Wiedemann syndrome.

11.4 SURVEILLANCE

11.4.1 SCREENING PROGRAMMES

It is recommended that families are offered regular screening, with perhaps one clinician or a genetic department monitoring and coordinating the programme [3]. DNA predictive testing by linked markers may be justified in families with a suitable structure. Screening programmes may comprise:

1. Ultrasound scans: these may be offered during pregnancy to detect cardiac tumours and developmental malformations, which may require early decisions about neonatal surgery, and to detect an extremely enlarged head which may necessitate operative delivery.
2. A detailed neonatal examination: this may

confirm the physical signs of a large head, cleft palate, or eye anomaly. X-rays may confirm bifid ribs or vertebral abnormalities. An echocardiogram is best performed early, as at least two cases have presented before 3 months of age with fibromas.
3. Six-monthly neurological examination: this may detect a deficit indicative of a medulloblastoma. Routine scanning with computed tomography (CT) or excessive use of X-rays is not recommended because of concerns about inducing skin malignancies. At 3 years the examinations could be reduced to annually until 7 years, after which a medulloblastoma is very unlikely. Although these examinations are of low sensitivity and specificity a parent will have contact with a specialist department should suspicious symptoms develop.
4. Annual dental screening: these may commence from about 8 years usually including an orthopantomogram of the jaw.
5. Annual examination of the skin: these are recommended at least annually from puberty, although if a lesion suddenly becomes aggressive, the patient needs open access to the specialist taking the main responsibility for treatment of the skin.

   Patients must be warned to inspect all areas of the body – BCCs have been reported on the vulva, and the mucosa of the anal sphincter, for instance. It is especially important to offer early treatment for lesions of the eyelids, nose, ears and scalp.

11.4.2 EXPOSURE TO SUNLIGHT

As sunlight may be one of the environmental agents promoting the appearance of BCCs, it is sensible to recommend basic sunscreening precautions, including the wearing of a wide-brimmed hat to offer some protection to the areas around the eyes.

Laboratory experiments with ultraviolet radiation have been inconclusive, but there is circumstantial evidence from a comparison of English and Australian studies: 4% of cases in North-West England [3] developed a BCC before the age of 20, compared with 47% in Australia (G. Chenevix-Trench, personal communication). However, the genetic background of the population itself may influence sensitivity to skin cancer [33]. A questionnaire study of 16 families in the US [34] did not find a strong relation between numbers of BCCs in white-skinned people and a history of lifetime sun exposure. In agreement with the literature, only two of their eight black-skinned patients reported a BCC. The distribution of BCCs in white-skinned patients differed from that of the general population: 35% of BCCs occurred on the trunk, compared with 10.5% in the general population. It was suggested that either frequent sun exposure is not essential for the development of BCCs, or patients may be susceptible to low levels of sun exposure.

11.5 TREATMENT

11.5.1 SKIN

(a) Local treatment

The most suitable form of treatment may vary depending on the type, size and site of the NBCC. Surgical excision, cryotherapy, curettage and diathermy, topical 5-fluorouracil and Moh's[35] microsurgery are all in use. The priorities are to ensure complete eradication of aggressive BCCs, and to preserve normal tissue to prevent disfigurement.

Some practitioners urge treatment of all lesions, while others reserve treatment for those with evidence of progression.

Some patients have many naevi which remain symptomless for long periods which can be kept under frequent review. Others have hundreds of aggressive BCCs. This could be due to different mutations of the gene, or exposure to a potentiating environmental factor.

Treatment may seem overwhelming and hopeless to patients with many hundreds of BCCs. A great deal of support may therefore be required, not least to encourage attendance at follow-up clinics and to accept early treatment.

(b) Systemic retinoids

There are a few reports of oral synthetic retinoids (etretinate, isotretinoin, and 13-*cis*-retinoic acid) preventing the development of new tumours, inhibiting the growth of existing tumours, and causing the regression of superficially invasive basal cell carcinomas.

In two reports [36, 37], etretinate at a dose of 1 mg/kg/day resulted in regression of 76% and 83% of lesions. Less aggressive surgery was required in a female patient, who received treatment with oral etretinate, initially at 1 mg/kg/day [38].

Isoretinoin (0.4 mg/kg/day) prevented the formation of the majority of new BCCs and reduced the rate of growth of existing lesions in twin males who had hundreds of lesions [39]. A child was managed for 10 years with a combination of topical 5-fluorouracil and etretinoin [40].

Potential teratogenicity and side effects such as chelitis, pruritus, peeling of the palms and soles, eczema and diffuse idiopathic skeletal hyperostosis [41] dictate that retinoids should be used in carefully controlled circumstances. Their long-term role in the management of the condition is still being assessed.

(c) Treatment by radiation

Radiotherapy should be avoided because of clinical evidence that new lesions appear in the irradiated field [15, 16]. Some families appear less clinically radiosensitive than others.

11.5.2 JAW CYSTS

As proliferating dental lamina and satellite cysts may occur in the fibrous wall of the primary cyst cavity, marsupialization may be successful only if no satellite cysts are left behind. Small single lesions with regular spherical outlines can usually be completely enucleated provided access is good. Stoelinga *et al.* [42] have recommended that the overlying mucoperiosteum should be excised for cysts close to the surface because of the possible origin of the cyst from basal cell proliferations. For the large multilocular lesions, excision and immediate bone grafting is the treatment of choice at the first operation.

11.6 LABORATORY FINDINGS

Several laboratories have sought evidence for chromosome fragility and DNA repair defects. Results have been conflicting; whether this reflects small sample size and perhaps suboptimal choice of controls, or true disease heterogeneity in cellular responses [43], may have to await molecular pathology studies when the gene has been isolated. Important clinical information (whether or not a patient shows clinical hypersensitivity to the induction of BCCs by irradiation) which might explain conflicting results is not given in most reports. There may also be differences betweeen different cell types: keratinocytes, for instance, from both Gorlin syndrome and normal donors are more resistant to ultraviolet C (UV-C) and X-rays than skin-derived fibroblasts [44]. In one patient with unilateral Gorlin syndrome where fibroblasts from the unaffected side could be used as control cells, there was no difference in X-ray, ultraviolet B (UV-B) or

UV-C radiation sensitivity compared with the affected side [45].

Overall, it appears likely that the cancer susceptibility is neither caused by nor manifests as chromosome instability, nor that increased cell killing is a major effect of the gene. It is interesting to note, however, that the syndrome maps to an area of chromosome 9 that is now known to contain genes for xeroderma pigmentosum (which results in cells being deficient in DNA repair) and Fanconi anaemia (in which hypersensitivity to DNA cross-linking agents results in chromosome fragility).

11.6.1 CHROMOSOMAL INSTABILITY

(a) Chromosome breaks

Spontaneous:
An increase in spontaneous breaks and rearrangements in fibroblasts of two of three patients was reported but later studies with additional patients failed to confirm chromosome instability [46]. Increased breaks and rearrangements were detected in the cultured lymphocytes of a 62-year-old female patient but her unaffected son also showed chromosome fragility [47].

Following irradiation:
Featherstone *et al.* [48] demonstrated a small but statistically significant increase in X-ray-induced chromosome aberrations in G0 lymphocytes in seven unrelated affected patients compared with controls. However, Nagasawa *et al.* failed to show either increased chromosome aberrations or single strand breaks in DNA in fibroblasts [49].

(b) Sister chromatid exchanges (SCEs)

Gao *et al.* [50] found baseline SCEs to occur nearly three times as frequently in the lymphocytes of four affected members of a family than in controls, and Romke *et al.* [51] demonstrated a small increase in both baseline and mitomycin C-induced SCEs in nine patients compared with nine unrelated controls. Nagasawa et al. [49] noted abnormally high SCE rates during repair of potentially lethal ultraviolet damage in two fibroblast lines.

Two studies found no evidence of increased SCEs. Sarto *et al.* [52] found that the frequencies of chromosomal aberrations induced by mitomycin C (MMC) and bleomycin, and sister-chromatid exchanges induced by MMC and 4-nitroquinoline *N*-oxide in lymphocytes of four patients were within normal ranges. Bale and colleagues [53] investigated aphidocolin-induced chromosome fragility and radiomimetic chemical-induced sister chromatid exchange in 20 affected individuals from five multiplex pedigrees, and 15 first- or second-degree unaffected relatives. No significant differences were noted for either chromosome fragility or SCE between the two groups.

11.6.2 CELL SURVIVAL

No differences were found between five patients and controls in the lethal effects of ionizing radiation [54–56]. However, Chan and Little [57] reported that five NBCCS fibroblast cell strains were slightly but significantly more sensitive to the cytotoxic effects of radiation than were six control strains studied in parallel, but the controls have been questioned [43].

Little *et al.* [43] found that overall, the X-ray response of cells from affected individuals showed no systematic difference from that of cells from non-affected relatives or cell bank controls for either cytotoxicity or chromosome breakage. One of four affected Gorlin syndrome patients showed a moderate degree of radiation hypersensitivity, whereas the remaining affected and non-affected individuals from the same family responded

normally. The response of cells from four other patients who had developed radiation-induced tumours also fell within the normal range. They suggest that isolated cases of *in vitro* radiation hypersensitivity probably do not relate to the underlying genetic disorder.

11.6.3 REPAIR OF POTENTIALLY LETHAL DAMAGE

An investigation of repair of potentially lethal damage (RPLD), measured by post-irradiation holding experiments, could detect no difference between fibroblasts from patients and from controls [48]. However, a different assay using two of the same fibroblast strains showed there was very little capacity for RPLD after gamma-irradiation. A third strain did show some repair capacity, indicating the possibility of heterogeneity [58].

11.6.4 ULTRAVIOLET RADIATION

Most experiments have been conducted with UV-C radiation (254 nm), a wavelength which is filtered out by the stratospheric ozone. Epidemiological and clinical studies indicate that UV-B radiation (280–320 nm), which reaches the surface of the earth in sunlight, is responsible for the induction of most skin cancers in humans. Ringborg *et al.* [59] found a 25% lower level of maximum DNA repair synthesis following UV-C exposure in peripheral lymphocytes from seven patients compared with 39 normal controls.

Fibroblasts have been found to have no differences in sensitivity [60] following UV-C, while others were more sensitive to UV-C [49]. However, Ananthaswamy *et al.* [61] have claimed a six-fold enhancement of sensitivity for NBCCS fibroblasts compared with normals to UV-B, but not to UV-C. The ionizing radiation response of both fibroblasts and lymphocytes from the patient was normal.

In a follow-up report [62], skin fibroblasts from NBCC patients were shown to be hypersensitive to killing by UV-B, but not UV-C radiation [62] compared with skin fibroblasts from normal individuals. The effect was not due to a defect in the excision repair of pyrimidine dimers.

11.6.5 RESPONSE TO PARATHORMONE

The hyporesponsiveness to parathormone suggested by studies using the Ellsworth–Howard test have not been confirmed by later studies [63] using cyclic AMP.

11.7 FUNCTION OF THE GENE

As so many organ systems can be affected, it is tempting to speculate that the underlying mechanism could be a structural chromosomal alteration affecting several genes – a contiguous gene syndrome. The variability between families could then be explained by the extent of the genetic material involved; however, this would not adequately explain the variation in severity (in type and extent of manifestations) between family members.

Alternative explanations include modifying genes at other loci, and the timing and frequency of mutations at a second locus. The mechanism underlying the variation in expression is unknown; its elucidation will be one of the most exciting consequences of the eventual isolation of the gene.

The natural history and clinical features of the syndrome suggest that it is more likely that a single gene is responsible – a gene active in the control of cell growth, and ubiquitously expressed.

Evidence has now been furnished that the gene is a tumour suppressor gene. BCCs from patients with Gorlin syndrome have been shown to lose heterozygosity for alleles at 9q22.3–31, the deleted alleles being those inherited from the unaffected parent [64].

The behaviour of the naevi fits the paradigm of Knudson's two-hit hypothesis [65]. Loss of function of the normal allele in a cell which already has a mutation (inherited or acquired) on the homologous chromosome allows development of a tumour because the negative control of the locus on cell growth is lost. This may result in the initial production of a naevus, and perhaps at least one further step is then required for the naevus to behave aggressively.

Other features of Gorlin syndrome, especially the malformations present at birth, however, do not fit easily into a loss of function model, and require further explanation. A gene dosage effect may be the cause of the congenital malformations and the variation in expression, both between and within families. The production of a mutant protein which inhibits the function of the remaining wild-type protein could promote tumorigenesis [66] and perhaps congenital malformations by the so-called dominant-negative effect [67].

11.8 THE SIGNIFICANCE OF CHROMOSOMAL REGION 9q22

Genes involved in DNA repair and chromosomal stability – Fanconi anaemia complementation group C (FACC), and xeroderma pigmentosum complementation group A (XPAC) – have been mapped to 9q22–31. Multiple self-healing squamous epitheliomata (ESS1) [68] has also been mapped to this area, raising the possibility that it is allelic to Gorlin syndrome. ESS1, an autosomal dominant disorder, has been mapped by haplotype studies [69] in families with common ancestry; the great majority of individuals have been of Scottish origin and their condition may be attributable to a single mutation. The skin tumours are invasive but then undergo spontaneous resolution over a period of months; there does not appear to be an increase in developmental anomalies as in

NBCCS (D.R. Goudie, personal communication).

As NBCCS, FACC, ESS1 and XPAC all map to the same region, it will be intriguing not only to discover the relationships of these syndromes and their genes – but also to see if they are caused by related gene(s), how the molecular pathology can explain the clinical features, and the modes of inheritance.

REFERENCES

1. Gorlin, R.J. and Goltz, R.W. (1960) Multiple nevoid basal-cell epithelioma, jaw cysts and bifid rib: a syndrome. *N. Engl. J. Med.*, **262**, 908–12.
2. Gorlin, R.J. (1987) Nevoid basal-cell carcinoma syndrome. *Medicine*, **66**, 96–113.
3. Evans, D.G.R., Ladusans, E.J., Rimmer, S., Burnell, L.D., Thakker, N. and Farndon, P.A. (1993) Complications of the naevoid basal cell carcinoma syndrome: results of a population based study. *J. Med. Genet.*, **30**, 460–4.
4. Rahbari, H. and Mehregan, A.H. (1982) Basal cell epithelioma (carcinoma) in children and teenagers. *Cancer*, **49**, 350–3.
5. Summerly, R. (1965) Basal cell carcinoma. An aetiological study of patients aged 45 and under with special reference to Gorlin's syndrome. *Br. J. Derm.*, **77**, 9–15.
6. Chudina, A.P., Savluchinskaia, L.A., Mikhailovskii A.V., and Briuzgin, V.V. (1989) Detection of basal-cell nevus syndrome in patients with multiple skin basiliomas. *Voprosy Onkologii*, **35**, 1166–9.
7. Shear M. (1983) *Cysts of the Oral Regions (A Dental Practitioner Handbook: No 23)*, 2nd edn, Wright, Bristol, p. 11.
8. Gorlin, R.J., Cohen, M.M. and Levin, L.S. (1990) Multiple nevoid basal cell carcinoma syndrome; in *Syndromes of the Head and Neck*, 3rd edn, Oxford University Press, Oxford, pp. 372–80.
9. Jones, K.L., Smith, D.W., Harvey, M.A., Hall, B.D. and Quan, L. (1975) Older paternal age and fresh gene mutation: data on additional disorders. *J. Pediatr.*, **86**, 84–8.
10. Howell, J.B. and Freeman, R.G. (1980) Structure and significance of the pits with their tumors in the nevoid basal cell carcinoma syndrome. *J. Am. Acad. Dermatol.*, **2**, 224–38.
11. Stoelinga, P.J., Cohen, M.M. and Morgan, A.F. (1975) The origin of keratocysts in the basal cell naevus syndrome. *J. Oral Surg.*, **33**, 659–63.
12. Etter, L.E. (1944) Osseous abnormalities of the thoracic cage seen in 40,000 consecutive chest photoroentgenograms. *Am. J. Roentgenol.*, **51**, 359–63.
13. Evans, D.G.R., Farndon, P.A., Burnell, L.D., Rao Gattamaneni, H. and Birch, J.M. (1991) The incidence of Gorlin syndrome in 173 consecutive cases of medulloblastoma. *Br. J. Cancer*, **64**, 959–61.
14. Burket, R.L. and Rauh, J.L. (1976) Gorlin's syndrome: ovarian fibromas at adolescence. *Obstet. Gynecol.*, **47**, S43–6.
15. Strong, L.C. (1977) Genetic and environmental interactions. *Cancer*, **40**, 1861–6.
16. Southwick, G.J. and Schwartz, R.A. (1979) The basal cell nevus syndrome: disasters occurring among a series of 36 patients. *Cancer*, **44**, 2294–305.
17. Bushby, K.M.D., Cole, T., Matthews, J.N.S. and Goodship, J.A. (1992) Centiles for adult head circumference. *Arch. Dis. Child.*, **67**, 1286–7.
18. Gailani, M.R., Keffell, D.J. and Bale, A.E. (1991) Evidence for a tumor suppressor gene on chromosome 9 in basal cell carcinomas of the skin. *Am. J. Hum. Genet.* supplement to volume 49, A454.
19. Reis, A., Kuster, W., Gebel, E. *et al.* (1992) Localisation of the gene for the naevoid basal cell carcinoma syndrome. *Lancet*, **339**, 617.
20. Farndon, P.A., Del Mastro, R.D., Evans, D.G.R. and Kilpatrick, M.W. (1992) Location of gene for Gorlin syndrome. *Lancet*, **339**, 581–2.
21. Gailani, M.R., Bale, S.J., Leffell, D.J., *et al.* (1992) Developmental defects in Gorlin syndrome related to a putative tumor suppressor gene on chromosome 9. *Cell*, **69**, 111–17.
22. Chenevix-Trench, G., Wicking, C., Berkman, J., Sharpe, H. and Hockey, A. (1993) Further localization of the gene for nevoid basal cell syndrome in 15 Australasian families: linkage and loss of heterozygosity. *Am. J. Hum. Genet.*, **53**, 760–7.
23. Povey, S., Smith, M., Haines, J. *et al.* (1992)

Report on the first international workshop on chromosome 9. *Ann. Hum. Genet.*, **56**, 167–221.

24. Povey, S., Armour J., Farndon, P. *et al.* (1994) Report on the third international workshop on human chromosome 9. *Ann. Hum. Genet.*, **58**, 177–250.

25. Kwiatkowski, D.J., Dib, C., Slaugenhaupt, S., Povey, S., Gusella, J.F. and Haines, J.L. (1993) An index marker map of chromosome 9 provides strong evidence for positive interference. *Am. J. Hum. Genet.*, **53**, 1279–88.

26. Bleiberg, J. and Brodkin, R.H. (1969) Linear unilateral basal cell nevus with comedones. *Arch. Dermatol.*, **100**, 187–90.

27. Rasmussen, J.E. (1975) A syndrome of trichoepitheliomas, milia and cylindromas. *Arch. Dermatol.*, **111**, 610–14.

28. Welch, J.P., Wells, R.S. and Kerr, C.B. (1968) Ancell–Spiegler cylindromas (turban tumours) and Brooke–Fordyce trichoepitheliomas: evidence for a single genetic entity. *J. Med. Genet.*, **5**, 29–35.

29. Viksnins, P. and Berlin, A. (1977) Follicular atrophoderma and basal cell carcinomas: the Bazex syndrome. *Arch. Dermatol.*, **113**, 948–51.

30. Michaelsson, G., Olsson, E. and Westermark, P. (1981) The Rombo syndrome. *Acta Dermatovener.*, **61**, 497–503.

31. Oley, C.A., Sharpe, H. and Chenevix-Trench, G. (1992) Basal cell carcinomas, coarse sparse hair, and milia. *Am. J. Med. Genet.*, **43**, 799–804.

32. Starink, T.M., van der Veen, J.P.W., Arwert, F. *et al.* (1986) The Cowden syndrome: a clinical and genetic study in 21 patients. *Clin. Genet.*, **29**, 222–33.

33. Howell, J.B. (1984) Nevoid basal cell carcinoma syndrome: profile of genetic and environmental factors in oncogenesis. *J. Am. Acad. Dermatol.*, **11**, 98–104.

34. Goldstein, A.M., Bale, S.J., Peck, G.L. and DiGiovanna, J.J. (1993) Sun exposure and basal cell carcinomas in the nevoid basal cell carcinoma syndrome. *J. Am. Acad. Dermatol.*, **29**, 34–41.

35. Mohs, F.E., Jones, D.L. and Koranda, F.C. (1980) Microscopically controlled surgery for carcinomas in patients with nevoid basal cell carcinoma syndrome. *Arch. Dermatol.*, **116**, 777–9.

36. Cristofolini, M., Zumiani, G., Scappni, P. *et al.* (1984) Aromatic retinoid in chemoprevention of the progression of nevoid basal cell carcinoma syndrome. *J. Dermatol. Surg. Oncol.*, **10**, 778–81.

37. Hodak, E., Ginzburg, A., David, M. *et al.* (1987) Etretinate treatment of the nevoid basal cell carcinoma syndrome. *Int. J. Dermatol.*, **26**, 606–9.

38. Sanchez-Conejo-Mir, J. and Camacho, F. (1989) Nevoid basal cell carcinoma syndrome: combined etretinate and surgical treatment. *J. Dermatol. Surg. Oncol.*, **15**, 868–71.

39. Goldberg, L.H., Hsu, S.H. and Alcalay, J. (1989) Effectiveness of isotretinoin in preventing the appearance of basal cell carcinomas in basal cell nevus syndrome. *J. Am. Acad. Dermatol.*, **21**, 144–5.

40. Strange, P.R. and Lang, P.G. Jr (1992) Long-term management of basal cell nevus syndrome with topical tretinoin and 5-fluorouracil. *J. Am. Acad. Dermatol.*, **27**, 842–5.

41. Theiler, R., Hubscher, E., Wagenhauser, F.J., Panizzon, R. and Michel, B. (1993) Diffuse idiopathic skeletal hyperostosis (DISH) and pseudo-coxarthritis following long-term etretinate therapy. *Schweiz. Med. Wochenschr.*, **123**, 649–53.

42. Stoelinga, P.J., Peters, J.H., van de Staak, W.J. and Cohen, M.M. (1973) Some new findings in the basal cell nevus syndrome. *Oral Surg.* **36**, 686–92.

43. Little, J.B., Nichols, W.W., Troilo, P., Nagasawa, H. and Strong, L.C. (1989) Radiation sensitivity of cell strains from families with genetic disorders predisposing to radiation-induced cancer. *Cancer Res.*, **49**, 4705–14.

44. Stacey, M., Thacker, S. and Taylor, A.M. (1989) Cultured skin keratinocytes from both normal individuals and basal cell naevus syndrome patients are more resistant to gamma-rays and UV light compared with cultured skin fibroblasts. *Int. J. Radiat Biol.*, **56**, 45–58.

45. Sharpe, G.R. and Cox, N.H. (1990) Unilateral naevoid basal cell carcinoma syndrome – an individually controlled study of fibroblast sensitivity to radiation. *Clin. Exp. Dermatol.*, **15**, 352–5.

46. Happle, R. (1981) Genetik der basalioma, in *Das Basaliom der Houfigste Tumor der haurt*, (eds F. Eichmann and U.W. Schnyder), Springer, Berlin, pp. 17–28.

47. Horland, A.A., Wolman, S.R., Reich, E. and Coz, R.P. (1975) Cytogenetic studies in patients with the basal cell nevus syndrome and their relatives. *Am. J. Hum. Genet.*, **27**, 47A.

48. Featherstone, T., Taylor, A.M. and Harden, D.G. (1983) Studies on the radiosensitivity of cells from patients with basal cell nevus syndrome. *Am. J. Hum. Genet.*, **35**, 58–66.

49. Nagasawa, F., Little, F.F., Burke, M.J. *et al.* (1984) Study of basal cell nevus fibroblasts after treatment with DNA damaging agents. *Basic Life Sci.*, **29B**, 775–85.

50. Gao, J., Zhang, Y., Xu, M. *et al.* (1985) Studies on the genetics of basal cell nevus syndrome in one family. *Chin. Med. J.*, **98**, 538–42.

51. Romke, C., Godde-Salz, E. and Grote, W. (1985) Investigations of chromosomal stability in the Gorlin–Goltz syndrome. *Arch. Dermatol. Res.*, **277**, 370–2.

52. Sarto, F., Mazzoti, D., Tomanin, R., Corsi, G.C., and Peserico, A. (1989) No evidence of chromosomal instability in nevoid basal cell carcinoma syndrome. *Mutat. Res.*, **225**, 21–6.

53. Bale, A.E., Bale, S.J., Murli, H., Ivett, J., Mulvihill, J.J. and Parry, D.M. (1989) Sister chromatid exchange and chromosome fragility in the nevoid basal cell carcinoma syndrome. *Cancer Genet. Cytogenet.*, **42**, 273–9.

54. Arlett, C.F. and Harcourt, S.A. (1980) Survey of radiosensitivity in a variety of human cell strains. *Cancer Res.*, **40**, 926–32.

55. Nagasawa, H., Little, J.B., Tsang, H.M., Saunders, E., Tesmer, J. and Strniste, G.F. (1992) Effect of dose rate on the survival of irradiated human skin fibroblasts. *Radiat. Res.*, **132**, 375–9.

56. Newton, J.A. Black, A.K., Arlett, C.F. and Cole, J. (1990) Radiobiological studies in the naevoid basal cell carcinoma syndrome. *Br. J. Dermatol.*, **123**, 573–80.

57. Chan, G.L. and Little, J.B. (1983) Cultured diploid fibroblasts from patient with the nevoid basal cell carcinoma syndrome are hypersensitive to killing by ionizing radiation. *Am. J. Pathol.*, **111**, 50–55.

58. Arlett, C.F. and Priestley, A. (1984) Deficient recovery from potentially lethal damage in some gamma-irradiated human fibroblast cell strains. *Br. J. Cancer (Suppl)*, **6**, 227–32.

59. Ringborg, U., Lambert, B., Landergan, J. and Lewensohn, R. (1981) Decreased UV-induced DNA repair synthesis in peripheral leukocytes from patients with the nevoid basal cell carcinoma syndrome. *J. Invest. Dermatol.*, **76**, 268–70.

60. Lehmann, A.R., Kirk–Bell, S., Arlett, C.F. *et al.* (1977) Repair of UV light damage in a variety of human fibroblast cell strains. *Cancer Res.*, **37**, 904–10.

61. Ananthaswamy, H.N., Applegate, L.A., Goldberg, L.H. *et al.* (1989) Skin fibroblasts from basal cell nevus patients are hypersensitive to killing by solar UVB radiation. *Photochem. Photobiol.*, **49**, 60S.

62. Applegate, L.A., Goldberg, L.H., Ley, R.D. and Ananthaswamy, H.N. (1990) Hypersensitivity of skin fibroblasts from basal cell nevus syndrome patients to killing by ultraviolet B but not by ultraviolet C radiation. *Cancer Res.*, **50**, 637–41.

63. Murphy, K.J. (1969) Subcutaneous calcification in basal cell carcinoma syndrome: response to parathyroid hormone and relationship to pseudohypoparathyroidism. *Clin. Radiol.*, **20**, 287–93.

64. Bonifas, J.M., Bare, J.W., Kerschmann, R.L., Master, S.P. and Epstein, E.H. (1994) Parental origin of chromosome 9q22.3-q31 lost in basal cell carcinomas from basal cell nevus syndrome patients. *Hum. Mol. Genet.*, **3**, 447–8.

65. Knudson, A.G. (1971) Mutation and cancer: statistical study of retinoblastoma. *Proc. Nat. Acad. Sci. USA*, **68**, 820–3.

66. Levine, A.J., Momand, J. and Finlay, C.A. (1991) The p53 tumour suppressor gene. *Nature*, **351**, 453–6.

66. Hastie, N.D. (1992) Dominant negative mutations in the Wilms tumour (WT1) gene cause Denys–Drash syndrome: proof that a tumoursuppressor gene plays a crucial role in normal genitourinary development. *Hum. Mol. Genet.*, **1**, 293–5.

68. Ferguson-Smith, M.A., Wallace, D.C., James, Z.H. and Renwick, J.H. (1971) Multiple selfhealing squamous epithelioma. *Birth Defects Original Article Series*, **VII**, 157–63.

69. Goudie, D.R., Yuille, M.A.R., Leversha, M.A., Furlong, R.A. and Carter, N. (1993) Multiple self-healing squamous epitheliomata (ESS1) mapped to chromosome 9q22-q31 in families with common ancestry. *Nature Genet.*, **3**, 165–9.

Chapter 12

Xeroderma pigmentosum, Cockayne syndrome and trichothiodystrophy: sun sensitivity, DNA repair defects and skin cancer

COLIN F. ARLETT and ALAN R. LEHMANN

12.1 INTRODUCTION

Xeroderma pigmentosum (XP) is a rare, autosomal recessive disease [1] with a combination of clinical, cellular and molecular features which initially generated an intellectually satisfying and simple association between defects in DNA repair, increased mutability and cancer proneness. As the study of XP patients has proceeded, however, interesting anomalies and unanticipated complexities have been uncovered. In particular, as a consequence of using XP as a model, two other, extremely rare but not cancer-prone, autosomal recessive diseases, Cockayne syndrome (CS) and trichothiodystrophy (TTD) [2] have extended the apparent relationship of DNA repair defects to a wide spectrum of associated clinical features. The relationship between the three conditions is complex – there are a few individuals with the features of both XP and CS, and mutations in one of the XP genes can give rise to individuals with XP alone, XP with CS, or TTD alone. In order to understand the relationship between DNA damage/repair and cancer revealed in XP, it is necessary to study all three conditions at the clinical, cellular and molecular levels.

12.2 CLINICAL OBSERVATIONS

12.2.1 XERODERMA PIGMENTOSUM

Comprehensive reviews of the clinical characteristics of XP are available [1]. The individuals are sun-sensitive and this is coupled with an abnormal erythemal response [3]. The dermatological features in unprotected individuals include, in sun-exposed areas, pigmented macules, achromic spots and

Genetic Predisposition to Cancer. Edited by R.A. Eeles, B.A.J. Ponder, D.F. Easton and A. Horwich. Published in 1996 by Chapman & Hall, London.
0 412 56580 3

telangiectasia followed, ultimately, by basal cell carcinoma (BCC), squamous cell carcinoma (SCC) and malignant melanoma. The survey by Kraemer *et al.* [4] of 830 published cases showed that: (i) individuals with the disease die about 30 years earlier than the US population as a whole; (ii) 50% of patients in the 10–14-year age group had skin cancers; and (iii) the median age for first skin neoplasms is approximately 50 years lower than in the normal population.

The role of sunlight in the induction of skin cancer in the normal human population is unambiguous – 97% of the BCC plus SCC are found on regions of the body which receive most direct sunlight. Conversely, protection by avoidance of sunlight can materially reduce the extent of cutaneous damage. Thus, patients with the cellular characteristics of XP (see below) but with no tumours or reduced skin damage may have been exposed to relatively little sunlight. There are, however, well-documented examples of such individuals who do not attempt to protect themselves from sunlight. The explanation for their relatively mild skin damage is not clear. In addition to increased skin cancer, XP patients have also been reported to have an increased incidence of some internal tumours [5].

Neurological defects were described in 20% of the patients reviewed by Kraemer *et al.* [4]. Here, of course no direct involvement of sunlight can be inferred. Progressive neurological degeneration results from premature neuronal death.

A number of other clinical abnormalities have been associated with XP. Impaired immune status has been reported. This includes a reduced response to recall antigens and DNCB antigens, a reduction in the ratio of T helper/suppressor cells and a reduced response to phytohaemagglutinin stimulation of lymphocytes. There is considerable variation among patients with regard to these effects. Natural killer (NK) cell number and function have been found to be reduced in some, but not all, XP patients [6, 7]. Indeed, in one interesting case, an individual aged 65 years with self-healing melanomas had reduced NK function on a per cell basis but greatly increased numbers of NK cells [8]. Turner *et al.* [9] have recently reported a case where intra-lesional α-interferon injection was effective in the treatment of melanomas in an XP patient. It is of interest that cells from such patients have a reduced capacity to mount a γ-interferon stimulation of ICAM-1 expression [10] following UV-B irradiation.

12.2.2 COCKAYNE SYNDROME

This rare disorder shows a pattern of inheritance consistent with a recessive status. In a review of 140 published cases Nance and Berry [11] suggested that the primary clinical hallmarks included neurodevelopmental delay and dwarfism, together with any three of the following: hearing loss, dental caries, pigmentary retinopathy (with or without cataract), characteristic facial appearance and photosensitivity (see also [12]). No increased incidence of skin cancer has been recorded.

As a consequence of the rarity of these patients there has been limited opportunity to investigate their immunological status. In two patients, adaptive cell-mediated immunity and NK cell function were within normal limits [6]. Amazingly, in the light of the rarity of both CS and XP there are reports of individuals with features of both syndromes. This provides a strong indication of a causal connection between these disorders.

12.2.3 TRICHOTHIODYSTROPHY

This rare autosomal recessive condition is characterized by sulphur-deficient brittle hair, ichthyosis, physical and mental retardation and abnormal facies [13]. The condition is extremely heterogeneous, and various forms have been given different acronyms, e.g. BIDS, IBIDS, PIBIDS, the latter denoting P(hotosensitivity), I(chthyosis), B(rittle hair), I(mpaired intelligence), D(ecreased fertility) and S(hort stature). In many, but not all, cases photosensitivity is recorded, but the ichthyosis precludes any attempt to assess monochromator tests. There are no reports of skin cancer in association with TTD. No defects were observed in the immune system of one patient studied [6].

12.3 CELLULAR AND BIOCHEMICAL REPAIR STUDIES

12.3.1 XERODERMA PIGMENTOSUM

The first indication of a cellular defect was recorded by Gartler [14] who reported hypersensitivity to the lethal effects of UV-C. In 1968 Cleaver made the major discovery that XP fibroblasts were defective in excision repair of UV-C damage [15]. This was followed shortly by the recognition of a so-called ('variant') form of XP which was clinically indistinguishable but competent in excision repair [16]. Variant fibroblasts were shown subsequently to be defective in daughter strand repair [17] and are minimally hypersensitive to the lethal effects of UV light. Excision-defective XP fibroblasts are also hypersensitive to the lethal action of many chemical carcinogens such as benzo(a)-pyrene or 4-nitroquinoline-1-oxide, which produce bulky lesions in DNA [18]. Hypersensitivity to the lethal action of 254 nm UV light is not limited to XP fibroblasts but has been recorded for lymphoblastoid lines and both unstimulated and stimulated T lymphocytes [19].

Nucleotide excision repair (NER) involves five steps: (i) the recognition of a lesion; (ii) incision of the damaged DNA strand on both sides of the lesion; (iii) removal of the damaged oligonucleotide; (iv) synthesis of new, replacement, DNA using the intact complementary strand as a template; and (v) ligation. The synthesis step (iv) of NER can be monitored conveniently by incorporation of ^{3}H thymidine into non S-phase or non-dividing cells. This is defined as 'unscheduled DNA synthesis' (UDS). Excision-defective XP cells have reduced UDS compared with normal cells at comparable UV dose levels.

NER can be divided into different branches. Damage in the transcribed strands of active genes is repaired most rapidly (transcription-coupled NER), and both strands of active genes are repaired more rapidly than the bulk DNA, which is repaired relatively slowly. These different branches of NER are under the control of different genes.

(a) Complementation groups

The ability of cell cultures from different XP patients to complement each other can be determined by fusing pairwise combinations and measuring levels of UDS in response to UV light (Figure 12.1). This has been extensively used as the basis of a genetic complementation test and to date seven excision-defective complementation groups, A–G, have been assigned to this disease [20]. The excision-proficient XP variants comprise about 20% of cases. In a study on six XP variant strains, only a single complementation group was identified [21].

When complementation studies were first performed, there was much discussion as to whether the various complementation groups represented separate genes or whether intragenic complementation was occurring. Subsequent investigations have identified chromosomal locations for most of the XP complementing genes (see Table 12.1) and show unequivocally that they represent different genes. The structure and function of these genes is described on pages 195–9. There is an uneven distribution of the complementation groups both on the basis of

CELL LINES

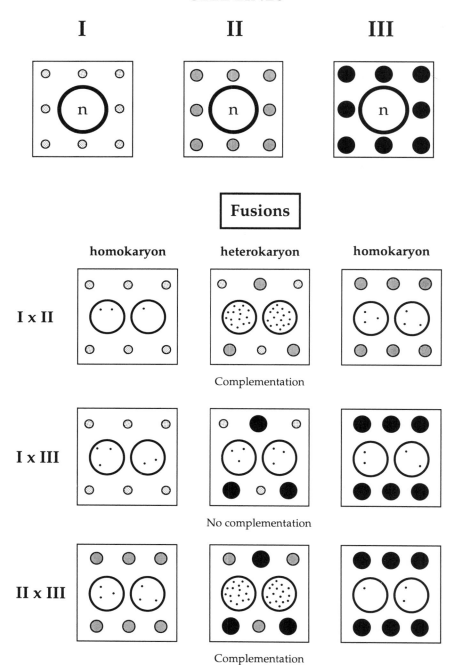

I **II** **III**

Fusions

homokaryon   heterokaryon   homokaryon

I x II

Complementation

I x III

No complementation

II x III

Complementation

their frequency and worldwide occurrence. Groups A, C, D and variant are the most common in Europe and the US, while in Japan groups A and variant are the most common, and groups C and D are rarely observed. The patients in the two known families in group B have the features of both XP and CS, and another four individuals with XP and CS are known, two in group D and two in group G [20].

The presence of DNA repair defects in XP cells has made them a fertile field for repair studies. The injection of T4 endonuclease can restore excision repair to some XP cells and reduce their hypersensitivity to the lethal action of UV light [22]. Similarly, unscheduled DNA synthesis was restored to cells of all complementation groups after microinjection of *Micrococcus luteus* ultraviolet endonuclease [23]. Thus, XP cells are defective at the endonuclease incision step, and this can also be demonstrated in a very rapid test, the single cell microgel assay in which XP cells, because of their defect in the incision step, respond negatively when compared with normal cells [24].

As reviewed in detail elsewhere [20, 25] and summarized in Table 12.1, cell strains from XPs of different complementation groups have different repair characteristics. XP-A cells in general have very low levels of UDS and are most sensitive to killing by UV (see also pages 195–6). XP-D and XP-C cells have significant levels of UDS but XP-C cells are more resistant than XP-D cells. Although the overall level of UDS is severely reduced in XP-C cells, they retain the normal ability to effect the the rapid transcription-coupled

repair of damage in the transcribed strands of active genes [26]. Retention of this crucial activity renders the cells relatively resistant compared with other XP groups. In contrast, the repair deficiency in the XP-D group [27] is distributed in both active and inactive genes, and the cells are relatively sensitive. In XP-F cells repair occurs at a low rate, but is fairly prolonged, so that much of the damage is eventually repaired, and the cells are relatively resistant to UV killing.

(b) Mutability

In vitro mutation experiments measuring UV-C-induced resistance to 6-thioguanine, 8-azaguanine or diphtheria toxin reveal that both excision-defective and excision-competent XP fibroblasts are hypermutable when compared with cells from normal individuals [28–30]. The cells are also hypersensitive to the induction of sister chromatid exchanges (SCE) [31] and chromosome aberrations by UV-C. They do not, however, have an elevated frequency of spontaneous SCE or chromosome aberrations [32].

Mutation spectrum analysis of 6-thioguanine-resistant (hprt⁻) mutants induced by UV-C in both untransformed and SV40-immortalized XP (complemention group A) fibroblasts [33, 34] has shown that the sites of the mutations could largely be assigned to dipyrimidine sequences on the transcribed strand. In contrast, in untransformed normal fibroblasts, although the sites of mutation were again at dipyrimidine sequences the presumptive damage was largely on the non-

Fig. 12.1 Cells, usually fibroblasts, have cytoplasm labelled with latex beads of different sizes (○, ◉, ●). They are fused with polyethylene glycol. Two classes of binuclear cells are produced, homokaryons and heterokaryons, the latter being identified by mixed cytoplasm. The extent of UDS (repair) is reflected as silver grain counts of ³H-thymidine in nuclear track emulsion over the nuclei following UV irradiation (∷∷∷). In the experiment shown in the diagram, donors I and III are in the same complementation group, whereas donor II is in a different group.

Table 12.1 Features of xeroderma pigmentosum (XP), Cockayne syndrome (CS) and trichothiodystrophy (TTD) patients and complementation groups

Complementation group	Clinical manifestations			Chromosomal location	Cellular repair characteristics		
	Skin cancer	Neurological changes	Occurrence[1]		Relative cellular sensitivity to UV-C[2]	Residual UDS[3]	Comments
XP-A	+	++	f	9q34.1	+++	<5	
XP-B	+/-	+++/+	vr	2q21	++	<10	Only three families, two with XP and CS, one with TTD
XP-C	+	+/-	f	3p	+	15–30	Deficient in global genome NER Normal transcription-coupled repair
XP-D	+	++/+	i	19q13.2	++	15–30	Includes patients with TTD, and XP with CS
XP-E	+/-	–	r-i	?11	o-+	>50	
XP-F	+/-	–	r-i	?16p13	o-+	15–30	Repair slow but prolonged
XP-G	+/-	+++/+	r	13q23-33	++	<10	Includes patients with XP and CS
XP-V	+	–	f		o-+	100	Defective in daughter-strand repair NER normal
CS-A	–	++	r		+	100	Defective in preferential repair of active genes Global genome NER normal
CS-B	–	++	f	10q11-21	+	100	Defective in preferential repair of active genes Global genome NER normal
TTD-A	–	++	vr		+-+	25	Defective in NER

[1] Relative occurrence: f, frequent; i, intermediate; r, rare; vr, very rare.
[2] Based on fibroblast survival curve experiments.
[3] Based largely on grain-counting experiments in fibroblasts, expressed as percent of normal cell response to UV-C. UDS, unscheduled DNA synthesis.

transcribed strand of the duplex [34]. This difference may be brought about by preferential repair of damage in the transcribed strand in normal cells. Mutation spectra have also been analysed in a shuttle vector pZ189 passaged in XP or normal cells [35]. A 100-fold increase in UV-C-induced mutant frequency was observed in the marker gene (*supF*) in XP cells and more GC → AT transitions and fewer GC → TA transversions were recorded than in normal cells. These spectra are again consistent with damage at dipyrimidine sites.

Measurement of the frequency of 6-thioguanine-resistant mutants among circulating T-lymphocytes from peripheral blood revealed an elevated mutant frequency for XP patients as a population, whether they were excision-competent or -defective [36]. Molecular spectra of these mutants from one excision-defective (complementation group C) and one excision-competent (variant) XP patient have been compared with five normal donors. Mutations from the excision-defective donor were similar to the normals being largely GC → AT transitions whereas in the variant approximately half the mutations were small deletions [37]. Although most of the mutations occurred at dipyrimidine sites, no strand bias was observed. These data suggested that the enhanced mutant frequency seen in T lymphocytes of XP patients was not generated by exposure to UV-B as cells pass through the skin, although a contribution from this source has not been ruled out. The molecular analysis of mutants from additional XP patients from more complementation groups may be necessary to establish this important point.

(c) Unusual responses

Examples exist of XP patients showing no or little skin cancer. In some cases this may result from relatively limited exposure to sunlight for particular individuals. In addition, secondary control mechanisms such as the enhancement of immune surveillance, or the absence of its suppression may also be important. Two siblings from complementation group B with symptoms of both XP and CS have limited neurological abnormalities, very mild cutaneous symptoms and a complete absence of skin tumours, even after 40 years of making no attempt at sun avoidance, even though their levels of NER are very low [38]. While T lymphocytes and fibroblasts from these individuals are hypersensitive to the lethal effects of UV-C and UV-B, there is no evidence for elevated mutant frequency in blood-derived lymphocytes. There are no data available for UV-induced mutant frequency in these individuals. Two other XP patients XP125LO and XP7NE, from complementation groups G and F respectively, are similarly normal in the mutant frequency amongst circulating T lymphocytes and are free of skin cancer, despite having low levels of NER [39]. In one fascinating case an XP patient has been shown to be a mosaic of normal and XP cells [40].

(d) Paradigm and prospects for management

Taken together the clinical and cellular features of XP present a convincing conjunction of observation and hypothesis. Thus the presence of sun sensitivity, leading to skin damage (including cancer) is correlated with defects in DNA repair and hypermutability, providing convincing support for the mutational theory of cancer induction. Perhaps the most important lesson to be learnt from the study of this disease is that these unfortunate individuals provide us all with a dramatic model of the consequences of excessive exposure to sunlight.

Several hypotheses have been proposed to account for the neurological abnormalities found in some XP patients (e.g. see [41]). We do not discuss these further in this chapter.

The defects in repair can be used to confirm clinical diagnoses which, if achieved early in the life of the individual, can establish a helpful UV light avoidance programme [41]. Successful prenatal diagnosis has also been performed in families with an affected child [43, 44].

As knowledge of XP has progressed, so various routes for its management have become apparent. Clinical observation of skin changes implicates solar irradiation in the aetiology of the disease. Thus, early diagnosis followed by rigorous protection from sunlight or damaging artificial light can, despite the obvious life-style disadvantage, achieve skin and ocular sparing [41]. Significant control of cancer and other skin changes has been achieved with retinoids [45–47]. Here, control is based upon tumour suppression and is believed to be a reflection of chemoprophylaxis of skin tumours in both non-XP and XP patients, and not by correcting any defect in DNA repair. A note of caution should be made with respect to a potential rebound effect as seen in one study [45], such that, following withdrawal of isotretinoin because of adverse side effects, an increase in tumour incidence was observed.

A treatment protocol based on knowledge of repair defects is currently undergoing development and is aimed at delivering an endonuclease repair enzyme via topical liposomes, thereby ameliorating defective excision repair. The possibility that immuno-surveillance is perturbed in XP patients has generated a report of a successful outcome of intralesional α-interferon injection of melanoma in one such patient [9].

12.3.2 COCKAYNE SYNDROME

Cockayne syndrome cells are hypersensitive to the lethal effects of UV-C, although, in general, this is not as marked as in excision-defective XP cells. Their sensitivities to other DNA-damaging agents are broadly similar to those of XP [48]. They are also hypersensitive to the induction of SCE [49]. Both excision repair and daughter strand repair are normal but cells from CS patients may be distinguished from normals by the failure of RNA synthesis to recover following UV irradiation [50]. The defect in recovery of post-ultraviolet RNA synthesis is used both as a confirmation of clinical diagnosis and for prenatal diagnosis [12, 51]. This defect, in combination with normal NER, has allowed the assignment of two complementation groups A and B in this syndrome. Complementation group B is more frequently encountered than A ([52] and unpublished observations of M. Stefanini and A.R. Lehmann).

Although excision repair, as assessed by UDS, is within normal limits in CS cells, the preferential repair of damage in active genes is impaired. All genes are repaired at the relatively slow rate at which the bulk of the DNA is repaired in normal cells. This accounts for the lack of recovery of RNA synthesis after UV exposure and is probably responsible for the increased hypersensitivity to the lethal effects of UV [53].

Considerable efforts have been expended in attempts to determine the mutability of CS cells, but they have been hampered by the tendency of CS fibroblasts to age rapidly on subculture and lose viability. Such data as do exist indicate hypermutability [54], an observation supported by studies of mutation induction in herpes simplex virus grown in lymphoblastoid cultures of CS [55].

The measurements of mutant frequencies in circulating T lymphocytes from CS patients are elevated in comparison with normal controls [56], an observation consistent with the assumption of hypermutability in CS cells.

12.3.3 TRICHOTHIODYSTROPHY

Investigations with fibroblast cultures from these patients have given complex results. The response of TTD cells to UV-irradiation is very heterogeneous [57, 58]. Cells from patients who are not photosensitive are indistinguishable from normal. Cells from photosensitive patients have a wide range of DNA repair capabilities. At one extreme are cell strains which have a very pronounced defect in UDS and are very sensitive to the lethal effects of UV. At the other extreme are two cell strains which are barely sensitive to UV. UDS levels are about 50% of normal and this is attributed to a specific deficiency in the ability of these cells to remove 6–4 photoproducts from their DNA [58]. In nearly all cases the repair deficiency appears to fall in the XP-D complementation group [59]. Very recently, however, cells from one patient, TTD1BR, with a severe repair deficiency, have been shown to complement not only XP complementation group D, but all other XP groups as well. This individual is therefore a representative of a new NER complementation group designated TTD-A [60]. A further family has been recently assigned to XP group B [61].

12.4 XP GENES AND THEIR PRODUCTS

12.4.1 CLONING PROCEDURES

Cloning of the XP genes can, in principle, be accomplished most simply by complementing the UV sensitivity of the XP cells using DNA-mediated gene transfer, and rescuing the complementing DNA. In practice this approach has proven to be extremely difficult because human cell lines are very poor recipients of transfected DNA [62] and only the *XPA* and *XPC* genes have been cloned by this means [63, 64].

A large number of UV-sensitive rodent mutants have been isolated in several laboratories. They have so far been assigned to 11 complementation groups [20] and isolation of the defective genes using gene transfer procedures has proven to be much easier, as the rodent cell-lines often are very efficient recipients for transfection [65]. Six human genes designated *ERCC1–6* have been isolated by their ability to correct the defects in rodent groups 1–6. Several of these genes have proven also to be XP genes [20, 25, 66]. The *XPB, D* and *G* genes have been isolated in this way. A third procedure for cloning XP genes has entailed the isolation of the encoded proteins. This has led to the cloning of the *XPC* gene and a candidate for the *XPE* gene [67, 68].

Determining the function of the individual XP proteins is being investigated by four different routes: (i) Expression and overproduction of the recombinant products of the cloned genes; (ii) *in vitro* complementation using a cell-free system for studying excision repair; (iii) homology to yeast genes; and (iv) the recent serendipitous discovery that several of the XP gene products have a second function as part of a basal transcription factor.

The development of an *in vitro* system for measuring nucleotide excision repair eluded scientists in the field for many years. In 1988 Wood and co-workers [69] successfully developed a system whereby repair of a UV-damaged plasmid could be assayed in cell-free extracts. Most of the repair activity could be attributed to excision of 6–4 photoproducts [70]. This repair activity was deficient in cells from XP groups A→G. Mixing of extracts from different XP complementation groups restored *in vitro* repair activity [71]. This assay for *in vitro* complementation has enabled several XP proteins to be purified.

Properties of the XP genes and their products are summarized in Table 12.2.

Table 12.2 Properties of products and excision-repair genes

Human gene	Cloned	Rodent group	S. cerevisiae homologue	S. pombe homologue	Size of gene (kb)	Size of product (amino acids)	Activity
XPA	+	–	RAD14		25 (6 exons)	273 (31 kDa)	Binds damaged DNA
XPB	+	ERCC3	RAD25	ERCC3^{SP}	45 (>14 exons)	782 (89 kDa)	Helicase. Part of TFIIH
XPC	+		RAD4			940 (125 kDa)	?
XPD	+	ERCC2	RAD3	RAD15	20 (23 exons)	760 (87 kDa)	Helicase. Part of TFIIH
XPE	?+					(127 kDa)	Binds damaged DNA
XPF	–	ERCC4	RAD1	RAD16			Binds to ERCC1 to give structure-specific endonuclease
XPG	+	ERCC5	RAD2	RAD13	32	1196 (133 kDa)	Structure-specific endonuclease
		ERCC1	RAD10	SWI10	15 (10 exons)	297 (33 kDa)	Binds to ERCC4
CSA	–						
CSB	–	ERCC6	RAD26		>85 (21 exons)	1493 (168 kDa)	?DNA helicase ⎱ Couple repair to transcription
TTDA	–						Part of TFIIH

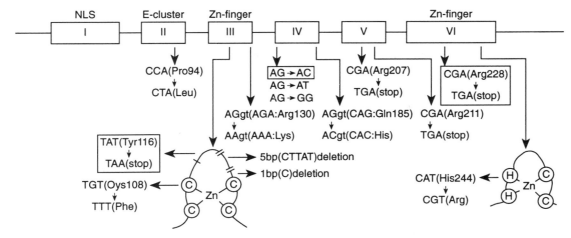

Fig. 12.2 Mutations in XP-A individuals. The top of the diagram shows the exon/intron structure of the gene. Mutations found in Japanese patients are boxed. The two zinc fingers are represented at the bottom. (Reproduced from [75] with permission of Elsevier and K. Tanaka.)

12.4.2 XPA

The *XPA* gene was isolated by transfection of immortalized XP-A cells with a mouse genomic library. In an experiment of heroic dimensions Tanaka and co-workers [63] eventually succeeded in identifying clones of mouse DNA which were able to correct the UV sensitivity of XP-A cells. This in turn led to the identification of the human *XP-A* gene [72]. The gene, located on chromosome 9q34.1 was 25 Kb in length with six exons [73]. It encodes a 31-kDa protein which has 33% sequence identity to the *Saccharomyces cerevisiae RAD14* product over a run of 130 amino acids in the middle of the gene. The 273-amino acid protein contains two zinc finger motifs, a C4 type in the middle of the protein and a C_2H_2 type close to the C-terminus [72, 73]. The XPA protein has also been purified from calf thymus, using the *in vitro* complementation assay [74]. It binds strongly and specifically to UV-irradiated DNA. The recombinant human protein has been studied in detail by Tanaka and co-workers [73, 75]. It also binds to UV-irradiated DNA better than to unirradiated DNA. Deletion of the N-terminal 58 amino acids did not affect the capability of the protein to restore DNA repair activity to XP-A cells, whereas the C-terminus was required for activity. Alteration of the C4 zinc finger by site-directed mutagenesis resulted in loss of much of the repair activity, which could be correlated with loss of DNA binding activity. Further studies showed that exon 1 contained a nuclear localization signal but was not essential for activity, whereas the remaining five exons were essential for activity but did not affect nuclear localization.

A survey of mutations in XP-A patients has been carried out by Tanaka and co-workers [75, 76]. In Japan more than 80% of XP-A patients are homozygous for a G→C substitution at the 3' splice acceptor site of intron 3 [76]. This results in two abnormally spliced forms of mRNA and no active protein. Several different mutations were found in the remaining Japanese patients and in Caucasian XP-As [75]. Their locations are shown in Figure 12.2. The mutations in exon 6 resulted in relatively less marked UV sensitivity and repair defect, and mild clinical symptoms. The other nonsense and frameshift mutations, the mutations affecting splicing and the missense mutation in the zinc finger motif in exon 3 all abolished repair activity and resulted in severe clinical symptoms.

In addition to these comprehensive studies by Tanaka and co-workers, others have attempted to clone the *XPA* gene and have encountered a significant problem with revertants of the XP phenotype to UV-resistance. Virtue has been made of necessity and exploitation of revertants has revealed the biological importance of 6–4 photoproducts. In one such revertant (XP129), UV-sensitivity was similar to that in normal cells despite the fact that most of the cyclobutane pyrimidine dimers appeared to remain unrepaired [77]. Further studies showed that 6–4 photoproducts were repaired normally and cyclobutane dimers in active genes were also repaired. The original mutation in XP12RO was recorded as a conversion of an arginine residue to a termination codon at position 207 (see Figure 12.2). In the revertant culture XP129, this codon has mutated to a glycine residue. The resulting product confers substrate specificity onto the NER pathway [78].

12.4.3 XPB

The *ERCC3* gene was isolated by virtue of its ability to correct the UV-sensitivity of a Chinese hamster cell line which had been assigned to rodent group 3. When a full-length *ERCC3* cDNA was transfected or microinjected into XP cell lines of different complementation groups, it specifically corrected the repair defect in an XP cell strain from group B, strongly suggesting that *ERCC3* was the *XPB* gene [79]. The 45 kb gene contains 14 exons, and the 2.5 kb cDNA encodes a predicted protein of 782 amino acids. The identity of *ERCC3* and *XPB* was confirmed by sequencing of the gene in one of the existing XP-B patients. A mutation,

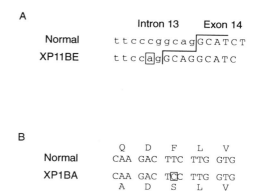

Fig. 12.3 Mutations in XP-B individuals. (a) XP11BE. Upper case, exon sequence; lower case, intron sequence. (b) XP1BA. The mutated bases are boxed. (Data from [39, 79].)

found in one allele of patient XP11BE, was a C→A transversion close to the acceptor site of the C-terminal intron 13 [79]. This caused aberrant splicing of the mRNA, resulting in a 4-base insertion, as shown in Figure 12.3. The C-terminal 42 amino acids, are therefore out of frame. This allele, inherited from the patient's mother is the only one expressed in this cell strain. In two brothers from a second XP-B family, who showed only very mild symptoms (see page 191), the causative mutation in the only expressed allele was a T→C transition resulting in a Phe to Ser change in exon 3 (Figure 12.3) [39].

12.4.4 XPC

The *XPC* gene was first cloned by transfection of an immortalized line with an Epstein–Barr virus-based cDNA library followed by selection for UV-resistance. One resistant cell line was obtained, from which the episomally maintained complementing plasmid was rescued. It contained a 3.5-kb insert which was able to complement fully and specifically the repair deficiency of XPC cell lines [64]. The mRNA encoded by this insert was absent or much reduced in four XP–C cell lines. The

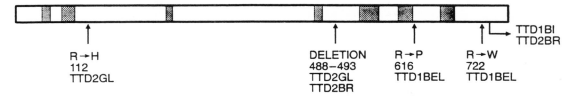

Fig. 12.4 Mutations in the *XPD* gene in four TTD individuals. The *XPD* gene is shown with the seven helicase domains shaded. The alterations in amino acid sequence are shown → represents a frameshift caused by a −G deletion. Designations such as TTD2GL refer to different cell strains. (Data from [89].)

sequence encoded by the insert contained an ORF of 823 amino acids. Recently however, using the *in vitro* complementation assay, an activity which was able to correct the DNA repair deficiency in XP-C extracts was purified by Hanaoka and co-workers [67]. It contained a large and a small subunit. Using oligonucleotide hybridization, the genes encoding these subunits were isolated. The gene encoding the large subunit was identical to that obtained by Legerski and Peterson [64], except that it was substantially longer at the 5′ end. This suggested that the open reading frame (ORF) was in fact considerably longer at the N-terminus, encoding a protein of approximately 940 amino acids. The smaller subunit was found to be a human homologue of the *S. cerevisiae RAD23* gene [67]. As yet, the precise enzymatic activity of the XPC protein has not been identified. Six mutations have been identified in five XP-C donors [80]. In contrast to mutations found in other XP genes, the majority of these mutations were frameshifts (two −2, one +3, one +83), the other two being base-changes.

12.4.5 XPD

The *ERCC2* gene, cloned by its ability to complement rodent group 2 mutants [81], was able to correct the UV sensitivity of XPD [82, 83] and TTD cells [84]. The *XPD* gene is highly homologous to the *RAD3* gene of *S. cerevisiae* and the *rad15* gene of *Schizosaccharomyces pombe* [81, 85]. The sequence of the encoded protein contains seven domains characteristic of DNA helicases, and indeed the RAD3 protein, and more recently the XPD protein have been shown to have ATP-dependent DNA helicase activity [86, 87]. Both yeast genes and the human gene have essential functions, which at least in *RAD3*, was separable from the repair function [88]. A variety of point mutations have been identified in TTD patients [89]. Their locations relative to the helicase domains are shown in Figure 12.4. A frameshift close to the C-terminus resulted in a mild deficiency in DNA repair, suggesting that the last 30 amino acid were not essential for repair ability. In contrast, several other mutations, which were found in highly conserved areas of the gene, resulted in very severe repair deficiencies [89].

12.4.6 XPE

In 1988 Chu and Chang reported that a protein which bound specifically to DNA damaged by UV light or cisplatin was absent in an XP-E cell strain [90]. This finding was reproduced in several other laboratories, but in an extensive survey this DNA binding activity was defective in only three out of 12 individuals assigned to the XPE group [91]. The purified UV-damaged DNA-binding protein has a molecular weight of 127 KDa, and is isolated complexed with a 41-kDa protein. When the purified protein was microinjected into an XP-E cell strain, which was lacking the binding activity, normal DNA repair synthesis was restored [92]. This demonstrated that the deficiency in this protein is indeed responsible for the repair defect. The 4.2-kB cDNA encoding the binding protein has recently been cloned and sequenced. It locates to chromosome 11 [68]. Until a mutation has been identified in this gene in an XP-E patient, it must still be regarded as a candidate gene.

12.4.7 XPF

Work on DNA repair genes from *S. cerevisiae* has shown that the products of the *RAD*1 and *RAD*10 genes interact to form a tight complex which has single-stranded exonuclease activity [93]. The human homologue of *RAD*10 is the *ERCC*1 gene. The *ERCC*1 gene is not able to correct the repair defect in cells from any of the human syndromes [94] and does not therefore correspond to any of the known XP, CS or TTD genes. Using the *in vitro* complementation assay it was found that the *ERCC*1 and *ERCC*4 gene products formed a tight complex, which also co-purified with the XP-F complementing activity [95, 96]. These results suggest that either the *XPF* gene may be identical to the *ERCC*4 gene, or that the XPF protein is closely associated with an ERCC1/ERCC4 complex.

12.4.8 XPG

The *XPG* gene was cloned independently in two different ways. Screening of a Xenopus cDNA library with serum from a patient with systemic lupus erythematosus resulted, by chance, in the isolation of a cDNA, whose predicted product showed sequence homology to that of *RAD*2, an excision repair gene from *S. cerevisiae*. The homologous human cDNA was isolated and was able to restore UV-sensitivity to an XPG cell line [97]. Independently the *ERCC*5 gene cloned by

MacInnes *et al.* [98] was found to be a human homologue of *RAD*2, and O'Donovan and Wood [99] showed by *in vitro* complementation that *XPG* and *ERCC*5 were identical. The *XPG* (*ERCC*5) gene is about 32 kb in length and encodes a protein of 1196 amino acids, which is homologous to the products of the *RAD*2 gene of *S. cerevisiae* and the *RAD*13 gene of *S. pombe* [97, 98]. The sequence identity between the three organisms is highest in two regions of about 70 amino acids close to the termini of the protein. The spacing between these two regions is also conserved between the three organisms, even though there is little similarity in the intervening sequence. These observations suggest that these two domains are crucial for the function of the proteins. The XPG protein has recently been purified and found to have structure-specific endonuclease activity [100]. The properties of the protein make it ideally suited to cleave a damaged DNA molecule on the 3' side of the damaged site.

12.4.9 EXCISION REPAIR AND TRANSCRIPTION – XPB, XPD AND TTD GENES

The product of the *XPB* (*ERCC*3) gene was discovered from an unexpected quarter. Its sequence, like that of the XPD protein, contained seven domains characteristic of DNA helicases, suggesting that the protein had helicase activity [79]. The *S. cerevisiae* homologue was found to be an essential gene, which apart from its role in excision repair, was involved in control of translation by permitting translation through an artificially induced stem-loop structure. The yeast gene was termed *SSL*2 [101] or *RAD*25 [102]. The *Drosophila* homologue of the *XPB* gene was found to be the '*haywire*' gene [103]. '*Haywire*' mutants, as well as being UV-sensitive, had CNS deficiencies and abnormalities in β-tubulins in sperm. The clue to the relationships between these complex phenotypes came from work on transcription factors.

The transcription factor TFIIH is involved in basal transcription and is part of a multifactor system whereby RNA polymerase II is loaded on to a promoter to initiate transcription. TFIIH itself is a complex protein comprised of a minimum of five different subunits. The 89-kDa subunit was purified, and found to have helicase activity [104]. Partial sequencing enabled the gene to be cloned. Sequencing of this gene revealed, most unexpectedly, that it was identical to the *XPB* (*ERCC*3) gene [104]. Subsequent studies showed that TFIIH, when microinjected into cells or added to cell extracts was able to restore repair activity not only to XP-B [105] but also to XP-D cells and to TTD-A cells [61]. These and other results [106, 107] provided compelling evidence that the products of the *XPD*, *XPB*, *TTDA* and other genes combine to form the TFIIH complex which has two separate roles, in basal transcription and in excision repair. This complex has two helicase activities, one 3′–5′ associated with the *XPB* gene [104], the other 5′–3′ with the *XPD* gene [87], although only the former (at least in yeast) appears to be necessary for the essential role in transcription [88].

12.4.10 SUMMARY

The current model for excision repair involves several interacting proteins. The XPA protein and the candidate XPE protein each bind specifically to UV-irradiated DNA and may be candidates for initiating excision repair. The XPA protein has recently been shown to bind *in vitro* to the ERCC1 protein [108, 109], which in turn is known to form a tight complex with the ERCC4 (XPF) protein (see earlier). It is likely therefore that the XPA protein, after binding to the DNA damage, is able to recruit the ERCC1/ERCC4 nuclease. The specificity of this nuclease is such that it could cleave 5′ to the damage [110], and as

discussed above it is likely that the XPG protein cleaves 3′ to the damage. The function of the helicase activities of the XPB and XPD proteins within the TFIIH complex may be to unwind the DNA in the damaged region and render it susceptible to cleavage by the above-mentioned nucleases. The role of the XPC protein is as yet uncertain.

12.5 RELATIONSHIP TO CLINICAL SYMPTOMS

In considering the relationship of DNA repair defects to the clinical features of XP, CS and TTD, we need to consider several questions:

1. What is the relationship of defective DNA repair to the clinical features of XP?
2. How can mutations in *XPB* (in two of the three known families), *XPD* and *XPG* (occasionally) result in the features of XP and CS?
3. How can mutations in *XPD* result in the features of XP alone, XP with CS or TTD?

Cellular and biochemical studies discussed on pages 189–91 demonstrated that in XP cells, defective excision or daughter strand repair is associated with UV-hypermutability of cultured fibroblasts. This has led to the hypothesis that a high frequency of sunlight-induced mutations in the skin of XP patients is the cause of the freckling and high incidence of skin cancer in these patients. The observations that a large proportion of basal and squamous cell carcinomas in normal individuals contain mutations in the *TP*53 gene with a spectrum characteristic of that produced by UV light [111], and that skin tumour cells from many XP patients also contain UV-type mutations in the *TP*53 gene [112] are consistent with this hypothesis. A sunlight-induced mutation in *TP*53 appears, therefore, to be a crucial event in skin carcinogenesis, and will occur at a greatly elevated frequency in XP patients. This hypothesis is neat, coherent and satisfactorily accounts for the skin abnormalities in XP. Less clear, however, is the explanation for the clinical features of TTD, and in particular the lack of freckling and skin cancer in TTD patients, even though the cultured fibroblasts have a repair deficiency, and in some cases UV mutability, indistinguishable from that in XP cells.

The brittle hair, ichthyosis and other features of TTD are not related in any obvious way to a DNA repair deficiency. The clue to their possible aetiology comes from the recent findings discussed on pages 198–9 that the gene products defective in the three known TTD complementation groups are probably all subunits of the transcription factor TFIIH. It is thus likely that the clinical features of TTD might result from subtle deficiencies in transcription, which are not manifest in cultured fibroblasts, but may have more marked effects in specific tissues, e.g. abnormal keratin expression in hairshaft cells, resulting in trichothiodystrophy [61, 113]. Mutations in the *XPD* gene can result in the clinical features either of XP or of TTD but not of both. We can therefore envisage that a mutation affecting the DNA repair capability of the TFIIH complex will result in XP, whereas mutations affecting transcription (and repair?) will result in TTD. A necessary but difficult to understand postulate of this hypothesis is that a defect affecting the transcription activity in TTD also prevents the development of skin cancer resulting from the UV hypermutability consequent upon the defect in DNA repair.

Cockayne's syndrome poses further problems. The disorder is associated with a specific deficiency in the ability to carry out the rapid repair of damage in the transcribed strand of active genes. The *CSB* gene has been cloned (see Table 12.2) and appears not to be essential. The features of XP and CS are found in both families in the rare XP-B group and in two families in each of the more

common XP-D and XP-G groups [20]. The yeast homologues of the *XPG* gene are not essential, whereas the essential XPB and XPD products are subunits of TFIIH. The latter would suggest that the features of CS may also result from a deficiency in transcription, as suggested for TTD. Indeed, the two disorders do appear to have some features in common, e.g. mental and physical retardation, cataracts, dental caries, abnormal facies. However, the specific hairshaft abnormalities seen in TTD have not been found in CS, nor has ichthyosis been reported. The neurological abnormalities in CS are progressive whereas this does not appear to be the case for TTD. Furthermore, any gene whose product is directly involved in basal transcription must be essential. A self-consistent explanation for the features of CS is therefore still lacking at the time of writing.

The rapid progress currently being made in cloning of DNA repair genes and understanding the precise roles of the gene products should help to unravel the complex interrelationships associated with the disorders discussed in this chapter. These studies are not only contributing to our understanding of the mechanisms of carcinogenesis, but the association of DNA repair proteins with transcription factors may reveal a new category of transcription-related disorders [61, 113].

ACKNOWLEDGEMENTS

We are indebted to B.A. Bridges for his helpful critical comments.

REFERENCES

1. Kraemer, K. H. and Slor, H. (1984) Xeroderma pigmentosum. *Clin. Dermatol.*, **2**, 33–69.
2. Lehmann, A. R. (1987) Cockayne's syndrome and trichothiodystrophy: defective repair without cancer. *Cancer Rev.*, **7**, 82–103.

3. Ramsay, C. A. and Giannelli, F. (1975) The erythemal action spectrum and deoxyribonucleic acid repair synthesis in xeroderma pigmentosum. *Br. J. Dermatol.*, **92**, 49–56.

4. Kraemer, K. H., Lee, M. M. and Scotto, J. (1987) Xeroderma pigmentosum. Cutaneous, ocular and neurologic abnormalities in 830 published cases. *Arch. Dermatol.*, **123**, 241–50.

5. Kraemer, K. H., Lee, M. M. and Scotto, K. (1984) DNA repair protects against cutaneous and internal neoplasia: Evidence from xeroderma pigmentosum. *Carcinogenesis*, **5**, 511–14.

6. Norris, P. G., Limb, G. A., Hamblin, A. S. *et al.* (1990) Immune function, mutant frequency and cancer risk in the DNA repair defective genodermatoses xeroderma pigmentosum, Cockayne's syndrome and trichothiodystrophy. *J. Invest. Dermatol.*, **94**, 94–100.

7. Gaspari, A. A., Fleisher, T. A. and Kraemer, K. H. (1993) Impaired interferon production and natural killer cell activation in patients with the skin cancer prone disorder, xeroderma pigmentosum. *J. Clin. Invest.*, **92**, 1135–42.

8. Anstey, A., Arlett, C. F., Cole, J. *et al.* (1991) Long term survival and preservation of natural killer cell activity in a xeroderma pigmentosum patient with spontaneous regression and multiple deposits of malignant melanoma. *Br. J. Dermatol.*, **125**, 272–8.

9. Turner, M.L., Moshell, A., Corbett, D.W. *et al.* (1993) Clearing of melanoma-in-situ with intralesional α-interferon in a patient with xeroderma pigmentosum. *J. Invest. Dermatol.*, **100**, 538.

10. Krutmann, J., Bohnert, E. and Jung, E.G. (1994) Evidence that DNA damage is a mediate in ultraviolet B radiation – Induced inhibition of human gene expression: Ultraviolet B radiation effects on intercellular adhesion molecule-1 (ICAM-1) expression. *J. Invest. Dermatol.*, **102**, 428–32.

11. Nance, M.A. and Berry, S.A. (1992) Cockayne syndrome: review of 140 cases. *Am. J. Med. Genet.*, **42**, 68–84.

12. Lehmann, A.R., Thompson, A.F., Harcourt, S.A., Stefanini, M. and Norris, P.G. (1993) Cockayne's syndrome; correlation of clinical features with cellular sensitivity of RNA synthesis to UV-irradiation. *J. Med. Genet.*, **30**, 679–82.

13. Itin, P.H. and Pittelkow, M.R. (1990) Trichothiodystrophy: review of sulfur-deficient brittle hair syndromes and association with the ectodermal dysplasias. *J. Am. Acad. Dermatol.*, **20**, 705–17.

14. Gartler, S.M. (1964) Inborn errors of metabolism at the cell culture level, in *Second International Conference on Congenital Malformations*, (ed. M. Fishbein), International Medical Congress, New York, p. 94.

15. Cleaver, J.E. (1968) Deficiency in repair replication of DNA in xeroderma pigmentosum. *Nature*, **218**, 652–6.

16. Cleaver, J.E. (1972) Xeroderma pigmentosum: variants with normal DNA repair and normal sensitivity to uv light. *J. Invest. Dermatol.*, **58**, 124–8.

17. Lehmann, A.R., Kirk-Bell, S., Arlett, C.F. *et al.* (1975) Xeroderma pigmentosum cells with normal levels of excision repair have a defect in DNA synthesis after UV-irradiation. *Proc. Natl Acad. Sci. USA*, **72**, 219–23.

18. Maher, V.M., McCormick, J.J., Grover, P. and Sims, P. (1977) Effect of DNA on the cytotoxicity and mutagenicity of polycyclic hydrocarbon derivatives in normal and xeroderma pigmentosum human fibroblasts. *Mutat. Res.*, **43**, 117–38.

19. Arlett, C.F., Lowe, J.E., Harcourt, S.A. *et al.* (1993) Hypersensitivity of human lymphocytes to UV-B and solar irradiation. *Cancer Res.*, **53**, 609–14.

20. Hoeijmakers, J.H.J. (1993) Nucleotide excision repair II: from yeast to mammals. *Trends Genet.*, **9**, 211–17.

21. Jaspers, N.G.J., Jansen-van De Kuilen, G. and Bootsma, D. (1981) Complementation analysis of xeroderma pigmentosum variants. *Exp. Cell Res.*, **136**, 81–90.

22. Tanaka, K., Sekiguchi, M. and Okada, Y. (1975) Restoration of ultraviolet-induced unscheduled DNA synthesis of xeroderma pigmentosum cells by the concomitant treatment with bacteriophage T4 endonuclease V and HVJ (Sendai virus). *Proc. Natl Acad. Sci. USA*, **72**, 4071–5.

23. De Jonge, A.J.R., Vermeulen, W., Klein, B. and Hoeijmakers, J.H.J. (1985) Microinjection

of *Micrococcus luteus* UV-endonuclease restores UV-induced unscheduled DNA synthesis in cells of 9 xeroderma pigmentosum complementation groups. *Mutat. Res.*, **150**, 99–105.

24. Green, M.H.L., Lowe, J.E., Harcourt, S.A. *et al.* (1992) UV-C sensitivity of unstimulated and stimulated human lymphocytes from normal and xeroderma pigmentosum donors in the Comet Assay: a potential diagnostic technique. *Mutat. Res.*, **273**, 137–44.

25. Weeda, G. and Hoeijmakers J.H.J. (1993) Genetic analysis of nucleotide excision repair in mammalian cells. *Semin. Cancer Biol.*, **4**, 105–17.

26. Venema, J., Van Hoffen, A., Karcagi, V., Natarajan, A.T., Van Zeeland, A.A. and Mullenders, L.H.F. (1991) Xeroderma pigmentosum complementation group C cells remove pyrimidine dimers selectively from the transcribed strand of active genes. *Mol. Cell. Biol.*, **11**, 4128–34.

27. Johnson R.T. and Squires S. (1992) The XP-D complementation group. Insight into xeroderma pigmentosum, Cockayne's syndrome, and trichothiodystrophy. *Mutat. Res.*, **273**, 97–118.

28. Maher, V.M. and McCormick, J.J. (1976) Effect of DNA repair on the cytotoxicity and mutagenicity of UV irradiation and of chemical carcinogens in normal and xeroderma pigmentosum cells, in: *Biology of Radiation Carcinogenesis*, (eds J.M. Yuhas, R.W. Tennant and J.B. Regan), Raven Press, New York, pp. 129–45.

29. Arlett, C.F. and Harcourt, S.A. (1983) Variation in response to mutagens amongst normal and repair- defective human cells, in *Induced Mutagenesis. Molecular Mechanisms and their Implications for Environmental Protection*, (ed. C.W. Lawrence), Plenum Press, New York, pp. 249–66.

30. Glover, T.W., Chang, C.-C., Trosko, J.F. and Li, S.S.-I. (1979) Ultraviolet light induction of diphtheria toxin-resistant mutants in normal and xeroderma pigmentosum human fibroblasts. *Proc. Natl Acad. Sci. USA*, **76**, 3982–6.

31. De Weerd-Kastelein, E.A., Keijzer, W., Rainaldi, G. and Bootsma, D. (1977) Induction of sister chromatid exchanges in xeroderma pigmentosum cells after exposure to ultraviolet light. *Mutat. Res.*, **45**, 253–61.

32. Marshall, R.R. and Scott, D. (1976) The relationship between chromosome damage and cell killing in UV-irradiated normal and xeroderma pigmentosum cells. *Mutat. Res.*, **36**, 397–400.

33. Dorado, G., Steingrimsdottir, H., Arlett, C.F. and Lehmann, A.R. (1991) Molecular analysis of UV-induced mutations in a xeroderma pigmentosum cell line. *J. Mol. Biol.*, **217**, 217–22.

34. McGregor, W.G., Chen, R.-H., Lukash, L., Maher, V.M. and McCormick, J.J. (1991) Cell cycle-dependent strand bias for UV-induced mutations in the transcribed strand of excision repair-proficient human fibroblasts but not in repair deficient cells. *Mol. Cell. Biol.*, **11**, 1927–34.

35. Bredberg, A., Kraemer, K.H. and Seidman, M.M. (1986) Restricted ultraviolet mutational spectrum in a shuttle vector propagated in xeroderma pigmentosum cells. *Proc. Natl Acad. Sci. USA*, **83**, 8273–7.

36. Cole, J., Arlett, C.F., Norris, P.G. *et al.* (1992) Elevated *hprt* mutant frequency in circulating T-lymphocytes of xeroderma pigmentosum patients. *Mutat. Res.*, **273**, 171–8.

37. Steingrimsdottir, H., Rowley, G., Waugh, A. *et al.* (1993) Molecular analysis of mutations in the *hprt* gene in circulating lymphocytes from normal and DNA-repair-deficient donors. *Mutat. Res.*, **294**, 29–41.

38. Scott, R.J., Itin, P., Kleijer, W.J., Kolb, K., Arlett, C. and Muller, H. (1993) Xeroderma pigmentosum–Cockayne syndrome complex in two, new patients: absence of skin tumors despite severe deficiency of DNA excision repair. *J. Am. Acad. Dermatol.*, **29**, 883–9.

39. Vermeulen, W., Scott, R.J., Potger, S. *et al.* (1994) Clinical heterogeneity within xeroderma pigmentosum associated with mutations in the DNA repair and transcription gene ERCC3. *Am. J. Hum. Genet.*, **54**, 191–200.

40. Chang, H.R., Ishizaki, K., Sasaki, M.S. *et al.* (1989) Somatic mosaicism for DNA repair capacity in fibroblasts derived from a group A xeroderma pigmentosum patient. *J. Invest. Dermatol.*, **93**, 460–5.

41. Kraemer, K.H. (1980) Xeroderma pigmentosum, in *Clinical Dermatology*. Vol. 4, (eds D.J. Demis, R.L. Dobson and J. McGuire), Harper and Row, Hagerstown, pp. 1–33.

42. Robbins, J.H. (1988) Defective DNA repair in xeroderma pigmentosum and other neurologic diseases. *Curr. Opin. Neurol. Neurosurg.*, **1**, 1077–83.

43. Halley, D.J.J., Keijzer, W., Jaspers, N.G.J. *et al.* (1979) Prenatal diagnosis of xeroderma pigmentosum (group C) using assays of unscheduled DNA synthesis and postreplication repair. *Clin. Genet.*, **16**, 137–46.

44. Ramsay, C.A., Coltart, T.M., Blunt, S., Pawsey, S.A. and Giannelli, F. (1974) Prenatal diagnosis of xeroderma pigmentosum. *Lancet*, **ii**, 1109–12.

45. Kraemer, K.H., DiGiovanna, J.J., Moshell, A.N., Tarone, R.E. and Peck, G.L. (1988) Prevention of skin cancer in xeroderma pigmentosum with the use of oral isotretinoin. *N. Engl. J. Med.*, **318**, 1633–7.

46. Strong, A. (1989) Xeroderma pigmentosum variant: prevention of cutaneous neoplasms with etretinate. *Retinoids*, **17**, 40–2.

47. Berth-Jones, J., Cole, J., Lehmann, A.R., Arlett, C.F. and Graham-Brown, R.A.C. (1993) Xeroderma pigmentosum variant: 5 years of tumor suppression by etretinate. *J.R. Soc. Med.*, **86**, 355–6.

48. Wade, M.H. and Chu, E.H.Y. (1979) Effects of DNA damaging agents on cultured fibroblasts derived from patients with Cockayne syndrome. *Mutat. Res.*, **59**, 49–60.

49. Marshall, R.R., Arlett, C.F., Harcourt, S.A. and Broughton, B.C. (1980) Increased sensitivity of cell strains from Cockayne's syndrome to sister-chromatid-exchange induction and cell killing by UV light. *Mutat. Res.*, **69**, 107–12.

50. Mayne, L.V. and Lehmann, A.R. (1982) Failure of RNA synthesis to recover after UV-irradiation: an early defect in cells from individuals with Cockayne's syndrome and xeroderma pigmentosum. *Cancer Res.*, **42**, 1473–8.

51. Lehmann, A.R., Francis, A.J. and Giannelli, F. (1985) Prenatal diagnosis of Cockayne's syndrome. *Lancet*, **i**, 486–8.

52. Lehmann, A.R. (1982) Three complementation groups in Cockayne syndrome. *Mutat. Res.*, **106**, 347–56.

53. Venema, J., Mullenders, L.H.F., Natarajan, A.T., Van Zeeland, A.A. and Mayne, L.V. (1990) The genetic defect in Cockayne's syndrome is associated with a defect in repair of uv-induced DNA damage in transcriptionally active DNA. *Proc. Natl Acad. Sci. USA*, **87**, 4707–11.

54. Arlett, C.F. and Cole, J. (1989) Photosensitive human syndromes and cellular defects in DNA repair, in *Ozone Depletion: Health and Environmental Consequences*, (eds R. Russell Jones and T. Wigley), Wiley and Sons Ltd, Chichester, pp. 147–60.

55. Henderson, E.E. and Long, W.K. (1981) Host cell reactivation of UV- and X-ray-damaged herpes simplex virus by Epstein-Barr virus (EBV)-transformed lymphoblastoid cell lines. *Virology*, **115**, 237–48.

56. Norris, P.G., Lehmann, A., Cole, J., Arlett, C.F., and Hawk, J.L.M. (1991) Photosensitivity and lymphocyte hypermutability in Cockayne's syndrome. *Br. J. Dermatol.*, **124**, 453–60.

57. Lehmann, A.R., Arlett, C.F., Broughton, B.C. *et al.* (1988) Trichothiodystrophy, a human DNA repair disorder with heterogeneity in the cellular response to ultraviolet light. *Cancer Res.*, **48**, 6090–96.

58. Broughton, B.C., Lehmann, A.R., Harcourt, S.A. *et al.* (1990) Relationship between pyrimidine dimers, 6–4 photoproducts, repair synthesis and cell survival: studies using cells from patients with trichothiodystrophy. *Mutat. Res.*, **235**, 33–40.

59. Stefanini M., Lagomarsini, P., Giliani, S. *et al.* (1993) Genetic heterogeneity of the excision repair defect associated with trichothiodystrophy. *Carcinogenesis*, **14**, 1101–5.

60. Stefanini, M., Vermeulen, W., Weeda, G. *et al.* (1993) A new nucleotide excision repair gene associated with the genetic disorder trichothiodystrophy. *Am. J. Hum. Genet.*, **53**, 817–21.

61. Vermeulen, W., Van Vuuren, A.J., Chipoulet, M. *et al.*, (1994) Three excision repair proteins in transcription factor BTF2(TFIIH). Evidence for the existence of a transcription syndrome.

Cold Spring Harbor Symp. Quant. Biol., **59**, 317–29.

62. Mayne, L.V., Jones, T., Dean, S.W. *et al.* (1988) SV40-transformed normal and DNA-repair-deficient human fibroblasts can be transfected with high frequency but retain only limited amounts of integrated DNA. *Gene*, **66**, 65–76.

63. Tanaka, K., Satokato, I., Ogita, Z., Uchida, T. and Okada, Y. (1989) Molecular cloning of a mouse DNA repair gene that complements the defect of group-A xeroderma pigmentosum. *Proc. Natl Acad. Sci. USA*, **86**, 5512–16.

64. Legerski, R. and Peterson, C. (1992) Expression cloning of a human DNA repair gene involved in xeroderma pigmentosum group C. *Nature*, **359**, 70–3.

65. Hoeijmakers, J.H.J., Odijk, H. and Westerveld, A. (1987) Differences between rodent and human cell lines in the amount of integrated DNA after transfection. *Exp. Cell Res.*, **169**, 111–19.

66. Hoeijmakers, J.H.J. and Bootsma, D. (1990) Molecular genetics of eukaryotic DNA excision repair. *Cancer Cells*, **2**, 311-20.

67. Masutani, C., Sugasawa, K., Yanagisawa, J. *et al.* (1994) Purification and cloning of a nucleotide excision-repair complex involving the xeroderma-pigmentosum group-C protein and a human homolog of yeast rad23. *EMBO J.*, **13**, 1831–43

68. Takao, M., Abramic, M., Moos, M. *et al.* (1993) A 127 KDa component of a UV-damaged DNA-binding complex, which is defective in some xeroderma-pigmentosum group-E patients, is homologous to a slime-mould protein. *Nucleic Acids Res.*, **21**, 4111–18.

69. Wood, R.D., Robins, P. and Lindahl, T. (1988) Complementation of the xeroderma pigmentosum DNA repair defect in cell-free extracts. *Cell*, **53**, 97–106.

70. Wood, R.D. (1989) Repair of pyrimidine dimer ultraviolet light photoproducts by human cell extracts. *Biochemistry*, **28**, 8287–92.

71. Biggerstaff, M. and Wood, R.D. (1992) Requirement for ERCC-1 and ERCC-3 gene products in DNA excision repair in vitro.

Complementation using rodent and human cell extracts. *J. Biol. Chem.*, **267**, 6879–85.

72. Tanaka, K., Naoyuki, M., Satokata, I. *et al.* (1990) Analysis of a human DNA excision repair gene involved in group A xeroderma pigmentosum and containing a zinc-finger domain. *Nature*, **348**, 73–6.

73. Miyamoto, I., Miura, N., Niwa, H., Miyazaki, J. and Tanaka, K. (1992) Mutational analysis of the structure and function of the xeroderma pigmentosum group A complementing protein. Identification of essential domains for nuclear localisation and DNA excision repair. *J. Biol. Chem.*, **267**, 12182–7

74. Robins, P., Jones, C.J., Biggerstaff, M., Lindahl. T. and Wood, R.D. (1991) Complementation of DNA repair in xeroderma pigmentosum group A cell extracts by a protein with affinity for damaged DNA. *EMBO J.*, **10**, 3913–21.

75. Tanaka, K. (1993) Analysis of DNA excision repair genes in XP, in *Frontiers of Photobiology*, (eds A. Shima, M. Ichahashi, Y. Fujiwara and H. Takebe), Excerpta Medica, Amsterdam, pp.293–302.

76. Satokata, I., Tanaka, K., Miura, N. *et al.* (1990) Characterization of a splicing mutation in group A xeroderma pigmentosum. *Proc. Natl Acad. Sci. USA*, **87**, 9908–12.

77. Cleaver, J.E., Cortes, F., Lutze, L.H., Morgan, W.F., Player, A.N. and Mitchell, D.L. (1987) Unique DNA repair properties of a xeroderma pigmentosum revertant. *Mol. Cell. Biol.*, **7**, 3353–7.

78. McDowell, L., Nguyen, T. and Cleaver, J.E. (1993) A single-site mutation in the *XPAC* gene alters photoproduct recognition. *Mutagenesis*, **8**, 155–61.

79. Weeda, G., Van Ham, R.C.A., Vermeulen, W., Bootsma, D., Van Der Eb, A. J. and Hoeijmakers, J.H.J. (1990) A presumed DNA helicase encoded by *ERCC-3* is involved in the human repair disorders xeroderma pigmentosum and Cockayne's syndrome. *Cell*, **62**, 777–91.

80. Li, L., Bales, E.S., Peterson, C.A. and Legerski, R.J. (1993) Characterization of molecular defects in xeroderma pigmentosum group C. *Nature Genet.*, **5**, 413–7.

81. Weber, C.A., Salazar, E.P., Stewart, S.A.

and Thompson, L.H. (1990) *ERCC-2*: cDNA cloning and molecular characterization of a human nucleotide excision repair gene with high homology to yeast RAD3. *EMBO J.*, **9**, 1437–48.

82. Gozukara, E.M., Parris, C.N., Weber, C.A. *et al.* (1994) The human DNA repair gene, *ERCC2* (XPD), corrects ultraviolet hypersensitivity and ultraviolet hypermutability of a shuttle vector replicated in xeroderma pigmentosum group D cells. *Cancer Res.*, **54**, 3837–44.

83. Flejter, W.L., McDaniel, L.D., Johns, D., Friedberg, E.C. and Schultz R.A. (1992) Correction of xeroderma pigmentosum complementation group D mutant cell phenotypes by chromosome and gene transfer: involvement of the human *ERCC2* DNA repair gene. *Proc. Natl Acad. Sci. USA*, **89**, 261–5.

84. Mezzina, M., Eveno, E., Chevallier Lagente, O. *et al.* (1994) Correction by the ERCC2 gene of UV sensitivity and repair deficiency phenotype in a subset of trichothiodystrophy cells. *Carcinogenesis*, **15**, 1493–8.

85. Murray, J.M., Doe, C., Schenk, P., Carr, A.M., Lehmann, A.R. and Watts, F.Z. (1992) Cloning and characterisation of the *S. pombe rad 15* gene, a homologue to the *S. cerevisiae RAD3* and human *ERCC2* genes. *Nucleic Acids Res.*, **20**, 2673–8.

86. Sung, P., Prakash, L., Matson, S.W. and Prakash, S. (1987) *RAD3* protein of *Saccharomyces cerevisiae* is a DNA helicase. *Proc. Natl Acad. Sci. USA*, **84**, 8951–5.

87. Sung, P., Bailly, V., Weber, C., Thompson, L.H., Prakash, L. and Prakash, S. (1993) Human xeroderma pigmentosum group D gene encodes a DNA helicase. *Nature*, **365**, 852–5.

88. Song, J.M., Montelone, B.A., Siede, W. and Friedberg, E.C. (1990) Effects of multiple *rad3* alleles on UV sensitivity, mutability, and mitotic recombination. *J. Bacteriol.*, **172**, 6620–30.

89. Broughton, B.C., Steingrimsdottir, H., Weber, C. and Lehmann, A.R. (1994) Mutations in the xeroderma pigmentosum group D DNA repair/transcription gene in patients with trichothiodystrophy. *Nature Genet.*, **7**, 189–94.

90. Chu, G. and Chang, E. (1988) Xeroderma pigmentosum group E cells lack a nuclear factor that binds to damaged DNA. *Science*, **242**, 564–7.

91. Keeney, S., Wein, H. and Linn, S. (1992) Biochemical heterogeneity in xeroderma pigmentosum complementation group E. *Mutat. Res.*, **273**, 49–56.

92. Keeney, S., Eker, A.P.M., Brody, T. *et al.* (1994) Correction of the DNA repair defect in xeroderma pigmentosum group E by injection of a DNA damage-binding protein. *Proc. Natl Acad. Sci. USA*, **91**, 4053–6.

93. Tomkinson, A.E., Bardwell, A.J., Bardwell, L., Tappe, N.J. and Friedberg, E.C. (1993) Yeast DNA repair and recombination proteins Rad1 and Rad10 constitute a single-stranded-DNA endonuclease. *Nature*, **362**, 860–2.

94. Van Duin, M., Vedeveldt, G., Mayne, L.V *et al.* (1989) The cloned human DNA excision repair gene *ERCC-1* fails to correct xeroderma pigmentosum complementation groups A through I. *Mutat. Res.*, **217**, 83–92.

95. Biggerstaff, M., Szymkowski, D.E. and Wood, R.D. (1993) Co-correction of the ERCC1, ERCC4 and xeroderma pigmentosum group F DNA repair defects *in vitro*. *EMBO J.*, **12**, 3685–92.

96. Van Vuuren, A.J., Appeldoorn, E., Odijk, H. *et al.* (1993) Evidence for a repair enzyme complex involving ERCC1 and complementing activities of ERCC4, ERCC11 and xeroderma pigmentosum group F. *EMBO J.*, **12**, 3693–701.

97. Scherly D., Nouspikel T., Corlet J., Ucla C., Bairoch A. and Clarkson S.G. (1993) Complementation of the DNA repair defect in xeroderma pigmentosum group G cells by a human cDNA related to yeast *RAD2*. *Nature*, **363**, 182–5.

98. MacInnes, M.A., Dickson, J.A., Hernandez, R.R. *et al.* (1993) Human *ERCC5* cDNA-cosmid complementation for excision repair and bipartite amino acid domains conserved with RAD proteins of *Saccharomyces cerevisiae* and *Schizosaccharomyces pombe*. *Mol. Cell. Biol.*, **13**, 6393–402.

99. O'Donovan A. and Wood R.D. (1993) Identical defect in DNA repair in xeroderma pigmentosum group G and rodent ERCC group 5. *Nature*, **363**, 185–8.

100. O'Donovan, A., Davies, A.A., Moggs, J.G., West, S.C. and Wood, R.D. (1994) XPG endonuclease makes the 3′ incision in human DNA nucleotide excision repair. *Nature*, **371**, 432–5.

101. Gulyas, K.D. and Donahue, T.F. (1992) SSL2, a suppressor of a stem–loop mutation in the *HIS4* leader encodes the yeast homolog of human *ERCC-3*. *Cell*, **69**, 1031–42.

102. Park, E., Guzder, S.N., Koken, M.H.M. *et al.* (1992) *RAD25 (SSL2)*, the yeast homolog of the human xeroderma pigmentosum group B DNA repair gene, is essential for viability. *Proc. Natl Acad. Sci. USA*, **89**, 11416–20.

103. Mounkes, L.C., Jones, R.S., Liang, B-C., Gelbart, W. and Fuller, M.T. (1992) A *Drosophila* model for xeroderma pigmentosum and Cockayne's syndrome: *haywire* encodes the fly homolog of *ERCC3*, a human excision repair gene. *Cell*, **71**, 925–37.

104. Schaeffer, L., Roy, R., Humbert, S. *et al.* (1993) DNA repair helicase: a component of BTF2 (TFIIH) basic transcription factor. *Science*, **260**, 58–63.

105. van Vuuren, A. J., Vermeulen, W., Ma, L. *et al.* (1994) Correction of xeroderma pigmentosum repair defect by basal transcription factor BTF2 (TFIIH). *EMBO J.*, **13**, 1645–53.

106. Schaeffer, L., Monocollin, V., Roy, R. *et al.* (1994) The ERCC2/DNA repair protein is associated with the class II BTF2/TFIIH transcription factor. *EMBO J.*, **13**, 2388–92.

107. Drapkin, R., Reardon, J. T., Ansari, A. *et al.* (1994) Dual role of TFIIH in DNA excision repair and in transcription by RNA polymerase II. *Nature*, **368**, 769–72.

108. Li, L., Elledge, S.J., Peterson, C.A., Bales, E.S. and Legerski, R.J. (1994) Specific association between the human DNA repair proteins XPA and ERCC1. *Proc. Natl Acad. Sci. USA*, **91**, 5012–16.

109. Park, C-H. and Sancar, A. (1994) Formation of ternary complex by human XPA, ERCC1, and ERCC4(XPF) excision repair proteins. *Proc. Natl Acad. Sci. USA*, **91**, 5017–21.

110. Bardwell, A.J., Bardwell, L., Tomkinson, A.E. and Friedberg, E.C. (1994) Specific cleavage of model recombination and repair intermediates by the yeast Rad1-Rad10 DNA endonuclease. *Science*, **265**, 2082–5.

111. Ziegler, A., Leffell, D.J., Kunala, S. *et al.* (1993) Mutation hotspots due to sunlight in the p53 gene of nonmelanoma skin cancers. *Proc. Natl Acad. Sci. USA*, **90**, 4216–20.

112. Dumaz, N., Drougar, C., Sarasin, A. and Daya-Grosjean, L. (1993) Specific UV-induced mutation spectrum in the p53 gene of skin tumors from DNA repair deficient xeroderma pigmentosum patients. *Proc. Natl Acad. Sci. USA*, **90**, 10529–33.

113. Bootsma D. and Hoeijmakers, J.H.J. (1993) Engagement with transcription. *Nature*, **363**, 114–15.

Part Four

The Common Cancers

Chapter 13

Genetics and the common cancers

RICHARD S. HOULSTON and JULIAN PETO

13.1 INTRODUCTION

The importance of inherited predisposition is now established for a number of common cancers and the mechanisms by which mutations in some genes leads to cancer are at least partially understood. The ability to identify susceptibles among cancer patients and in the general population provides a basis for estimating the contribution of each such gene to overall cancer incidence. These powerful techniques will continue to dominate cancer research for many years, and not only in the field of genetic susceptibility. The same genes are often lost or mutated somatically in the multi-step evolution of cancer in non-susceptibles and may therefore be targets for novel screening and treatment methods. Most cancer susceptibility genes so far discovered are rare and highly penetrant, and known genes cause only a small proportion of all cancers. There is also suggestive evidence for the existence of more common but less penetrant genes which cause a larger proportion of all cancers, but such genes may prove very difficult to detect. They will rarely give rise to enough cancers in a single family for linkage analysis to succeed, and they may

not even give rise to a detectably increased risk in relatives of cancer patients.

In this chapter we review the evidence on the role of genes of high and low penetrance in the aetiology of the common cancers, and discuss the practical implications of this knowledge.

13.2 INHERITED CANCER SYNDROMES

A large number of inherited cancer syndromes have been recognized for many years. Many have an associated phenotype such as polyps in adenomatous polyposis coli, so that gene carriers are identifiable, even if they have not developed cancer. The inherited basis of such cancer syndromes is incontrovertible because the cancers or associated phenotypic abnormalities are rare in the general population and expression within families is consistent with Mendel's laws. McKusick [1] lists several hundred inherited disorders for which neoplasia is a major feature or complication, but the great majority are rare. The frequency of some of these syndromes is not accurately known, but it is

Genetic Predisposition to Cancer. Edited by R.A. Eeles, B.A.J. Ponder, D.F. Easton and A. Horwich. Published in 1996 by Chapman & Hall, London.
0 412 56580 3

likely that in total they are responsible for less than 1% of cancers in the UK. Nine of the more common 'classical' inherited cancer syndromes are listed in Table 13.1 [2].

Recent molecular studies have demonstrated a Mendelian basis for several hereditary syndromes with no associated phenotype conferring increased risk of one or more common cancers. These include the Li–Fraumeni syndrome due to mutations in the *TP*53 gene [3, 4], breast and breast–ovarian cancer families due to the recently cloned *BRCA*1 gene on chromosome 17q22 [5], breast cancer families linked to the *BRCA*2 gene on chromosome 13 [6], and some hereditary non-polyposis colorectal cancer (HNPCC) families caused by mutations in genes located on chromosomes 2, 3 and 7 [7–10]. The genetic basis of such syndromes was often questioned in the past on the grounds that even very striking familial clusters of a common cancer could be due to ascertainment bias. This is a statistical fallacy. For example, a family with three sisters affected with breast cancer before the age of 45 would be expected to occur by chance less than once every 10 years in the whole of Britain, and a family with four or more such sisters less than once every 1000 years.

13.3 FAMILIAL CLUSTERING OF COMMON CANCERS

For many common cancers, first-degree relatives of patients are at increased risk for cancer at the same site. This has been recognized for many years, but for most cancers there are still too few systematic studies to provide precise estimates of these familial risks, particularly for relatives of younger patients. Some cohort studies have been conducted, but most estimates of familial cancer risks have been from case-control studies. Tables 13.2–13.5 give published estimates of risks to relatives of affected cases for a number of common cancers. Where available, estimates

subdivided by age are also shown. Estimates from earlier case-control studies may be somewhat inflated by under-reporting of affected relatives by controls, but in most recent studies this bias is minimized by systematic questioning about each relative. For those sites where numerous reports have been published only the largest or most recent is presented. For first-degree relatives (parents, siblings and children) of patients with most common cancers the risk of developing cancer at the same site is generally increased by two- to five-fold above that in the general population. Such apparently moderate increases in risk could be due to a shared environment or a polygenic mechanism, but Table 13.6 shows that if they are caused by single genes the genetic effect must be substantial. For example, if a dominant gene confers a three-fold increase in risk in siblings, the risk in a susceptible individual has to be at least 21-fold higher than in a non-susceptible, and for a recessive gene the risk ratio must be at least 26. Table 13.6 also shows that a moderate familial risk is consistent with a wide range of gene frequencies and genetic effects. Even assuming that a single gene causes all familial cases, the underlying genetic model cannot therefore be inferred from the relative risks in first-degree relatives. A higher risk in siblings than in parents suggests a recessive model, but the gene frequency cannot be estimated without substantial numbers of families with three or more cases, which are rare in most population-based studies. Common susceptibility genes can never confer substantially increased risks in relatives, since the frequency of such a gene among relatives of cancer patients will not be very much higher than in the general population. For this reason common susceptibility genes are extremely difficult to detect.

The distribution of age at diagnosis in susceptible individuals is likely to differ from that in non-susceptibles for two reasons: first,

Table 13.1 Clinical features and estimates of cancer caused by mendelian cancer syndrome. (Adapted from [2].)

Syndrome	Tumour	Associated phenotype	Lifetime risk (%)	Frequency	Cancers/ year in UK
Adenomatous polyposis coli	Colon	Colonic polyps, retinal pigment hypertrophy, desmoid tumours, jaw osteomas	90	1/8000	70
Hereditary retinoblastoma	Retina Bone[1]	–	>90	1/40 000	15
MEN type 2	Phaeochromocytoma Medullary thyroid cancer	Mucosal neuromata, marfanoid habitus	60	1/50 000	10
Neurofibromatosis type 1	Neurofibrosarcoma	Café au lait patches	5–10	1/3000	10–20
Neurofibromatosis type 2	CNS tumour CNS tumours	Neurofibromata	5–10	1/35 000	<1
Ataxia telangiectasia	Leukaemia[2]	Cerebellar ataxia, telangiectases	?	1/300 000	<5%
Xeroderma pigmentosum	Skin tumours	–	?	1/250 000	<5
Fanconi's anaemia	AML	Radial defects	10	<1/20 000	<5
Von Hippel–Lindau	Cerebellar haemangiomas Renal cell tumours	Renal/pancreatic/epididymal cysts	99	1/53 000	10

[1] Also an excess of osteosarcomas, melanoma, bladder, and lung tumours in adult life.
[2] Also predisposes to breast cancer, possibly 7% of cases.

Table 13.2 Familial risks of lung, colorectal and stomach cancer in relatives of cancer probands. (see Reference appendix for reference details.)

Study	Risk	95% C.l.
Lung cancer		
Tokuhhata and Lilienfeld, 1963 [1]	2.6	
Tokuhhata and Lilienfeld, 1963 [2]	2.4	1.1–4.8
Lynch *et al.*, 1986 [3]	~2-fold	
Ooi *et al.*, 1986 [4]	2.4	
Samet *et al.*, 1986 [5]	5.3	2.2–12.8
Gao *et al.*, 1987 [6]	1.1	0.6–2.3
Tsugane *et al.*, 1987 [7]	No association	
Wu *et al.*, 1988 [8]	3.9	2.0–7.6
Horwitz *et al.*, 1988 [9]	2.3	0.7–7.3
McDuffie *et al.*, 1989 [10]	2.0	1.4–2.9
McDuffie *et al.*, 1991 [11]	2.0	1.2–3.4
Osann, 1991 [12]	1.9	0.7–5.6
Shaw *et al.*, 1991 [13]	1.8	1.3–2.5
Lee, 1993 [14]	1.3	0.9–1.8
Goldgar *et al.*, 1994 [15]	2.6	2.1–3.1
Colorectal cancer		
Woolf, 1958 [16]	3.3	1.5–7.1
Macklin, 1960 [17]	3.2	2.2–4.5
Lovett, 1976 [18]	3.5	2.5–4.8
Duncan and Kyle, 1982 [19]	8.0	1.0–60.9
Maire *et al.*, 1984 [20]	5.3	2.3–12.3
Kune *et al.*, 1987 [21]	1.8	1.6–2.0
Ponz de Leon *et al.*, 1987 [22]	7.0	3.9–19.8
Bonnelli *et al.*, 1988 [23]	2.4	1.5–3.6
Stephenson *et al.*, 1991 [24]	4.6	1.8–11.5
Sondergaard *et al.*, 1991 [25]	1.9	1.5–2.0
case <50; relative <49	5.5	2.7–10.2
case <50; relative 50+	1.5	1.1–2.1
case 50–59; relative <49	2.4	0.8–5.6
case 50–59; relative 50+	1.7	1.4–2.0
St John *et al.*, 1993 [26]	2.1	1.4–3.1
case <45	3.7	1.5–9.1
case 45–54	1.8	0.9–3.8
case >55	1.8	1.0–3.1
1 case	1.8	1.2–2.7
2+ cases	5.7	1.7–19.3
Goldgar *et al.*, 1994 [15]		
colon:	2.7	2.3–3.1
case <60	4.0	2.1–6.4
rectum:	1.8	1.1–2.7
case <60	8.0	2.1–17.8

Table 13.2 Continued

Study	Risk	95% C.l.
Stomach cancer		
Macklin, 1960 [17]	2.6	1.9–3.4
Zangheri *et al.*, 1990 [27]	3.1	
LaVeehia *et al.*, 1991 [28]	2.7	1.9–3.7
Goldgar *et al.*, 1994 [15]	2.1	1.0–3.6

those susceptible may have a different underlying disease process. Such heterogeneity could, for example, account for differences in the age–incidence curves seen in different populations for Hodgkin's lymphoma. An important special case is where susceptibility to cancer is due to a germline mutation in a tumour suppressor gene, as in adenomatous polyposis coli. A simple multi-stage model in which this mutation is a necessary step which occurs somatically in the development of non-hereditary cancer would predict that the non-susceptible to susceptible incidence ratio for an adult tumour will be proportional to age. Secondly, cancers caused by a gene conferring a high lifetime risk will tend to be younger at diagnosis than sporadic cases, as the proportion of surviving susceptibles will fall progressively with increasing age. If tumours develop earlier in susceptibles, for whatever reason, the relative risk in relatives of affected cases will be greatest in young relatives of young cases. This pattern of risk is exhibited by many common cancers, including breast, colon, prostate, bladder and melanoma (Tables 13.2–13.5).

13.3.1 GENETIC MODELS OF PREDISPOSITION TO COMMON CANCERS

Genetic models of familial cancer can be formally tested using segregation analysis. This involves comparing the observed pattern of disease incidence in each pedigree with that predicted by different models. Table 13.7 lists published segregation analyses of breast, colorectal, lung and ovarian cancer pedigrees. The

Table 13.3 Familial risks of breast cancer in relatives of cancer probands. (see Reference appendix for reference details.)

Study	Risk	95% C.l.
Female breast cancer		
Adami *et al.*, 1980 [29]	1.7	1.3–2.1
case <50	2.3	1.0–6.2
case 50–64	1.7	1.1–2.5
case 65+	1.7	1.2–2.3
Bain *et al.*, 1980 [30]	2.0	1.7–2.4
mother: case <40	3.2	1.5–6.7
case 40–44	1.6	0.8–3.0
case 45–49	1.5	1.0–2.3
case 50–55	1.9	1.4–2.5
sister: case <40	8.4	1.5–26.3
case 40–44	3.1	1.3–7.6
case 45–49	2.5	1.4–4.6
case 50–55	2.2	1.6–3.2
Briton *et al.*, 1982 [31]	2.1	1.7–2.6
case <40	5.3	1.4–20.5
case 40–44	1.9	0.8–4.1
case 45–49	1.5	0.9–2.6
case 50–54	2.1	1.3–3.2
case 55–59	2.2	1.3–3.7
case >60	2.2	1.5–3.2
Sattin *et al.*, 1985 [32]	2.3	1.9–2.7
case 20–39	4.0	2.7–5.8
case 40–44	2.2	1.5–3.3
case 45–54	1.9	1.6–2.4
mother and sister	13.6	4.1–44.8
Ottman *et al.*, 1986 [33]		
case <40 unilateral	2.4	0.5–10.9
case 41–50 unilateral	0.9	0.3–2.9
case 51–64 unilateral	1.3	0.6–3.0
case <41 bilateral	10.5	4.0–27.2
case 41–50 bilateral	3.8	1.6–9.3
Dupont and Page, 1987 [34]	2.3	1.6–3.4
Negri *et al.*, 1988 [35]	2.0	1.7–2.3
Bouchardy *et al.*, 1990 [36]	2.6	1.6–4.3
Houlston *et al.*, 1991 [37]	1.9	1.2–2.7
case <45	3.9	1.7–7.6
case 45–54	1.3	0.3–3.2
case 55+	1.6	0.8–2.7
bilateral case	6.4	1.3–18.8
Tulinius *et al.*, 1992 [38]	2.3	2.0–2.6
case <45	3.0	2.3–3.7
case 45–54	2.2	1.7–2.7
case >54	1.8	1.4–2.3
bilateral	4.4	3.4–6.5

Table 13.3 Continued

	Risk	95% C.l.
Peto *et al.*, 1994 [39]	1.85	1.6–2.1
case <40; relative <40	5.1	2.2–9.9
relative 40–49	2.3	1.3–3.0
case 40–50; relative <40	5.5	2.2–11.4
relative 40–49	1.9	1.0–3.3
relative 50–59	1.6	1.0–2.5
case 50–58; relative <40	1.9	0.2–6.7
relative 40–49	2.3	1.2–3.9
relative 50–59	2.0	1.3–3.0
Goldgar *et al.*, 1994 [15]	1.8	1.7–2.0
case <50	3.7	2.5–5.2
Male breast cancer (male probands)		
Casagrande *et al.*, 1988 [40]		
female relative	1.8	0.7–4.5
Rosenblatt *et al.*, 1991 [41]		
male relative	4.0	0.4–40.1
female relative	2.4	1.5–4.0
Anderson and Badzioch, 1992 [42]		
female relative	1.9	1.2–2.8

majority of these studies have found evidence for major dominant genes predisposing to these cancers.

Segregation analysis of cancer families ascertained within population-based studies can in principle provide estimates of both gene frequency and age-specific cancer incidence for susceptibles and non-susceptibles. For example in the CASH case-control study of breast cancer a dominant gene with a frequency of 0.0033 provided the most parsimonious model, conferring a risk of 14% by age 40, 38% by age 50 and 67% by age 70. The postulated gene accounted for 26% of breast cancer cases by age 40, 15% by age 50 and 8% by age 70 [14]. It is now known, however, that two major genes (*BRCA*1 and *BRCA*2), as well as AT heterozygotes and the rare Li–Fraumeni (*TP*53) syndrome, contribute to this overall excess risk.

One feature of familial breast cancer risk which is not readily explained by a dominant model is the higher risk reported in sisters of breast cancer cases than in their

Table 13.4 Familial risks of uterine, ovarian and prostate cancer in relatives of cancer probands. (see Reference appendix for reference details.)

Study	Risk	95% C.l.
Uterine cancer		
Schildkraut *et al.*, 1989 [43]	2.7	1.6–4.8
Goldgar *et al.*, 1994 [15]	1.3	0.9–1.8
case <60	1.8	0.7–3.4
Ovarian cancer		
Hildreth *et al.*, 1981 [44]	18.2	4.8–69.0
Cramer *et al.*, 1983 [45]	11.3	8.9–
Booth *et al.*, 1986 [46]	7.8	0.9–69.4
Schildkraut *et al.*, 1989 [43]	2.8	1.6–4.9
case <45; relative <45	2.0	0.4–9.4
case <45; relative >45	2.2	0.6–7.7
case >45; relative >45	4.9	2.4–10.1
Koch *et al.*, 1989 [47]	2.6	1.1–1.6
Easton *et al.*, 1996 [48]	2.2	1.6–3.1
case <40; relative <50	4.8	0.7–3.3
case <40; relative >50	1.2	0.6–2.2
case >40; relative <50	6.5	2.4–14.0
case >40; relative >50	2.1	1.0–3.7
Goldgar *et al.*, 1994 [15]	2.1	1.0–3.4
Prostate cancer		
Morganti, 1956 [49]	11.0	1.4–83.9
Steele, 1971 [50]	2.5	0.5–12.1
Krain, 1974 [51]	6.1	1.4–26.8
Schuman *et al.*, 1977 [52]	2.3	0.6–8.4
Cannon *et al.*, 1982 [53]	2.4	
case <65; relative <65	6.0	
relative 65–79	2.8	
case >65; relative <65	2.8	
relative 65–79	2.0	
Meikle, 1985 [54]	4.0	2.0–7.2
Steinberg *et al.*, 1990 [55]	2.0	1.2–3.3
1 case	2.2	1.4–3.5
2 cases	4.9	2.0–12.3
3 cases	10.9	2.7–43.1
Spitz *et al.*, 1991 [56]	2.4	1.3–4.5
Ghadirain *et al.*, 1991 [57]	8.7	2.0–38.2
Goldgar *et al.*, 1994 [15]	2.2	2.1–2.4
case <60	4.1	2.0–7.1

Table 13.5 Familial risks of melanoma, non-medullary thyroid, testicular and pancreatic, bladder and renal cancers in relatives of cancer probands. (see Reference appendix for reference details.)

Study	Risk	95% C.l.
Melanoma		
Holman and Armstrong, 1984 [58]	2.8	1.7–4.9
Green *et al.*, 1985 [59]	2.1	1.0–4.5
Cristofolini *et al.*, 1987 [60]	7.8	0.9–71.3
Holly *et al.*, 1987 [61]	1.7	0.4–6.4
Osterlind *et al.*, 1988 [62]	1.5	0.7–2.9
Goldgar *et al.*, 1994 [15]	2.1	1.4–2.9
case <50	6.5	3.0–11.7
Non-medullary thyroid cancer		
Stoffer *et al.*, 1986 [63]	4.7	2.0–9.3
Ron *et al.*, 1991 [64]	5.2	0.2–544
Goldgar *et al.*, 1994 [15]	8.6	4.7–13.7
Testicular		
Forman *et al.*, 1992 [65]	9.8	2.8–16.7
Pancreas		
Ghadirian *et al.*, 1991 [66]	14.0	1.9–103.3
Goldgar *et al.*, 1994 [15]	1.3	0.4–2.6
Bladder		
Kantor *et al.*, 1985 [67]	1.5	1.2–1.8
case <45	2.7	0.8–8.9
case 45–64	1.7	0.2–2.4
case 65+	1.5	1.0–2.2
Renal		
Mellemgaard *et al.*, 1994 [68]	4.1	1.5–10.8
Goldgar *et al.*, 1994 [15]	5.1	1.0–12.5

mothers in some studies (for example, [28]). If real, this could be due to shared lifestyle factors among sisters, anticipation, reduced fertility in female carriers, or the presence of co-dominant or recessive susceptibility genes. In principle, risks to second-degree and more distant relatives provide useful additional evidence on the mode of inheritance, since for a simple dominant gene the excess relative risk (R-1) reduces by a factor of two for each degree of relationship [29].

213

Table 13.6 Dominant and recessive gene models causing specific relative risk in siblings of affected cases. Tabulated values are the ratios of risks in susceptible to non-susceptible individuals. (From [2].)

		Relative risk to sibling			
	Gene frequency	*1.5*	*2*	*3*	*5*
Dominant gene model	0.001	25	35	50	74
	0.01	10	14	21	35
	0.05	6	10	21	35
	0.1	6	13	280	–
	0.2	10	–	–	–
Recessive gene model	0.01	143	203	289	414
	0.05	30	44	64	96
	0.1	16	24	36	60
	0.5	8	35	–	–

However, in practice this approach is unlikely to be helpful even for common cancers, since complete unbiased data on second- and third-degree relatives are rarely available.

In addition to the highly penetrant genes causing colorectal cancer which have been identified by linkage, such as the *APC* and HNPCC genes, segregation studies have suggested the presence of more common genes with lower penetrance predisposing to colorectal cancer in the general population [23, 24]. Cannon-Albright *et al.* [23] fitted a dominant model with a gene frequency of 0.19 and a lifetime penetrance of 0.4 for adenomas or colorectal cancer in susceptible individuals. This model implies that most, and perhaps all, adenomas arise through inherited predisposition, although the confidence limits were wide [23].

Few segregation analyses of familial cancer have incorporated data on environmental risk factors. In an analysis of lung cancer Sellers *et al.* [25] fitted a model in which lung cancer risk is increased both by genetic susceptibility and by smoking. The observed pattern of familial aggregation was compatible with the inheritance of a co-dominant gene conferring an increased susceptibility to lung cancer.

While segregation analysis can provide some support for the presence of major genes predisposing to a specific cancer, it has never established a previously unsuspected mode of inheritance. Furthermore, the predictions of single and multiple gene models are virtually identical and can be distinguished only through genetic linkage.

13.3.2 DETECTION OF SUSCEPTIBILITY GENES

Genetic linkage analysis of multiple case families has proved a powerful method for detecting predisposing genes, leading to the localization of the *BRCA1* gene on chromosome 17 predisposing to both breast and ovarian cancer [30, 31], the *BRCA2* gene on chromosome 13 predisposing to breast cancer [6], genes on chromosomes 2 and 3 predisposing to colorectal cancer [32, 33] and a gene for melanoma on chromosome 9p [34].

The most direct evidence for genetic susceptibility is the observation that mutations in a particular gene occur in the germline of cancer patients. Identification of susceptibility genes has been achieved for adenomatous polyposis coli (the *APC* gene on chromosome 5q) [35], HNPCC (the *hMSH*2, *hMLH*1, *hPMS*1 and *hPMS*2 genes on chromosomes 2p, 3p and 7q) [7–10] and for the Li–Fraumeni

Table 13.7 Segregation analyses of breast, colon, lung, ovarian and prostate cancers. (see References for details.)

Authors	Dominant model (except*)			
	No. of families	Gene frequency	Lifetime penetrance	Comments
Breast cancer				
Population-based studies				
Jacobsen pedigrees				
Williams and Anderson 1984 [11]	200	0.0076	0.57	Possible enrichment of pre-menopausal onset
Iselius et al., 1992 [12]	200	0.0092	0.78	Specific mortality neglected. Incorporating specific mortality. Probands aged <55 years
CASH study				
Newman et al., 1988 [13]	1579	0.0006	0.82	
Claus et al., 1991 [14]	4730	0.003	0.95	
Others				
Iselius et al., 1992 [15]	254	0.029	0.79	Enrichment of premenopausal onset
Bilateral cases				
Goldstein et al., 1987 [16]	286	0.0014	?	All breast cancer cases
	252	0.00092	?	Premenopausal cases only. Evidence of non-mendelian transmission
Selected families				
Bishop and Gardner 1980 [17]	1	0.0056	0.84	Large family, ascertainment and prevalence ignored
Go et al., 1983 [18]	18	?	0.95	10 families with dominant inheritance
Cannon et al., 1986 [19]	16	0.0134	0.8	At least three affected cases in each pedigree
Bishop et al., 1988 [20]	9	0.009	0.84	Correction made for ascertainment
Iselius et al., 1991 [15]	670	0.003	0.83	254 consecutive pedigrees + 416 high-risk families
Colorectal cancer				
Burt et al., 1985 [21]	1	0.003		Large single multiple case family
Bailey-Wilson et al., 1986 [22]	11	0.054	0.7	HNPCC families
Cannon-Albright et al., 1988 [23]	34	0.19	0.4	Large extended families
Houlston et al., 1991 [24]	209	0.006	0.64	
Lung cancer				
Sellers et al., 1990 [25]	337	0.052*		
Ovarian cancer				
Houlston et al., 1991 [26]	518	0.0015	0.79	Ascertainment through consultand; potential bias
Prostate cancer				
Carter et al., 1992 [27]	691	0.003	0.88	Enrichment for younger cases

*Co-dominant model of inherited susceptibility favoured

syndrome (the *TP*53 gene on chromosome 17p) [3, 4].

Once a gene has been identified, its frequency and penetrance, and hence the contribution to overall cancer incidence, can be estimated from population-based studies of gene carriers. Families used for linkage cannot be used to estimate gene frequency because they have usually been selected for the occurrence of multiple cases, but they can be used to estimate penetrance by maximizing the LOD score over all possible penetrance functions. Using this method, Easton and co-workers [36] estimated the penetrance of breast or ovarian cancer in female carriers of the *BRCA*1 gene to be 59% by age 50 and 82% by age 70. A detailed review of linkage is presented in Chapter 2.

The frequency of a deleterious gene and its contribution to overall cancer incidence cannot be estimated solely from linkage studies without population-based data on familial risk. In the case of *BRCA*1, where linkage studies suggested that nearly all high-risk breast–ovarian families were the result of *BRCA*1, an estimate was obtained by assuming that the excess risk of ovarian cancer observed in a population-based study of relatives of breast cancer patients was entirely due to *BRCA*1. The overall gene frequency was thus estimated to be 0.0007 [36].

13.3.3 FAMILIAL ASSOCIATIONS BETWEEN COMMON CANCERS

A number of dominantly inherited susceptibility genes cause cancer at several sites. These include clustering of adenocarcinomas of the colorectum and endometrium in HNPCC families, the association of soft tissue sarcomas, leukaemia, brain and breast tumours in the Li–Fraumeni syndrome and clustering in *BRCA*1 families of cancers of the breast and ovary, with smaller risks for colon and prostate cancer. Whether population-based studies could reliably detect associations between cancers caused by such rare genes is unclear. Only a small relative risk would be expected, and the risk for other cancers is usually less than that for the primary site.

A large number of epidemiological studies have examined the risk to relatives for cancer at the same site as the proband, but few have systematically examined the risk of cancer at other sites. Rather than present a myriad of published multi-site associations, Tables 13.8 and 13.9 detail the results of Goldgar *et al* [37] who carried out a systematic study of the clustering of cancer at 28 distinct sites using the Utah population database. Strong familial relationships were seen in this study between breast, colon and prostatic cancer. A recent analysis of a large series of breast and ovarian cancer families linked to the *BRCA*1 locus showed significantly elevated risks for both colon and prostatic cancer among gene carriers [38].

Environmental and behavioural risk factors which are similar within families may account for some observed associations, such as the familial clustering seen for cancers at smoking related sites (lung, lip, cervix). Clustering of cancers of the female genitalia, lip and oral cavity may reflect a common viral aetiology. An increased risk of soft tissue cancers among relatives of breast cancer probands presumably reflects in part the Li–Fraumeni syndrome. However, the only evidence of the HNPCC complex of cancers was seen in relatives of young uterine cancer probands. In addition to these previously reported associations between cancer sites, highly significant excesses of thyroid cancer and non-Hodgkin's lymphoma were seen in relatives of breast cancer probands, suggesting a hitherto unrecognized inherited association. Relationships were also identified between ovarian and pancreatic cancer and between colorectal cancer and leukaemias.

Table 13.8 Familial relative risks in first-degree relatives of cancer probands with gastrointestinal, urogenital and haemopoietic, soft tissue tumours and melanoma. (From [37].)

Proband site	Second site	Risk
Probands with gastrointestinal cancers		
Rectum	Colon	2.0*
Early rectum	Colon	3.5*
Colon	Prostate	1.3*
Colon	Breast	1.2*
Rectum	Prostate	1.3*
Early colon	Lung	1.7**
Colon	Granulocytic	1.7**
	leukaemia	1.4**
Early colon	Breast	1.8**
Colon	Anus	1.3**
Colon	Lung	1.8**
Early colon	Melanoma	2.0**
Rectum	Lymphatic leukaemia	2.2***
Early colon	Granulocytic	2.5***
	leukaemia	2.4***
Pancreas	Gall bladder	
Stomach	Female genitals	
Probands with urogenital tract cancers		
Prostate	Colon	1.3*
Prostate	Non-Hodgkin's	1.2**
Prostate	Rectum	1.3**
Early prostate	Rectum	2.0**
Prostate	Brain/CNS	1.3***
Early bladder	Lymphatic leukaemia	3.6***
Early bladder	Cervix	2.3***
Testis	Myeloma	3.7***
Testis	Bladder	2.4***
Probands with haemopoietic, soft tissue tumours and melanoma		
Early NHL	Prostate	1.6*
Non-Hodgkin's	Prostate	1.3**
Melanoma	Brain/CNS	1.7**
Granulocytic	Colon	1.7**
leukaemia		
Lymphatic	Rectum	2.0**
leukaemia	Granulocytic	3.2***
Soft tissue	leukaemia	
Lymph	Thyroid	2.4***
Soft tissue	Thyroid	2.8***

CNS, central nervous system; NHL, non-Hodgkin's lymphoma.
***P<0.05, **P<0.01, *P<0.001.

Table 13.9 Familial relative risks in first-degree relatives of cancer probands with female reproductive cancers and other cancers. (From [37].)

Proband site	Second site	Risk
Probands with gastrointestinal cancers		
Breast	Colon	1.4*
Breast	Colon	1.2*
Breast	Thyroid	1.7*
Early breast	Colon	1.7*
Breast	Non-Hodgkin's	1.4*
Early breast	Non-Hodgkin's	1.9*
Ovary	Lip	2.2**
Cervix	Lung	1.6**
Early breast	Prostate	1.4**
Ovary	Pancreas	2.1**
Cervix	Colon	1.5**
Early uterine	Colon	1.6**
Early uterine	Female genitals	2.9***
Female genitals	Oral cavity	3.0***
Female genitals	Stomach	2.6***
Female genitals	Lip	2.5***
Ovary	Soft tissue cancers	2.2***
Probands with cancers at other sites		
Thyroid	Breast	1.7*
Larynx	Lip	3.5*
Lung	Lip	1.7*
Early brain/CNS	Pancreas	4.7*
Brain/CNS	Prostate	1.3**
Lung	Cervix	1.6**
Larynx	Lung	2.1**
Brain	Stomach	1.9**
Brain	Melanoma	1.6**
Early brain	Stomach	3.6**
Lip	Ovary	1.9**
Thyroid	Prostate	1.4**
Lung	Colon	1.3**
Oral cavity	Female genitals	3.0***
Thyroid	Lymphatic leukaemia	2.7***
Thyroid	Soft tissue cancers	2.9***
Lip	Female genitals	2.3***
Larynx	Thyroid	3.0***

CNS, central nervous system.
***P<0.05, **P<0.01, *P<0.001.

13.4 GENES OF LOW PENETRANCE PREDISPOSING TO CANCER

The preceding sections of this chapter have been largely confined to the inherited cancer syndromes due to highly penetrant genes which cause remarkable multiple case families. With the possible exception of HNPCC, such genes are likely to account for only a small proportion of common cancers. There may also be predisposing genes of lower penetrance which account for a larger proportion of cancers. Less penetrant genes will rarely produce large numbers of cancers in a family, but if they cause a high proportion of cancers of a particular type they may be detectable by linkage analysis of affected pairs of siblings, particularly if the mode of inheritance is recessive, as the examples of Hodgkin's disease and nasopharyngeal carcinoma have demonstrated [39]. Another way in which such genetic effects might be detected is through an associated phenotypic or molecular marker of susceptibility. Examples of established or suspected susceptibility markers include candidate gene complexes such as cytochrome p450, clinically detectable lesions such as naevi, colorectal adenomas, benign fibrocystic breast disease or palmar keratoses, metabolic markers such as slow acetylation, and markers of DNA repair efficiency or chromosomal instability detectable by cellular assay or DNA analysis.

13.4.1 METABOLIC POLYMORPHISMS

A number of biochemical pathways involved in the handling of drugs and carcinogens show polymorphic variation. One subfamily of the cytochrome p450 system responsible for the metabolism of debrisoquine is encoded by the *CYP*2D6 locus. Approximately 10% of the population are homozygotes and show an impaired ability to metabolize debrisoquine. Several studies have demonstrated that poor metabolizers are at a lower risk of lung and bladder cancers, suggesting

that this p450 subfamily influences the metabolism of carcinogens important in the aetiology of these cancers [40, 41]. Similar observations have been made for the metabolic system involved in activation of arylamine carcinogens. About 25–30% of the population are rapid acetylators. Among workers exposed to the carcinogen benzidine, Cartwright *et al.* [42] found a 16.7-fold increased risk of urinary tract cancers in slow acetylators compared with rapid acetylators.

13.4.2 BENIGN LESIONS

Case-control studies have shown that melanoma risk is strongly correlated with the number of skin melanocytic naevi [43]. A twin study carried out by Easton *et al.* [44] strongly suggests that naevus prevalence and hence melanoma risk has a genetic component. The intraclass correlation in monozygotic twins was 0.83, whereas there was little or no correlation in dizygotic twins. Further evidence of genetic susceptibility to naevi was found by Goldgar *et al.* [45] in studies of families of melanoma cases.

Palmar keratoses are known to be strongly associated with bladder cancer [46]. Cuzick *et al.* [47] found that keratoses were significantly more frequent in first-degree relatives of relatives of bladder cancer cases (odds ratio 5.7), particularly if the case also had keratoses (odds ratio 9.2). Spouses of cases also had an increased, but smaller, risk of bladder cancer, especially if the case had keratoses (odds ratio 4.3) [46]. These results clearly implicate genetic, as well as environmental, factors in the aetiology of keratoses.

13.4.3 DNA REPLICATION AND REPAIR GENES

Some classical inherited diseases such as Fanconi anaemia, ataxia telangiectasia, xeroderma pigmentosum and Bloom's syndrome which are associated with increased cancer

Table 13.10 Dominant low-penetrance genetic models giving a relative risk of 2 in siblings

Carrier frequency	Proportion of cancers in carriers (%)	Risk ratio (susceptibles: non-susceptibles)	Relative risk (susceptibles: general population)	Penetrance by age 70 in susceptibles	
				Female breast or male lung (population risk = 5%)	Prostate or colon (population risk = 1–2%)
0.02	22	14	11.0	0.43	0.12
0.1	53	10	5.3	0.24	0.06
0.2	76	13	3.8	0.18	0.04

risk involve chromosome instability or DNA replication or repair defects. Other important cancer susceptibility genes are also of this type. A normal function of the *TP53* gene is either to induce cell cycle arrest or to induce apoptosis in response to DNA damage, and inactivation of the HNPCC genes on chromosomes 2, 3 and 7 is associated with somatic instability of di- and tri-nucleotide repeats. The recently discovered p16 cell cycle regulator gene (*CDKN2*) on chromosome 9, originally located by linkage in familial melanoma, is deleted or mutated in a high proportion of cancers at many sites [48]. If p16 inactivation leads to uncontrolled cell division it is also likely to increase the risk of other mutations. The possibility that other 'mutator' genes of this general class might be detectable phenotypically is suggested by the recent report that 42% of breast cancer patients exhibit lymphocyte radiation sensitivity, while only 9% of the general population do so [49]. If this effect is hereditary, the lifetime breast cancer risk must be about 40% in the 9% who are susceptible and 5% in non-susceptibles, to give the overall national rate of 8%. If due to a Mendelian mechanism, this would imply a relative risk of only 1.5–2 in first-degree relatives of cancer patients and about 3 in monozygotic twins (Table 13.6). These figures are in the range of the risks seen in relatives of breast cancer patients above the age of 50. The evidence is thus consistent with almost half of all breast cancers occurring in the 9% who are susceptible. This effect, if real, is not due to a single gene. Most *A-T* heterozygotes exhibit high radiation sensitivity in the test, but they do not constitute 9% of the population. They do, however, have a relative risk of the order of 5 for breast cancer [50].

13.4.4 LINKAGE ANALYSIS OF PHENOTYPIC MARKERS

Highly penetrant genes such as *BRCA1* may cause a substantial proportion of cancers at young ages, but they are unlikely to cause a high proportion of all cancers. As the preceding example shows, however, less penetrant genes could well do so. The relative risk in first-degree relatives is of the order of 1.5–2 at older ages for most common cancers. The range of dominant low-penetrance models consistent with a relative risk of 2 in siblings is shown in Table 13.10. (The range of models would be similar for a relative risk of 1.5.) This shows that the ratio of cancer risk in susceptibles to that in the general population cannot exceed about 5 if 50% of all cancers occur in susceptibles, when about 10% of the population must be at high risk. A dominant gene carried by 1 in 50 of the population would cause a risk 11 times that in the general population, and would cause 22% of all cancers. Within this range, such genes would rarely produce striking multiple case families except possibly for lung or breast

219

cancer, where an 11-fold increase in risk would correspond to a penetrance by age 70 of 43%. For colon cancer, for example, where the cumulative risk in the general population is only 1.2% by age 70, an 11-fold increase in risk in susceptibles would correspond to a penetrance of only 12%. The example of nasopharyngeal cancer shows that such a gene could be detected from affected sibling pairs if a single locus accounts for most of the genetic risk, particularly if the mode of inheritance is recessive. Multiple case families would be rare, however, and linkage would fail if several different genes act similarly (heterogeneity). Such a gene might, however, be readily detectable by linkage in a single large family if carriers exhibit a phenotype such as the lymphocyte sensitivity in breast cancer affecting 9% of the population described earlier or the susceptibility to adenomas in colon cancer modelled by Cannon-Albright *et al.* [23], who suggested that about 35% of the population have a lifetime risk of adenoma development of 40%. Whether many such genes exist is a major unanswered question. If they do, and they cause a substantial proportion of all cancers, their identification would be of great practical importance. There may also be susceptibility genes which are carried by the majority of the population, but these could not cause a detectably increased risk in relatives, and they would have such low penetrance that their discovery would be of scientific rather than immediate clinical value. In the extreme case of the polymorphic *CYP*2D6 locus, where more than 90% of the population are at high risk, even if poor metabolizers were totally immune from lung cancer the resulting relative risk to first-degree relatives would be only 1.02 [2].

13.5 CONCLUSIONS

Studies of multiple case families have led to the identification of highly penetrant genes

predisposing to colon, breast and ovarian cancer and melanoma. Such genes account for most striking multiple case families and a substantial proportion of cancers diagnosed below age 45, although they cause a much smaller proportion of older cases. The large risks observed in relatives of young patients suggest the existence of genes predisposing to other common cancers. With the possible exception of ovarian cancer, however, most of the familial risk in first-degree relatives of older cancer patients is probably not due to highly penetrant genes. A major unanswered question in cancer genetics is whether a substantial proportion of all cancers arise in susceptible individuals as a result of genes of lower penetrance. If so, such genes may be detectable by linkage analysis of sibling pairs or phenotypic markers.

The ability to identify a large number of individuals with a lifetime risk for a particular cancer of the order of 20–50% would present a number of practical opportunities and ethical difficulties. Phenotypic or genetic tests might be offered routinely as an adjunct to screening for cancers such as breast, colon and prostate, extending the ethical difficulties of obtaining fully informed consent for genetic testing to the general population. There would also be important implications for industrial and environmental exposure to carcinogens. Susceptible individuals can perhaps be excluded from certain occupations or persuaded to give up smoking, but if identified individuals in the general population suffer much higher than average risks from carcinogenic agents such as ionizing radiation it could be argued that much more stringent environmental limits must be introduced. The discovery of identifiable susceptibility genes such as those predisposing to HNPCC has already raised these ethical quandaries, but they have yet to be resolved.

The study of cancer genetics has given rise to a succession of statistical fallacies during the 60 years since Cramer [51] noted that the overall cancer rate varies much less than the rates for individual sites between different countries, and inferred that a certain fixed proportion of all populations must be cancer-prone. The low relative risks seen in relatives of cancer patients were mistakenly believed to be inconsistent with the effects of penetrant mendelian genes, familial clusters of common cancers which could not possibly have arisen by chance were often ascribed to ascertainment bias by those sceptical of the importance of genetic susceptibility in carcinogenesis, while genetic enthusiasts advanced the illogical argument that genetics must play a dominant role, as not all heavy smokers develop lung cancer. The statistical pitfalls of modern genetic epidemiology are more subtle. The results described earlier illustrate the importance of formal modelling in an area where the predictions of even the simplest genetic models can be somewhat counterintuitive.

REFERENCES

MAIN TEXT

1. McKusick, V.A. (1994) Mendelian inheritance in man: catalogues of autosomal dominant inheritance, autosomal ressive inheritance and X-linked phenotypes.The Johns Hopkins University Press, Baltimore and London.
2. Easton, D.E. and Peto, J. (1990) The contribution of inherited predisposition to cancer incidence. *Cancer Surv.*, **9**, 395–416.
3. Malkin, D., Li, F.P., Fraumeni, J.F. Jr. *et al.* (1990) Germline p53 mutations in a familial syndrome of breast cancer, sarcomas and other neoplasms. *Science*, **250**, 1233–5.
4. Srivastava, S., Zou, Z. Q., Pirollo, K., Blatter, W. and Chang, E.W. (1990) Germline transmisssion of a mutated p53 gene in a cancer family with Li–Fraumeni syndrome. *Nature*, **348**, 747–9.
5. Miki, Y., Swensen, J., Schattuck-Eidens, D. *et al.* (1994) Isolation of BRCA1, the 17q-linked breast and ovarian cancer susceptibility gene. *Science*, **266**, 66–71.
6. Wooster, R., Neuhausen, S., Manigion, J. *et al.* (1994) Localisation of a breast cancer susceptibility gene (BRCA2) to chromosome 13q by genetic linkage analysis. *Science*, **265**, 2088–90.
7. Bronner, C.E., Baker, S.M., Morrison, P.T. *et al.* (1994) Mutation in the DNA mismatch repair gene homologue hMLH1 is associated with hereditary nonpolyposis colon cancer linked to chromosome 3p. *Nature*, **368**, 258–61.
8. Leach, F.S., Nicolaides, N.C., Papadopoulos, N. *et al.* (1993) Mutations of a mutS homolog in hereditary nonpolyposis colorectal cancer. *Cell*, **75**, 1215–25.
9. Papadopoulos, N., Nicolaides, N.C., Wei, Y.-F. *et al.* (1994) Mutation of the mutL homolog associated with hereditary colon cancer. *Science*, **263**, 1625–9.
10. Nicolaides, N.C., Papadopoulos, N., Lu, B. *et al.* (1994) Mutations of two PMS homologues in hereditary nonpolyposis colon cancer. *Nature*, **371**, 75–80.
11. Williams, W.R. and Anderson, D.E. (1984) Genetic epidemiology of breast cancer: segregation analysis of 200 Danish pedigrees. *Genet. Epidemiol.*, **1**, 7–20.
12. Iselius, L., Littler, M. and Morton, N.E. (1992) Transmission of breast cancer – a controversy resolved. *Clin. Genet.*, **42**, 211–17.
13. Newman, B., Austin, M.A., Lee, M. and King, M-C. (1988) Inheritance of human breast cancer: evidence for autosomal dominant transmission in high risk families. *Proc. Natl Acad. Sci. USA*, **85**, 3044–8.
14. Claus, E.B., Risch, N. and Thompson, W.D. (1991) Genetic analysis of breast cancer in the cancer and steroid hormone study. *Am. J. Hum. Genet.*, **48**, 232–41.
15. Iselius, L., Slack, J., Littler, M. and Morton, N.E. (1991) Genetic epidemiology of breast cancer in Britain. *Ann. Hum. Genet.*, **55**, 151–9.
16. Goldstein, A.M., Haile, R.W.C., Marazita, M.L. and Paganni-Hill, A. (1987) A genetic epidemiologic investigation of breast cancer in families with bilateral breast cancer. I. Segregation analysis. *J. Natl Cancer Inst.*, **78**, 911–18
17. Bishop, D.T. and Gardner, E.J. (1980) Analysis of the genetic predisposition to cancer in individual pedigrees, in *Cancer Incidence in Defined Populations*, Banbury Report 4, Cold

Genetics and the common cancers

Spring Harbor Laboratory Press, New York, pp. 389–406.

18. Go, R.C.P., King, M-C., Bailey-Wilson, J., Elston, R.C. and Lynch, H.T. (1983) Genetic epidemiology of breast and associated cancers in high-risk families. I. Segregation analysis. *J. Natl Cancer Inst.*, **71**, 455–61.

19. Cannon-Albright, L.A., Bishop, D.T. and Skolnick, M.H. (1986) Segregation and linkage analysis of breast cancer in the Dutch and Utah families. *Genet. Epidemiol.*, **1** (Suppl.), 43–8.

20. Bishop, D.T., Cannon-Albright, L., McLellan, T., Gardner, E.J. and Skolnick, M.H. (1988) Segregation and linkage analyisis of nine Utah breast cancer pedigrees. *Genet. Epidemiol.*, **5**, 151–69.

21. Burt, R.W., Bishop, T., Cannon, L.A., Dowdle, M.A., Lee, R.G. and Skolnick, M.H. (1985) Dominant inheritance of adenomatous colonic polyps and colorectal cancer. *N. Engl. J. Med.*, **312**, 1540–4.

22. Bailey-Wilson, J.E., Elston, R.C., Schuelke, G.S. *et al.* (1986) Segregation analysis of hereditary non-polyposis colorectal cancer. *Genet. Epidemiol.*, **3**, 27–38.

23. Cannon-Albright, L.A., Skolnick, M.H., Bishop, D.T., Lee, R.G. and Burt, R.W. (1988) Common inheritance of susceptibility to colonic adenomatous polyps and associated colorectal cancers. *N. Engl. J. Med.*, **319**, 533–7.

24. Houlston, R.S., Collins, A., Slack, J. and Morton, N.E. (1992) Dominant genes for colorectal cancer are not rare. *Ann. Hum. Genet.*, **56**, 99–103.

25. Sellers, T.A., Bailey-Wilson, J.E., Elston, R.C. *et al.* (1990) Evidence for mendelian inheritance in the pathogenesis of lung cancer. *J. Natl Cancer Inst.*, **82**, 1272–9.

26. Houlston, R.S., Collins, A., Slack, J. *et al.* (1991) Genetic epidemiology of ovarian cancer: segregation analysis. *Ann. Hum. Genet.*, **55**, 291–9.

27. Carter, B.S., Beaty, T.H., Steinberg, G.D., Childs, B. and Walsh, P.C. (1992) Mendelian inheritance of prostate cancer. *Proc. Natl Acad. Sci. USA*, **89**, 3367–71.

28. Ottman, R., Pike, M.C., King, M.-C., Casagrande, J.T. and Hendersen, B.E. (1986) Fam-

ilial breast cancer in a population based series. *Am.J. Epidemiol.*, **123**, 15–21.

29. Risch, N. (1990) Linkage strategies for genetically complex multilocus traits, I. Multilocus models. *Am. J. Hum. Genet.*, **46**, 222–8.

30. Hall, J.M., Lee, M.K., Morrow, J. *et al.* (1990) Linkage analysis of early onset familial breast cancer to chromosome 17q21. *Science*, **250**, 1684–9.

31. Easton, D.F., Bishop, T., Ford, D., Cockcroft, G.P. and the Breast Cancer Linkage Consortium. (1992) Genetic linkage analysis in familial breast and ovarian cancer: results from 214 families. *Am. J. Hum. Genet.*, **52**, 678–701.

32. Lindbolm, A., Tannergaard, P., Werelius, B. and Nordenskjoid, B. (1993) Genetic mapping of a second locus predisposing to hereditary non-polyposis colon cancer. *Nature Genet.*, **5**, 279–82.

33. Peltomaki, P., Aaltonen, L.A., Sistonen, P. *et al.* (1993) Genetic mapping of a locus predisposing to human colorectal cancer. *Science*, **260**, 810–12.

34. Cannon-Albright. L.A., Goldgar, D.E., Meyer, L.J. *et al.* (1992) Assignment of a locus for familial melanoma, MLM, to chromosome 9p13-p22. *Science*, **258**, 1148–52.

35. Nishisho, I., Nakamura, Y., Miyoshi, Y. *et al.*, (1991) Muations of chromosome 5q21 genes in FAP and colorectal cancer patients. *Science*, **253**, 665–9.

36. Easton, D., Ford, D. and Peto, J. (1994) Inherited susceptibility to breast cancer. *Cancer Surv.*, **18**, 95–113.

37. Goldgar, D.E., Easton, D.E., Cannon-Albright, L.A. and Skolnick, M.H. (1994) A systematic population based-assessment of cancer risk in first degree relatives of cancer probands. *J. Natl Cancer Inst.*, **86**, 200–9.

38. Ford, D., Easton, D.F., Bishop, D.T., Narod, S., Golgar, D.E. and the Breast Cancer Linkage Consortium. (1994) Risks of cancer in BRCA1-mutation carriers. *Lancet*, **343**, 692–5.

39. Lu, S., Day, N.E., Degos, L. *et al.* (1990) Linkage of a nasopharyngeal carcinoma susceptibility locus to the HLA region. *Nature*, **346**, 470–1.

40. Ayesh, R., Idle, J.R., Rithcie, J.C., Crothers, M.J. and Hetzel, M.R. (1984) Metabolic oxi-

dation phenotypes as markers for susceptibility to lung cancer. *Nature*, **312**, 169–70.

41. Gough, A.C., Miles, J.S., Spurr, N.K. *et al.* (1990) Identification of the primary gene defect at the cytochrome P450 CYP2D locus. *Nature*, **347**, 773–5.

42. Cartwright, R.A., Glasan, R.W., Rogers, H.J. *et al.* (1982) Role of N-acetyltransferase phenotypes in bladder cancinogenesis: a pharmaco-genetic epidemiological approach to bladder cancer. *Lancet*, **2**, 842–6.

43. Swerdlow, A.J. and Green, A. (1987) Melanocytic naevi and melanoma: an epidemiological perspective. *Br. J. Dermatol.*, **117**, 137–46.

44. Easton, D.F, Cox, G.M., Macdonald, A.M. and Ponder, B.A.J. (1991) Genetic susceptibility to naevi – a twin study. *Br. J. Cancer*, **64**, 1164–7.

45 Goldgar, D.E., Cannon-Albright, L.A., Meyer, L.J., Peipkorn, M.W., Zone, J.J. and Skolnick, M.H. (1992) Inheritance of nevus number and size in melanoma/DNS kindreds. *Cytogenet. Cell. Genet.*, **59**, 200–2.

46. Cuzick, J., Harris, R. and Mortimer, P.S. (1983) Palmar keratoses and bladder cancer. *Lancet*, **i**, 530–3.

47. Cuzick, J., Babiker, A., de Stovola, B.L., McCance, D., Cartwright, R. and Glashan, R.W. (1990) Palmar keratoses in family members with bladder cancer. *J. Clin. Epidemiol.*, **43**, 1421–6.

48. Kamb, A., Gruis, N.A., Weaver-Feldhaus, J. *et al.* (1994) A cell cycle regulator potentially involved in genesis of many tumor types. *Science*, **264**, 436–40.

49. Scott, D., Spreadborough, A., Levine, E. and Roberts, S.A. (1994) Genetic predispisition to breast cancer. *Lancet*, **344**, 1444.

50. Easton, D. (1994) Cancer risks in A-T Heterozygotes. *Int. J. Radiat. Biol.*, **66**, 5177–82.

51. Cramer, W. (1934) The prevention of cancer. *Lancet*, **1**, 1–5.

TABLES 13.2–13.5 ONLY

1. Tokuhuta, G. and Lilienfeld, A. (1963) Familial aggregation of lung cancer among hospital patients. *Public Health Rep.*, **78**, 277–83.

2. Tokuhuta, G. and Lilienfeld, A. (1963) Familial aggregation of lung cancer in humans. *J. Natl Cancer Inst.*, **30**, 289–312.

3. Lynch, H.T., Schuelke, G.S., Kimberling, W.J. *et al.* (1986) Genetics and smoking-associated cancers: a study of 485 families. *Cancers*, **56**, 939–51.

4. Ooi, W., Elston, R., Chen, V., Bailey-Wilson, J. and Rothschild, H.J. (1986) Increased familial risk for lung cancer. *J. Natl Cancer Inst.*, **76**, 217–22.

5. Samet, J., Humble, C. and Pathak, D. (1986) Personal and family history of respiratory disease and lung cancer risk. *Am. Rev. Respir. Dis.*, **134**, 466–70.

6. Gao, Y.T., Blot, W., Zhen, G. *et al.* (1987) Lung cancer among Chinese women. *Int. J. Cancer*, **40**, 604–9.

7. Tsugane, S., Watanabe, S., Suginmura, H., Arimoto, H., Shimosato, Y. and Suemasu, K. (1987) Smoking, occupation and family history in lung cancer patients under fifty years of age. *Jpn. J. Clin. Oncol.*, **17**, 309–17.

8. Wu, A.H., Yu, M.C., Thomas, D.C., Pike, M.C. and Henderson, B.E. (1988) Personal and family history of lung disease as risk factors for adenocarcinma of the lung. *Cancer Res.*, **48**, 7279–84.

9. Horwitz, R., Smaldone, L. and Viscoli, C. (1988) An ecogenetic hypothesis for lung cancer in women. *Arch. Intern. Med.*, **148**, 2609–12.

10. McDuffie, H.H., Dosman, J.A. and Klaassen, D.J. (1989) Cancer genes and agriculture in *Principles of Health and Safety in Agriculture*, (eds J.A., Dosman and D.W. Cockcroft), CRC Press, Boca Raton, Florida pp. 258–61.

11. McDuffie, H.H., Klassen, D.J. and Dosman, J.A. (1991) Clustering of cancer in families of patients with primary lung cancer. *J. Clin. Epidemiol.*, **44**, 69–76.

12. Osann, K. (1991) Lung cancer in women: the importance of smoking, family history of cancer, and medical history of respiratory disease. *Cancer Res.*, **51**, 4893–7.

13. Shaw, G., Falk, R., Pickle, L., Mason, T. and Buffler, P. (1991) Lung cancer risk associated with cancer in relatives. *J. Clin. Epidemiol.*, **44**, 429–37.

14. Lee, P.N. (1993) Epidemiological studies relating family history of lung cancer to risk of the disease. *Indoor Environment*, **2**, 129–42.

15. Goldgar, D.E., Easton, D.E., Cannon-Albright, L.A. and Skolnick, M.H. (1994) A systematic population based-assesment of cancer risk in first degree relatives of cancer probands. *J. Natl Cancer Inst.*, **86**, 200–9.

16. Woolf, C.M. (1958) A genetic study of carcinoma of the large intestine. *Am. J. Hum. Genet.*, **10**, 42–7.

17. Macklin, M.T. (1960) Inheritance of cancer of the stomach and large intestine in man. *J. Natl Cancer Inst.*, **24;** 551–71.

18. Lovett, E. (1976) Family studies in cancer of the colon and rectum. *Br. J. Surg.*, **63**, 13–18.

19. Duncan, J.L. and Kyle, J. (1982) Family incidence of carcinoma of the colon and rectum in North-East Scotland. *Gut*, **23**, 169–71.

20. Maire, P., Morichau-Beachant, M., Drucker, J., Barboteau, J. and Matuchansky, C. (1984) Familial occurrence of cancer of the colon and rectum: results of a 3-year case control survey. *Gastroenterol. Clin. Biol.*, **8**, 22–7.

21. Kune, G.A., Kune, S. and Watson, L.F. (1987) The Melborne Colorectal cancer study. *Dis. Colon Rectum*, **30**, 600–6.

22. Ponz de Leon, M., Antonioli, A., Ascari, A., Zangheri, G.A. and Sachetti, C. (1987) Incidence and familial occurrence of colorectal cancer and polyps in a health care district of Northern Italy. *Cancer*, **60**, 2848–59.

23. Bonnelli, L., Martines, H., Conio, M., Bruzzi, P. and Aste, H. (1988) Family history of colorectal cancer as a risk factor for benign and malignant tumours of the large bowel. A case-control study. *Int. J. Cancer*, **41**, 513–17.

24. Stephenson, B.M., Finan, P.J., Gascoyne, J., Garbett, F., Murday, V.A. and Bishop, D.T. (1991) Frequency of familial colorectal cancer. *Br. J. Surg.*, **78**, 1162–6.

25. Sondergaard J.O., Bulow, S. and Lynge, E. (1991) Cancer incidence among parents of patients with colorectal cancer. *Int. J. Cancer*, **47**, 202–6.

26. St John, D.J., McDermott, F.T., Hopper, J.L., Debney, E.A., Johson, W.R. and Hughes, E.S.R. (1993) Cancer risk in relatives of patients with common colorectal cancer. *Ann. Intern. Med.*, **118**, 785–90.

27. Zangheri, G., DiGregorio, C., Sacchetti, C. *et al.* (1990) Familial occurrence of gastric cancer in the 2-year exerience of a population-based registry. *Cancer*, **66**, 2047–51.

28. LaVecchia, C., Negri, E., Franceschi, S. and Gentile, A. (1991) Family history and risk of stomach and colorectal cancer. *Cancer*, **70**, 50–5.

29. Adami, H.O., Hansen, J., Jung, B. and Rimsten, A. (1980) Familiarity in breast cancer: a case control study in a Swedish population. *Br. J. Cancer*, **42**, 71–7.

30. Bain, C., Speizer, F.E., Rosner, B., Belanger, C. and Hennekens, C.H. (1980) Family history of breast cancer as a risk indicator for the disease. *Am. J. Epidemiol.*, **111**, 301–8.

31. Brinton, L.A., Hoover, R. and Fraumeni, J.F. Jr. (1982) Interaction of familial and hormonal risk factors for breast cancer. *J. Natl Cancer Inst.*, **69**, 817–22.

32. Sattin, R.W., Rubin, G.L., Webster, L.A. *et al.* (1985) Family history and the risk of breast cancer. *JAMA*, **253**, 1908–13.

33. Ottman, R., Pike, M.C., King, M.-C., Casagrande, J.T. and Hendersen, B.E. (1986) Familial breast cancer in a population based series. *Am. J. Epidemiol.*, **123**, 15–21.

34. Dupont, W.D. and Page, D.L. (1987) Breast cancer risk associated with proliferative disease, age at first birth, and a family history of breast cancer. *Am. J. Epidemiol.*, **125**, 769–79.

35. Negri, E., La Vecchia, C., Bruzi, P. *et al.* (1988) Risk factors for breast cancer: pooled results from three Italian case-control studies. *Am. J. Epidemiol.*, **128**, 1207–15.

36. Bouchardy, C., Le, M.G. and Hill, C. (1990) Risk factors for breast cancer according to age at diagnosis in a French case-contol study. *J. Clin. Epidemiol.*, **43**, 267–75.

37. Houlston, R.S., McCarter, E., Parhboo, S., Scurr, J. and Slack, J. (1991) Family history and risk of breast cancer. *J. Med. Genet.*, **29**, 154–7.

38. Tulinius, H., Sigvalsason, H., Olafsdottir, G. and Tryggvadottir, L. (1992) Epidemiology of breast cancer in families in Iceland. *J. Med. Genet.*, **29**, 158–64.

39. Peto, J., Easton, D.F., Matthews, F.E., Ford, D. and Swerdlow, A.J. (1996) Cancer mortality in relatives of women with breast cancer: The OPCS study. *Int. J. Cancer*, In Press.

40. Casagrande, J.T., Hanish, R., Pike, M.C. *et al.* (1988) A case-control study of male breast cancer. *Cancer Res.*, **48**, 1326–30.

41. Rosenblatt, K.A., Thomas, D.B., McTiernan, A. *et al.* (1991) Breast cancer in men: aspects of familial aggregation. *J. Natl Cancer Inst.*, **83**, 849–53.

42. Anderson, D.E. and Badzioch, M.D. (1992) Breast cancer risks in relatives of male breast cancer patients. *J. Natl Cancer Inst.*, **84**, 1114–17.

43. Schildkraut, J.M., Risch, N. and Thompson, W.D. (1989) Evaluating the genetic association among ovarian, breast and endometrial cancer: evidence for a breast ovarian relationship. *Am. J. Hum. Genet.*, **45**, 521–9.

44. Hildreth, N.G., Kelsey, S.L., LiVolsi, V. *et al.* (1981) An epidemiologic study of epithelial carcinoma of the ovary. *Am. J. Epidemiol.*, **114**, 398–405.

45. Cramer, D.W., Hutchinson, G.B., Welch, W.R., Scully, R.E. and Ryan, K.J. (1983) Determinants of ovarian cancer risk, I: reproductive experiences and family history. *J. Natl Cancer Inst.*, **71**, 711–16.

46. Booth, M.A. (1986) *Aspects of the Epidemiology of Ovarian Cancer*. PhD Thesis, University of London.

47. Koch, M., Gaedke, H. and Jenkins, H. (1989) Family history of ovarian cancer: a case-control study. *Int. J. Epidemiol.*, **18**, 782–5.

48. Easton, D.E., Matthews, F.E., Ford, D., Swerdlow, A.J. and Peto, J. (1996) Cancer mortality in relatives of women with ovarian cancer. The OPCS Study. *Int. J. Cancer* (in press).

49. Morganti, G., Gianferrari, L., Cresseri, A., Arrigoni, G. and Glovati, G. (1956) Recherches clinico-statistiques et genetiques sur les neoplasies de la prostate. *Acta Genet.*, **6**, 304–5.

50. Steele, R., Lees, R.E., Kraus, A.S. and Rao, C. (1971) Sexual factors in the epidemiology of cancer of the prostate. *J. Chron. Dis.*, **24**, 29–37.

51. Krain, L.S. (1974) Some epidemiologic variables in prostatic carcinoma in California. *Prev. Med.*, **3**, 154–9.

52. Schuman, L.M., Mandel, J., Bauer, H., Scarlett, J. and McHugh, R. (1977) Epidemiologic study of prostatic cancer: preliminary report. *Cancer Treat. Rep.*, **61**, 181–6.

53. Cannon, L., Bishop, D.T., Skolnick, M., Hunt, S., Lyon, J.L. and Smart, C.R. (1982) Genetic epidemiology of prostate cancer in the Utah geneology. *Cancer Surv.* **1**, 47–69.

54. Meikle, A.W., Smith J.A. and West, D.W. (1985) Familial factors affecting prostatic cancer risk and plasma sex-steroid levels. *Prostate*, **6**, 121–8.

55. Steinberg, G.D., Carter, B.S. Beaty, T.H., Childs, B. and Walsh, P.C. (1990) Family history and the risk of prostate cancer. *Prostate*, **17**, 337–47.

56. Spitz, M.R., Currier, R.D., Fueger, J.J., Babaian, J. and Newell, G.R. (1991) Familial patterns of prostate cancer: a case control analysis. *J. Urol.*, **146**, 1305–7.

57. Ghadrain, P., Cadotte, M. and Perret, C. (1991) Familial aggregation of cancer of the prostate in Quebec: The tip of the Iceberg. *Prostate*, **19**, 43–52.

58. Holman, C.D.J. and Armstrong, B.K. (1984) Pigmentary traits, ethnic origin, benign nevi and family history as risk factors for cutaneous malignant melanoma. *J. Natl Cancer Inst.*, **2**, 257–66.

59. Green, A., MacLennan, R. and Siskind, V. (1985) Common acquired naevi and the risk of malignant melanoma. *Int. J. Cancer*, **35**, 297–300.

60. Cristofolini, M., Franceschi, S., Tasin, L. *et al.*, (1987) Risk factors for cutaneous malignant melanoma in a Northern Italian population. *Int. J. Cancer*, **39**, 150–4.

61. Holly, E.A., Kelly, J.W., Shpall, S.N. and Chius, S.-H. (1987) Number of melanocytic nevi as a major risk factor for malignant melanoma. *J. Am. Acad. Dermatol.*, **17**, 459–68.

62. Osterlind, A., Tucker, M.A., Hou-Jensen, K., Stone, B.J., Engholm, G. and Jensen, O.M. (1988) The Danish case-control study of cutaneous malignant melanoma. I. Importance of host factors. *Int. J. Cancer*, **42**, 200–6.

63. Stoffer, S., Van Dyke, D.L., Vaden Bach, V. and Weiss, L. (1980) Familial papillary carcinoma of the thyroid. *Am. J. Med. Genet.*, **25**, 775–82.

64. Ron, E., Kleinerman, R.A., LiVolsi, V.A. and Fraumeni, J.F. Jr. (1991) Familial nonmedullary thyroid cancer. *Oncology*, **48**, 309–11.

65. Forman, D., Oliver, R.T.D., Brett, A.R. *et al* (1992) Familial testicular cancer: a report of the UK family register, estimation of risk and an HLA Class 1 sib-pair analysis. *Br. J. Cancer*, **65**, 255–62.

66. Ghadirian, P., Boyle., Simard, A., Baillargeon, J., Maisonneuve, P. and Perret C. (1991) Reported family aggregation of pancreatic cancer within a population-based case-control study in the Franchophone Community in Montreal, Canada. *Int. J. Pancreatol.*, **10**, 183–96.

67. Kantor, A.E., Hartage, P., Hoover, R.N. and Fraumeni, J.F. (1985) Familial and environ-mental interactions in bladder cancer risk. *Int. J. Cancer*, **35**, 703–6.

68. Mellemgaard, A., Engholm, G., McLaughton, J.K. and Olsen, J.H. (1994) Risk factors for renal cell carcinoma in Denmark. I. Role of socioeconomic status, tobacco use, beverages, and family history. *Cancer Causes and Control*, **5.2**, 105–13.

Chapter 14

Familial breast cancer

DAVID E. GOLDGAR, MICHAEL R. STRATTON and
ROSALIND A. EELES

14.1 INTRODUCTION

Breast cancer has been recognized for over 100 years as having a familial component [1]. More recently, a number of epidemiological investigations have attempted to quantify the risks of breast cancer associated with a positive family history. Attempts have also been made to examine whether the pattern of related individuals with breast cancer are consistent with the effects of a single gene of large effect, shared environmental effects, many genes acting in an additive manner, or most likely, a combination of two or more of these effects. In addition to this statistical and observational evidence for the role of genes in the development of breast cancer, a number of specific genes have been identified as playing a role. Perhaps the most notable of these genes is *BRCA*1, which was identified through genetic linkage studies and localized to the long arm of chromosome 17 [2]. Because *BRCA*1 has been extensively studied, it is the subject of a separate chapter (Chapter 15) in this book. However, the *BRCA*1 gene accounts for, at most, half (and probably less) of all familial breast cancer. In this chapter, we will begin by examining the epidemiological evidence for familial risks in breast cancer, then discuss the results of statistical analyses of breast cancer families for the presence of major genetic effects, and describe specific genes other than *BRCA*1 which influence breast cancer risk. We will also present evidence that additional genes exist, as yet unmapped, which account for a substantial proportion of familial breast cancer.

14.2 FAMILIAL RISK OF BREAST CANCER

Evidence that women with a positive family history of breast cancer are at increased risk for developing the disease has been accumulating for over 50 years; virtually every study in which this question has been examined has found significantly elevated relative risks to female relatives of breast cancer patients. However, the magnitude of these risks has varied considerably according to the number and type of affected relatives, age at diagnosis of the proband(s), laterality, and the overall study design. Table 14.1 summarizes the results from approximately 40 such studies. Most studies have found relative risks between 2 and 3 for first-degree relatives of

Genetic Predisposition to Cancer. Edited by R.A. Eeles, B.A.J. Ponder, D.F. Easton and A. Horwich. Published in 1996 by Chapman & Hall, London.
0 412 56580 3

Table 14.1 Estimates of relative risks for breast cancer. (Modified and updated from [3].)

Relative affected, status of proband	Estimate of relative risk	Reference	Study type[1]
Mother	18	Martynova, 1936 [4]	II
Mother	3	Jacobsen, 1946 [5]	I
Sister	3	Jacobsen, 1946 [5]	I
Mother	2	Penrose *et al.*, 1948 [6]	I
Sister	3	Penrose *et al.*, 1948 [6]	I
Mother	2	Smithers, 1948 [7]	I
Sister	3	Woolf, 1955 [8]	I
Mother	2	Woolf, 1955 [8]	
Sister	2	Anderson VE *et al.*, 1958 [9]	II
Sister	3	Macklin, 1959 [10]	IV
Mother	2	Murphy and Abbey, 1959 [11]	I
Mother	2	Macklin, 1959 [10]	IV
Sister, premenopausal proband	5	Anderson DE, 1971 [12]	IV
Sister, postmenopausal proband	2	Anderson DE, 1971 [12]	IV
First-degree relative	2	Anderson DE, 1972 [13]	IV
First-degree relative, premenopausal proband	3	Anderson DE, 1972 [13]	IV
First-degree relative, premenopausal bilateral proband	9	Anderson DE, 1972 [13]	IV
First-degree relative, bilateral proband	5	Anderson DE, 1972 [13]	IV
Sister and mother affected, pre-menopausal bilateral proband	47–51	Anderson DE, 1974 [14]	IV
Sister and mother affected, pre-menopausal bilateral proband	39	Anderson DE, 1976 [15]	IV
Sister	3	Tulinius *et al.*, 1980 [16]	I
First-degree relative	2	Brinton *et al.*, 1982 [17]	III
Mother and sister affected	14	Sattin, 1985 [18]	III
First-degree relative	2	Sattin, 1985 [18]	III
Second-degree relative	2	Sattin, 1985 [18]	III
Sister, bilateral proband <50 years	6	Ottman *et al.*, 1986 [19]	III
Sister, bilateral proband <40 years	10.5	Ottman *et al.*, 1986 [19]	III
Sister, unilateral proband <40 years	2.4	Ottman *et al.*, 1986 [19]	III
First-degree relative	2	Negri *et al.*, 1988 [20]	III
First-degree relative, proband with P2 + DY mammographic pattern	6	Saftlas *et al.*, 1989 [21]	III
Sister	2	Carter *et al.*, 1989 [22]	V
Mother	2	Carter *et al.*, 1989 [22]	V
First-degree relative	2	Schildkraut *et al.*, 1989 [23]	I
First-degree relative ≤45 years, proband ≤45 years	3	Schildkraut *et al.*, 1989 [23]	I
First-degree relative ≤45 years, proband >45 years	3.3	Schildkraut *et al.*, 1989 [23]	I
First-degree relative >45 years, proband ≤45 years	2	Schildkraut *et al.*, 1989 [23]	I

Table 14.1 Continued

First-degree relative >45 years, proband >45 years	1.5	Schildkraut *et al.*, 1989 [23]	I
First-degree relative, proband >55 years	1.8	Mettlin *et al.*, 1990 [24]	I
First-degree relative >55 years, proband >55 years	1.9	Mettlin *et al.*, 1990 [24]	I
Two or more first-degree relatives	3.3	Mettlin *et al.*, 1990 [24]	I
First-degree relative, bilateral proband >55 years	2.3	Mettlin *et al.*, 1990 [24]	I
First degree relative	2	Claus *et al.*, 1990 [25]	III
First-degree relative, proband >55 years	1.6	Houlston *et al.*, 1992 [26] I	
First-degree relative, proband <55 years	2.3	Houlston *et al.*, 1992 [26]	I
First-degree relative, proband <45 years	3.8	Houlston *et al.*, 1992 [26]	I
First-degree relative, bilateral proband	6.4	Houlston *et al.*, 1992 [26]	I
First-degree relative	2.3	Tulinius *et al.*, 1992 [27]	I
Second-degree relative	1.7	Tulinius *et al.*, 1992 [27]	I
First-degree relative	2.4	Slattery and Kerber, 1993 [28]	III
Second-degree relative	1.8	Slattery and Kerber, 1993 [28]	III
Mother	2	Slattery and Kerber, 1993 [28]	III
First-degree relative	1.8	Goldgar *et al.*, 1994 [29]	I
Two or more first-degree relatives	2.7	Goldgar *et al.*, 1994 [29]	I
Male breast cancer			
Sister, male proband	2.5	Casagrande *et al.*, 1988 [30]	III
Mother, male proband	1	Casagrande *et al.*, 1988 [30]	III
First-degree female relative, male proband	1.8	Casagrande *et al.*, 1988 [30]	III
Male, family history in male relatives	4	Rosenblatt *et al.*, 1991 [31]	I
Mother, male proband	2.3	Rosenblatt *et al.*, 1991 [31]	I
Sister, male proband	2.2	Rosenblatt *et al.*, 1991 [31]	I
First-degree relative, male proband	2.3	Rosenblatt *et al.*, 1991 [31]	I
Mother, male proband	1.4	Anderson and Badzioch, 1992 [32]	I
Sister, male proband	2.1	Anderson and Badzioch, 1992 [32]	I
Daughter, male proband	2.9	Anderson and Badzioch, 1992 [32]	I

I, Ratio of observed frequencies in cancer families to expected frequencies in the general population; II, ratio of observed rate of cancer in relatives of cases to observed rate of cancer in relatives of selected controls; III, odds ratio from case-control study with non-cancer controls; IV, odds ratio from case-control study with cancer controls; V, relative risk from prospective study.

breast cancer patients selected without regard to age at diagnosis or laterality.

In one of the first studies of familial breast cancer in a population-based series [19], sisters of unilateral breast cancer cases diagnosed at age 50 or younger did not show significantly increased risk; however, sisters of unilateral patients diagnosed at age 40 or younger did appear to have increased risk (relative risk = 2.4).

In a comprehensive population-based study of familial cancer using the Utah Population Database, Goldgar *et al.* [29] studied the incidence of breast and other cancers among 49 202 first-degree relatives of 5559 breast cancer probands diagnosed before age 80. This study estimated a relative risk of 1.8 in relatives of these breast cancer probands. When the age criteria was reduced to early-onset cancer (diagnosed before age 50), the relative risk of breast cancer among first-degree relatives increased to 2.6 and the risk for early-onset breast cancer among these relatives was 3.7 (95% C.I. 2.8–4.6). Similarly, when the risk to subsequent relatives in families with two affected sisters was considered, the risk increased to 2.7 with a particularly high risk of 4.9 to breast cancers diagnosed before age 50. When the study was extended to examine only second-degree relatives of early-onset probands, the relative risk estimate decreased to 1.4 (95% C.I. 1.1–1.8) for all breast cancer, and 1.7 (95% C.I. 0.9–2.8) for early-onset breast cancer. Similarly, when cousins of early-onset probands were considered, the overall familial relative risks were 1.2 for all breast cancer cases, and 1.5 (95% C.I. 1.1–2.0) for those diagnosed before the age of 50.

Although most studies have shown the risk to relatives of early-onset probands to be higher than that for probands diagnosed after age 50 or for relatives of all probands, one study [24] found a higher relative risk (1.8) among probands diagnosed over the age of 55 than that for probands diagnosed at an earlier age.

Perhaps the largest population-based study of familial breast cancer is the one done as part of the Cancer and Steroid Hormone (CASH) case-control study of 4730 probands with breast cancer diagnosed between the ages of 20 and 54. The risk of breast cancer in the first-degree relatives of these women compared with controls was 2.1 [23]. From this large data set, Claus *et al.* [33] estimated age-specific risks as a function of the age at diagnosis of the proband and the number of affected relatives. Some of these data (reproduced from [25]) are shown in Figure 14.1. For example, a woman with a sister affected at age 50 has an estimated lifetime risk of 3.6

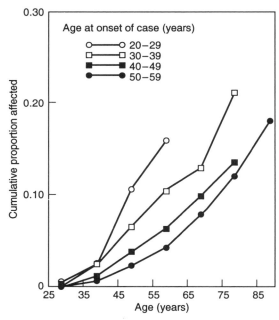

Fig. 14.1 Cumulative proportion of breast cancer cases occurring in first-degree relatives of cases by age of case. (Reproduced from [25], with permission.)

(95% C.I. 2.1–6.1), while a woman at age 50 with a mother and a sister affected has an estimated lifetime risk of 17.1 (95% C.I., 9.4–31.3).

In addition to the relationship between age at diagnosis and the magnitude of the familial component of breast cancer (which was discussed above), other investigators have examined the role of other factors with respect to family history. Ottman *et al.* [19] found larger familial effects among relatives of young bilateral probands compared with young probands with unilateral breast cancer. Similar findings have been reported by Anderson [14].

The issue of relationship of histology to familial breast cancer is less clear. Claus *et al.* [34] extensively reviewed the more recent literature, which continues to show no consistent picture. Some studies have found that lobular carcinoma is more often associated with a positive family history [35]. However, Lagios *et al* [36] found that cases with tubular carcinoma more frequently reported a positive family history than other histological subtypes. Multicentricity was also found to be positively associated with family history [37]. Other studies have shown conflicting reports of correlation between family history and subtypes or found no differences [38–40]. In the CASH study, Claus *et al* [34] found that cases with lobular carcinoma *in situ* were significantly more likely to have a mother or sister affected with breast cancer.

Another feature which conveys strong familial risk of breast cancer is the occurrence of breast cancer in a male. It has been estimated that female relatives of probands with male breast cancer have a two- to three-fold increased risk of breast cancer [31, 32].

14.3 FAMILIAL ASSOCIATIONS OF BREAST AND OTHER CANCERS

A number of studies, including those described earlier, have found increased risks for other cancers among relatives of breast cancer probands. The most commonly reported sites have been ovarian, uterine, prostate and colon cancer. However, most of these studies have only examined risks at selected sites in relatives. The study by Goldgar *et al*. [29] examined risks to all other sites among such probands. Statistically significant familial associations were found between breast cancer and cancers of the prostate (relative risk = 1.2, $P<0.0001$), colon (1.35, $P<0.0001$), thyroid (1.7, $P<0.001$) and non-Hodgkin's lymphoma (1.4, $P<0.001$). When the analysis was confined to relatives of the 1145 probands diagnosed before age 50, the risks for colon cancer and non-Hodgkin's lymphoma were increased, with familial relative risks of 1.7 ($P<0.001$) and 1.9 ($P<0.001$) respectively. In this study, there did not appear to be an increased risk of ovarian cancer among the relatives of breast

cancer probands (70 observed, 68 expected). There was a slightly increased frequency of ovarian cancer among relatives of the early-onset breast cancer cases (17 observed, 11.3 expected, relative risk = 1.5) but this difference was not statistically significant.

Perhaps the most consistently identified familial association of other cancers with breast cancer is prostate cancer. In addition to the comprehensive study of familial cancer association described previously, a number of other investigators have also observed significant associations between breast cancer and prostate cancer. Using the Utah Genealogy, Cannon *et al*. [41] found that among all pairs of individuals in which one member of the pair had prostate cancer and the other breast cancer, there was a significantly higher average degree of relatedness between the affected pair than among cohort-matched control pairs. Tulinius *et al*. [27], in a similar population-based study of the Iceland genealogies and cancer registry, found a significantly increased risk of prostate cancer in all relatives of women with breast cancer, a relative risk of 1.5 in first-degree relatives, and 1.3 in second-degree relatives. More recently, Anderson and Badzioch [32] reported a greater than two-fold risk of familial breast cancer when prostate cancer is also in the family history. Analysis of a subset of the Breast Cancer Linkage Consortium (BCLC) families suggests that the *BRCA*1 locus confers increased risks of prostate cancer (relative risk 3.33) and colon cancer (relative risk 4.11) [42].

Other studies have also shown relationships between breast cancer and ovarian, colon and uterine cancers, although the results have not been consistent across studies. For example, in a case-control study of 4730 breast cancer probands diagnosed between the ages of 20 and 54 in the CASH data set, Thompson and Schildkraut [43] found a significant odds ratio of 1.9 (95% C.I. 1.1–2.0) for ovarian cancer among relatives of the older probands (e.g. diagnosed after age 44), but a smaller, statistically non-significant increased risk of ovarian cancer among relatives of the younger probands (odds ratio 1.5). Nelson *et al.* [44], in a population-based study of 41 837 women aged 55–69 years, examined the family history of cancer in 1431 women who reported a personal history of breast cancer. The study found no association between personal history of breast cancer and a family history of ovarian cancer in first-degree relatives (odds ratio 1.1).

Anderson and Badzioch [45] found an association between breast and ovarian cancer only in relatives of bilateral breast cancer probands; none was found among unilateral breast cancer probands. In an Italian case-control study conducted from 1983–1989, Parazzinni *et al.* [46], conversely, found a significantly elevated risk of ovarian cancer in women with a family history of breast cancer (overall risk 1.6). Undoubtedly, the majority of the association between breast and ovarian cancer detected in these population studies is due to the *BRCA1* gene, which is known to be involved in a large proportion of extended kindreds with clearly inherited susceptibility to breast and ovarian cancer.

14.4 IMPLICATIONS OF MAJOR GENES IN BREAST CANCER AETIOLOGY

Because of the increased risk of breast cancer in relatives of breast cancer cases and the existence of families with unusual clusters of breast cancer cases, genes have been recognized as playing an important role in breast cancer aetiology [47]. Numerous investigators have examined the evidence for genetic inheritance [33, 48] in breast cancer families ascertained from a variety of population and non-population-based sources and concluded that the data were most consistent with autosomal dominant inheritance for a major susceptibility locus with high, but not complete, lifetime penetrance in genetically

susceptible women. The genetic models arising from these studies also implied that there was a non-negligible risk of breast cancer among women who did not carry this genetic susceptibility, and that because the risks to gene carriers was not 100%, there must be other genetic or environmental effects which influence risk.

In 1986, the fourth Genetic Analysis Workshop examined segregation and linkage analysis in several large data sets of breast cancer families. These workshops were conceived as a way of bringing together many different genetic epidemiologists with a variety of approaches to tackle a common problem. The group analysed data consisting of 200 families of sequential breast cancer probands in the Danish Cancer Registry from 1942–1945 collected by Jacobson *et al.*, 18 Nebraskan families ascertained in a variety of ways by Henry Lynch *et al.*, 16 two- to five-generation pedigrees collected in the Netherlands by Cleton *et al.*, and nine families ascertained from the Utah Genealogy by Skolnick *et al.*, (families and data are described by Bailey-Wilson *et al.* [49]). The results of these analyses are summarized in reports [50, 51] and confirmed the presence of an autosomal dominant susceptibility locus or loci acting to increase breast cancer susceptibility, at least in a subset of familial breast cancer.

More recently, Claus *et al.* [33] analysed a large data set collected as part of the CASH study and demonstrated a rare dominant susceptibility allele for breast cancer. The estimated frequency of the allele which conferred increased susceptibility to breast cancer was 0.003, implying a carrier rate in the general population of 6/1000. The estimated increased risk due to this susceptibility allele ranged from almost 100-fold in women in their 20s to a modest two-fold increase in women in their 80s. However, it must be recognized that the results of any segregation analysis of breast cancer families is likely to reflect the effects of a number of different susceptibility loci, given that it is extremely unlikely that all familial breast cancer is due to a single locus. Thus, the estimates of gene frequency derived from such analyses would represent the sum of the allele frequencies of a number of specific susceptibility loci. Similarly, the penetrance estimates are an average of the effects of each individual susceptibility locus. Confirmation of the existence of one or more loci which contribute to familial breast cancer and elucidation of the effects of individual loci, can come only through local-ization of such genes to specific chromosomal regions by linkage analysis of breast cancer families, or through identification of germ line mutations of specific candidate loci in familial breast cancer patients.

14.5 GENE MAPPING STUDIES IN FAMILIAL BREAST CANCER

A number of possible linkages between genetic markers and familial breast cancer have been reported in the past. The first such linkage was found between polymorphism at the glutamate-pyruvate transaminase (GPT) locus on chromosome 10 [52]. Later, Skolnick *et al.* [53] reported an initial linkage of a single kindred to the ABO blood group locus on chromosome 9q. The LOD score reached a maximum value of 3.0 before subsequent observations in new cases of breast cancer in the family reduced the strength of this evidence. These findings illustrate the diffi-culty in linkage analysis of complex traits, and demonstrate the need for confirmation in multiple families by different investigators. In spite of these difficulties, the existence of a specific gene, denoted *BRCA1*, conferring increased susceptibility to breast cancer, was confirmed in late 1990 with the finding of linkage between early-onset breast cancer and a specific marker (D17S74) on the long arm of chromosome 17 [2] (see also Chapter 15).

14.6 OTHER GENES CONFERRING INCREASED RISK OF BREAST CANCER

Aside from *BRCA1*, there are a number of specific genes which have been associated with an increased risk of breast cancer. The most striking of these genes is the *TP*53 tumour suppressor locus on chromosome 17p (see Chapter 8). Although mutations in this gene are commonly found in many types of tumours, germline *TP*53 mutations are most often associated with the Li–Fraumeni syndrome (LFS) in which families typically exhibit multiple affected members with child-hood cancers, primarily sarcomas and brain tumours [54] in addition to very early-onset breast cancer, often diagnosed before age 30. It has been estimated that 50–60% of Li–Fraumeni families are due to germline *TP*53 mutations in the coding region of the gene [55]. However, in families which have some of these characteristics but do not fulfil the classical definition of LFS, only 10% are attributable to germline *TP*53 mutations [55]. However, overall, germline *TP*53 mutations account for only a small (<1%) proportion of early-onset breast cancers and a negligible fraction of familial breast cancer in general. For example, Borreson *et al.* [56] screened 237 women with early-onset breast cancer and found only two germline *TP*53 mutations; both cases belonged to families with some features seen in the Li–Fraumeni syndrome. Sidransky *et al.* [57] examined 126 cases and found only one patient with breast cancer diagnosed before age 40 to have germline *TP*53 mutations; again, this case came from a Li–Fraumeni-like family.

Ataxia-telangiectasia (A-T) is an autosomal recessive disorder associated with a high incidence of cancer (61–184-fold), particularly lymphomas and leukaemias, but also prim-ary carcinomas of other organs, including the breast [58]. It has been reported that indivi-duals who carry one copy of the abnormal *A-T* gene are also at an increased risk (relative risk 5.1) for breast cancer [58]. It should be noted that this paper generated a great deal of controversy; the results were questioned on the basis of methodological issues of control groups and radiation exposure assessment, which could reduce the risk reported [59, 60]. If this result is true and the *A-T* gene frequency is as high as some estimates have indicated, the *A-T* locus could account for a substantial proportion of the observed familial relative risk (see Chapter 9). In a test of a number of early-onset breast cancer families which were not linked to *BRCA1*, no evidence of linkage to the *A-T* region of chromosome 11 was found [61]. However, if the *A-T* gene has moderate penetrance, it may not cause the dramatic familial clusters needed for linkage analysis, but may still make an important contribution to genetic breast cancer.

Other previously identified genes which might be biologically plausible candidates for breast cancer, include the oestrogen receptor (*ESR*) and the *HRAS1* locus. The *ESR* locus on chromosome 6q is a biological candidate in a region frequently lost in tumours [62] for which possible genetic linkage in a single postmenopausal breast cancer family has been reported [63]. The LOD score for this family with *ESR* was only 1.85, indicating a suggestive but not conclusive indication of linkage in this family. In a test of candidate gene loci in a set of *BRCA1*-unlinked breast cancer and breast–ovarian families, no evidence of linkage to the *ESR* locus was found; however, it should be noted that these families were selected primarily for premenopausal breast cancer. Further studies in older-onset families will be necessary to either confirm or disprove the involvement of the oestrogen receptor gene in familial breast cancer.

A recent study [64] showed a small but significant elevated risk of 2.29 for breast cancer associated with certain rare variants at a minisatellite locus located in the three prime untranslated region of the *HRAS* oncogene locus on the distal short arm of chromosome 11. The authors of this study hypothesize that *HRAS1* minisatellite mutations interfere with regulatory mechanisms governing the control of gene expression.

14.7 THE SEARCH FOR ADDITIONAL BREAST CANCER SUSCEPTIBILITY GENES

Based on genotypings at a series of marker loci surrounding the *BRCA1* locus, it was estimated from the BCLC data set that 45% of families with breast cancer only and virtually 100% of breast cancer families which also had at least one case of ovarian cancer were linked to 17q. Among those breast cancer families in which the average age at diagnosis was less than 45, it was estimated that two-thirds were due to the *BRCA1* locus [65]. However, it must be recognized that these estimates of heterogeneity are based on a set of families that were highly selected. Accurate estimates of the proportion of familial breast cancer due to *BRCA1* must await the mutation screening studies of the *BRCA1* gene. Although the BCLC found that virtually all families in which breast and ovarian cancer were present were due to *BRCA1*, the lower 95% confidence limit for this estimate was 0.79. Since the consortium data were submitted, at least 10 breast/ovarian cancer families have been identified which appear to be unlinked to *BRCA1* [66]. Interestingly, in families of breast cancer or breast–ovarian cancer studied thus far, which also include one or more cases of male breast cancer, all but two have proven to be unlinked to the *BRCA1* region of 17q [67]. One such example is shown in Figure 14.2. A genomic search which involved typing over 250 genetic markers localized the gene in this family to 13q12-13 [68]. This gene has been named *BRCA2* and has recently been cloned [69].

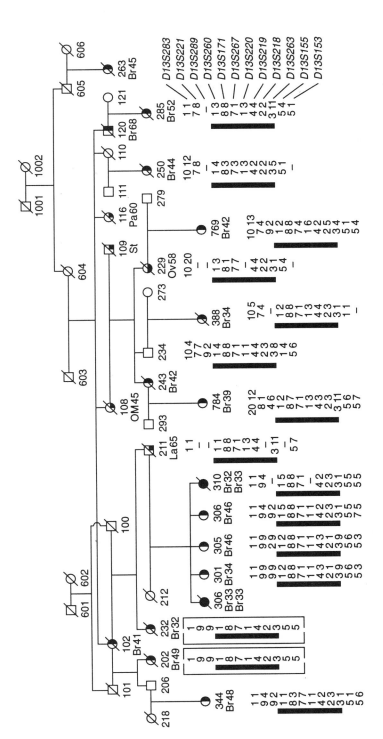

Fig. 14.2 Breast cancer family linked to chromosome 13. Haplotypes are shown below the typed cases. ●, ■, represent breast cancer; ◑, represents ovarian cancer. La, laryngeal cancer; Pa, pancreatic cancer; St, stomach cancer; OM, ocular melanoma. (Reproduced from [68], with permission.)

Familial breast cancer

14.8 SUMMARY

It is well established that a positive family history is the strongest epidemiological risk factor known for breast cancer, stronger than any known reproductive, hormonal or dietary factors. Although a common family environment could account for some portion of the observed familiality, there is substantial evidence that the majority of this familial effect is due to the action of a number of specific genes. This evidence comes from several sources: the observation that there is an increased risk to more distant relatives of breast cancer probands who do not share common environments; the results of segregation analyses which show that the pattern of familiarity is consistent with the actions of dominant high penetrant susceptibility loci; and, most convincingly, the cloning of two such susceptibility genes, *BRCA*1, and *BRCA*2. There is evidence for at least one further high-risk dominant gene. The role of specific, known genes such as *A-T* and *HRAS* which seem to be associated with a moderately increased breast cancer risk remains to be clarified.

REFERENCES

1. Broca, P.P. (1866) *Traites des Tumeurs.* Asselin, Paris, France.
2. Hall, J.M., Lee, M.K., Newman, B. *et al.* (1990) Linkage of early-onset familial breast cancer to chromosome 17q21. *Science,* **250,** 1684–9.
3. Cannon-Albright, L.A., Bishop, D.T., Goldgar, C. and Skolnick, M.H. (1991) Genetic predisposition to cancer, in *Important Advances in Oncology,* (eds V.T. DeVita Jr., S. Hellman and S.A. Rosenberg), J.B. Lippincott, Philadelphia, pp. 39–55.
4. Martynova, R.P. (1936) On the genetics of breast cancer in women. *Proc. Maxim-Gorky Res. Inst.,* **4,** 159–73.
5. Jacobsen, O. (1946) *Heredity and Breast Cancer,* H.K. Lewis, London.
6. Penrose, L.S., Mackenzie, J.H. and Karn, M.N. (1948) A genetical study of human mammary cancer. *Ann. Eugenics,* **14,** 234–66.
7. Smithers, D.W. (1948) Family histories of 459 patients with cancer of the breast. *Br. J. Cancer,* **2,** 163–7.
8. Woolf, C.M. (1955) Investigations on genetic aspects of carcinoma of the stomach and breast. *University of California Publications in Public Health,* **2,** 265–73.
9. Anderson, V.E., Goodman, H.O. and Reed, S.C. (1958) *Variables Related to Human Breast Cancer,* University of Minnesota Press, Minneapolis.
10. Macklin, M.T. (1959) Comparison of the number of breast-cancer deaths observed in relatives of breast-cancer patients, and the number expected on the basis of mortality rates. *J. Natl Cancer Inst.,* **22,** 927–51.
11. Murphey, D.P. and Abbey, H. (1959) *Cancer in Families. (A study of the relatives of 200 Breast Cancer Probands.)* Harvard University Press, Cambridge.
12. Anderson, D.E. (1971) Some characteristics of familial breast cancer. *Cancer,* **28,** 1500–4.
13. Anderson, D.E. (1972) A genetic study of human breast cancer. *J. Natl Cancer Inst.* **48,** 1029–34.
14. Anderson, D.E. (1974) Genetic study of breast cancer: identification of a high risk group. *Cancer,* **34,** 1090–7.
15. Anderson, D.E. (1976) Genetic predisposition to breast cancer. *Rec. Res. Cancer Res.,* **57,** 10–20.
16. Tulinius, H., Day, N.E. Sigvaldason, H. *et al.* (1980) A population-based study on familial aggregation of breast cancer in Iceland, taking some other risk factors into account, in *Genetic and Environmental Factors in Experimental and Human Cancer,* (eds H.V. Gelboin *et al.*), Japan Scientific Society Press, Japan, pp. 303–12.
17. Brinton, L.A., Hoover, R.N. and Fraumeni, J.F. (1982) Interaction of familial and hormonal risk factors for breast cancer. *J. Natl Cancer Inst.,* **69,** 817–22.
18. Sattin, R.W., Rubin, G.L., Webster, L.A. *et al.* (1985) Family history and the risk of breast cancer. *JAMA,* **253,** 1908–13.
19. Ottman, R., Pike, M.C., King, M-C., Casagrande, J.T. and Henderson, B.E. (1986) Familial breast cancer in a population based series. *Am. J. Epidemiol.,* **123,** 15–21.

20. Negri, E., La Vecchia, C., Bruzzi, P. *et al.* (1988) Risk factors for breast cancer: pooled results from three Italian case-control studies. *Am. J. Epidemiol.*, **128**, 1207–15.

21. Saftlas, A.F., Wolfe, J.N., Hoover, R.N. *et al.* (1989) Mammographic parenchymal patterns as indicators of breast cancer risk. *Am. J. Epidemiol.*, **129**, 518–26.

22. Carter, C.L., Jones, D.Y., Schatzkin, A. and Brinton, L.A. (1989) A prospective study of reproductive, familial and socioeconomic risk factors for breast cancer using NHANES I data. *Public Health Rep.*, **104**, 45–50.

23. Schildkraut, J.M., Risch, N. and Thompson, W.D. (1989) Evaluating genetic association among ovarian, breast, and endometrial cancer: evidence for a breast/ovarian cancer relationship. *Am. J. Hum. Genet.*, **45**, 521–9.

24. Mettlin, C., Croghan, I., Natarajan, N. and Lane, W. (1990) The association of age and familial risk in a case-control study of breast cancer. *Am. J. Epidemiol.*, **131**, 973–83.

25. Claus, E.B., Risch, N. and Thompson, W.D. (1990) Age of onset as an indicator of familial risk of breast cancer. *Am. J. Epidemiol.*, **131**, 961–72.

26. Houlston, R.S., McCarter, E., Parbhoo, S. *et al.* (1992) Family history and risk of breast cancer. *J. Med. Genet.*, **29**, 154–7.

27. Tulinius, H., Egilsson, V., Olafsdottir, G.H. and Sigvaldsson, H. (1992) Risk of prostate, ovarian and endometrial cancer among relatives of women with breast cancer. *Br. Med. J.*, **305**, 855–7.

28. Slattery, M.L. and Kerber R.A. (1993) A comprehensive evaluation of family history and breast cancer risk. *JAMA*, **270**, 1563–8.

29. Goldgar, D.E., Easton, D.F., Cannon-Albright, L.A. and Skolnick, M.H. (1994) Systematic population-based assessment of cancer risk in first degree relatives of cancer probands. *J. Natl Cancer Inst.*, **86**, 1600–7.

30. Casagrande, J.T., Hanisch, R., Pike, M.C. *et al.* (1988) A case-control study of male breast cancer. *Cancer Res.*, **48**, 1326–30.

31. Rosenblatt, K.A., Thomas, D.B., McTiernan, A. *et al.* (1991) Breast cancer in men: aspects of familial aggregation. *J. Natl Cancer Inst.*, **83**, 849–53.

32. Anderson, D.E. and Badzioch, M.D. (1992) Breast cancer risks in relatives of male breast cancer patients. *J. Natl Cancer Inst.*, **84**, 1114–17.

33. Claus, E.B., Risch, N. and Thompson, W.D. (1991) Genetic analysis of breast cancer in the cancer and steroid hormone study. *Am J. Hum. Genet.* **48**, 232–42.

34. Claus, E.B., Risch, N. and Thompson, W.D. (1993) Relationship between breast histopathology and family history of breast cancer. *Cancer*, **71**, 147–53.

35. Erdreich, L.S., Asal, N.R. and Hoge, A.F. (1980) Morphologic types of breast cancer: age, bilaterality, and family history. *South. Med. J.*, **73**, 28–32.

36. Lagios, M.D., Rose, M.E. and Margolin, F.R. (1980) Tubular carcinoma of the breast: association with multicentricity, bilaterality and family history. *Am. J. Clin. Pathol.*, **73**, 25–30.

37. Lagios, M.D. (1977) Multicentricity of breast carcinoma demonstrated by routine correlated serial subgross and radiographic examination. *Cancer*, **40**, 1726–34.

38. Lynch, H.T., Albano, W.A., Heieck, J.J. *et al.* (1984) Genetics, biomarkers, and control of breast cancer: a review. *Cancer Genet. Cytogenet.*, **13**, 43–92.

39. Rosen, P.P., Lesser, M.L., Senie, R.T. and Kinne, D.W. (1982) Epidemiology of breast carcinoma. III. Relationship of family history to tumor type. *Cancer*, **50**, 171–9.

40. Burki, N., Buser, M., Emmons, L.R. *et al.* (1990) Malignancies in families of women with medullary, tubular, and invasive ductal breast cancer. *Eur. J. Cancer Clin. Oncol.*, **26**, 295–303.

41. Cannon, L., Bishop, D.T., Skolnick, M.H. *et al.* (1982) Genetic epidemiology of prostate cancer in the Utah Mormon genealogy. *Cancer Surv.*, **1**, 1–12.

42. Ford, D., Easton, D.F., Bishop, D.T., Narod, S.A., Goldgar D.E. and the BCLC (1994) Risks of cancer in BRCA1-mutation carriers. *Lancet*, **343**, 692–5.

43. Thompson, W.D. and Schildkraut, J.M. (1991) Family history of gynaecological cancers: relationship to the incidence of breast cancer to age 55. *Int. J. Epidemiol.*, **20**, 595–602.

44. Nelson, C.L., Sellers, T.A., Rich, S.S. *et al.* (1993) Familial clustering of colon, breast, uterine and ovarian cancers as assessed by family history. *Genet. Epidemiol.*, **10**, 235–44.

45. Anderson, D.E. and Badzioch, M.D. (1993) Familial breast cancer risks: Effects of prostate and other cancers. *Cancer*, **72**, 114–19.

46. Parazzinni, F., Franceschi, S., Vecchia, C. and Fasoli, M. (1991) The epidemiology of ovarian cancer. *Gynecol. Oncol.*, **43**, 9–23.

47. Lynch, H.T., Guirgis, H.A., Albert, S. *et al.* (1974) Familial association of carcinoma of the breast and ovary. *Surgery*, **138**, 717–24.

48. Bishop, D.T., Albright, L.C., McClellan, T., Gardner, E.J. and Skolnick, M.H. (1988) Segregation and linkage analysis of nine Utah breast cancer pedigrees. *Genet. Epidemiol.*, **5**, 151–69.

49. Bailey-Wilson, J.E., Cannon, L.A. and King, M.-C. (1986) Genetic analysis of human breast cancer: a synthesis of contributions to GAW IV. *Genet. Epidemiol. (Suppl.)*, **1**, 15–35.

50. King, M.-C., Cannon, L.A., Bailey-Wilson, J.E. *et al.* (1986) Genetic analysis of human breast cancer: literature review and description of family data in workshop. *Genet. Epidemiol. (Suppl.)*, **1**, 3–13.

51. Cannon, L.A., Bishop, D.T. and Skolnick, M.H. (1986) Segregation and linkage analysis of breast cancer in the Dutch and Utah families. *Genet. Epidemiol.*, **3**(1), 43–6.

52. King, M.-C., Go, R.C.P., Elston, R.C. *et al.* (1980) Allele increasing susceptibility to human breast cancer may be linked to the glutamate-pyruvate transaminase locus. *Science*, **208**, 406–8.

53. Skolnick, M.H., Thompson, E.A., Bishop, D.T. and Cannon, L.A. (1984) Possible linkage of a breast cancer susceptibility locus to the ABO locus: sensitivity of LOD scores to a single new recombinant observation. *Genet. Epidemiol.*, **1**, 363–73.

54. Li, F.P. and Fraumeni, J.F. (1969) Soft tissue sarcomas, breast cancer and other neoplasms: a familial syndrome? *Ann. Intern. Med.*, **71**, 747–60.

55. Birch, J.M., Hartley, A.L., Tricker, K.J. *et al.* (1994) Prevalence and diversity of constitutional mutations in the p53 gene among 21 Li–Fraumeni families. *Cancer Res.*, **54**, 1298–304.

56. Borreson, A.L., Anderson, T.I., Garber, J. et al. (1992) Screening for germ line TP 53 mutations in breast cancer patients. *Cancer Res.*, **52**, 3234–6.

57. Sidransky, D., Tokino, T., Helzlsouer, K. *et al.* (1992) Inherited p53 mutations in breast cancer. *Cancer Res.*, **52**, 2984–6.

58. Swift, M., Reitnauer, P.J., Morrell, D. and Chase, C.L. (1991) Incidence of cancer in 161 families affected by ataxia telangiectasia. *N. Engl. J. Med.*, **325**, 1831–6.

59. Wagner, L.K. (1992) Correspondence: risk of breast cancer in ataxia-telangiectasia. *N. Engl. J. Med.*, **326**, 1358–9.

60. Land, C.E. (1992) Correspondence: risk of breast cancer in ataxia-telangiectasia. *N. Engl. J. Med.*, **326**, 1359–60.

61. Wooster, R., Ford, D., Mangion, J. *et al.* (1993) Absence of linkage to the ataxia-telangiectasia locus in familial breast cancer. *Hum. Genet.*, **92**, 91–4.

62. Fuqua, S.A., Chamness, G.C. and McGuire, W.L. (1993) Estrogen receptor mutations in breast cancer. *J. Cell Biochem.*, **51**, 135–9.

63. Zuppan, P., Hall, J.M., Lee, M.K., Ponglikitmongko, M. and King, M.-C. (1991) Possible linkage of the estrogen receptor gene to breast cancer in a family with late-onset disease. *Am. J. Hum. Genet.*, **48**, 1065–8.

64. Krontiris, T.G., Devlin, B., Karp, D.D., Robert, N.J. and Risch, N. (1993) An association between the risk of cancer and mutations in the HRAS1 minisatellite locus. *N. Engl. J. Med.*, **329**, 517–23.

65. Easton, D.F., Bishop, D.T., Ford, D. and Crockford, G.P. (1993) Genetic linkage analysis in familial breast and ovarian cancer – Results from 214 families. *Am. J. Hum. Genet.*, **52**, 678–701.

66. Narod, S.A., Ford D., Devilee P. *et al.* (1995) An evaluation of genetic heterogeneity in 145 breast–ovarian cancer families. *Am. J. Hum. Genet.* **56**, 2254–64.

67. Stratton, M.R., Ford, D., Seal, S. *et al.* (1994) Familial male breast cancer is not linked to the BRCA1 locus on chromosome 17q. *Nature Genet.*, **7**, 103–7.

68. Wooster, R., Neuhausen, S., Mangion, J. *et al.* (1994) Localization of a breast cancer susceptibility gene, BRCA2, to chromosome 13q12–13. *Science*, **265**, 2088–90.

69. Wooster, R., Bignell, G., Swift, S. *et al.* (1995) Identification of the *BRCA2* gene. *Nature*, **378**, 789–92.

Chapter 15

The breast–ovarian cancer syndrome and *BRCA*1

DEBORAH FORD and DOUGLAS F. EASTON

15.1 INTRODUCTION

Previous chapters have presented evidence that both breast and ovarian cancer exhibit familial clustering, consistent in some families with inheritance of a high risk gene. Over the past 5 years a number of the genes responsible for inherited predisposition to breast and/or ovarian cancer have been identified or localized. In particular, *BRCA*1 [1], *BRCA*2 [2], the ataxia-telangiectasia gene [3,4], the *TP*53 gene [5,6] and the androgen receptor gene [7] are now known to increase susceptibility to breast cancer. *BRCA*1 [8], *BRCA*2 [2] and the genes responsible for hereditary non-polyposis colorectal cancer syndrome [9–13] increase susceptibility to ovarian cancer. These genes differ dramatically in terms of the risks of cancer which they confer, the cancer phenotypes with which they are associated and their gene frequencies.

In this chapter we consider the breast and ovarian cancer predisposition gene *BRCA*1. We discuss in particular the mutations in the gene which have been identified to date, the risks a mutation in *BRCA*1 confers, the

frequency of *BRCA*1 mutations and the proportion of cancers which may be attributable to *BRCA*1 mutations. (The *BRCA*2, *AT*, *TP*53 and *HNPCC* genes are dealt with in other chapters.)

15.2 LINKAGE TO CHROMOSOME 17q

In 1990 Hall *et al.* [1] reported the first convincing localization of a breast cancer gene by genetic linkage. In an analysis based on 23 families they obtained a two-point LOD score of 3.28 at a recombination fraction θ of 0.14 from D17S74, a marker on chromosome 17q21, with an estimated 40% of families linked. Analysis by age showed that linkage evidence was restricted to families with a mean age of diagnosis of less than 46 years; the maximum LOD score was 5.98 at θ=0.001 in this subgroup. (For a discussion of LOD scores, see Chapter 2.) Families with older cases either showed evidence against linkage or were uninformative for linkage depending on the genetic model used [14].

Confirmation of linkage to 17q21 was

Genetic Predisposition to Cancer. Edited by R.A. Eeles, B.A.J. Ponder, D.F. Easton and A. Horwich. Published in 1996 by Chapman & Hall, London.
0 412 56580 3

obtained by Narod *et al.* [8] in three of five breast–ovarian cancer families. Figure 15.1 (a) shows one of these families with D17S74 typing (by kind permission of Henry Lynch). The maximum LOD score for the five families combined was 3.03, corresponding to a θ of 0.10 and a linked proportion of 0.6. There was no trend in this study between positive linkage and age of onset and all families contained multiple cases of ovarian cancer in addition to breast cancer. This breast and ovarian cancer locus became known as *BRCA1* [15].

Following these two publications, an international collaborative group known as the Breast Cancer Linkage Consortium (BCLC) was established to pursue linkage to *BRCA1* and other loci. This consortium now includes virtually all groups conducting breast cancer linkage and the remainder of this chapter draws heavily on results from the BCLC. A common set of six polymorphic genetic markers on 17q was recommended for typing across all families, and data on 214 families from 13 research groups was submitted to the BCLC. The BCLC was able, in this study, to demonstrate overwhelming evidence for linkage of breast and ovarian cancer to 17q, to localize *BRCA1* more precisely, to define the extent of genetic heterogeneity and to characterize linked and unlinked families, and to estimate the penetrance of *BRCA1* [16].

Multipoint linkage analysis in the BCLC data set was able to localize the position of *BRCA1* to an interval bounded by the proximal marker D17S250 and by the distal marker D17S588. This interval has a genetic length of 18.0 cM in females and 8.3 cM in males. The best estimate for the position of the gene was some 19.2 cM (sex-averaged) proximal to D17S74, the marker to which linkage had originally been reported [16]. Subsequent data convincingly localized *BRCA1* to an interval of < 2 cM bounded by D17S857 and D17S78 [17].

15.3 THE CLONING OF *BRCA*1

The *BRCA*1 gene has recently been identified by positional cloning, some 4 years after its initial localization [18]. It is composed of 22 coding exons distributed over more than 100 kb of genomic DNA and encodes a protein of 1863 amino acids. Interestingly, *BRCA*1 shows little homology to any previously identified genes, so its function is as yet unclear. However, the amino terminal region of this protein contains a zinc finger domain, a motif found in many nucleic acid binding proteins, suggesting that BRCA1 may regulate gene expression.

Germline mutations were initially detected in five of eight families which demonstrated linkage to *BRCA*1 [18] and in four of 44 breast and ovarian tumours [19]. Mutations were subsequently reported in 80 patient samples by an international collaboration [20]. Sixty-three mutations, 38 of which were distinct, were identified through a complete screen of the *BRCA*1 gene. Three specific mutations appeared to be relatively common, occurring eight, seven and five times respectively. The two most common mutations were then found in 17 additional patients using targeted screening. The majority of alterations were frameshift or nonsense mutations which truncate the protein product. In addition there were a number of missense mutations. Not all *BRCA*1-linked families, however, are due to alterations in the coding sequence, since a number of families with clear evidence of linkage have not revealed any abnormalities, even when the entire coding sequence has been examined by direct sequencing. The collaborative study also identified a mutation in a splice site, and a family with an inferred regulatory mutation (where the copy of *BRCA*1-linked to the disease was not transcribed into RNA). Since a variety of methods have been used to identify mutations, the true proportions of

240

Fig. 15.1 Two breast–ovarian cancer families. Symbols are: □ indicate males; ○ females; upper half shading, breast cancer; B is bilateral breast cancer; lower half shading, ovarian cancer; left hand lower quarter shading, other cancers. The age of diagnosis in affected individuals is given. In unaffected individuals the age stated is age of death or current age. Abbreviations for other cancers: LU, lung; LK, leukaemia; LA, larynx; HO, Hodgkin's disease; ST, stomach; UT, uterus; EY, eye. (a) IARC 2090 is a breast–ovarian cancer family consistent with linkage to *BRCA1*. The typing shown is for D17S74, the marker to which linkage was originally reported. (b) CRC 186 contains breast and ovarian cancer and includes one male breast cancer case. Typing of markers which flank *BRCA1* demonstrates that the family is inconsistent with linkage to *BRCA1*. This family has recently been shown to be linked to *BRCA2*.

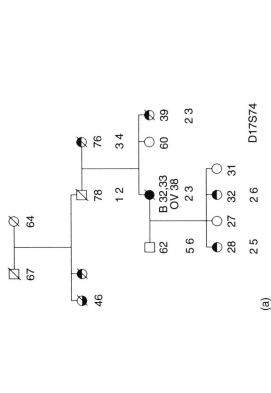

(a)

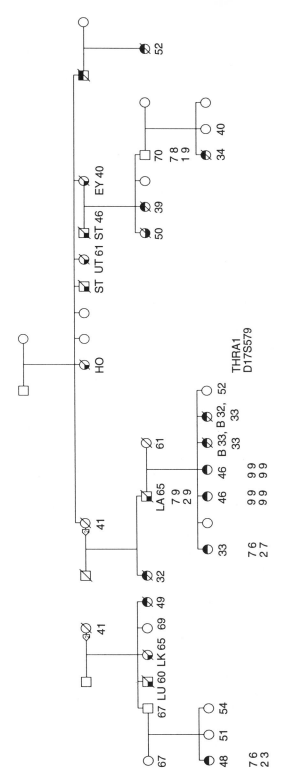

(b)

mutations of different types are not yet known. As of December 1995, over one hundred germline *BRCA*1 mutations have been reported to the international database, BIC.

The fact that many mutations are clearly inactivating suggests that *BRCA*1 acts as a tumour suppressor gene. Under this model, cancers in *BRCA*1-linked families result from the inheritance of an inactivating mutation in one copy of the gene followed by a somatic loss of the non-mutant (wild-type) gene on the other chromosome. Support for this hypothesis is provided by the fact that loss of heterozygosity on 17q in breast and ovarian tumours in *BRCA*1 families invariably involves the wild-type chromosome [17, 21].

Under the model for inherited cancer syndromes first proposed by Knudson [22] (and shown to be correct for a number of syndromes including retinoblastoma [23] and familial adenomatous polyposis [24, 25]), *BRCA*1 alterations should also be important events (somatically) in the development of non-hereditary (sporadic) cancer. Under this model, hereditary cancer would occur at an earlier age, on average, than sporadic, cancer, loss of heterozygosity would be seen in sporadic tumours and the remaining copy of *BRCA*1 should contain an inactivating mutation. Breast cancers in *BRCA*1-linked families do occur at an earlier age than in the population, though the effect is not so clear for ovarian cancer, and loss of heterozygosity is observed in a high proportion (30–70%) of sporadic breast and ovarian tumours [26, 27]. However, the evidence for inactivating mutations in sporadic breast and ovarian tumours is limited. Futreal *et al.* [19] examined 32 breast and 12 ovarian cancer tumours (selected for loss of heterozygosity at *BRCA*1) for mutations in the coding region of *BRCA*1. They detected four mutations, three in breast cancers and one in an ovarian cancer, but all four mutations were germline alterations and occurred in early-onset cases. Two of the breast cancer cases had an affected first-degree

relative found retrospectively in their medical records; one case had a mother with ovarian cancer and the second patient had a sister with breast cancer diagnosed at age 34. Although Merajver *et al.* [28] have recently reported somatic mutations in four out of 47 ovarian cancers, no somatic mutations in breast cancer have been reported to date. There are also no reports of homozygous deletions or translocations affecting *BRCA*1 in tumours. The evidence thus far, therefore, suggests that *BRCA*1 may not be critical in the development of the majority of breast and ovarian cancers.

15.4 GENETIC HETEROGENEITY

In the BCLC study a clear distinction was apparent between breast–ovarian families and families containing breast cancer only. All families with at least one case of ovarian cancer were estimated to be linked, with a lower 95% confidence interval of 0.79 on the proportion linked. In contrast only an estimated 45% of families with breast cancer only were linked (95% C.I. 25–66%). There was some suggestion in the breast cancer families of the age-effect observed by Hall *et al.* [1]; an estimated 67% of families with an average age of diagnosis of < 45 years were linked (LOD score 6.56) compared with 19% of families with age at diagnosis of between 45 and 54 (LOD score 0.40) and 38% of families with age at diagnosis of 55 or more (LOD score 0.08). There was also some evidence to suggest that the families with larger numbers of cases were more likely to be linked. These results are consistent with a model under which *BRCA*1 mutations confer a high penetrance, which includes a risk of ovarian cancer in addition to breast cancer, so that families with only two or three cases of breast cancer, or with higher average age at onset may be due to other genes with lower penetrance.

Since the original BCLC study, some breast–ovarian families have been reported which are inconsistent with linkage to

BRCA1 [29]. A pattern that has emerged, however, is that it is those families with male breast cancer, some of which also contain ovarian cancer, which are unlinked to BRCA1. A recent analysis of 132 breast–ovarian cancer families with no male breast cancer confirmed that the majority, although possibly not all, of these are due to BRCA1 [29]. Overall, an estimated 88% of families were linked (95% C.I. 74–97%) and in the subgroup of 81 families with at least two ovarian cancers 92% of families were linked (95% C.I. 76–100%). There are few families which contain multiple cases of ovarian cancer but no breast cancer, but all the evidence suggests that most, if not all, of these families are also caused by BRCA1. Steichen-Gersdorf *et al.* [30] studied nine families with at least three cases of ovarian cancer and no cases of breast cancer diagnosed below age 50. Seven of the nine families were completely consistent with linkage to BRCA1.

In the original BCLC study only five families with any case of male breast cancer were included and evidence for or against linkage to BRCA1 was inconclusive. More recently, Stratton *et al.* [31] have studied 22 families, each containing at least one male breast cancer case. Of these, 12 also contained ovarian cancer. Figure 15.1(b) shows one such family. Overall no evidence for linkage to BRCA1 was seen in the families containing male breast cancer. The best estimate of the proportion of linked families was zero with an upper 95% confidence limit of 0.18. For the subgroup of families containing one or more ovarian cancer cases the estimate of the proportion of linked families was again zero with an upper limit of 0.29; this differed significantly from the BCLC estimate of 0.88 (95% C.I. 0.74–0.97) for the proportion of linked breast–ovarian cancer families with no male cases ($P<0.001$). For the families containing male and female breast cancer cases, but no ovarian cancer, an

estimated 0% were linked (95% C.I. 0–37%); this was also significantly different from the estimated 45% linked (95% C.I. 25–66%) for families containing female breast cancer only ($P=0.03$). Several families containing male breast cancer, including the family shown in Figure 15.1(b), are now known to be due to BRCA2 [2].

It should be noted that all ovarian cancers due to BRCA1 appear to be invasive epithelial tumours; there is no evidence that BRCA1 can cause borderline or germ cell tumours, or benign cysts. Equally, there is no evidence that BRCA1 mutations result in lobular or ductal carcinoma *in situ* of the breast. There is some suggestion that BRCA1 linked ovarian cancers are more likely to be serous than mucinous [32].

15.5 RISKS OF CANCER IN BRCA1 MUTATION CARRIERS

15.5.1 BREAST AND OVARIAN CANCER

For the purposes of genetic counselling of BRCA1 families, it is essential to provide estimates of the age-specific risks of breast and ovarian cancer in mutation carriers. In the future it should be possible to estimate these cancer risks directly by studying gene carriers identified through large population-based studies but, in the meantime, estimates can be derived from linkage studies. The overall penetrance can be estimated by maximizing the LOD score over all possible penetrance functions. Using this method, Easton *et al.* [16] estimated the overall risk of either breast or ovarian cancer to be 59% by age 50 and 82% by age 70.

More recently Easton *et al.* [33] have completed a study on 33 families collected by the BCLC which contained at least four cases of ovarian cancer or breast cancer diagnosed before age 60 and which had a posterior probability of linkage to BRCA1 of at least 90%. In this subset of families the overall

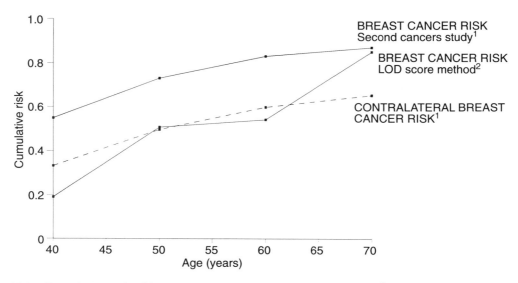

Fig. 15.2 Cumulative risk of breast cancer in *BRCA1* mutation carriers. [1]Estimated from the observed risk of a contralateral breast cancer in carriers. [2]Estimated by maximization of the LOD score over the penetrance function.

penetrance estimates were very similar to those obtained above (62% by age 50 and 95% by age 70). Estimates of the disease-specific risks were then obtained by dividing the estimated overall incidence rate in each decade by the numbers of first breast and ovarian cancers respectively in that decade as a proportion of all cancers. Assuming no heterogeneity of risk between families the breast cancer risk conferred by *BRCA1* was estimated to be 51% by age 50 and 85% by age 70 (Figure 15.2). The corresponding estimates for ovarian cancer were 23% by age 50 and 63% by age 70 (Figure 15.3).

In the same study details of all second breast cancers and ovarian cancers following a first breast cancer, and age of death or when status was last known were collected [33, 34]. Using these data it was therefore possible to estimate directly the risk of contralateral breast cancer in women already affected with breast cancer by standard cohort analysis. Second breast cancers occurring within 3

years of the first breast cancer were ignored on the basis that some of these might not be true primary cancers. Twenty-six second breast cancers occurred during follow-up, leading to an estimated contralateral breast cancer risk of 50% by age 50 and 65% by age 70 (Figure 15.2). Assuming that there is no individual variation in risk due to other genetic or environmental factors, an independent estimate of the breast cancer risk in gene carriers was obtained by doubling the incidence rates, i.e. allowing for the fact that only one breast was at risk. The estimated first breast cancer risk was 73% by age 50 and 87% by age 70 (Figure 15.2). The ovarian cancer risk was estimated similarly. Twenty-three ovarian cancers occurred during follow-up, resulting in an estimated cumulative risk of ovarian cancer of 29% by age 50 and 44% by age 70 (Figure 15.3).

The estimated age-specific penetrances derived from the second cancer data were higher than those derived from the maximum

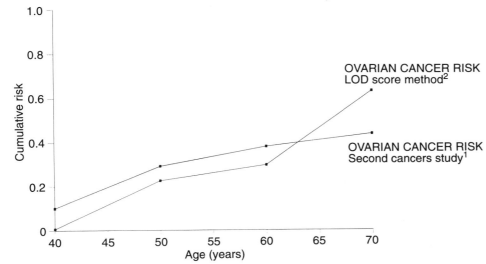

Fig. 15.3 Cumulative risk of ovarian cancer in *BRCA*1 mutation carriers. [1]Estimated from the observed risk of an ovarian cancer in a carrier previously affected with breast cancer. [2]Estimated by maximization of the LOD score over the penetrance function.

LOD score method; in particular, the cumulative risks by age 60 (though not by age 70) based on the second cancer data were significantly higher than those based on the maximum LOD score method. However, both methods confirm that the overall life-time penetrance is close to 100%; the estimated risk of either cancer was 95% by age 70 using the maximum LOD score method and 93% by age 70 using the second cancer data. Additionally, the second cancers study confirms that *BRCA*1 mutation carriers previously affected with one cancer have a high risk of developing a second breast or ovarian cancer and need to be managed accordingly.

As predicted by the segregation analyses, the age-specific incidence of breast cancer in *BRCA*1 mutation carriers follows a very different pattern from that seen in the general population. The relative risk based on the contralateral breast cancer data declined significantly with age from over 200-fold below age 40 to 15-fold in the 60–69-year age group. Such a dramatic decline suggests that there may be important mechanistic differences

between breast cancers caused by *BRCA*1 and sporadic breast cancers. Some decline in the relative risk was also apparent from the maximum LOD score method. The results for ovarian cancer are, however, somewhat ambiguous. The relative risk based on the second cancer data declined significantly, although the decline was not so dramatic as for breast cancer, but there was no trend in the relative risk for ovarian cancer based on the maximum LOD score method.

15.5.2 HETEROGENEITY OF OVARIAN CANCER RISK BETWEEN FAMILIES

The above results assume that the risks of breast and ovarian cancer are the same in all families. In fact, simple inspection of the families suggests that this is not the case. Some of the large linked families contain no cases of ovarian cancer (for example, family 1901 reported by Goldgar *et al.* [35] contains 10 breast cancers and no ovarian cancers), while other families contain more ovarian cancers than breast cancers (for example, the

245

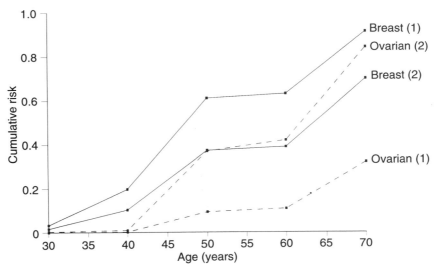

Fig. 15.4 Cumulative risks of breast cancer and ovarian cancer in *BRCA1* mutation carriers, allowing for allelic heterogeneity with two susceptibility alleles (1 and 2).

family reported by Milner *et al.* [36] contains three breast cancers and eight ovarian cancers). Although some of this heterogeneity must be due to ascertainment differences (some families being ascertained on the basis of multiple cases of breast cancers and some on the basis of multiple cases of ovarian cancer), most of the families have been extended extensively beyond their initial ascertainment, and it therefore seems unlikely that ascertainment bias could explain the whole effect.

Easton *et al.* [33] have shown that the observed patterns of disease risks are much better explained by a model with two different *BRCA1* susceptibility alleles, one conferring a cumulative breast cancer risk of 91% by age 70 and an ovarian cancer risk of 32%, the other conferring a breast cancer risk of 70% and an ovarian cancer risk of 84% (Figure 15.4). Under this model, the second allele, conferring a high ovarian cancer risk was estimated to account for 29% of *BRCA1* mutations and the first allele (with a lower ovarian cancer risk), the remaining 71%. The

major difference between this model and the homogeneity model (above) is in the estimated ovarian cancer risk; the model was not a significant improvement over a model in which the breast cancer risks are assumed to be the same for both alleles. Under this latter model, the cumulative breast cancer risk was estimated to be 76% by age 70, and the cumulative ovarian cancer risk 26% and 85% respectively for alleles 1 and 2, with allele 1 accounting for only 11% of *BRCA1* mutations and allele 2, the remainder. There was significant evidence that, though the type 1 allele conferred a lower ovarian cancer risk than the type 2 allele, this risk was above general population risk.

Some independent evidence for this allelic heterogeneity comes from the risk of ovarian cancer in individuals already affected with breast cancer. The second ovarian cancer risk was two-fold higher in families with a posterior probability of greater than 50% of being due to type 2 mutations than in the remaining type 1 families (cumulative risks by age 70, 58% and 35% respectively). A two-fold difference in risk is, however, considerably lower than the 10-fold difference predicted by the heterogeneity model and does suggest that the difference in ovarian cancer risk between families may have been exaggerated in the heterogeneity analysis. As described above, the proportion of type 1 versus type 2 alleles is also imprecise, with 29% of mutations being type 2 under the best fitting model, compared with only 11% of mutations under the model in which the breast cancer risks are the same for both type 1 and type 2 mutations.

Now that BRCA1 has been cloned it may prove possible to resolve the issue of heterogeneity by examining the disease phenotypes associated with different types of mutations. However, it appears that large numbers of families will be required. In the collaborative survey of mutations in BRCA1 reported by Schattuck-Eidens *et al.* [20] there was not a statistically significant difference in the distribution of the BRCA1 mutational spectra among low and high prevalance ovarian cancer families.

It is conceivable that there are BRCA1 mutations which confer a much lower overall risk of cancer than suggested here and do not usually generate the large multiple-case families suitable for linkage. If such mutations exist, then the estimates presented here would only be relevant to the 'high-risk' type families; however these are the families which are currently being counselled on the basis of linkage data in clinics.

15.5.3 CLUSTERING OF BREAST AND OVARIAN CANCERS

If the risks of breast and/or ovarian cancer in BRCA1 carriers are modified by other genes or by environmental factors one would expect to see clustering of breast–ovarian cancer within families; i.e. the risk of breast cancer (and possibly ovarian cancer) would be higher in close relatives of breast cancer

cases than in more distant relatives. Similarly, the risk of ovarian cancer in relatives of ovarian cases would diminish with degree of relationship. It is not possible to consider the overall risks of breast and ovarian cancer in relatives because of ascertainment biases. Easton *et al.* [33] have, however, investigated the possibility that the site-specific risks might be determined by modifying genetic or environmental effects by examining the risk of ovarian cancer as a proportion of the risk of either cancer. While there was some slight suggestion that the proportion of ovarian cancers was higher among first-degree relatives of ovarian cases than among more distant relatives, there was no corresponding effect for breast cancer and the overall conclusion was that there was no detectable modifying effect.

15.5.4 INCREASED RISKS OF COLON AND PROSTATE CANCER IN BRCA1 MUTATION CARRIERS

For the subset of 33 families with a high probability of linkage to BRCA1 (for further details see page 243) information was obtained, where possible, for all breast and ovarian cases and their first-degree relatives, on date of birth, cancer incidence and date of death or age at which status was last known. Standard cohort analysis was used to examine the risks of cancers other than breast and ovarian cancer [34].

Overall, 87 cancers were observed compared with 69.3 expected. Weighted estimates for the relative risks of site-specific cancers in BRCA1 carriers compared with the general population were computed by assigning each individual a probability of being a carrier using any typing information available and taking into account affection status, age and sex. There were statistically significant excesses of colon cancer ($P=0.002$) and prostate cancer ($P=0.006$), but no significant excesses (or deficits) for any other sites.

The maximum likelihood estimate of the relative risk of colon cancer in carriers compared with the general population was 4.11 (95% C.I. 2.36–7.15). The absolute risk of colon cancer in gene carriers is therefore of the order of 6% by age 70, compared with between 1 and 2% in non-carriers. Although there was some suggestion of a higher risk in females (relative risk 6.74) compared with males (2.10), this difference was non-significant. There was no evidence to support a higher relative risk at young ages.

The maximum likelihood estimate of the relative risk of prostate cancer in carriers compared with the general population was 3.33 (95% C.I. 1.78–6.20). There was some suggestion that the relative risk of prostate cancer in BRCA1 carriers is higher in the European families than in the American families, though this difference did not quite reach statistical significance (relative risks 8.49 and 2.48 respectively, $P=0.06$). Since the incidence of prostate cancer is three-fold higher in the US than in England and Wales (the majority of the European families were from the UK and cancer rates for England and Wales were used as the population rates for this group), the absolute risk of prostate cancer is similar in the two populations and is approximately 8% by age 70. BRCA1 families have, until now, presumably received similar surveillance for prostate cancer as the general population, so one interpretation of this finding would be that BRCA1 causes an increased risk of clinically significant prostate cancer but not asymptomatic (screen detected) disease. There was no suggestion of a higher relative risk at young ages.

Given that there are increased risks of colon and prostate cancer, an interesting issue is whether or not the risks are homogeneous across families. There were five families with multiple cases of colon cancer, and the 17 colon cancers which were in individuals with non-zero probabilities of being BRCA1 carriers occurred in just 11 of the 33 families, suggesting some heterogeneity of colon cancer risk. While a formal test for clustering of colon cancers within families was non-significant ($P=0.17$), there was some evidence that the excess colon cancer was greatest in families with a low ovarian cancer risk (see page 246 for definition). Nine of the families which contained colon cancers in individuals with non-zero probabilities of being carriers were families with a posterior probability of greater than 50% of being due to type 1 mutations and only two of the families were type 2 families; this led to an estimated relative risk of colon cancer in type 1 families of 6.40 (95% C.I. 3.59–11.40) and a corresponding estimate for type 2 families of 1.11 (95% C.I. 19–6.40; test for difference, $P=0.06$). In contrast, only one family in the set contained two prostate cancers (both in carriers) and this family was a particularly large one. There was no suggestion that the risk of prostate cancer differed with ovarian cancer risk. Clearly, as with the heterogeneity of ovarian cancer risk between families (discussed on pages 245–7), any difference in the risks of colon and/or prostate cancer between families may be resolved if the spectrum of BRCA1 mutations can be correlated with the distribution of phenotypes seen in the families.

15.6 ESTIMATES OF THE GENE FREQUENCY OF *BRCA1*

At the present time there are no direct estimates of the gene frequency of BRCA1 (that is, estimates obtained by mutation testing in large population based series of samples). However, Ford *et al.* [37] have obtained indirect estimates by combining the penetrance estimates of BRCA1 (allowing for heterogeneity) with the results of two population-based studies of cancer mortality in the relatives of breast and ovarian cancer cases [38, 39]. Since the linkage studies suggest that nearly all high-risk breast–

ovarian cancer families are due to *BRCA*1, a reasonable estimate of the gene frequency can be obtained by assuming that the excess risk of ovarian cancer in relatives of breast cancer patients and the breast cancer excess in relatives of ovarian cancer patients are both entirely accounted for by *BRCA*1. In the study of cancer mortality in the first-degree relatives of breast cancer cases, 49 ovarian cancer deaths below age 70 were observed compared with 33.7 expected at national rates, that is, an excess of 15.3 deaths. If the excess deaths were entirely accounted for by *BRCA*1, the overall gene frequency of *BRCA*1 would be 0.00064. In the companion study of cancer mortality in the first-degree relatives of ovarian cancer cases, 45 breast cancer deaths in females were observed under age 70 compared with 33.6 expected, giving an estimated gene frequency of 0.00052. The best estimate of the gene frequency, taken as the inverse variance weighted mean of the two estimates, is 0.0006 (95% C.I. 0.0002–0.001) [37]. Thus, the frequency of *BRCA*1 mutation carriers in the general population is probably low. Based on a gene frequency estimate of 0.0006, only one in 833 women is carrying the mutation. Even taking the upper 95% confidence limit the carrier frequency would only be one in 500 women. Although this estimated gene frequency has been based on the results from just two population studies, it is interesting to note that other studies have obtained similar estimates for the relative risk of ovarian cancer in the relatives of breast cancer patients and vice versa. Ford *et al.* [37] obtained a pooled estimate of 1.32 (95% C.I. 1.17–1.48) from nine studies, or 1.60 (95% C.I. 1.24–2.07) for the risk of ovarian cancer in relatives of young breast cancer patients based on four studies. Therefore the above estimate is similar to that which might be obtained if data from all such population-based studies could be included. These figures could, however, be an overestimate if some of the excess

risk of ovarian cancer in the relatives of breast cancer patients (or vice versa) is not due to *BRCA*1, or an underestimate if there are mutations which increase susceptibility to either breast or ovarian cancer but not both. Claus *et al.* [40], as a result of their segregation analysis of the Cancer and Steroid Hormone (CASH) Study, estimated the combined gene frequency of all breast cancer genes to be 0.0033, which is five times as large as the gene frequency estimate for *BRCA*1 given above. This difference can be explained because firstly a gene frequency of 0.0006 would not explain all excess familial breast cancer in the CASH study and secondly, the penetrance of *BRCA*1 is higher than the penetrance estimated by the CASH model; hence, the gene frequency would have to be lower.

The frequency of *BRCA*1 mutations could be higher in certain isolated populations as a result of founder effects. It has been noted that one particular mutation (185delAG) occurs almost exclusively in Ashkenazi Jews [41], and the frequency of this mutation has been estimated as 0.9% (95% C.I. 0.4–1.8%) [42].

15.7 THE CONTRIBUTION OF *BRCA*1 TO BREAST AND OVARIAN CANCER INCIDENCE

On the basis of a gene frequency of 0.0006 and the estimated penetrance of *BRCA*1 (allowing for heterogeneity), the estimated proportion of breast cancer cases in the general population due to *BRCA*1 would be 5.3% below age 40, 2.2% between the ages of 40 and 49 and 1.1% in the group aged 50 to 70. The corresponding estimates for ovarian cancer are 5.7% below age 40, 4.6% between the ages of 40 and 49 and 2.1% in the group aged 50 to 70.

To examine the contribution of *BRCA*1 to familial breast and ovarian cancer Ford *et al.* [37] have modelled the effect of *BRCA*1 in their own mortality-based studies [38, 39]. In the study of cancer mortality in relatives of breast cancer patients, 185 breast cancer deaths were observed under age 70 in females compared with 95.7 expected at national rates, an excess of 89.3 deaths. If the gene frequency of *BRCA*1 is assumed to be 0.0006 and the cumulative incidence of breast cancer is predicted up to age 70, from the estimated penetrance of *BRCA*1, 30% of the overall observed excess of familial breast cancer is explained by *BRCA*1. Even if the *BRCA*1 gene frequency were 0.001, only 49% of the excess familial risk would be explained. There were marked deficits in the predicted numbers of breast cancer only families with two or more cases of breast cancer (110.5 predicted and 163 observed with two cases of breast cancer; 3.3 predicted and 10 observed with three or more cases of breast cancer). These observations, while imprecise, are consistent with BCLC results which suggest that only a minority of families with two or three breast cancers aged under 60 are linked to *BRCA*1.

In the study of cancer mortality in relatives of ovarian cancer patients, if the effect of *BRCA*1 is modelled in the same way, an estimated 57% of the excess ovarian cancer risk is explained by *BRCA*1. The discrepancy between observed and predicted ovarian cancer deaths (30 versus 22.3) was, however, barely statistically significant. It is therefore possible that *BRCA*1 accounts for nearly all familial clustering of ovarian cancer. Now that *BRCA*1 has been cloned, it should be possible to define the contribution of *BRCA*1 to familial ovarian (and breast) cancer much more precisely, by mutation testing in affected relative pairs.

15.8 CONCLUSIONS

The localization of *BRCA*1 and its subsequent cloning have been major steps forward towards understanding inherited susceptibility to breast and ovarian cancer. Since *BRCA*1 accounts for almost all large breast–ovarian cancer families, and a substantial fraction of all familial breast and ovarian cancer, the cloning of *BRCA*1 may have implications for a very large number of families. It is already possible to identify women in families linked to *BRCA*1 and to counsel them on the basis of linkage data and reasonably precise estimates of cancer risk. Now that *BRCA*1 has been cloned it may not be long before direct testing for *BRCA*1 mutations becomes practical on a routine basis in high-risk women. However, it is already clear that mutations are widely scattered throughout the gene and a significant proportion occur outside the coding sequence; thus, testing on a large scale is likely to be laborious and it will be difficult to exclude the presence of a mutation. This, combined with the rarity of *BRCA*1 mutations, makes it unlikely that testing in the general population will be useful, other than for research purposes.

At present, risk estimates for *BRCA*1 mutation carriers are only available from linkage studies. While the overall risk of breast or ovarian cancer in gene carriers is fairly well estimated and is close to 100% life-time, the disease-specific risk estimates, particularly the ovarian cancer risk, are less precise, largely because of the heterogeneity of risk between families. The excess risks of colon and prostate cancer, while highly significant in the BCLC study, cannot yet be regarded as firmly established. However, further evidence either way should be accrued from prospective follow-up of gene carriers. The absolute risks of these cancers in gene carriers (about 6% and 8% respectively by age 70) are probably too low to justify any particular preventative strategy; however, this could alter if these cancers are found to be associated with particular *BRCA*1 mutations.

Another important issue is whether or not the risks of breast and ovarian cancer in *BRCA*1 carriers are substantially modified by other risk factors. In this respect studies of *BRCA*1 carriers in countries with a low risk of breast and ovarian cancer (e.g. Japan), may be worthwhile. Goldgar *et al.* [43] have presented some evidence to suggest that parity and age at first birth have little effect on breast cancer risk in *BRCA*1 carriers. From a practical point of view the most important risk factor is oral contraceptive use. In the general population, long-term oral contraceptive use is known to reduce substantially the risk of ovarian cancer but to increase the risk of breast cancer at young ages; hence, its use in *BRCA*1 carriers might cause a marked increase or decrease in overall cancer risk. An epidemiological study is currently being conducted by the BCLC in order to address these issues.

REFERENCES

1. Hall, J.M., Lee, M.K., Morrow, J. *et al*, (1990) Linkage analysis of early onset familial breast cancer to chromosome 17q21. *Science*, **250**, 1684–9.

2. Wooster, R., Neuhausen, S., Manigion, J. *et al.* (1994) Localisation of a breast cancer suceptibility gene (BRCA2) to chromosome 13q by genetic linkage analysis. *Science*, **265**, 2088–90.

3. Gatti, R.A., Berkel, I., Boder, E. *et al.* (1988) Localisation of an ataxia-telangiectasia gene to chromosome 11q22–23. *Nature*, **336**, 577–80.

4. Swift, M., Morrell, D., Massey, R.B. and Chase, C.L. (1991) Incidence of cancer in 161 families affected with ataxia-telangiectasia. *N. Engl. J. Med.*, **325**, 1831–6.

5. Li, F.P., Fraumeni, J.F. Jr., Mulvihill, J.J. *et al.* (1988) A cancer family syndrome in twenty-four kindreds. *Cancer Res.*, **48**, 5358–62.

6. Malkin, D., Li, F.P., Strong, L.C. *et al.* (1990) Germline p53 mutations in a familial syndrome of breast cancer, sarcomas and other neoplasms. *Science*, **250**, 1233–8.

7. Wooster, R., Mangion, J., Eeles, R. *et al.* (1992) A germline mutation in the androgen receptor in two brothers with breast cancer and Reifenstein syndrome. *Nature Genet.*, **2**, 132–4.

8. Narod, S.A., Feunteun, J., Lynch, H.T. *et al.* (1991) Familial breast–ovarian cancer locus on chromosome 17q12–23. *Lancet*, **338**, 82–3.

9. Watson, P. and Lynch, H.T. (1993) Extracolonic cancer in hereditary nonpolyposis colorectal cancer. *Cancer*, **71**, 677–85.

10. Bronner, C.E., Baker, S.M., Morrison, P.T. *et al.* (1994) Mutation in the DNA mismatch repair gene homologue hMLH1 is associated with hereditary nonpolyposis colon cancer linked to chromosome 3p. *Nature*, **368**, 258–61.

11. Leach, F.S., Nicolaides, N.C., Papadopoulos, N. *et al.* (1993) Mutations of a mutS homolog in hereditary nonpolyposis colorectal cancer. *Cell*, **75**, 1215–25.

12. Papadopoulos, N., Nicolaides, N.C., Wei, Y.F. *et al.* (1994) Mutation of the mutL homolog associated with hereditary colon cancer. *Science*, **263**, 1625–9.

13. Nicolaides, N.C., Papadopoulos, N., Liu, B. *et al.* (1994) Mutations of two PMS homologues in hereditary nonpolyposis colon cancer. *Nature*, **371**, 75–80.

14. Margaritte, P., Bonaiti-Pellie, C., King, M-C. and Clerget-Darpoux, F. (1992) Linkage of familial breast cancer may not be restricted to early onset disease. *Am. J. Hum. Genet.*, **50**, 515–19.

15. Solomon, E. and Ledbetter, D.H. (1991) Report of the Committee on the Genetic Constitution of Chromosome 17. *Cytogenet. Cell Genet.*, **58**, 686–738.

16. Easton, D.F., Bishop, D.T., Ford, D., Crockford, G.P. and the Breast Cancer Linkage Consortium (1993) Genetic linkage analysis in familial breast and ovarian cancer: results from 214 families. *Am. J. Hum. Genet.*, **52**, 678–701.

17. Kelsell, D.P., Black, D.M., Bishop, D.T. and Spurr, N.K. (1993) Genetic analysis of the BRCA1 region in a large breast/ovarian family: refinement of the minimal region containing BRCA1. *Hum. Mol. Genet.*, **2**, 1823–8.

18. Miki, Y., Swensen, J., Schattuck-Eidens, D. *et al.* (1994) Isolation of BRCA1, the 17q-linked breast and ovarian cancer susceptibility gene. *Science*, **266**, 66–71.

19. Futreal, P.A., Liu, Q., Schattuck-Eidens, D. *et al.* (1994) BRCA1 mutations in primary breast and ovarian carcinomas. *Science*, **266**, 120–2.

20. Schattuck-Eidens, D., McClure, M., Simard, J. *et al.* (1995) A collaborative survey of 80 mutations in the BRCA1 breast and ovarian cancer susceptibility gene. *JAMA*, **273**, 535–41.

21. Smith, S.A., Easton, D.F., Evans, D.G.R. and Ponder, B.A.J. (1992) Allele losses in the region 17q12–21 in familial breast and ovarian

cancer involve the wild-type chromosome. *Nature Genet.*, **2**, 128–31.

22. Knudson, A.G. Jr (1971) Mutation and cancer: statistical study of retinoblastoma. *Proc. Natl Acad. Sci. USA*, **68**, 820–3.

23. Huang, H-JS., Yee, J.K., Shew, J.Y. *et al.* (1988) Suppression of the neoplastic phenotype by replacement of the RB gene in human cancer cells. *Science*, **242**, 1563–6.

24. Groden, J., Thliveris, A., Samowitz, W. *et al.* (1991) Identification and characterization of the familial adenomatous polyposis coli gene. *Cell*, **66**, 589–600.

25. Kinzler, K.W., Nilbert, M.C., Su, L.K. *et al.* (1991) Identification of FAP locus genes from chromosome 5q21. *Science*, **253**, 661–5.

26. Cornelis, R.S., Devilee, P., Van Vliet, M. *et al.* (1993) Allele loss patterns on chromosome 17q in 109 breast carcinomas indicate at least two distinct target regions. *Oncogene*, **8**, 781–5.

27. Jacobs, I.J., Smith, S.A., Wiseman, R.W. *et al.* (1993) A deletion unit on chromosome 17q in epithelial ovarian tumors distal to the familial breast/ovarian cancer locus. *Cancer Res.*, **53**, 1218–21.

28. Merajver, S.D., Pham, T.M., Caduff, R.F. *et al.* (1995) Somatic mutations in the BRCA1 gene in sporadic ovarian tumours. *Nature Genet.*, **9**, 439–43.

29. Narod, S.A., Ford, D., Devilee, P. *et al.* (1995) An evaluation of genetic heterogeneity in 145 breast-ovarian cancer families. *Am. J. Hum. Genet.*, **56**, 254–64.

30. Steichen-Gersdorf, E., Gallion, H.H., Ford, D. *et al.* (1994) Familial site-specific ovarian cancer is linked to BRCA1 on 17q12–21. *Am. J. Hum. Genet.*, **55**, 870–5.

31. Stratton, M.R., Ford, D., Neuhausen, S. *et al.* (1994) Familial male breast cancer is not linked to BRCA1. *Nature Genet.*, **7**, 103–7.

32. Narod, S.A. (1994) Genetics of breast and ovarian cancer. *Br. Med. Bull.*, **50**, 656–76.

33. Easton, D.F., Ford, D., Bishop, D.T. and the Breast Cancer Linkage Consortium (1995) Breast and ovarian cancer incidence in BRCA1 mutation carriers. *Am. J. Hum. Genet.*, **56**, 265–71.

34. Ford, D., Easton, D.F., Bishop, D.T., Narod, S.A., Goldgar, D.E. and the Breast Cancer Linkage Consortium (1994) Risks of cancer in BRCA1 mutation carriers. *Lancet*, **343**, 692–5.

35. Goldgar, D.E., Cannon-Albright, L.A., Oliphant, A. *et al.* (1993) Chromosome 17q linkage studies of 18 Utah breast cancer kindreds. *Am. J. Hum. Genet.*, **52**, 743–8.

36. Milner, B.J., Allan, L.A., Kelly, K.F. *et al.* (1993) Linkage studies with 17q and 18q markers in a breast/ovarian cancer family. *Am. J. Hum. Genet.*, **52**, 761–6.

37. Ford, D., Easton, D.F. and Peto, J. (1995) Estimates of the gene frequency of BRCA1 and its contribution to breast and ovarian cancer incidence. *Am. J. Hum. Genet.* **57**, 1457–62.

38. Peto, J., Easton, D.F., Matthews, F.E., Ford, D. and Swerdlow, A.J. Cancer mortality in relatives of breast cancer patients. *Int. J. Cancer*, (in press).

39. Easton, D.F., Matthews, F.E., Ford, D., Swerdlow, A.J. and Peto, J. Cancer mortality in relatives of ovarian cancer patients. *Int. J. Cancer*, (in press).

40. Claus, E.B., Risch, N. and Thompson, W.D. (1991) Genetic analysis of breast cancer in the Cancer and Steroid Hormone study. *Am. J. Hum. Genet.*, **48**, 232–41.

41. Tonin, P., Serova, O., Lenoir, G. *et al.* (1995) BRCA1 mutations in Ashkenazi Jewish women. *Am. J. Hum. Genet.*, **57**, 189.

42. Struewing, J.P., Abeliovich, D., Peretz, T. *et al.* (1995) The carrier frequency of the BRCA1 185delAG mutation is approximately 1 percent in Ashkenazi Jewish individuals. *Nature Genet.*, **11**, 198–200.

43. Goldgar, D.E., Fields, P., Lewis, C.M. *et al.* (1994) A large kindred with 17q-linked breast and ovarian cancer: genetic, phenotypic and genealogical analysis. *J. Natl Cancer Inst.*, **86**, 200–9.

Chapter 16

Screening for breast cancer in high-risk populations

JOCELYN CHAMBERLAIN

16.1 INTRODUCTION

The purpose of screening for breast cancer is to detect and treat potentially lethal cancers at a time when they are still curable. Thus the benefit of screening is a reduction in the risk of death from breast cancer. This benefit must be weighed against several potential disadvantages. These include advancing the date of diagnosis of low malignancy cancers which would still have been curable if left until symptomatic presentation, anxiety and unnecessary biopsies in women with false positive results, radiation hazard from mammography and, last but not least, the very considerable resource costs of providing a screening and diagnostic follow-up service.

Focusing screening on high-risk populations can be regarded from two angles. First, from the public health point of view, limiting screening to high-risk individuals is appealing because the high-risk group is normally only a small fraction of the average-risk population, and thus costs are less and the disadvantages are incurred by a much smaller number of people than would be the case with general population screening. However, unless the relative risk is extremely

high and/or the prevalence of the risk group in the population is moderately high, restricting screening to high-risk populations will have little impact in control of the disease [1]. In the case of breast cancers, by combining several risk factors (e.g. family history, late age at first birth) it has been shown that to include 67% of breast cancers one would have to screen 79% of women [2]. Moreover, identification of this large risk group would entail setting up some form of pre-screening organization, thus adding to costs. Therefore, public health authorities have tended to opt for screening the whole average-risk population, selected only by age, for reasons discussed further below.

The second viewpoint on screening high-risk groups is that of the high-risk individuals themselves. If screening can reduce their risk of dying from breast cancer then it is desirable that they be offered it. As an alternative to prophylactic bilateral mastectomy, or chemoprophylaxis (if shown to be an effective means of primary prevention), screening may seem to be a less radical option. In offering it to women or responding to their requests for it, it is most important that they

Genetic Predisposition to Cancer. Edited by R.A. Eeles, B.A.J. Ponder, D.F. Easton and A. Horwich. Published in 1996 by Chapman & Hall, London.
0 412 56580 3

should understand that it will not reduce their risk of **developing** breast cancer. Indeed, it will increase that risk, by diagnosing their cancer earlier than would otherwise happen and possibly by diagnosing indolent cancers that might never have surfaced in their lifetime. (In the US, where screening is widespread, it is often advocated as the solution to that country's increasing breast cancer incidence but it is more likely to be one cause of the increase.) The women must understand that its purpose is to reduce their risk of **dying** from breast cancer.

The remainder of this chapter will review current scientific evidence on the benefit of screening for breast cancer, and its application to women who are at risk by virtue of a confirmed family history.

16.2 THE EFFECT OF SCREENING ON BREAST CANCER MORTALITY

Screening for breast cancer in the general population has been more thoroughly evaluated than screening for any other condition in adult life. Five randomized controlled trials have compared the death rate from breast cancer over periods ranging from 7 to 18 years among average-risk women aged from 40 to 74 who have been invited for mammography screening compared with women who have not. All have found 20–30% fewer breast cancer deaths in the women who have been offered screening, although these reductions have not always been statistically significant [3–7]. Three of the trials were in Sweden and a meta-analysis of these and one additional ongoing Swedish trial concluded that there was a statistically significant 24% reduction in breast cancer deaths resulting from periodic mammography screening [8]. In addition, one non-randomized geographical comparison of districts in which screening was or was not, provided [9], three retrospective case-control studies [10–12], and one study in which an artificial popula-

tion matched to a screened population was modelled [13], have all reached conclusions consistent with those shown by the randomized trials, that screening does confer a reduced risk of dying from breast cancer.

Two further randomized controlled trials in Canada [14] have compared different intensities of screening. One randomized volunteer 50–59-year-old women to a group screened annually by physical examination, or to a group screened annually by physical examination and mammography and found no significant difference in breast cancer mortality after 7 years. The second randomized 40–49-year-old women into a group which had a single physical examination and a group which was offered mammography and physical examination annually for 3 or 4 years, and again found no significant difference in breast cancer mortality after 7 years. In the younger women there were in fact more breast cancer deaths in the annually screened group than the control group who only had one examination at entry, although this difference was not statistically significant. These Canadian trials in volunteer women differ in several respects from the other population-based trials. First, neither had an unscreened control group. Second, the women who participated were at somewhat higher risk of developing breast cancer than the general Canadian population but – perhaps because of their greater awareness and the fact that the control groups were partially screened – were at lower risk of dying from breast cancer. This lowered the statistical power of the trials. Third, in the 40–49-year-old trial, the randomization process by chance resulted in a higher prevalence of advanced breast cancers detected at entry in the mammography plus physical examination group than in the physical examination alone group, and these cases largely account for the excess deaths in the former group. Finally, the quality of mammography in the early years of this trial has been criticized, although little is known about mammographic quality in other trials, and the interval cancer rate was not exceptionally high.

A recent overview [15] of the prospective trials, excluding the Canadian studies, concluded, like the Swedish overview, that the risk of breast cancer death in women offered screening relative to controls was 0.76.

Other aspects of screening which have been studied include the sensitivity of different screening modalities, the frequency with which routine rescreening is repeated, and the effectiveness of screening different age groups.

16.2.1 SENSITIVITY OF DIFFERENT SCREENING MODALITIES

The two main screening tests which have been studied in screening well women are physical examination and mammography. Thermography has been shown to have low levels of both sensitivity and specificity, and ultrasound fails to detect tumours <1 cm in diameter. Newer imaging methods such as magnetic resonance imaging (MRI) and positron emission tomography (PET) are not yet feasible on a large scale.

The original randomized controlled trial conducted 30 years ago in New York [3] found that physical examination detected 67% of screen-detected cancers and mammography 55%, both tests being positive in only 22% of cases. Some cancers also presented symptomatically in women who had previously screened negative (interval cancers) and these comprised 25% of all cancers in screened women. Improvements in mammography since that time, including use of the mediolateral oblique view with compression, have led to greatly improved sensitivity [16]. A recent British study in which physical examination and oblique view mammography were both used, found that 94% of screen-detected cancers were positive on mammography compared with only 65%

positive on clinical examination [17]. Many screening programmes now omit physical examination on the grounds that the marginal extra yield does not justify the cost.

16.2.2 FREQUENCY OF ROUTINE SCREENING

The frequency with which routine screening should be repeated has been studied in one of the Swedish trials [18]. The rate at which interval cancers presented in different time periods after a negative screen was compared with the expected incidence of breast cancer in unscreened women, derived from the control group of the trial. Of breast cancers expected to arise in the first 12 months after a negative screen in 50–69-year old women, 13% were interval cancers, implying that the remaining 87% had been detected by previous screening. Between 12 and 23 months after a negative screen, interval cancers comprised 32% of the expected incidence, and 24 to 29 months after a negative screen, 45% were interval cases. These findings have led most authorities to recommend a 2-year interval between routine screens for women aged over 50.

16.2.3 THE EFFECTIVENESS OF SCREENING WOMEN OF DIFFERENT AGES

With the exception of the two Canadian trials, the research studies outlined above have enrolled women over a fairly broad age-band from age 40–45 up to age 65–74. When mortality analyses have been performed within age groups, it has been found that the benefit of screening is concentrated among women aged 50–69 when first screened. Among women aged 70 or over, response to screening invitations drops off and it is assumed that the lower compliance in this age group accounts for the lesser effect on mortality.

Table 16.1 Odds ratios of breast cancer death in intervention groups compare with control groups

Trial	Duration of follow-up (years)	Odds ratio (95% C.I.)	
		Age <50 at trial entry	Age ≥50 at trial entry
New York, HIP [3]	18	0.78 (0.52–1.18)	0.80 (0.59–1.08)
Swedish Overview [8]	5–13	0.87 (0.63–1.20)	0.75 (0.65–0.87)
Edinburgh [7]	10	0.87 (0.46–1.65)	0.85 (0.63–1.13)
UKTEDBC [9]	10	0.74 (0.54–1.01)	0.83 (0.68–1.01)
Canada NBSSS [14][1]		1.36 (0.84–2.21)	0.97 (0.62–1.52)

[1] Control groups were partially screened.

The disappointing finding of a lesser effect among women aged under 50 when first screened is a cause of much concern, not least because of its implications for women in high-risk families. It is generally assumed that the cut-off age of 50 is a crude marker for age at menopause. One of the difficulties in interpreting results for women aged under 50 in individual trials is the relative rarity of breast cancer death in this age group in control women. With so few deaths, the sample size required to show a statistically significant difference is much greater than any individual trial could supply. Nevertheless, the finding of a smaller or even negligible effect in younger women has been consistent. One overview of results from individual trials, with a cut-off follow-up period of 10 years, reached the conclusion that screening had no effect (relative risk of breast cancer death in those offered screening compared with controls 0.98 [19]). This analysis also drew attention to a non-significant excess number of breast cancer deaths in the intervention groups during the first few years, not only in the Canadian study but also in some of the other trials.

More recently the meta-analysis of five Swedish trials [8] with follow-up periods ranging from 5 to 13 years, found that women aged under 50 when first invited for screening had a risk of breast cancer death 13% lower than control women in the same age group, although with 95% confidence intervals extending from 37% reduction to 20% excess, this finding is far from statistically significant. Comparable risks in women of older age groups are shown in Table 16.1. This meta-analysis also looked at cumulative breast cancer mortality over time and showed that while a mortality advantage for women over 50 when first screened appeared 4–5 years after entry, for younger women it took longer, not appearing until 8 years from entry. The original trial in New York had similar findings, showing no effect up to 9 years from entry, at ages 40–44, but after 18 years the mortality reduction was 22%, no different from that in other age groups (Table 16.1) although none was statistically significant. This analysis was restricted to deaths among women whose breast cancer was diagnosed within 5 years from entry (when the youngest age group would still not have attained the age of 50) and hence avoids the uncertainty in other trials of whether the same deaths could have been avoided by screening at a later point, perhaps after age 50.

The two UK trials [7,8] which enrolled women from age 45 are unusual in that, with a 10-year follow-up, they show no difference in effect between younger women and older women. It is of interest that the underlying breast cancer mortality rate in UK women and in the control group of the New York trial 30 years ago, is considerably higher than that in Sweden, Canada or the US today. One may speculate that where underlying risk of breast cancer death is high, the scope for a positive effect of screening, even at relatively young ages, is greater.

One of the reasons why screening is less effective in younger women is that both mammography and physical examination are less sensitive in premenopausal breasts, presumably because of the greater density of glandular tissue compared with fatty tissue which is more prevalent in postmenopausal breasts. In the Swedish two-counties trial the average interval between screens in women aged 40–49 at entry was 22 months. An analysis of the rate at which interval cancers arose after a negative screen [18] showed that in these younger women interval cancers comprised 38% of the expected (control group) incidence in the first year after screening, rising to 68% in the second year. This lower sensitivity in younger women is consistent with the finding that the ratio of prevalence (yield of cancers at first screen) to control group incidence is lower in women under 50 than in older women. This implies that the average lead time (the time by which diagnosis of cancer is advanced) gained by screening younger women is less than that in older women. One possible reason may be that, because of breast density, the earliest signs of cancer are not visible on the mammogram. Another may be that new cancers arise and develop to the symptomatic stage more quickly in younger women.

If this were true it would imply that the natural history of breast cancer differed with age, with faster growth rates in the young. Analyses of stage-specific survival rates from population-based cancer registries support the hypothesis that breast cancers in very young women are faster growing [20], but those in premenopausal women in their 40s have a better prognosis than either younger women or postmenopausal women [20, 21]. Whatever the reason for the high rate of interval cancers in young women, the consequence is that if screening is proved to be effective in young women it will need to be repeated more frequently – even annual screening will miss a fair number of cancers.

Uncertainty about the level of benefit, if any, which could be achieved by annual screening can only be resolved by a randomized controlled trial, designed with a sufficient sample size to be reasonably certain of showing a statistically significant reduction in mortality if one is truly present. One such trial, sponsored by the UK Coordinating Committee for Cancer Research, has recently been started (S.M. Moss, personal communication). A total of 195 000 women aged 40–41 are being allocated randomly into an intervention group (65 000) or a control group (130 000). Women in the intervention group are being invited for two-view mammography screening every year for 7 years. When they reach age 50 women in both groups will enter the routine UK screening programme. It has been estimated that (assuming 70% acceptance of screening) this trial will have 80% power to show a mortality reduction of 20%, significant at the 5% level, 10 years after trial entry. For a smaller mortality reduction a greater number of women would need to be studied. Various European and North American groups are considering joining this trial, or variants of it, such as starting screening at different ages. Whether the conclusion is positive or negative it is particularly important to quantify the level of mortality reduction (if any) which could be achieved by screening women in their fourth decade. However, such trials are very expensive and there is controversy among cancer research funding agencies about their scientific priority.

16.3 DISADVANTAGES OF SCREENING AVERAGE-RISK WOMEN

Postulated adverse effects of screening on the health of screened women may be physical

257

and psychological, and may arise from the screening test procedure, from the additional investigations required to discern true positives from false positives, and from the early diagnosis of breast cancer itself. In addition to these health effects, population-based screening programmes are very expensive in resources.

16.3.1 DISADVANTAGES OF THE SCREENING PROCESS

(a) Risk of radiogenic cancers

Mammography subjects the breast to a dose of ionizing radiation which may be potentially carcinogenic. Follow-up studies of women who received massive doses of radiation either for medical reasons or as a result of fall-out from atomic explosions, have established that they have an increased risk of subsequent breast cancer, the excess risk being inversely related to age at exposure, and increasing gradually over a 10-year period, after which the increased risk is constant [22]. Extrapolations from the very high doses received by these women to the very small doses of current mammography (mean absorbed dose per exposure of 0.5–3 mGy) have been used to estimate the risk of induction of breast cancer by screening. An estimate [23] using American breast cancer incidence rates has calculated that 21 radiation-induced breast cancers would occur per million women screened at age 50, compared with the underlying lifetime incidence of some 80 000 breast cancers per million. If 50 000 of the latter were destined to die from their cancer, and if screening were to reduce this risk of death by 25% then the ratio of deaths avoided to cancers induced would be nearly 600 to 1. For women screened at age 40 the risk of radiogenic breast cancer is greater (78 cancers per million women) and since the benefit of screening in terms of reducing mortality is unproven, the

benefit-to-risk ratio is unknown. The favourable balance, at least for the over-50s, is very reassuring but does not detract from the need for screening units to monitor their dosage levels on a routine basis to ensure that radiation is kept down to the lowest level compatible with good image quality.

(b) Discomfort and pain

Obtaining a good image of the whole breast necessitates compressing the breast against the X-ray plate. This is uncomfortable, particularly for women with small breasts. A large multicentre survey of 1847 screened women in the US reported that 39% experienced mild discomfort, 10% moderate or severe discomfort but only 1% experienced pain [24]. A similar UK study of 597 screened women found that 35% had some level of discomfort, and 6% pain. However, a majority of women ranked mammography as less unpleasant than other preventive procedures, including cervical smears and dental check-ups [25].

(c) Anxiety

There is no evidence to support the hypothesis that inviting or encouraging women to attend for screening heightens their awareness of their vulnerability to breast cancer to the extent of morbid levels of anxiety. One study found no difference in psychiatric morbidity between women attending for screening and an age-matched sample of women in the general population [26]. Nor does there seem to be any difference in psychiatric morbidity between attenders and non-attenders for screening [27].

16.3.2 DISADVANTAGES OF FALSE POSITIVE RESULTS

Since the purpose of screening is not to make a definitive diagnosis but to sort out those who probably have the disease from those who probably do not [28], it is inevitable that there will be some false positives. Where the prevalence of disease is low, even though the test may have high specificity, the number of false positives is likely to exceed the number of true positives, giving the test a low predictive value. At first screening, around 5–7% of women will have suspicious mammographic or clinical findings necessitating referral for a diagnostic work-up, of whom only one-tenth will be found to have cancer [29]. On routine re-screening the proportion referred is lower but so is the cancer detection rate. Thus the positive predictive value of screening average risk women is around 10%.

The diagnostic procedures for women with a positive screening test include clinical examination, imaging by further mammography and by ultrasound, and fine-needle aspiration cytology. The combination of these diagnostic modalities enables a firm diagnosis to be made in the great majority of referred women, with less than 1% of screened women requiring excision biopsy [30]. Nevertheless, in the controlled trials it has been shown that the absolute rate of benign biopsies in a population offered screening is several times greater than in a control population, particularly during the period when women are having their first screen [29].

As well as the physical morbidity consequent on excision biopsy, the notification of a positive screening test result and of the need for further tests inevitably causes anxiety about the outcome. Although anecdotal reports of worry, sometimes amounting to panic, abound, there has been little formal investigation of this side effect of screening. One study compared anxiety and depression levels in women attending for further investigation after a suspicious mammogram with those in women attending for routine screening, and with a third group of unscreened women referred because of breast symptoms

[31]. Anxiety levels were higher in the symptomatic group than in the women with suspicious screening mammograms, and higher in the latter than in women attending for routine screening. However, 3 months later anxiety in the women with false positive screening mammograms was no different from that in women who had been screened and found negative. Another study found that 6 weeks after screening there was no significant increased anxiety in women who had had to undergo further investigation of a suspicious mammogram, nor in those who had a benign biopsy [32].

16.3.3 DISADVANTAGES OF ADVANCING THE DATE OF DIAGNOSIS OF BREAST CANCER

Only a minority (10–20%) [33] of women with screen-detected cancer will benefit from the cure of an otherwise lethal cancer within the period of follow-up of the controlled trials. Of the remainder, some will already be metastatic and will die regardless of screening; these tend to be cancers detected at the first screen and deaths among breast cancers detected at routine re-screening are substantially fewer [34]. Of greater concern is the relatively large number of patients who, if their cancer had not been detected at screening, would have survived anyway. Assuming that indolent slow-growing tumours spend longer than aggressive tumours in the phase when they are presymptomatic but detectable, screening will selectively detect cancers with an inherently good prognosis – so-called length – or duration-biased sampling. Early diagnosis of these cancers does not confer any prognostic benefit but may permit less radical treatment than would have been required had the cancer progressed to the symptomatic stage. There are, however, no data to test this hypothesis.

(a) Psychological morbidity

If detection by screening benefits only a small proportion of cancer patients, does it do the remainder any harm? These women inevitably go through the distress and anxiety which accompanies a diagnosis of cancer. It is postulated that, because the change from well-woman to breast cancer patient is more abrupt in screen-detected patients than symptomatic patients, psychological adjustment to the diagnosis is more difficult, although again this hypothesis has not been tested. One study in a population with a screening programme compared anxiety and depression levels in breast cancer patients 1 year or more from diagnosis, and in age-matched women without breast cancer from the same population. Psychological morbidity was significantly less in the breast cancer patients than the controls, and the method of detection of cancer (screen-detected case, interval case or unscreened case) made no difference to anxiety and depression levels [35]. Thus on present evidence there seems little reason to suspect that long-term psychological harm is caused by advancing the date of diagnosis, although other social disadvantages, such as high life insurance and health insurance premiums may result.

(b) Over-diagnosis

Possibly included among the women with screen-detected cancer is an unknown proportion in whom the cancer would not otherwise have surfaced within the woman's lifetime. This is thought to be particularly likely in cases of ductal carcinoma-*in-situ* (DCIS) which comprise 15–20% of screen-detected cancers. Studies of biopsied women originally diagnosed as benign but who, on histological review, had DCIS, have found that about one-quarter develop invasive cancer (sometimes metastatic) in the same breast during a follow-up of up to 10 years

[36]. One autopsy study in Denmark of the breast tissue of 110 women aged under 55 who had died of other causes, found one previously undiagnosed breast cancer (prevalence nine per 100) and 15 previously undiagnosed instances of DCIS (prevalence 14%) [37]. The median age of these women was 45 and this prevalence of *in-situ* cancer exceeded the cumulative life-time risk of breast cancer in Danish women. There is clearly a dilemma here in that the evidence points **both** to the invasive and metastatic potential of DCIS, **and** to its potential for remaining latent. In the Danish study, the breast specimens were X-rayed before the histology result was known and seven of the 15 DCIS cases were positive on X-ray.

The question of the extent of over-diagnosis of latent carcinoma could be resolved by follow-up of controlled trials of screening until the number of breast cancers was equal in intervention group and control group, or until all subjects had died. In the original Health Insurance Plan study, screening ceased in the fourth year after entry and within 3 years the cumulative number of breast cancers in the control group equalled that in the intervention group, indicating that there had been no element of over-diagnosis [3]. However, mammography at that time was much less sensitive and did not detect *in-situ* cancers, which occurred in equal numbers in both groups. A more recent study in the Netherlands in which screening by both mammography and clinical examination was used found 11% more cancers in a screened population than in geographic controls [38]. However, they noted that in the first birth cohort of women invited to be screened, incidence was at first higher than in a comparable birth cohort in the control population, but 8–12 years after the start of the screening programme there were more cancers diagnosed in the control population. This suggests that the extra cancers detected by screening in the early years would have presented symptomatically several years later.

The accumulating evidence that screening reduces mortality means that such natural experiments are no longer feasible since women originally in the control groups of trials are now being offered screening, and therefore any element of over-diagnosis will be present in both groups. The Swedish two-counties trial addressed this problem by comparing the annual incidence of breast cancer in the intervention group, after excluding cancers detected at the first screen, with the annual incidence in the control group before they were offered screening [4]. They found that the two groups were equal and concluded that any element of over-diagnosis was limited to the first (prevalence) screen when most of the *in-situ* disease was diagnosed. They also suggested that over-diagnosis was almost entirely concentrated in women aged under 50, although its extent requires further research.

16.4 BALANCE OF BENEFITS AND DISADVANTAGES

In summary, current evidence suggests that for average-risk women aged over 50 a screening programme which is taken up by 65% or more of the eligible population will reduce breast cancer deaths by about one-quarter. For those women who accept screening the reduction in risk is of course, greater – of the order of 40%. The disadvantages of screening (apart from cost) occur mainly at the first screen and are small once a woman is in a routine re-screening programme. On this basis, many developed countries which can afford it now provide a mammography screening programme for women aged 50 to 65 or 70.

For younger women, the reduction in risk

of breast cancer death is certainly less than that in women over 50, but it is still not quantified, no trial so far having established a statistically significant result in this age group. If a reduction in risk does occur it is likely to take several years after the start of screening to emerge. Moreover, some of the disadvantages, namely radiation hazard and over-diagnosis, although rare, are probably more common in younger women than older. Also, the poor sensitivity of mammography in premenopausal women dictates that screening should be repeated annually, thus at least doubling the cost. For all these reasons the ratio of benefit-to-cost is less favourable in premenopausal women, and even if trials do show a mortality reduction of perhaps 15–20%, the balance may not be deemed sufficiently favourable to set up a public health screening programme. However, it remains important to try to quantify these issues further in order to provide accurate information to individual women who seek screening, and in particular to those of them at high risk.

16.5 IMPLICATIONS FOR WOMEN AT INHERITED RISK OF BREAST CANCER

The fact that family history of breast cancer leads to increased risk is now widely known, and many women may request screening because they have an affected relative. As discussed elsewhere in this book, construction of an accurate pedigree, including age at diagnosis of affected first-degree relatives, bilaterality, and other malignancies, enables a much more accurate estimate of risk to be made. This narrows down the number of women at high risk and enables reassurance to be given to the remainder that they are not in fact at above-average risk. The process of defining the truly high-risk group will shortly become much more precise when it becomes possible to test for mutations in genes such as *BRCA*1 and *BRCA*2.

Should the policy for screening these clearly defined high-risk women differ from that for average-risk women? The principal questions arising from the evidence on screening average-risk women concern the age at which screening should start, and the frequency with which it should be repeated.

16.5.1 AGE OF STARTING SCREENING

In women with an inherited susceptibility to cancer, the age at onset of the disease is much younger than in sporadic cases in the average-risk population, and it has been estimated that most of the excess risk of familial breast cancer occurs before age 50 [39]. It has been suggested that high-risk women should start to be screened 5–10 years before the earliest age at diagnosis of affected family members, although as has been shown earlier, there is no proof that screening women below 50 reduces their risk of breast cancer death.

It may be postulated that, because the breast tissue of high-risk women has already been subjected to an early oncogenic 'hit', familial breast cancers will behave in a similar way to sporadic breast cancers, arising a decade or two later from more recent oncogenic events, and that therefore screening for familial breast cancer at young ages will have comparable benefits to screening for sporadic breast cancer after age 50. There is no evidence to support this hypothesis and it takes no account of the poorer sensitivity of mammography in premenopausal women, which is presumably the same for high-risk as for average-risk women. Thus, at present, there is no reason to believe that screening young high-risk women will be more effective than screening young average-risk women, and the disadvantages probably apply equally to both groups.

16.5.2 FREQUENCY OF ROUTINE SCREENING

The frequency with which screening needs to be repeated depends on the growth rate of the disease and the sensitivity of the test.

(a) Growth rate of familial breast cancer

If familial breast cancer were faster-growing than sporadic breast cancer, screening would need to be repeated at shorter intervals. Stage-specific survival rates can be used as a marker for different rates of growth. As already noted, survival rates in breast cancer patients below 40 (among whom a high proportion are familial) are worse than in women over 40 [20]. Nevertheless, studies comparing the survival of patients with affected first-degree relatives [40] or those probably carrying the *BRCA*1 gene [41] with the survival of age-matched sporadic breast cancer patients, have shown that familial breast cancers have a better prognosis. If the familial cases had been diagnosed by screening, this would lead to a spurious survival advantage because of lead-time and length-biased sampling, but screening was not thought to be a confounding factor in either of the above studies. Thus, on the basis of growth rates, there is no reason why high-risk women should be screened any more frequently than average-risk women.

(b) Sensitivity of screening

As already noted, sensitivity is markedly worse in premenopausal women. Therefore, if screening is offered to high-risk premenopausal women it should be repeated routinely at intervals no longer than 1 year and in informing such women of a negative screening result they should be warned about the possibility of an interval cancer arising before the next screen is due. For postmenopausal women, sensitivity is much better and a 2-year interval between routine tests is as appropriate for high-risk as for average-risk women.

16.5.3 RESEARCH PROSPECTS TO MEASURE THE BENEFITS OF SCREENING YOUNG HIGH-RISK WOMEN

It is frustrating to clinicians advising premenopausal high-risk women, that the benefits of screening are so hedged with uncertainty. In theory, the best way of resolving this would be to conduct a randomized controlled trial of screening within a population of high-risk women, comparable to those described above in average-risk women. However, this would be impracticable because the size of the high-risk population is small, and the sample size required to show a reduction in mortality could not be achieved without a large multinational recruitment. Moreover, obtaining informed consent to randomization would be difficult, and it is likely that many women would not adhere over several years, to the screening or non-screening arm to which they had been allocated.

A compromise solution, which would throw further light on the value of screening, would be to compare interim indicators of screening effectiveness in premenopausal high-risk women, with those in average-risk premenopausal women participating in controlled research trials. These interim indicators include the prevalence-to-incidence ratio, the proportional incidence of interval cancers (as a measure of sensitivity), and the trends in stage-specific incidence since the start of screening. Such comparisons would necessitate modelling an estimate of the underlying incidence of breast cancer in high-risk women in the absence of screening. To conduct such a study the organization and quality of screening offered to high-risk women should approximate to that in trials of

screening average-risk women. If and when any significant mortality difference emerges from trials in average-risk women, comparison of the interim indicators in high-risk and average-risk women could be used to model the effect of screening high-risk women on their subsequent breast cancer mortality. To this end, the UKCCCR has endorsed a study which will record data from the screening of women at increased risks (H. Cuckle, personal communication). Unfortunately accumulation of this proxy evidence of benefit will still take some 10 years to accumulate.

16.6 GUIDELINES FOR CURRENT PRACTICE

Screening for postmenopausal high-risk women should be provided, as for average-risk women over 50. However, given present uncertainty over the extent to which screening can improve prognosis, should it be provided for premenopausal high-risk women who actively request it, and should it be offered to those who do not?

A possible additional benefit of screening, unrelated to reduced risk of death, is the reassurance which a negative result may provide. A perception of vulnerability to breast cancer has been shown to be a moderately important factor encouraging attendance for screening [42]. For high-risk women, particularly those who have been classified as at risk after full investigation, their heightened awareness may cause considerable anxiety. They, and their medical advisers, may seek screening with the aim of showing that they do **not** have detectable cancer at that point in time. The reassurance this gives must, however, be tempered with caution about imperfect sensitivity. Even for women found by screening to have cancer there may be some reassurance value in ending a period of uncertainty, particularly if the cancer is at a very early stage. This reassurance value of screening is, however, still speculative and further psychological research is required in this area.

The preferred screening advice to be given to premenopausal high-risk women should enable them to make an informed decision about whether they should enter a regular screening programme or not. This entails educating them about the uncertainty as to whether, and by how much, it can reduce their risk of breast cancer death, about its relatively poor sensitivity, and about its possible harmful side effects. The women themselves, taking account of its reassurance value to them, can then participate in the decision.

Where a decision is made in favour of screening, every effort should be made to ensure that the woman is screened by a mammography screening unit with an inbuilt quality assurance programme, and which can recall her at annual intervals.

16.6.1 ATAXIA TELANGIECTASIA GENE CARRIERS

This subgroup of women at inherited risk of cancer not only has a high risk of breast cancer but also increased radiosensitivity [43]. For this reason routine screening by mammography may be contraindicated in relatives of known ataxia telangiectasia patients, particularly those aged under 50.

16.7 CONCLUSION

Screening, as a form of management for women at inherited high risk of breast cancer, is not the panacea it may at first appear. This is because the majority of these women are premenopausal, and the major component of their increased risk occurs before age 50. Screening, the purpose of which is to reduce the risk of breast cancer death, is of uncertain benefit in women aged under 50 and some of its unwanted side effects are more common in this age group

than in older women. Mammography screening is contraindicated in premenopausal women who are at high risk by virtue of a family history of ataxia telangiectasia, because of its radiation risk.

For the remainder, the decision of whether or not to be screened should be taken by the woman herself, after she has been fully informed of current evidence on the benefits and side effects. For those who opt for screening, it should be performed annually and the women alerted to the possibility of cancer developing in the interval between screens.

For high-risk women aged over 50, the benefit of screening is clear and its side effects are less. These women should be encouraged to participate in a general population screening programme, at the same frequency as that advised for average-risk women.

There is no case at present for actively seeking out premenopausal women with an inherited risk of breast cancer on the assumption that screening will improve their prognosis.

REFERENCES

1. Hakama, M. (1984) Selective screening by risk groups, in *Screening for Cancer*, (eds P.C. Prorok and A.B. Miller), UICC, Geneva, pp. 70–80.
2. Shapiro, S., Goldberg, J., Venet, L. and Strax, P. (1973) Risk factors in breast cancer – a prospective study, in *Host Environment Interactions*, (eds R. Doll and I. Vodopija), International Agency for Research on Cancer, Lyon, France, pp. 169–82.
3. Shapiro, S., Venet, W., Strax, P. and Venet, L. (1988) Current results of the breast cancer screening randomized trial: The Health Insurance Plan (HIP) of Greater New York Study, in *Screening for Breast Cancer*, (eds A. Miller and N. Day), Hans Huber, Toronto.
4. Tabar, L., Fagerberg, G., Duffy, S.W., Day, N.E., Gad, A. and Grontoft, O. (1992) Update of the Swedish two-county program of mammographic screening for breast cancer. *Radiol. Clin. N. Amer.*, **30**, (1), 187–210.

5. Anderson, I., Aspegren, K., Janzon, L. *et al.* (1988) Mammographic screening and mortality from breast cancer: the Malmo screening trial. *Br. Med. J.*, **297**, 943–48.

6. Frisell, J., Eklund, G., Hellstrom, L., Lidbrink, E., Rutqvist, L.-E. and Somell, A. (1991) Randomised study of mammography – preliminary report on mortality in the Stockholm trial. *Breast Cancer Res. Treat.*, **18**, 49–56.

7. Alexander, F.E., Anderson, T.J., Muir, B.B. *et al.* (1994) The Edinburgh Randomised Trial of Breast Cancer Screening: results after 10 years of follow-up. *Br. J. Cancer*, **70**, 542–8.

8. Nystrom, N., Rutqvist, L.-E., Wall, S. *et al.* (1993) Breast cancer screening with mammography: overview of Swedish randomised trials. *Lancet*, **341**, 973–8.

9. UK Trial of Early Detection of Breast Cancer Group. (1993) Breast cancer mortality after 10 years in the UK trial of early detection of breast cancer. *The Breast*, **2**, 13–20.

10. Collette, H.J.A., de Waard, F., Rombach, J.J., Collette, C. and Day, N.E. (1992) Further evidence of benefits of a non-randomised breast cancer screening programme: the DOM project. *J. Epidemiol Community Health*, **46**, 382–6.

11. Verbeek, A.L.M., Hendricks, J.H.C.L., Holland, R., Mravunac, M., Sturmans, F. and Day, N.E. (1984) Reduction in breast cancer mortality through mass screening with modern mammography. (First results of the Nijmegan Project 1975–81). *Lancet*, **i**, 1222–4.

12. Palli, D., del Turco, M.R., Buiatti, E. *et al.* (1986) A case-control study of the efficacy of a non-randomized breast cancer screening program in Florence (Italy). *Int. J. Cancer*, **38**, 501–4.

13. Morrison, A., Brisson, J. and Khalid, N. (1988) Breast cancer incidence and mortality in the Breast Cancer Detection Demonstration Project. *J. Natl Cancer Inst.*, **80**, 1540–7.

14. Miller, A.B., Baines, C.J., To, T and Wall, C. (1992) Canadian National Breast Screening Study. *Can. Med. Assoc. J.*, **147**, 1459–88.

15. Wald, N., Chamberlain, J. and Hackman, A. (1993) Report of the European Society for Mastology. Breast Cancer Screening Evaluation Committee. *The Breast*, **2**, 209–16.

16. Lundgren, B. and Jacobson, S. (1976) Single view mammography. *Cancer*, **38**, 1124–9.

17. Moss, S.M., Coleman, D.A., Ellman, R. *et al.* (1993) Interval cancers and sensitivity in the screening centres of the UK Trial of Early Detection of Breast Cancer. *Eur. J. Cancer*, **29A**, 225–58.

18. Tabar, L., Fagerberg, G., Day, N.E. and Holmberg, L. (1987) What is the optimum interval between mammographic screening examinations? *Br. J. Cancer*, **55**, 547–51.

19. Elwood, J.L.M., Cox, B and Richardson, A.K. (1993) The effectiveness of breast cancer screening by mammography in younger women. *Online J. Curr. Clin. Trials*, **32**.

20. Adami, H.O., Malker, B., Holmberg, L., Persson, I. and Stone, B. (1986) The relation between survival and age at diagnosis in breast cancer. *N. Eng. J. Med.*, **315**, 559–63.

21. De la Rochefordiere, A., Asselain, B., Campana, F. *et al.* (1993) Age as a prognostic factor in premenopausal breast cancer. *Lancet*, **341**, 1039–43.

22. National Institutes of Cancer. (1985) *Ad hoc Working Group to develop radio-epidemiological tables*, DHHS Publication No. NIH 852748, US Government Printing Office, Washington, DC.

23. Gohagen, J.K., Darby, W.P., Spitnagel, E.L., Monsees, B.S. and Tome, A.E. (1986) Radiogenic breast cancer effects of mammographic screening. *J. Natl Cancer Inst.*, **77**, 71–6.

24. Stomper, P.C., Kopans, D.B., Sadowsky, N.L. *et al.* (1988) Is mammography painful? A multicentre survey. *Arch. Intern. Med.*, **148**, 521–4.

25. Rutter, D.R., Calnan, M., Vaile, M.S.B., Field, S. and Wade, K.A. (1992) Discomfort and pain during mammography: description, prediction and prevention. *Br. Med. J.*, **305**, 443–5.

26. Dean, C., Roberts, M.M., French, K. and Robinson, S. (1986) Psychiatric morbidity after screening for breast cancer. *J. Epidemiol. Community Health*, **40**, 71–5.

27. Hunt, S.M., Alexander, F. and Roberts, M. (1988) Attenders and non-attenders at a breast screening clinic: a comparative study. *Public Health*, **102**, 3–10.

28. Wilson, J.M.G. and Jungner, G. (1968) *Principles and Practice of Screening for Disease*, Public Health Papers 34, World Health Organization, Geneva.

29. UK Trial of Early Detection of Breast Cancer Group. (1992) Specificity of screening in United Kingdom trial of early detection of breast cancer. *Br. Med. J.*, **304**, 346–9.

30. Chamberlain, J., Moss, S.M., Kirkpatrick, A.E., Michell, M. and Johns, L. (1993) National Health Service breast screening programme results for 1991–2. *Br. Med. J.*, **307**, 353–6.

31. Ellman, R., Angeli, N., Christians, A., Moss, S., Chamberlain, J. and Maguire, P. (1989) Psychiatric morbidity associated with screening for breast cancer. *Br. J. Cancer*, **60**, 781–4.

32. Bull, A.R. and Campbell, M.J. (1991) Assessment of the psychological impact of a breast screening programme. *Br. J. Radiol.*, **64**, 510–15.

33. Tabar, L., Fagerberg, G., Duffy, S.W. and Day, N.E. (1989) The Swedish two county trial of mammographic screening for breast cancer: recent results and calculation of benefit. *J. Epidemiol. Community Health*, **43**, 107–14.

34. UK Trial of Early Detection of Breast Cancer Group. (1988) First results on mortality reduction in the UK Trial of Early Detection of Breast Cancer. *Lancet*, **i**, 411–16.

35. Ellman, R. and Thomas, B.A. (1995) Is the quality of life of long-term survivors of breast cancer impaired? *J. Med. Screening*, **2**, 5–9.

36. Page, D.L., Dupont, W.D., Rogers, L.W., Landenberger, M. (1982) Intraductal carcinoma of the breast: follow-up after biopsy only. *Cancer*, **49**, 751–8.

37. Nielsen, M., Thomson, J.L., Primdahl, S., Dyreborg, U and Anderson, J.A. (1987) Breast cancer and atypia among young and middle-aged women: a study of 110 medico-legal autopsies. *Br. J. Cancer*, **56**, 814–19.

38. Peeters, P.H.M., Verbeek, A.L.M., Straatman, H. *et al.* (1989) Evaluation of overdiagnosis of breast cancer in screening with mammography: results of the Nijmegen Programme. *Int. J. Epidemiol.*, **28**, 295–9.

39. Houlston, R.S., McCarter, E., Parbhoo, S., Scurr, J.H. and Slack, J. (1992) Family history and risk of breast cancer. *J. Med. Genet.*, **29**, 154–7.

40. Ruder, A.M., Moodie, P.F., Nelson, N.A. and Choi, N.W. (1988) Does family history of breast cancer improve survival among patients with breast cancer? *Am. J. Obstet. Gynecol.*, **158**, 963–8.

41. Porter, D.E., Dixon, M., Smythe, E. and Steel, C.M. (1993) Breast cancer survival in BRCA1 carriers. *Lancet*, **341**, 184–5.

42. Calnan, M. and Chamberlain, J. (1984) Explaining participation in programmes for the early detection of breast cancer: a comparative analysis. *Rev. Epidem. et Santé Publ.*, **32**, 376–82.

43. Swift, M., Morell, D., Massey, R.B. and Chase, C.L. (1991) Incidence of cancer in 161 families affected by ataxia telangiectasia. *N. Engl. J. Med.*, **325**, 1831–6.

Chapter 17

The management of women with a high risk of breast cancer

I. The role of prophylactic tamoxifen

TREVOR J. POWLES and MARY E.R. O'BRIEN

17.1 INTRODUCTION

The search for genes which predispose to inherited breast cancer has intensified with the cloning of the *BRCA*1 and *BRCA*2 genes. This presents doctors with a new dilemma in the management of healthy women, at very high risk but with no clinical evidence of a disease. For many years we have been able to identify an increased risk of developing breast cancer because of a family history and this has encouraged us to develop clinical trials of intervention strategies for these people. Clearly, the problems of conducting these trials will become more difficult when we are able to identify subgroups of healthy women at very high risk, in whom randomized clinical trials may be unacceptable. On the other hand, offering them untested treatments such as mastectomy, ovarian ablation or even tamoxifen is confounded by the risks

that these interventions may be either ineffective or unnecessary.

We therefore started a programme in 1986 to examine the efficacy of tamoxifen for the prevention of breast cancer in high-risk women identified by a very strong family history. No doubt many of these women will in fact have genetic abnormalities when the genes are identified and can be evaluated. We would then be able to evaluate retrospectively whether we can in fact prevent breast cancer in such women at a genetic risk. There is obviously the theoretical possibility that the series of events which allow the initiation and promotion of a breast cancer may be such that the very high risk of initiation would allow expression of clinical cancers independent of any hormone promotion. In such women an endocrine intervention might be ineffective and it is therefore essential that the trials are undertaken in order to clarify this.

Genetic Predisposition to Cancer. Edited by R.A. Eeles, B.A.J. Ponder, D.F. Easton and A. Horwich. Published in 1996 by Chapman & Hall, London.
0 412 56580 3

17.2 EXPERIMENTAL AND CLINICAL BASIS FOR TAMOXIFEN USE

Tamoxifen has been shown capable of inhibiting the oestrogen-dependent proliferation of MCF7 cells *in vitro* [1]. Tamoxifen has some agonist properties and is also able to stimulate cell replication in suitably developed MCF7 cell lines in the absence of oestrogen. *In vivo*, tamoxifen will inhibit the promotion by oestrogen of experimental tumours in mice and in rats [2, 3].

Tamoxifen has been in use for clinical treatment of advanced breast cancer since 1971 [4] and as adjuvant therapy for treatment of patients with primary breast cancers since 1974. Over 4 million women have received treatment with very low clinical toxicity.

The use of tamoxifen as adjuvant therapy after primary treatment of operable breast cancer has been reported to reduce the risk of development of a new primary cancer in the contralateral breast, in three separate randomized trials. The Stockholm group used tamoxifen 40 mg/day and after a median follow-up of 7 years there were 47 cancers in the contralateral breast in the untreated women compared with only 29 in the treated women ($P = 0.03$) [5]. The NSABP used tamoxifen 20 mg/day and reported 55 second cancers in the contralateral breast in the untreated group compared with only 28 in the tamoxifen-treated group ($P = 0.001$) [6]. Similarly, the Cancer Research Campaign reported 18 contralateral cancers in the control group compared with only seven in the tamoxifen-treated group ($P = 0.02$) [7]. However, two studies using tamoxifen 20 mg/day for 2 years have failed to show a decrease in the incidence of contralateral breast cancer, one being a study from Denmark [8] and the other from the Christie Hospital, Manchester [9]. The Scottish trial using tamoxifen 20 mg/day for 5 years has shown a reduction in contralateral breast

cancer but at this stage it is not statistically significant [6, 10].

A meta-analysis of all adjuvant clinical trials indicated overall a 39% ($P < 0.00001$) reduction in the risk of contralateral breast cancer [11]. For these reasons tamoxifen was considered the best option for a clinical trial of endocrine intervention to reduce breast cancer incidence in those at increased risk of the disease.

17.3 DURATION OF TREATMENT AND DOSAGE

The results from animal carcinogenesis experiments, together with the epidemiological data of cancer incidence in Japan after the atomic bomb explosions in 1945 indicate that breast cancer in humans may have a long latent period extending from 10–30 years. The incidence of breast cancer in the western world seems to peak at about 55 and continues through to old age, indicating that much of the initiation and promotion of breast cancer occurs at about or before the menopause when oestrogen levels are comparatively high. This would indicate that endocrine intervention should probably start before the menopause, preferably after childbirth which may in itself have a protective effect.

At this stage there are no human clinical data to indicate how long tamoxifen should be used in order to achieve maximum effect. *In vivo* experimental data indicate that tamoxifen may only be cytostatic and hold tumour development for as long as the drug is used. However, clinical adjuvant data indicate that the reduction in risk of relapse continues up to at least 10 years, even though tamoxifen was used for only about 2 years [11]. A similar effect may occur in endocrine promotion of human breast cancer, and hence at present it would seem best to administer tamoxifen for at least 5 years in order to maximize any possible preventive effect.

The issue of tamoxifen dosage will become more important if the drug proves to be effective. The acute side effects, as well as (presumably) any long-term unknown risks, particularly of carcinogenesis, are each likely to be less at a dose of 10 mg/day than with 20 or 40 mg/day. Whether a 10 mg/day dose is optimal is unclear but some clinical data indicate that it is as effective as 20 mg/day in the reduction of mastalgia in patients with benign mammary dysplasia [12]. However, at the time our pilot prevention programme started, we opted for the most commonly used therapeutic dose of 20 mg/day.

17.4 TAMOXIFEN PREVENTION TRIALS

Over 2000 healthy women have now been entered into the ongoing Royal Marsden Hospital feasibility double-blind randomized trial. Women were considered to be at high risk if they had a strong family history of breast cancer. The eligibility criteria required included a first-degree relative who had breast cancer < 45 years of age, or one first-degree relative with bilateral breast cancer at any age, or more than two relatives with breast cancer – one of whom was first-degree. Participants were usually over the age of 40 years and not at risk of pregnancy. Eligible participants were required to give informed, written consent and undergo clinical assessment and mammography to exclude carcinoma before randomization to either tamoxifen 20 mg/day or placebo.

The tamoxifen and placebo groups are matched for age, menopausal status, family history and relative risk of breast cancer. Acute toxicity and compliance assessed in the first 1242 women indicate a low incidence for acute toxicity with a significant increase in hot flushes (34% versus 17%) and vaginal discharge (12% versus 4%) in pre- and postmenopausal women randomized to tamoxifen versus placebo. There was a marginal increase in menstrual period irregularities in women randomized to tamoxifen (14%) versus placebo (9%) although there was no evidence of tamoxifen-induced amenorrhoea or early menopause. There was no evidence of an increased incidence of nausea, vomiting, headaches, mood change and weight gain in women given tamoxifen [13–15].

The predicted compliance at 5 years is high for tamoxifen 75%, and placebo 80%. The marginally lower (P <0.025) compliance for tamoxifen can be attributed in part to toxicity, with 97 (16%) of participants on tamoxifen stopping medication because of toxicity (mostly hot flushes) compared with 52 (8%) on placebo. This would indicate that only 45 out of 613 participants stopped tamoxifen because of therapeutic toxicity.

Safety monitoring, including clotting, lipid profile and bone density, was undertaken to exclude potential harmful antioestrogenic effects of tamoxifen. Measurement of clotting factors pre-treatment and at 6 months indicate a significant reduction in the fibrinogen/AT3 ratio caused by a significant fall in fibrinogen in both pre and postmenopausal women (P <0.005) with only a small (<10%) fall in AT3 in postmenopausal women. There was a similar fall in protein S, mostly occurring in postmenopausal women (P <0.05) with no detectable change in protein C, suggesting that there was not a risk of increased coagulation on tamoxifen.

Monitoring of plasma total cholesterol showed a fall of about 10–15% in participants on tamoxifen compared with pre-treatment levels and this was maintained for 5 years. There was a significant but smaller fall in total cholesterol on placebo.

Sequential measurement of age-corrected bone mineral content by single photon absorption, now continued up to 5 years, showed no evidence of accelerated bone loss due to tamoxifen.

Annual ovarian screening using transvaginal ultrasound detected no cases of ovarian cancer. However, there was a significant increase ($P<0.025$) in the risk of detecting benign ovarian cysts in premenopausal women on tamoxifen for more than 3 months compared with placebo. Similarly, there was an increased likelihood of detecting fibroids in premenopausal and postmenopausal women on tamoxifen for 1–2 years ($P<0.001$) when compared with placebo. There was no associated increased likelihood of requiring laparotomy or laparoscopy for women given tamoxifen compared with placebo, although the number of women requiring hysterectomy is marginally more in the former case (29) than in the latter (16).

Of all women randomized in this trial, only 37 have been lost to follow-up for more than 18 months. There has been one non-malignant death and one pregnancy. Other prevention trials using tamoxifen in healthy women are now underway in the US, Italy, the UK and Australia.

17.5 POTENTIAL ADVERSE EFFECTS OF TAMOXIFEN

There is a current area of debate about the potential harmful effects of the partial agonist activity of tamoxifen on the uterus and liver.

Tamoxifen has experimental carcinogenic potential in rats (but not mice), and will cause liver cancers at low doses with features indicating a genotoxin rather than an oestrogenic promoter. Adduct formation indicating potential DNA damage due to tamoxifen has been identified in the rat liver at these low dose levels [16]. In women who have had primary breast cancer, the clinical data at present indicate no increased risk of liver cancer in women given tamoxifen 20 mg/day for up to 5 years. Although many of these women started tamoxifen more than 10 years ago, the median follow-up is relatively short for identification of an increased risk of solid tumours and further careful epidemiological follow-up is required.

Tamoxifen probably has an oestrogenic effect on the endometrium in postmenopausal women causing endometrial hyperplasia with a consequential increased risk of carcinoma. At the higher dose of 40 mg/day, tamoxifen has been reported to increase the risk of endometrial cancer about six-fold [17]. At the lower dose of 20 mg/day an increased risk of endometrial cancer of about 2–3-fold is likely [18], although reports of increased risk in randomized trials have not so far been published. Screening by transvaginal ultrasound for endometrial thickening in postmenopausal women, together with aspiration biopsies and possible progestin therapy, may be required if such a risk is established, at a dose level of 20 mg/day.

Visual disturbances have been reported as a specific type of retinopathy and keratopathy associated with relatively high doses of tamoxifen [19, 20]. At the more conventional dose of 20 mg/day, there is conflicting evidence of any drug-related retinopathy [21, 22]. The condition arising at higher dosages is usually reversible if diagnosed early. This indicates a need for ophthalmic evaluation of any woman taking tamoxifen at any dose level and who complains of visual symptoms.

Occasional acute liver toxicity [23] accompanied by agranulocytosis [24] and the risk of thromboembolism [25] have been reported in patients receiving tamoxifen but any cause and effect relationship has not been established.

Finally, there is a possibility that an unexpected toxicity may appear after long-term tamoxifen use. However, on balance the potential benefits of the drug at this time seem to far outweigh any potential risks. If tamoxifen proves to be effective in preventing breast cancer it may be used widely in women at increased risk of the disease. Identification of those individuals at increased risk of breast cancer by genetic, endocrine and environmental means, would clearly improve the risk–benefit ratio.

17.6 FUTURE DEVELOPMENTS OF TAMOXIFEN AS A CHEMOPREVENTIVE AGENT

Women have now become accustomed to the use of contraception in the form of tablets or by injection or implant. Oral contraceptives (OC) in themselves can decrease the incidence of cancer of the ovary and cancer of the endometrium [26, 27]. The influence of OCs on the incidence of breast cancer remains controversial with studies showing no effect [28], or a small increase in incidence [29]. The possibility of developing an OC combined with tamoxifen or similar agent such as toremifene is attractive. It is possible that such a combination could be developed as an effective OC which would prevent the subsequent development of breast cancer.

Similarly, hormone replacement therapy (HRT) combined with tamoxifen could be developed to prevent breast cancer. We have used tamoxifen combined with HRT for control of menopausal symptoms in patients with breast cancer [30], and have included women on HRT in our prevention trial with no evidence of any adverse interaction or activation of disease. The development of oral combinations of HRT and OC with tamoxifen or similar drugs has the attraction of involving women who already accept and are compliant on regular oral medication for another reason.

17.7 CONCLUSIONS

Experimental and clinical evidence indicate that tamoxifen may protect a substantial proportion of women who might develop breast cancer. Our initial feasibility and pilot trial indicated high acceptance and compliance for a trial in women with an increased risk of breast cancer because of a family history. This has now extended into large multicentre national trials involving tens of thousands of women. Should tamoxifen

prove to be effective at preventing breast cancer it will be important to be able to identify more effectively such groups of women at high risk of developing the disease and to be able to show retrospectively that tamoxifen is effective in such individuals. Careful integration of the genetic risk programme and the tamoxifen prevention programme will be required.

Integration of chemoprevention with agents such as tamoxifen given in combination with HRT and OCs would encourage extension of a prevention strategy into large populations of healthy women already receiving medication.

Ultimately, evaluation of the benefits of the use of tamoxifen or similar agents and associated risks will be obtained only from carefully controlled clinical trials. This is an opportunity to test whether it is possible to prevent a disease which afflicts over half a million women each year throughout the world. The risks of using any new medication in otherwise healthy, albeit at increased risk, women must be evaluated carefully to avoid unacceptable harm. At present, it appears that the estimated potential benefits of using tamoxifen in healthy women at increased risk of breast cancer because of a family history, may far outweigh any actual or potential risks.

REFERENCES

1. Lippman, M.E. Bolan, G. and Huff, K.K. (1976) The effects of androgens and antiandrogens on hormone-responsive human breast cancer in long-term tissue culture. *Cancer Res.*, **36**, 4595–601.
2. Jordan, V.C. (1990) Long-term adjuvant tamoxifen therapy for breast cancer: the prelude to prevention. *Cancer Treat. Rev.*, **17**, 15–36.
3. Gottardes, M.M. and Jordan, V.C. (1987) Antitumour actions of keoxifene and tamoxifen in the N-nitrose-methylurea-induced rat mammary carcinoma model. *Cancer Res.*, **47**, 4020–4.

4. Ward, H.W.C. (1973) Antioestrogen therapy for breast cancer. A trial of tamoxifen at low dose levels. *Br. Med. J.*, **1**, 13–15.

5. Rutqvist, L.E., Cedermark, B. Glas, U. *et al.* (1991) Contralateral primary tumors in breast cancer patients in a randomized trial of adjuvant tamoxifen therapy. *J. Natl Cancer Inst.*, **83**, 1299–306.

6. Fisher, B. and Redmond, C. (1991) New perspective on cancer of the contralateral breast: a marker for assessing tamoxifen as a preventive agent. *J. Natl Cancer Inst.*, **83**, 1278–80.

7. CRC Adjuvant Breast Trial Working Party (1988) Cyclophosphamide and tamoxifen therapy as adjuvant therapies in the management of breast cancer. *Br. J. Cancer*, **57**, 604–7.

8. Andersson, M., Storm, H.H, and Mouridsen, H.T. (1991) Incidence of new primary cancers after adjuvant tamoxifen therapy and radiotherapy for early breast cancer. *J. Natl Cancer Inst.*, **83**, 1013–17.

9. Ribeiro, G. and Swindell, R. (1988) The Christie Hospital adjuvant tamoxifen trial – status at 10 years. *Br. J. Cancer*, **57**, 601–3.

10. Stewart, H.J. (1991) Adjuvant systemic therapy for operable breast cancer. *Br. Med. Bull.*, **47(2)**, 343–56.

11. EBCTCG. (1992) Systemic treatment of early breast cancer by hormonal, cytotoxic, or immune therapy. *Lancet*, **339**, 1–15, 71–85.

12. Fentiman, I.S., Caleffi, M., Hamed, H. *et al.* (1988) Dosage and duration of tamoxifen treatment for mastalgia; a controlled trial. *Br. J. Surg.*, **75**, 845–6.

13. Powles, T.J., Hardy, J.R., Ashley, S.E. *et al.* (1989) A pilot trial to evaluate the acute toxicity and feasibility of tamoxifen for prevention of breast cancer. *Br. J. Cancer*, **60**, 126–31.

14. Powles, T.J., Tillyer, C.R., Jones, A.L. *et al.* (1990) Prevention of breast cancer with tamoxifen – an update on the Royal Marsden Hospital pilot programme. *Eur. J. Cancer*, **26**, 680–4.

15. Powles, T.J., Jones, A.L., Ashley, S.E. *et al.* (1994) The Royal Marsden Hospital pilot tamoxifen chemoprevention trial. *Breast Cancer Res. Treat.*, **31**, 73–82.

16. Han, X. and Liehr, J.G. (1992) Induction of covalent DNA adducts in rodents by tamoxifen. *Cancer Res.*, **52**, 1360–3.

17. Fornander, T., Rutquist, L.E., Cedermark, B. *et al.* (1989) Adjuvant tamoxifen in early breast cancer: Occurrence of new primary cancers. *Lancet*, **21**, 117–20.

18. Van Leeuwen, F.E., Benraadt, J., Coebergh, J.W.W. *et al.* (1994) Risk of endometrial cancer after tamoxifen treatment of breast cancer. *Lancet*, **343**, 448–52.

19. Kaiser-Kupfer, M.I. and Lippman M.E. (1978) Tamoxifen retinopathy. *Cancer Treat. Rep.*, **62**, 315–20.

20. McKeown, C., Swartz, M., Blom, J. *et al.* (1981) Tamoxifen retinopathy. *Br. J. Ophthalmol.*, **65**, 177–9.

21. Longstaff, S., Sigurdsson, H. and O'Keeffe, M. (1989) A controlled study of the ocular effects of tamoxifen in conventional dosage in the treatment of breast carcinoma. *Eur. J. Cancer Clin. Oncol.*, **25 (12)**, 1805–8.

22. Pavlidis, N., Petris, C., Briassoulis, E. *et al.* (1992) Clear evidence that long-term low-dose tamoxifen treatment can induce ocular toxicity. *Cancer*, **69**, 2961–4.

23. Blackburn, A., Amiel, S., Millis, R. and Rubens, R. (1984) Tamoxifen and liver damage. *Br. Med. J.*, **289**, 288.

24. Ching, C.K., Smith, P.G., Long, R.G. (1992). Tamoxifen-associated hepatocellular damage and agranulocytosis. *Lancet* **339**: 940.

25. Lipton, A., Harve, H. and Hamilton, R. (1984) Venous thrombosis as a side effect of tamoxifen treatment. *Cancer Treat. Rep.*, **68**, 887–9.

26. Weiss, N.S. and Sayvets, T. (1980) Incidence of endometrial cancer in relation to the use of oral contraceptives. *N. Engl. J. Med.*, **302**, 551–4.

27. Rosenberg, L., Shapiro, S., Slone, D. *et al.* (1982) Epithelial ovarian cancer and combination oral contraceptives. *JAMA*, **247**, 3210–12.

28. Wiseman, R.A. (1983) Oral contraceptives and breast cancer rates. *Lancet*, **2**, 1415–16.

29. Pike, M.C., Henderson, B.E., Krailo, M.D. *et al.* (1983) Breast cancer in young women and use of oral contraceptives: possible modifying effect of formulation and age at use. *Lancet*, **2**, 926–9.

30. Powles, T.J., Hickish, T., Casey, S. *et al.* (1993) Hormone replacement after breast cancer. *Lancet*, **342**, 60–1.

II. The controversy of prophylactic mastectomy

TIMOTHY I. DAVIDSON and NIGEL P.M. SACKS

17.8 INTRODUCTION

The controversy surrounding the operation of prophylactic mastectomy, usually with immediate reconstruction, has been of interest to surgeons and oncologists for a number of decades. In other areas of cancer management, prophylactic surgery has an established role, for example in patients with the multiple endocrine neoplasia (MEN 2) syndrome and raised serum calcitonin levels, prophylactic total thyroidectomy is advocated to avoid the development of medullary thyroid carcinoma [1]. Prophylactic colectomy is routinely advised in patients with familial adenomatous polyposis (FAP) syndrome to avoid the inevitable progression of colonic adenomas to invasive carcinomas [2]; in patients with total ulcerative colitis with severe dysplasia on biopsy, the high risk of large bowel cancer is an additional reason for advising proctocolectomy in severely affected patients.

The debate over the role of prophylactic surgery in women considered to be at high risk of breast cancer revolves around three main issues. The first is identifying which subgroup of women will have an acceptable cost/benefit ratio in relation to subsequent risk of breast cancer development to justify offering them prophylactic mastectomy. The second centres on the debate regarding which surgical technique should be used, subcutaneous or total mastectomy. The third unresolved issue is whether prophylactic mastectomy can adequately remove all breast tissue and so prevent the subsequent development of invasive breast cancer in all patients.

It is worthwhile remembering that the practice of subcutaneous mastectomy initially arose as an alternative to the Halsted radical mastectomy. This remained the standard operation for carcinoma of the breast until the acceptance of the modified radical mastectomy, and more recently, breast-conserving surgery. It is easy to imagine how a contour-saving operation which also preserved the nipple–areolar complex would be welcomed by women with a strong family history, borderline lesions or early breast cancer, who

Genetic Predisposition to Cancer. Edited by R.A. Eeles, B.A.J. Ponder, D.F. Easton and A. Horwich. Published in 1996 by Chapman & Hall, London.
0 412 56580 3

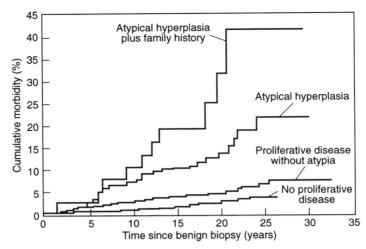

Fig. 17.1 Cumulative breast cancer incidence. The absolute risk of subsequent development of breast cancer according to type of histological lesion biopsied, and family history of breast cancer in a first-degree relative. (Reproduced with permission from [6].)

were at high risk of being disfigured by radical mastectomy should an invasive cancer subsequently be diagnosed. Subcutaneous mastectomy with reconstruction fulfilled this need, although coincidently in the past two decades the cosmetic morbidity from breast cancer surgical treatment has improved dramatically.

17.9 INDICATIONS FOR PROPHYLACTIC MASTECTOMY

There is as yet no consensus among surgeons, oncologists or epidemiologists on the absolute indications for prophylactic mastectomy, so for the time being we must state that there are none. The most common **relative** indications that have been proposed are specific premalignant proliferative lesions such as lobular carcinoma *in situ* or atypical lobular or ductal hyperplasia, a strong family history of breast cancer, contralateral invasive breast cancer or a combination of more than one of these factors [3].

17.9.1 BORDERLINE OR PREMALIGNANT LESIONS

The histological factors for subsequent development of breast cancer have in recent years been clarified [4–6] and borderline lesions can be stratified according to the degree of risk; when proliferative lesions with cellular atypia occur in the presence of a strong family history of breast cancer, this risk becomes disproportionately high (Figure 17.1). It would seem intuitive that with an increasing postulated relative risk in an individual, the option of prophylactic mastectomy should be more strongly considered.

However, the problem remains of the threshold **when** to advise surgery (Table 17.1]). For example, should a woman with a five-fold relative risk of developing breast cancer be counselled to consider prophylactic mastectomy while a woman with relative risk of two– or three-fold that of the age-matched population be counselled against this form of surgery? The ultimate decision to undergo surgery rests with the patient herself after

274

Table 17.1 Factors affecting the relative risk of breast cancer in later life. (From [7].)

Factor	Relative risk
Family history	
Primary relative with breast cancer	1.2–3.0
Premenopausal	3.1
Premenopausal and bilateral	8.5–9.0
Postmenopausal	1.5
Postmenopausal and bilateral	4.0–5.1
Menstrual history	
Age at menarche, 12	1.3
Age and menopause, 55 with 40 menstrual years	1.48–2.0
Pregnancy	
First child after age 35	2.0–3.0
Nulliparous	3.0
Other neoplasms	
Contralateral breast cancer	5.0
Cancer of the major salivary gland	4.0
Cancer of uterus	2.0
Benign breast disease	
Atypical lobular hyperplasia	4.0
Lobular carcinoma *in situ*	7.2
Previous biopsy	1.86–2.13

appropriate counselling in the light of all the information available to her.

17.9.2 FAMILIAL BREAST CANCER

Equally contentious is the issue of prophylactic mastectomy in a healthy woman with presumed normal breasts but where there is a strong family history of breast cancer. The relative risk to an individual woman depends on the number of members in her family affected by breast cancer, whether they are first- or second-degree relatives, the age at which the relatives were affected and whether the breast cancers were bilateral (Table 17.1). Fuer *et al.* [8] using surveillance, epidemiology and end result (SEER) data have tabulated the eventual risk of developing and dying from breast cancer over given time intervals, so that when counselling women with a family history of breast cancer some attempt can be made to quantify the degree of relative risk for an individual patient.

It is estimated that less than 10% of cases of breast cancer are due to an inherited predisposition. The location of the *BRCA1* breast cancer gene has recently been identified and the gene has now been cloned [9]. Once available, the genetic test to detect carriers of the the *BRCA1* gene will provide the potential for identifying accurately, in a small group of women at least, those women who have a sufficiently high risk/benefit ratio to justify prophylactic mastectomy. However, even though most *BRCA1* carriers will develop breast cancer within decades, some will never do so, so it is inevitable that some patients will be offered and will undergo unnecessary surgery. In addition, *BRCA1* is not the only breast cancer gene (see Chapter 14) and will not account for all the families with a history of inherited breast cancer.

17.9.3 SOCIAL ATTITUDES TO PROPHYLACTIC SURGERY

There is undoubtedly a cultural element affecting the degree of acceptability of prophylactic surgery in members of breast cancer families. In severely affected families in the US, the majority of reatives at risk have chosen surgery; it must be remembered that many have already seen several close relatives die of breast cancer. To date, a far smaller minority of women in the UK have chosen this option. The willingness of many North American women to undergo mastectomy for benign breast conditions such as mastalgia, as well as the large number of woman in the US opting for cosmetic breast surgery, may possibly reflect the extent to which these treatment choices are surgeon-driven in a society where private health care is dominant.

The choice is ultimately made by the patient in every case, after suitable counselling and after the best assessment of risk has been presented and discussed [10]. One of the most potent arguments in favour of prophylactic surgery is of course the lack of a proven alternative. It must be borne in mind that there is **no** evidence of benefit in terms of survival or even improved detection of early breast cancer in these high-risk groups of women from either intensive screening at an earlier age [10] or the use of chemopreventative agents such as tamoxifen [11] or retinoids [12].

17.10 SURGICAL TECHNIQUE

Once the patient who has been considered for prophylactic surgery has decided to proceed with the operation, the choice needs to be made as to the type of operation that is most appropriate. It must be remembered that the surgical aim is mastectomy with reconstruction, **not** an operation primarily to enhance the appearance of the breast [13]. The goal of preventing subsequent breast cancer in the high-risk woman has to be balanced against a good lasting cosmetic result in someone who is, at the time of surgery, usually a young woman with apparently normal breasts. The two options are subcutaneous mastectomy and total mastectomy, with immediate or delayed reconstruction.

While the breast is a subcutaneous organ, the difference between the two operations is largely one of the underlying surgical aim. Subcutaneous mastectomy is an operation designed to decrease the volume of breast tissue to minimize subsequent risk of breast cancer development. Interestingly, however, reduction in the volume of breast tissue in experimental animals does not lead to reduced risk of breast cancer [14]. The aim in

total mastectomy on the other hand is to remove **all** breast tissue with the intent of avoiding any subsequent breast cancer development.

17.10.1 TECHNIQUE FOR SUBCUTANEOUS MASTECTOMY

The surgical techniques for subcutaneous mastectomy have been widely reviewed [3, 15–17]. Whether the operation is performed by a general surgeon with an interest in oncological and breast surgery, or by a plastic surgeon with an interest in reconstruction, is immaterial, so long as the operator is well trained in the technical requirements for this demanding operation.

The most appropriate skin incision is dependent to some extent on the size of the breasts. An 8–12 cm inframammary incision is often adequate in small-sized breasts. In larger breasts we favour an 'S'-shaped incision that includes the upper third of the areola and extends laterally to allow the operator to clear the upper breast quadrants more easily (Figure 17.2). In pendulous breasts that necessitate skin reduction, a skin incision similar to that for reduction mammoplasty can be performed (Figure 17.3) and up to one-third of patients will need reduction of the skin envelope to achieve the best cosmetic results.

From these various incisions the skin is dissected off the gland to include as much of the breast tissue as possible, including the axillary tail. Ideally, over 95% of breast tissue should be cleared. A small amount of glandular tissue has to be left beneath the nipple to assure continued vascularity of the nipple–areolar complex. The tissue under the nipple–areolar complex can be examined histologically for atypical epithelial change to determine whether sacrifice of the nipple–areolar complex is prudent. After removal of the bulk of the glandular tissue, remaining islands of breast tissue may be identified and

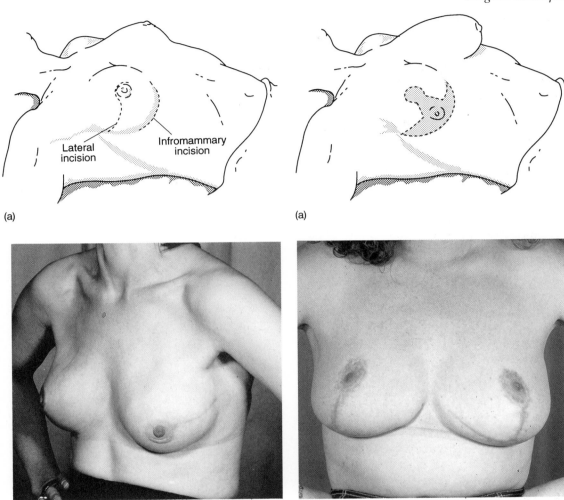

(a)

(b)

Fig. 17.2 (a) Skin incisions for subcutaneous mastectomy showing inframammary and lateral S-shaped incisions. (b) Postoperative appearances following bilateral subcutaneous mastectomy and subpectoral implants via lateral skin incisions.

Fig. 17.3 (a) Skin incisions for subcutaneous mastectomy with marking pattern as for reduction mammoplasty. (b) Postoperative result following bilateral subcutaneous mastectomy with skin reduction and subpectoral implants.

removed by everting the skin envelope of the breast. Particular care must be taken to include the entire axillary tail of the breast (including if desired a sample of the low axillary lymph nodes) and this may prove technically impossible through a small inframammary incision.

Immediate reconstruction involves the fashioning of a submuscular pocket deep to the pectoralis major muscle. This may be approached through an oblique incision in the pectoralis major muscle, or between the serratus anterior and pectoralis major muscles laterally. A large pocket is created with

277

blunt dissection and a textured silicone gel prosthesis is implanted. In those patients where the volume of the submuscular pocket is not initially adequate, a tissue expander or expander prosthesis (such as the Becker type prosthesis) can be used instead of a fixed-volume implant. The volume of this prosthesis can rapidly be increased over a period of weeks by injecting saline via a laterally placed subcutaneous filling port which is subsequently removed.

Early and long-term complications of subcutaneous mastectomy are not inconsiderable and those reported in a number of series have been reviewed [18, 19]. Acute complications include flap and/or nipple loss, haematoma, implant exposure and infection, and occur in up to 20% of patients in some series. Some years ago the most frequent long-term complication was capsular contracture secondary to subcutaneous placement of the prosthesis. However, with subpectoral placement of the implant this complication is very much rarer now, although displacement of the prosthesis, usually in an upward direction, may occur and need later correction. The use of textured silicone prostheses has to a large extent reduced the problem of late migration of the implant. The most serious (though rare) long-term complication of course remains the development of carcinoma in residual breast tissue, an indication that the surgery has failed to achieve its objective in that individual patient [20].

17.10.2 TECHNIQUE FOR TOTAL MASTECTOMY

With a total mastectomy the entire breast gland is removed, together with a small ellipse of skin bearing the nipple-aerolar complex (Figure 17.4). The breast tissue including the axillary tail can then be dissected from the skin flaps under direct vision and the likelihood of leaving residual islands of breast tissue is less than with subcutaneous

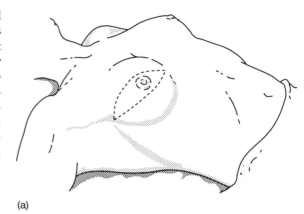

(a)

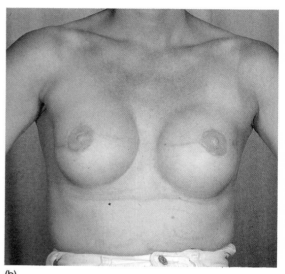

(b)

Fig. 17.4 (a) Skin incision for total mastectomy. (b) Postoperative result following bilateral total mastectomy with subpectoral implants and nipple–areolar complex reconstruction.

mastectomy. Reconstruction of the breast mound is performed the same way as for subcutaneous mastectomy, with a prosthesis inserted into the submuscular pocket deep to the pectoralis major muscle.

Nipple–areolar reconstruction can be performed immediately or as a second-stage procedure and a variety of techniques have been described. Nipple projection is obtained by forming local flaps such as the skate or tripod flaps [21] in the central areolar area. The areola can be reconstructed using a full-thickness skin graft from the inner medial thigh, or a good result can be achieved with tattooing.

The disadvantages of total mastectomy as opposed to subcutaneous mastectomy include the inevitable shortcomings of the reconstructed nipple with loss of nipple sensation, less nipple projection, and the presence of a central linear mammary scar which will remain cosmetically obtrusive. The advantages are more complete clearance of breast tissue, particularly the axillary tail and avoidance of the risk associated with retention of the nipple–areolar complex.

In both subcutaneous and total mastectomy techniques, delayed reconstruction with insertion of a submuscular prosthesis after a period of several months is an alternative approach to immediate reconstruction and is favoured by some authors, particularly in patients with large breasts and excessive redundant skin which might shrink in the interim. With either technique, the cosmetic results are variable even in the hands of expert surgeons. Excellent results can be achieved, although it is important when counselling women to show good, average and bad results.

17.10.3 WHICH TECHNIQUE TO CHOOSE?

To evaluate the efficacy of subcutaneous and total mastectomy procedures in reducing subsequent breast cancer, prospective studies of both operations with follow-up times in excess of 10–15 years are required. These data are unlikely to become available and opinion remains divided. The advocates of total mastectomy cite the high incidence of complications associated with subcutaneous mastectomy as a major factor. Secondly, there is concern about the 10–15% of breast

tissue not removed by subcutaneous mastectomy [22] although other authors assess this figure to be lower [16].

The third area of objection is the retention or the nipple–areolar complex and the anxiety that this may be a site of subsequent breast cancer [23]. While there have been several reported cases of subsequent invasive cancer following prophylactic subcutaneous mastectomy [24] its exact incidence is unknown. This is because of poor follow-up, variation in the patient population undergoing surgery and the lack of any prospective study addressing this fundamental issue. We would advocate total mastectomy if the indication was *in-situ* carcinoma (LCIS or DCIS) or if the patient expressed anxiety about the risk of cancer development in the retained nipple–areolar complex.

Advocates of subcutaneous mastectomy believe that the operation is a good 'risk-reducing' operation for the precancerous breast, despite small amounts of breast tissue remaining at the periphery and that the degree of compromise in this surgical procedure carries a minimal additional risk which is more than compensated for by the more cosmetically acceptable result. When performing the operation of subcutaneous mastectomy, we favour the lateral incision in order to reduce to a minimum the amount of breast tissue left behind.

17.11 PSYCHOSOCIAL AND PSYCHOSEXUAL SEQUELAE

The psychological effects of prophylactic surgery have largely been ignored. A woman who is fearful of developing breast cancer, and who may have seen close relatives die from this disease, may indeed become mentally crippled by her anxiety. Women at high risk of breast cancer need expert counselling and likewise those undergoing prophylactic surgery need psychological support, even after they have accepted the idea of surgery and have undergone mastectomy and reconstruction. There is little doubt that the inherent psychosexual problems known to be associated with mastectomy can indeed be reproduced by prophylactic mastectomy and reconstruction [25].

Postoperative difficulties in accepting the surgical result, sexual dysfunction and high levels of depression and anxiety have all been observed following surgery, related in some cases to specific personality characteristics [26]. Among the variables suggested as being of importance in predicting adverse psychological reactions after surgery, previous psychiatric treatment and insufficient social support may be relevant. One year after surgery, the majority of patients rate their marital relations as similar to their preoperative situation, but almost half of patients undergoing subcutaneous mastectomy change their sexual habits regarding their breasts after surgery.

More recently too, attention has been drawn to the psychological consequences for women of silicone implants which have proved to be of major concern in the US [27]. While the relationship between silicone gel prostheses and systemic ill health (in particular, connective tissue disease) remains a major litigation issue in the US, there is no scientific evidence to implicate implants in many of the disorders postulated and no evidence that the prosthetic material itself might have a carcinogenic role. Current guidelines for the use of silicone breast implants in the UK reflect this viewpoint [28].

17.12 CONCLUSIONS

In summary, the concept of prophylactic mastectomy and reconstruction is appealing but it remains flawed both in terms of its cosmetic and psychological morbidity, and its ability to guarantee absolute freedom from breast cancer in every patient. There is no doubt that this form of surgery should be undertaken only by surgeons with the relevant expertise and training in this field, and expert counselling for patients is required at every stage.

The results of the ongoing tamoxifen and retinoid chemoprevention studies are awaited with great interest and these should prove of major relevance to the role of prophylactic mastectomy in the future. It may well be that our imminent ability to screen for breast cancer genetic markers will accurately identify a subgroup of women at suitably high risk to justify this procedure and will produce a consensus among surgeons, oncologists and epidemiologists on the indications for prophylactic surgery in breast cancer.

REFERENCES

1. Robbins, J., Merino, M.J., Boice, J.D. Jr. *et al.* Thyroid cancer: a lethal endocrine neoplasm. *Ann. Intern. Med.*, **115**, 133.
2. Herrea–Irbelas, L. (1987) Familial polyposis coli. *Semin Oncol.*, *3*, 66–139.
3. Wapnir, I.L., Rabinowitz, B. and Greco, R.S. (1990) A reappraisal of prophylactic mastectomy. *Surg. Gynecol. Obstet.*, **171**, 171–84.
4. McDivitt, R.W., Stevens, J.A., Lee, N.C., Wingo, P.A., Rubin, G.L. and Gersell, D. (1992) Histologic types of benign breast disease and the risk for breast cancer. *Cancer*, **69**; 1408–14.
5. Page, D.L. (1990) Benign neoplastic disease – pathological considerations for high risk, in *Benign Breast Disease*, (eds I. Taylor and J.A. Smallwood), Edward Arnold, London, pp. 109–20.
6. Page, D.L. and Dupont, W.D. (1990) Anatomic markers of human pre-malignancy and breast cancer. *Cancer*, **66**, 1326–35.
7. Evans, D.G., Fentiman, I.S., McPherson, K., Asbury, D., Ponder, B.A. and Howell, A. (1994) Familial breast cancer. *Br. Med. J.*, **308**, 183–7.
8. Fuer, J.E., Lap-Ming, W., Boring, C., Flanders, D., Timmel, M.J. and Tong, T. (1993), The lifetime risk of developing breast cancer., *J. Natl Cancer Inst.*, **85**, 892–7.
9. Miki, Y., Swenson, J., Shattuck-Eidens, D. *et*

al. (1994) A strong candidate for the breast and ovarian cancer susceptibility gene BRCA1. *Science*, **266**, 66–71.

10. Garber, J.E., Henderson, I.C., Love, S.M. and Gelman, R.S. (1991) Management of high-risk groups, in *Breast Diseases*, 2nd edn, (eds J.R. Harris, S. Hellman, I.C. Henderson and D.W. Kinne), Lippincott, Philadelphia, pp. 152–63.

11 Powles, T.J., Tilyer C.R., Jones, A. *et al.* (1990) Prevention of breast cancer with tamoxifen – an update of the Royal Marsden pilot programme. *Eur. J. Cancer, 26*; 680–4.

12. Veroniesi, U., De-Palo, G., Costa, A., Formelli, F., Marubini, E. and Del-Vecchio, M. (1992) Chemoprevention of breast cancer with retinoids. *Monogr. Natl Cancer Inst.*, **12**, 93–7.

13. Eng, C., Stratton, M., Ponder, B. *et al.* (1994) Familial cancer syndromes. *Lancet*, **343**, 709–13.

14. Wong, J.H., Jackson, C.F., Swanson, J.S. *et al.* (1986) Analysis of the risk reduction of prophylactic partial mastectomy in Sprague-Dawley rats with 7,12-dimethylbenzathracene-induced breast cancer. *Surgery*, **99**, 67–71.

15. Horton, C.E. and Dascombe, W.H. (1988) Total mastectomy: indications and techniques. *Clin. Plast. Surg.*, **15**, 677–87.

16. Woods, J.E. (1983) Subcutaneous mastectomy: current state of the art. *Ann. Plast. Surg.*, **11**, 541–50.

17. Hobby, J.A. (1990) Plastic surgery techniques for non-malignant breast disease, in *Benign Breast Disease*, (eds J.A. Smallwcod and I. Taylor), Edward Arnold. London, pp.155–79.

18. Slade, L.C. (1984) Subcutaneous mastectomy: acute complications and long term follow up. *Plast. Reconstr. Surg.*, **73**, 84–8.

19. Fisher, J., Maxwell, G.P. and Woods, J. (1988) Surgical alternatives in subcutaneous mastectomy reconstruction., *Clin. Plast. Surg.*, **15**, 667–76.

20. Goodnight, J.E.Jr, Quagliana, J.M. and Morton, D.L. (1984) Failure of subcutaneous mastectomy to prevent the development of breast cancer., *J.Surg.Oncol.*, **26**, 198–201.

21. Georgiade, G.S. and Georgiade, N.G. (1986) Breast reconstruction, in *Rob & Smith's Operative Surgery*, 4th edn, (eds H. Dudley, D. Carter and R.C.G. Russell), Butterworths, London, pp.669–86.

22. Goldman, L.D. and Goldwyn, R.M. (1973) Some anatomical considerations of subcutanous mastectomy. *Plast. Reconstr. Surg.*, **51**, 501–3.

23. Parry, R.G. and Cochran, T.C. (1977) When is there nipple involvement in carcinoma of the breast? *Plast. Reconstr. Surg.*, **59**, 535–7.

24. Pennisi, V.R. and Capozzi, A. (1989) Subcutaneous mastectomy data: a final statistical analysis of 1500 patterns. *Aesth. Plast. Surg.*, **13**, 15–21.

25. Reuven, K. and Snyderman, M.D. (1984) Prophylactic mastectomy: pros and cons. *Cancer*, **53**, 803–8.

26. Meyer, L. and Ringberg, A. (1986) A prospective study of psychiatric and psychosocial sequelae of bilateral subcutaneous mastectomy. *Scand. J. Plast. Reconstr. Surg.*, **20**, 101–7.

27. Hatcher, C., Brooks, L. and Love, C. (1993) Breast cancer and silicone implants: psychological consequences for women. *J.Natl Cancer Inst.*, **85**, 1361–5.

28. Calman, K.C. (1993) Silicone gel breast implants. Chief Medical Officer, Department of Health, PL/CMO(93) 2.

Chapter 18

Psychological distress associated with genetic breast cancer risk

KATHRYN M. KASH

18.1 INTRODUCTION

It is estimated that one in every eight American women will develop breast cancer during her lifetime [1]. The risk is not evenly distributed in the population and is two to three times higher in the woman who has a first-degree relative with breast cancer, when compared with one who has a negative family history [2, 3]. There is also some evidence that for women with a first-degree relative with bilateral premenopausal breast cancer [2, 4] or unilateral breast cancer under the age of 40 [5–7] the risk is even greater.

Women at genetic risk for breast cancer need modifications to their screening guidelines [8, 9]. One suggestion is that women with a first-degree relative with premenopausal breast cancer should have mammograms and clinical breast examinations at an earlier age (e.g. age 35) [10]. There are special surveillance programs in the US (e.g. The Strang Cancer Prevention Center and Memorial Sloan-Kettering Cancer Center in New York City, The Johns Hopkins Onco-

logy Center in Baltimore, Maryland, and the University of California Medical Center in Los Angeles, California) that advocate mammograms every year after the age of 40 and clinical breast examinations by a qualified health care practitioner every 4–6 months for women with family histories of breast cancer. While there is no proven primary prevention for breast cancer, secondary prevention in the form of early detection or other treatment options currently offer the best chance against premature morbidity and mortality.

With the increased media attention focused on the importance of the early detection of breast cancer, more women have begun to recognize the need for breast cancer screening and to look for places (programmes, clinics, doctors) where they can obtain quality breast care. As women learn about their family history of breast cancer, they begin to speculate about their own risk. Without adequate information, many women overestimate their risk and become quite fearful that they too could develop breast cancer. The psychological consequences for these women

Genetic Predisposition to Cancer. Edited by R.A. Eeles, B.A.J. Ponder, D.F. Easton and A. Horwich. Published in 1996 by Chapman & Hall, London.
0 412 56580 3

can be overwhelming and can lead to low-ered adherence to the recommended screening guidelines [11, 12]. Thus, adherence to breast cancer screening poses a major problem for women at genetic risk who need timely screening.

18.2 GENETIC RISK

In the absence of clinical testing for the breast cancer gene, there needs to be a method for identifying women who are most likely to be at increased risk due to genetic factors. Two recent risk assessment systems derived by Gail *et al.* [13] and Claus *et al.* [7, 14, 15], have received acceptance in establishing breast cancer risk. They differ from earlier systems in that they are models based on large data sets rather than empirical analyses.

The Gail model factors in epidemiological risks (age at menarche, parity, number of breast biopsies) and family history to arrive at relative and absolute risks based on age of the consultand. It tends to underestimate risk due to family history since it only counts up to two first-degree relatives and does not recognize affected second-degree relatives as contributing to risk; affected paternal line family members are also ignored.

The Claus model is based solely on family history and age(s) at diagnosis of affected relative(s) with cumulative risks calculated for up to two affected relatives, first- and/or second-degree. The model assumes the existence of a rare dominant allele responsible for breast cancer predisposition. Neither the Gail nor the Claus model provides a fit for every positive family history. The Gail model is useful when family history is not striking and other risk factors are present. Its most notable application is in determining eligibility for the National Surgical Adjuvant Breast and Bowel Project (NSABP) Breast Cancer Prevention Trial, in which 16 000 North American women are randomized to either 20 mg of tamoxifen, or placebo, twice a day for 5 years.

Table 18.1 Psychological issues in women at genetic risk of breast cancer

Anxiety about developing breast cancer
Sense of vulnerability
Fear of disfigurement or death
Guilt
Misconceptions and myths
Powerless or lack of control
Denial or passive behaviour
Isolated and alone

18.3 PSYCHOLOGICAL ISSUES

Women who are at high risk of developing breast cancer because of their strong family histories are also at higher risk for psychological distress [11, 12, 16]. Women who have the above-described family histories of breast cancer suffer the negative psychological sequelae of their genetic risk status (Table 18.1). There are many issues for high-risk women who live with fear, anxiety and uncertainty every day of their lives. The first and most overwhelming issue for women is their **anxiety** about developing breast cancer. Anxiety peaks at certain points in their lives, for example, when a woman reaches the age her mother or sister developed breast cancer. At that age a woman becomes concerned that she too will develop breast cancer and die of the disease. Another peak in anxiety occurs when a woman has the same number of children as her mother did when she developed breast cancer. Some women magically believe if they have fewer children, they will be protected against breast cancer.

A woman's **sense of vulnerability** leads to an overestimation of risk which in turn heightens their subjective certainty of developing breast cancer. Data from other studies indicate that a substantial number of women with a family history of breast cancer have a heightened perception of risk [17, 18]. In particular, the study done in the UK, where the risk is 1 in 12 women, found that over 45% overestimated their risk for breast cancer and only 11% correctly identified their risk. Over 80% of 503 women in our study overestimated their risk of developing breast cancer; some by as much as four times greater than their actual risk. Some 15% of women in our study provided an accurate perception of their risk and 5% underestimated their risk. Underestimation most frequently occurred when a woman had a very high risk (35–50%) and had not received risk counselling. Frequently women report that they are '100% sure' that they will get breast cancer, as well as describing themselves as 'walking time bombs.' In other words, women at genetic risk do not wonder **if** they will get breast cancer but **when** it will appear.

The fear of **disfigurement** or **death** is a common theme and is sometimes worse for women who were young when their grandmothers, mothers and sisters developed the disease and died. Fears, such as having 'mutilating' surgery for breast cancer, are prevalent in their thinking. Many women remember the radical Halsted mastectomies of 20 years ago and believe this type of surgery will be performed on them if they develop breast cancer.

Variations in **guilt** are pervasive in women at high risk. Some women feel guilty because they were not there for their relatives, either physically or emotionally. Other women suffer guilt because they may have passed a gene to their daughters. Many women feel guilty because they are so worried and concerned about breast cancer and yet they are healthy. Women who do not develop breast cancer while other relatives have the disease experience 'survivor guilt.'

The **misconceptions** and **myths** about breast cancer are overwhelming for many women. Some of these have been passed from one generation to the next. One myth is, 'if you get hit in the breast, you will develop breast cancer.' A misconception about breast cancer is if 'you have fibrocystic breasts, this leads to breast cancer.' Yet another misconception is that 'if you have surgery for breast cancer, it spreads.'

Frequently, women who have strong family histories of breast cancer feel **powerless** about the disease. Women think they have a gene, they cannot control it, and breast cancer is their destiny. In addition, they felt helpless when their mothers and sisters had breast cancer and feel hopeless about avoiding the disease themselves. In other words, a woman's sense of self-efficacy regarding the prevention of breast cancer is lacking.

Another psychological issue for women at high risk is their **passivity** and their use of **denial** regarding breast cancer, and in particular, adherence to screening. Women frequently make statements, such as, 'If I don't think about breast cancer, I can't get it' or 'I just don't want to know if I have breast cancer.' Sometimes women join a surveillance programme and, after having two negative mammograms and clinical breast examinations, feel protected and postpone future screening dates.

Finally, one of the major issues surrounding all the above concerns is that women feel **isolated and alone**. Women stated that their surviving relatives are reluctant to discuss breast cancer with them. Generally, women feel no one else knows how they are feeling. Their friends are not interested in discussing their 'obsession' with breast cancer.

Studies have found that levels of psychological distress, such as greater cancer anxiety [11], more intrusive thoughts [19], and higher perceived susceptibility [16], led to a decrease in mammograms, clinical breast examination (CBE), and breast self-examination (BSE).

18.4 HIGH-RISK CLINIC – EXPERIENCE FROM THE STRANG CANCER PREVENTION CENTER

To qualify for the Strang Breast Surveillance Program, women must fall into one of four categories for increased risk for breast cancer: (i) two or more first-degree relatives (mother, sister, daughter) with breast cancer diagnosed before age 60; (ii) a first-degree relative with bilateral premenopausal breast cancer; (iii) a mother and maternal grandmother with breast cancer before age 60; or (iv) a first-degree relative with unilateral breast cancer diagnosed under the age of 40. These criteria were selected to include women whose lifetime risk for developing breast cancer based on their family histories is between 17 and 50% [15]. Family history and a detailed personal health history are collected, a pedigree is drawn, and the genetics counsellor, in conjunction with the geneticist, makes the final determination regarding programme entry.

Standard care in the Strang Breast Surveillance Program is provided as follows. The screening guidelines for the women are: (i) a baseline mammogram when aged 10 years younger than the age at which the relative developed breast cancer, but not before age 30, one mammogram between the ages of 30 and 34, a mammogram every 18–24 months from ages 35–39 (based on family history), and a yearly mammogram from age 40; (ii) to have a clinical breast examination every 6 months by the nurse practitioner or a physician; and (iii) to be taught breast self-examination (BSE) and given monthly reminder stickers to put on their calendars. Patients receive risk counselling, instructions in BSE, a clinical breast examination every 6 months and mammography according to risk and age. Women are sent cards 2 months in advance to remind them that it is time for an appointment (either clinical breast examination or mammogram, or both). It should be noted that most clinics in the UK practise annual mammography from age 35 or 5 years younger than the youngest case, usually not offering mammogram before age 30. In the Strang Program, 503 women, were enrolled and completed a questionnaire regarding health beliefs and behaviours, social support, and psychological distress. The assessment measures used were as follows.

1. Brief symptom inventory (BSI). The BSI [20] is a brief form of a symptom check-list that is used to reflect psychological symptom patterns of psychiatric and medical patients. Each item was rated on a 5-point scale of distress (0–4), ranging from 'not at all' to 'extremely'. Like the check-list, the BSI was scored on nine symptom dimensions and three global indices of distress. The reliability of the BSI has been demonstrated by internal consistency ($r=0.77$ to 0.90) and the test–retest reliability ($r=0.80$ to 0.90) for all scales. Internal consistency was 0.92 for the total BSI.

2. Taylor manifest anxiety scale (TMAS). The TMAS [21] consists of 28 items scored true or false, and was used to measure the manifest or trait anxiety of normal and psychiatric populations. The internal consistency was 0.85.

3. Social support. The perceived quality of social support was assessed by the Interpersonal Support Evaluation List (ISEL) [22]. The ISEL is a 40-item self-report scale that measures four major **functional** components of **perceived** social support: tangible (or instrumental); appraisal (or confidant); self-esteem; and belonging (or companionship). Each item was scored as true or false. The reliability of the ISEL by internal consistency was 0.87.

4. Cancer-related anxiety and helplessness scale (CAHS): This is a 12-item self-report inventory that assessed the women's general cancer anxiety and sense of helplessness. Items for this scale used a 4-point forced-choice format ranging from 'strongly agree' to 'strongly disagree'. This scale has been used in two other studies: 440 non-cancer patients from four community hospitals [23], and participants in a high-risk breast screening programme

Table 18.2 Factors predicting mammography

	Discriminant function[1]	
	Coefficient	P
Psychological distress	−0.78	0.006

Percent of cases correctly classified = 84%.
[1] This examines two dichotomous variables, i.e. adherence to or non-adherence to mammography. The maximum value is −1.0 (or +1.0 if it were a positive relationship).

Table 18.3 Factors predicting clinical examination adherence

	Discriminant function	
	Coefficient	P
Cancer anxiety	−0.65	0.005
Psychological distress	−0.47	0.05

Percent of cases correctly classified = 71%.

[11]. Internal consistency reliability was 0.78.

5. Health Belief Model questionnaire (HBMQ): The HBMQ is a series of face-valid questions, covering the major motivational determinants of preventive health behaviour postulated by the Health Belief Model [24, 25]. They assess perceived susceptibility to disease; severity of disease; benefits of intervention; risks of intervention; and practical obstacles to intervention. Questions were anchored for the women with respect to breast cancer and the breast cancer screening programme. The questionnaire has been found to have good reliability and validity [11].

The following is a summary of our findings. While 52% came in for regular clinical breast examinations, only 27% performed breast self-examination monthly. In women over age 40, less than half (46%) came in for yearly mammograms. For all three methods of early detection, greater cancer anxiety and psychological distress were significant predictors of poor adherence.

A discriminant function analysis found a negative relationship between psychological distress and adherence to regularly scheduled mammograms (Table 18.2). In other words, a high level of psychological distress is associated with a lower adherence to

Table 18.4 Factors predicting breast self-examination (BSE)

	Regression coefficient (r)[1]	P
Previous BSE performance	0.47	0.0001
Education	−0.19	0.0022
Cancer anxiety	−0.18	0.0030
Age	0.13	0.0190
Barriers and social support (more social support and fewer barriers)	−0.13	0.0115

[1] Change in distress score per unit change in explanatory variable.

mammography. We also examined adherence to the 6-month clinical examination by a nurse practitioner or physician. Some 52% adhered to this schedule, while 48% delayed coming for their follow-up examination between 6 months to 2 years. A discriminant function analysis found a negative relationship between cancer anxiety and psychological distress and regular clinical breast examination (Table 18.3). The most powerful predictor of adherence to regular clinical breast examination was cancer anxiety (discriminant function coefficient −0.65). For breast self-examination, a multiple regression analysis revealed the best predictors for adherence to monthly breast self-examination (Table 18.4). High performance of breast self-examination before coming to

Table 18.5 Factors predicting psychological distress

	Regression coefficient $(r)^1$	P
Perceived barriers	0.83	0.0001
Barriers and social support (little social support and many barriers)	−0.72	0.0001
Social desirability	−0.31	0.0019
Perceived risk	0.12	0.0288

[1] Change in distress score per unit change in explanatory variable.

the breast cancer screening programme was the best predictor ($P < 0.0001$) and high anxiety predicted poorer adherence with monthly breast self-examination ($P < 0.003$). We also found that younger ($P<0.01$), well-educated women ($P<0.002$) were less likely to perform monthly BSEs.

A multiple regression analysis revealed that women with the highest psychological distress levels had more barriers ($P<0.0001$) to screening, as well as an interaction effect of low social support and more barriers ($P<0.0001$) and a higher perception of risk ($P<0.03$) (Table 18.5). Over 28% of high-risk women were defined as having a level of psychological distress consistent with the need for counselling.

This study was the first to examine psychological distress and anxiety as predictors of adherence to all three screening behaviours in high-risk women. Based on this study and other studies in the literature, we found that there were several key variables related to screening adherence and quality of life. Barriers to screening were a major reason why women did not engage in any breast cancer prevention behaviours. Some of these barriers are the fear that 'something' would be found on examination and coming to the centre for an examination reminded them of their relative's (mother and/or sister) struggle

with breast cancer. Cognitive deficits, in terms of lack of knowledge, and breast cancer misbeliefs, contributed to poor adherence to screening. Most importantly, anxiety or emotional distress not only interfered with adherence to screening, but affected quality of life negatively, in that many women needed psychological counselling.

From the data above it appeared that overestimation of risk and subsequent emotional distress in women at genetic risk for breast cancer led to a decrease in adherence to screening. The emotional distress may also diminish a woman's quality of life, if the fear of developing breast cancer interferes with goal-directed behaviours and problem-solving activities. This information compelled us to intercede with women at genetic risk for breast cancer and develop an intervention that can help to improve quality of life and increase adherence to breast cancer screening.

18.5 CONCLUSIONS

In summary, we have conducted a study investigating the psychological and health behaviours of women at genetic risk of breast cancer and found that anxiety interfered with all three breast cancer screening behaviours. High breast self-examination performance before coming to the programme was the best predictor of current breast self-examination, and high anxiety predicted poor adherence to monthly breast self-examination. Women reporting more barriers to screening, fewer social supports, and low social desirability had more psychological distress. Higher anxiety was directly related to poor mammogram, clinical breast examination and breast self-examination adherence. Levels of psychological distress in high-risk women were 0.5–1 standard deviation above the mean for normal women in the population. One of our most striking findings was that high-risk women's scores were similar to those of women who were Hodgkin's disease and leukaemia survivors. These high levels of distress greatly interfered with their quality of life. This research led us to focus on strategies, particularly group interventions, that may help women cope with being at genetic risk for breast cancer. From the pilot groups we were able to help women estimate their risk accurately, increase their knowledge of breast cancer, and improve their adherence to screening behaviours. We are presently conducting a large randomized trial investigating this treatment modality.

REFERENCES

1. American Cancer Society (1995) *Cancer Facts and Figures*, American Cancer Society, Atlanta, GA.
2. Sattin, R.W., Rubin, G.L., Webster, L.A *et al.* (1985) Family history and the risk of breast cancer. *JAMA*, **253**, 1908–13.
3. Williams, W.R. and Osborne, M.P. (1987) Familial aspects of breast cancer: an overview, in *Breast Diseases*, (eds J.R. Harris, S. Hellman, I.C. Henderson and D.W. Kinne), J.B. Lippincott, Philadelphia, pp. 109–20.
4. Anderson, D.E. (1972) A genetic study of human breast cancer. *J.Natl Cancer Inst.*, **48**, 1029–34.
5. Bain, C., Speizer, F.E., Rosner, B. *et al.* (1980) Family history of breast cancer as a risk indicator for the disease. *Am. J. Epidemiol*, **111**, 301–8.
6. Mettlin, C., Croghan, I., Natarajan, N. *et al.* (1990) The association of age and familial risk in a case-control study of breast cancer. *Am. J. Epidemiol*, **131**, 973–83.
7. Claus, E.B., Risch, N. and Thompson, W.D. (1990) Age of onset as an indicator of familial risk of breast cancer. *Am. J. Epidemiol.*, **131**, 961–72.
8. Mettlin, C. (1992) Breast cancer risk factors. *Cancer*, **69**, 1904–10.
9. Woolf, S.H. (1992) United States Preventive Services Task Force recommendations on breast cancer screening. *Cancer*, **69**, 1913–18.
10. King, M.C., Rowell, S. and Love, S.M. (1993) Inherited breast and ovarian cancer: what are the risks? What are the choices? *JAMA*, **269**, 1975–80.
11. Kash, K.M, Holland, J.C, Miller, D.G and Halper, M.S (1992) Psychological distress and surveillance behaviors of women with a family history of breast cancer. *J. Natl Cancer Inst.*, **84**, 24–30.
12. Lerman, C., Rimer, B., Trock, B. *et al.* (1990) Factors associated with repeated adherence to breast cancer screening. *Prev. Med.*, **19**, 279–90.
13. Gail, M.H., Brinton, L.A., Byar, D.P. *et al.* (1989) Projecting individualized probabilities of developing breast cancer for white females who are being examined annually. *J. Natl Cancer Inst.*, **81**, 1879–86.
14. Claus, E.B., Risch, N. and Thompson, W.D. (1991) Genetics analysis of breast cancer in the cancer and steroid hormone (CASH) study. *Am. J. Hum. Genet.*, 48, 232–42.
15. Claus, E.B., Risch, N. and Thompson, W.D. (1994) Autosomal dominant inheritance of early-onset breast cancer. *Cancer*, **73**, 643–51.
16. Alagna, S.W., Morokoff, P.J., Bevett, J.M. and Reddy, D.M. (1987) Performance of breast self-examination by women at high risk for breast cancer. *Women & Health*, **12**, 29–46.
17. Stefanek, M. (1990) Counseling women at high risk for breast cancer. *Oncology*, **4**, 27–33.
18. Evans, D.G.R., Burnell, L.D., Hopwood P. *et al.* (1993) Perception of risk in women with a family history of breast cancer. *Br. J. Cancer*, **67**, 612–14.
19. Lerman, C., Daly, M., Sands, C. *et al.* (1993) Mammography adherence and psychological distress among women at risk for breast cancer. *J. Natl Cancer Inst.*, **85**, 1074–80.
20. Derogatis, L.R. and Spencer, P. (1982) The Brief Symptom Inventory (BSI). (Available directly from Dept of Medical Psychology, Johns Hopkins University School of Medicine, Baltimore, MD, USA.) Administration Scoring and Procedures manual–I., Baltimore: copyrighted manuscript.
21. Taylor, J.A. (1953) A personality scale of manifest anxiety. *J. Abnorm. Social Psychol.*, **48**, 285–90.
22. Cohen, S., Mermelstein, R.J., Kamarck, T. *et al.* (1985) Measuring the fundamental components of social support. In *Social Support: Theory, Research, and Application* (eds I.G. Sarason and

B. Sarason), Martinus Niijhoff, The Hague, Holland, pp. 73–94.

23. Schottenfeld, D. and Kerner, J. (1984) *Final Report: Cancer Control Development Grant*, (National Cancer Institute Grant CA 16402), Bethesda, MD: NCI.

24. Rosenstock, I.M. (1966) Why people use health services. *Millbank Memorial Fund Quarterly*, **44**, 94–127.

25. Becker, M.H. (ed) (1974) *The Health Belief Model and Personal Health Behavior*, Charles B. Slack, Inc. Thorofare, NJ.

Chapter 19

Familial ovarian cancer

BRUCE A.J. PONDER

19.1 GENETIC EPIDEMIOLOGY

The lifetime risk of epithelial ovarian cancer for a woman in the UK is about 1 in 80. Some families in which there are two ovarian cancers, or an ovarian cancer and another common cancer at a young age in close relatives will be expected to occur by chance. However, population-based epidemiological studies show that there is a significant excess risk of cancer at several sites in the relatives of ovarian cancer patients (Table 19.1). This familial clustering must arise from some combination of inherited and environmental effects.

Table 19.1 Cancer mortality in first-degree relatives of ovarian cancer. (From [1].)

	Observed	Expected	Relative risk	P
Ovary	35	15.72	2.22	<0.0001
Breast	60	47.04	1.28	=0.08
Colorectal	80	59.43	1.35	<0.01
Stomach	69	47.22	1.46	<0.01

The origin of the familial clustering can be studied by 'segregation analysis'. In ovarian cancer, as in other common cancers, this analysis suggests that the observed familial clustering is best explained by the effects of an uncommon, highly penetrant dominant gene. Segregation analysis looks at the pattern of cancers in an unselected series of families, and asks whether the pattern is best accounted for by genetic effects, environment, chance, or some mixture of these; and if genetic effects, whether dominant or recessive. The process can be understood in non-mathematical terms by the following illustration. Consider the risks of ovarian cancer to a woman who is a close relative (mother, sister) of an isolated ovarian cancer case, and to another woman who is a close relative of a case in a family where two relatives are already affected. If the familial effect were due to a weak predisposition spread fairly uniformly over the population of cases of ovarian cancer, then the risk to the woman who has two affected relatives will not be very much higher than the risk to the woman with only one affected relative – some families will have two affected cases by chance, but the same level of risk will be operating overall. However, if the observed familial clustering is due to a strong predisposition which is present in only a minority of cases, this minority will be heavily represented among the families where there are

Genetic Predisposition to Cancer. Edited by R.A. Eeles, B.A.J. Ponder, D.F. Easton and A. Horwich. Published in 1996 by Chapman & Hall, London.
0 412 56580 3

two or more affected women. The risk to a further woman in such a family will be much higher than that in a family with only one case, where quite probably no predisposition is operating at all.

Analysis of a population-based series of ovarian cancers has shown that the risk of ovarian cancer by age 70 in a woman with one affected relative is about 1 in 30, or three times the general population risk; whereas the risk to a woman with two affected close relatives is of the order of 1 in 4 [2, 3]. Risks of this magnitude are very seldom due to environmental exposures, and the most probable conclusion is that much of the family clustering is due to strong genetic predisposition operating in a few families.

Consistent with this, roughly one or two in each 100 unselected patients with ovarian cancer are found to give an extensive family history of the disease; and the pedigrees which are obtained are those that would be expected to result from predisposition by a single, strong, dominantly inherited gene (Figure 19.1).

At least three distinct clinical patterns of familial ovarian cancer can be recognized. The most common is ovarian cancer in association with breast cancer (Figure 19.1(a); see also Chapter 15); but there are also families in which ovarian cancer is associated with cancers of the colon and rectum, endometrium and stomach, and possibly other sites such as urothelium and pancreas as part of the 'family cancer' or 'Lynch II' syndrome (Figure 19.1(b)) [4], and others in which the predisposition appears to be specific to ovarian cancer (Figure 19.1(c)). How closely these clinical patterns will conform to genetic differences, remains to be seen: 'site-specific' ovarian cancer in particular may prove not to be distinct, but to be one end of a spectrum of involvement of ovarian cancer in other clinical syndromes.

It is important to realize that strong predisposing genes of the sort that result in striking familial aggregations of cancer probably account for well under 5% of the total ovarian cancer incidence. The possibility that there are also more common predisposing genes of weaker effect, rarely giving rise to multiple case families but of much greater potential importance in terms of total numbers, will be discussed below.

19.2 MOLECULAR GENETICS

The proof that genetic predisposition is responsible for familial clustering comes from genetic linkage studies, which demonstrate co-inheritance of the disease with a specific genetic marker in a set of families. To date, three genetic loci have been associated with inherited predisposition to ovarian cancer: (i) the *BRCA*1 locus on chromosome 17q12 (see Chapter 15); (ii) the *BRCA*2 locus on chromosome 13q12-13 (see Chapter 14) and (iii) the *h-MSH*2 locus on chromosome 2p [5].

19.2.1 THE *BRCA*1 LOCUS

Predisposition at this locus probably accounts for just under half of families with multiple cases of breast cancer, but a majority of families in which breast cancer is associated with epithelial ovarian cancer. The predisposing gene has been cloned, and appears to act as a tumour suppressor [6]. A combined analysis of over 200 breast and breast–ovarian families by the International Breast Cancer Consortium has provided useful information about the age-specific risks of breast and ovarian cancer in *BRCA*1 gene carriers, which can be applied to the management of families. These are described in detail in Chapter 15.

Inspection of the pedigrees of families linked to the *BRCA*1 locus suggests that there is variation between families in the risks of breast and ovarian cancer, either one or the other cancer being predominant. Analysis of the linkage consortium families confirms this (Chapter 15). A more recent analysis of nine

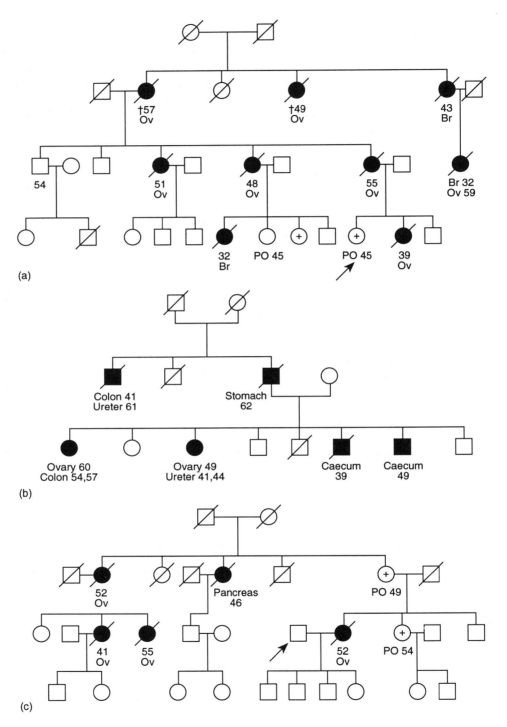

(a)

(b)

(c)

families with three or more cases of epithelial ovarian cancer, but no breast cancer before the age of 50, indicates that the majority of these families are also due to predisposition at the BRCA1 locus [7]. Thus, apparently 'site-specific' ovarian cancer families may be part of the same BRCA1 spectrum, and women in these families may be at increased risk of breast as well as of ovarian cancer. To date, however, there is no evidence of a connection between the position or type of mutations in the BRCA1 gene, and the proportion of breast or ovarian cancers in the family [8].

19.2.2 THE *h-MSH*2 LOCUS

This locus on chromosome 2p16 was identified by genetic linkage in families with non-polyposis colon cancer occurring as part of the 'family cancer' or Lynch II syndrome [5, 9]. It was noted that tumour DNA samples from some of these families showed a striking instability in the (CA)n repeat sequence which were used as polymorphic markers for genetic analysis. This suggested the possibility that a mutation in a DNA repair gene might be responsible for the predisposition; which led to the identification of the *h-MSH*2 gene, which is the human counterpart of a repair gene already well characterized in yeast [5, 10] see also Chapter 21. To the extent that ovarian cancer is part of the 'cancer family' syndrome, mutations in this gene will predispose to ovarian cancer: how-

ever, the proportion of ovarian cancer families or of apparently isolated ovarian cancers which can be attributed to the gene is yet to be determined. The *h-MSH*2 gene is part of a family of genes with related functions, which suggests that other members of the family may also be involved in predisposition in some cases: there is evidence for this, for colorectal cancer at least, at a locus on chromosome 3p [11, 12].

19.3 CLINICAL IMPLICATIONS: THE MANAGEMENT OF OVARIAN CANCER FAMILIES

19.3.1 EVALUATION OF THE FAMILY HISTORY

Until it is possible to search directly for mutations in predisposing genes, recognition of inherited risk of ovarian cancer will necessarily be based entirely on the family history. An accurate and complete history, with confirmation of all relevant diagnoses (by pathology review where possible since many cases are recalled by relatives simply as abdominal cancer) is essential. This takes time and practice, and experience suggests that it is rarely achieved in a busy routine surgical clinic.

For purposes of clinical management, several different types of family history can be distinguished:

1. One close relative (mother, sister) with epithelial ovarian cancer; no other cancers in close relatives. Epidemiological data (see above) suggest that such a history confers a roughly three-fold increased risk, corresponding to a 1 in 30 chance of ovarian cancer by age 70. In contrast to breast cancer, the age at which the affected relative was diagnosed seems *not* to have much effect on risk.
2. Two close relatives with ovarian cancer; no other cancers in close relatives. The

Fig. 19.1 Familial ovarian cancer (a) Family with ovarian and breast cancer. Ov 55, Br 43, ages at diagnosis of ovarian or breast cancer; 57, age at death; + PO, prophylactic oophorectomy; ↑, case seeking genetic advice. (b) Cancer family syndrome. Including two cases of ovarian cancer. (c) Family with 'site-specific' ovarian cancer. The significance of the pancreatic cancer is unknown at present.

question here is how likely this is to be a coincidence. Current epidemiological data suggest that about half such families (perhaps more if the cases are young, less if they are old) will be the result of a strong inherited predisposition. The unaffected relative at risk therefore has a $1/2 \times 1/2 = 1/4$ chance of having inherited the putative predisposing gene. This translates to a roughly 10–15% lifetime risk of ovarian cancer, depending on the penetrance of the gene.

3. Ovarian cancer associated with other cancers in close relatives. Epidemiological data indicate a familial association between ovarian cancer and breast, colo-rectal, endometrial, urothelial, gastric and possibly other (e.g. prostate) cancers; but other cancers (e.g. cervix, bronchus) seem not to be associated. As expected, one of the 'associated' cancers in a close relative, especially if diagnosed at a young age (e.g. below 50 years), increases the risk to other family members; whereas the presence of cancers which have no familial association (e.g. cervix) presumably does not. Precise identification of the cancers other than ovarian cancer in the family is therefore crucial in determining both the presence of increased familial risk and the spectrum of cancers likely to be involved.

4. Multiple-case families. Three or more epithelial ovarian cancers, or two ovarian cancers plus young-onset 'associated' cancers (breast, colorectal, endometrial, gastric, urothelial) in close relatives. In these families, predisposition by a strong dominantly inherited gene is likely. The risks of different cancers in relatives may to some extent be inferred from the existing pattern in the family: for example, whether this suggests 'cancer family syndrome' or 'breast–ovarian' cancer. However, except possibly in extensive breast–ovarian cancer families, the genetic and epidemiological data to make accurate estimates of the risks of different cancers still do not exist.

19.3.2 SCREENING AND PREVENTION

(a) Screening

No screening method for ovarian cancer has yet been shown to be effective [13]. Ideally, therefore, screening should only be carried out as part of a research programme which will allow evaluation of the results. In practice, this may not always be possible. The current recommendation of the UK Cancer Family Study Group is that screening is normally only justifiable on clinical grounds for women at higher risk – that is, those with either two first-degree relatives or one first-degree and one second-degree, both with epithelial ovarian cancer, or one with ovarian cancer and one with young-onset breast or colorectal cancer. Until evidence of efficacy is available, women with only one affected relative should only be offered screening as part of a formal research study.

Screening should consist of ultrasound scanning, preferably using a vaginal probe, and accompanied by a clinical examination to include the other sites at risk in ovarian cancer families. A yearly interval is currently used, but there are few data to support this. Abnormalities on the scan may be evaluated further by repeat ultrasound scanning, serum markers (e.g. CA 125) or colour Doppler blood-flow scanning as appropriate, before exploratory surgery. There are no formal data relating to the sensitivity or specificity of ultrasound screening in women with a strong family history of ovarian cancer; however, a small number of interval ovarian cancers have occurred within 6 months of ultrasound screening in the series currently being compiled by the UK Familial Ovarian Cancer Study. Measurement of serological markers (currently CA 125, but others may soon be available) may be used in conjunction with ultrasound screening. The relatively low sensitivity of serological markers suggests, however, that in a small population of women at high risk the more sensitive ultrasound techniques used alone are the most appropriate choice. Combination with CA 125 as a first-line screen will probably not provide much improvement in sensitivity, but will lead to reduced specificity and positive predictive value.

The age at which screening should start is also controversial. Data from the breast–ovarian families in the Consortium studies (see Chapter 15) suggest that the risk of ovarian cancer is low before the age of 30; of the 389 proven epithelial ovarian cancers in families with at least two affected close relatives in the UK Familial Ovarian Cancer Study (unpublished), fewer than 2% were diagnosed below the age of 30, and only 7% before the age of 40. Currently, most clinics recommend screening from about the age of 25, but this could possibly be raised to about 30; since the risk persists until at least age 70 (see Chapter 15; Figure 15.4), screening may be continued until that age.

(b) Prevention

Currently there is no medical preventive treatment available or under trial for ovarian cancer. Data from the general population indicate that oral contraceptive use may protect, and so the use of oral contraceptives has been suggested for young women at risk because of their family history; but this may increase the risk of breast cancer, which is already high in some families.

Prophylactic oophorectomy should be considered as an alternative to screening once a woman has completed her family. Most clinicians feel that it is probably appropriate only for women whose family history suggests a substantial risk – which would not include most women with only one affected relative. In premenopausal women, hormone

replacement therapy is recommended following oophorectomy, to reduce mortality and morbidity from cardiovascular disease and osteoporosis. Extrapolation from studies in the population as a whole suggests that combined therapy with oestrogen and progesterone carries a higher breast cancer risk than does unopposed oestrogen, but unopposed oestrogen causes a substantial risk of endometrial cancer. For this reason, salpingo-oophorectomy combined with total hysterectomy and replacement with low-dose oestrogen alone is usually recommended in the UK (although practice seems to vary between countries). The formal laparotomy also provides the opportunity to carry out a thorough inspection of the pelvic and abdominal cavities, including peritoneal washings and biopsies, for occult disease. In older women, hormone replacement therapy may not be needed, and laparoscopic removal of the ovaries without hysterectomy is recommended by some gynaecologists. Although there are no data about the morbidity associated with oophorectomy at a young age in this situation, at a recent meeting of the UK Familial Ovarian Cancer Study Group, most gynaecologists said that they would be reluctant to consider prophylactic oophorectomy below the age of 35 years.

The efficacy of prophylactic oophorectomy remains unproven. Several cases have been reported of cancers resembling ovarian cancer which are presumed to have arisen from the peritoneal mesothelium following oophorectomy [14]. A prospective multicentre study is currently in progress, to determine the incidence of both ovarian and breast cancer in women in high-risk families and to compare women who have had oophorectomy with those who have not. It is very difficult to estimate the risk of post-oophorectomy 'ovarian' cancer from current data, but it may be a few percent. The consensus is that, despite this presently unknown risk, prophylactic oophorectomy is probably the most effective means available now to reduce the chance of death from ovarian cancer in women at high risk.

(c)   Genetic testing

A family history of ovarian cancer can probably result from inheritance of one of several genes. It is clearly necessary to know which gene is present in a given family, before one can predict the inheritance in unaffected family members. In the case of *BRCA*1 mutations, which are probably the most numerous, the gene has recently been identified [15]. Direct testing for mutation is theoretically possible and, in principle, individuals can be tested regardless of the availability of affected family members. Testing must, however, be approached cautiously. The variation in risks of breast and ovarian cancer between different *BRCA*1 linked families (see Chapter 15) already suggests that there may be different risks associated with different mutant alleles although these are not evident from the first *BRCA*1 mutation data and this variation might affect not only the risks of cancers at different sites, but the risks of cancer by a given age. Until many families with different degrees of family history have been studied, it will not be safe to assume that the implications of a *BRCA*1 mutation in a woman with, say, only one affected relative is the same as in a large family. A similar caveat must apply to testing for mutations in other genes, such as *h-MSH*2.

REFERENCES

1. Easton, D.F., Matthews, F.E., Ford, D., Swerdlow, A.J. and Peto, J. (1995) Cancer risks to relatives of ovarian cancer patients. *Int. J. Cancer*, (in press).
2. Ponder, B.A.J., Easton, D. and Peto, J. (1990) Risk of ovarian cancer associated with a family history, in *Ovarian Cancer* (eds, F. Sharp, W.D. Mason and R.E. Leake), Chapman & Hall, London, pp. 3–6.
3. Schildkraut, J.M. and Thompson, W.D. (1988) Familial ovarian cancer: a population-based control study. *Am. J. Epidemiol.*, **128**, 456–66.
4. Lynch, H.T., Kimberley, W., Albano, W.A. *et al.* (1988) Hereditary non polyposis colonic cancer (Lynch syndrome I and II). 1. Clinical description of resource. *Cancer*, **56**, 939–51.
5. Fishel, R., Lescoe, M.K., Rao, M.R.S. *et al.* (1993) The human mutation gene homologue MSH2 and its association with hereditary nonpolyposis colon cancer. *Cell*, **75**, 1027–36.
6. Smith, S.A., Easton, D.F., Evans, D.G.R. and Ponder B.A.J. (1992) Allele losses in the region 17q12–21 in familial breast and ovarian cancer involve the wild-type chromosome. *Nature Genet.*, **2**, 128–31.
7. Steichen-Gersdorf, E., Gallion, H.H., Ford, D. *et al.* (1994) Familial site-specific ovarian cancer is linked to BRCA1 on 17q12–21. *Am. J. Hum. Genet.*, **55**, 870–5.
8. Shattinck., Evans, D. (1995) A collaborative survey of 80 mutations in the BRCA1 breast and ovarian cancer susceptibility gene. *JAMA*, **273**, 535–41.
9. Peltomaki, P., Aaltonen L.A., Sistonen, P. *et al.* (1993) Genetic mapping of a locus predisposing to human colorectal cancer. *Science*, **260**, 810–12.
10. Leach, F.S., Nicolaides, N.C., Papadopoulos, N. *et al.* (1993) Mutations of a *mutS* homolog in hereditary colon cancer. *Cell*, **75**, 1215–25.
11. Papadopoulos, N., Nicolaides, N.C., Wei, Y.-F. *et al.* (1994) Mutation of a *mutL* homolog in hereditary colon cancer. *Science*, **263**, 1625–9.
12. Bronner, C.E., Baker, S.M., Morrison, P.T. *et al.* (1994) Mutation in the DNA mismatch repair gene homologue *hMLH1* is associated with hereditary non-polyposis colon cancer. *Nature*, **368**, 258–61.
13. Austoker, J. (1994) Screening for ovarian prostate and testicular tumours. *Br. Med. J.*, **309**, 315–20.
14. Tobacman, J.K., Greene, M.H., Tucker, M.A. *et al.* (1982) Intra-abdominal carcinomatosis after prophylactic oophorectomy in ovarian-cancer-prone families. *Lancet*, **ii**, 795–7.
15. Miki, Y., Swensen, J., Shattuck-Eidens, D. *et al.* (1994) Isolation of BRCA1, the 17q linked breast and ovarian cancer susceptibility gene. *Science*, **266**, 56–70.

Chapter 20

Familial colon cancer syndromes and their clinical management

VICTORIA A. MURDAY, D. TIMOTHY BISHOP and
NIGEL R. HALL

20.1 INTRODUCTION

A family history of colorectal cancer increases the risk to an individual of developing the disease. This is presumably due to shared environmental factors within families as well as genetic factors. In general, the risk depends upon the extent of the family history with a stronger family history implying a greater risk.

In a few families, the risk is obviously transmitted as an autosomal dominant trait (see Chapter 1) with many family members in each generation developing colorectal cancer or other cancers and the risk being passed on average to one-half of their offspring. Such families are clearly due to a single gene (that is, within a family, one aberrant gene is sufficient to explain the increased risk) although different families may be due to separate genes. These families are a major concern in a clinical setting because of the high risk of cancer, especially as the cancers often occur at a young age or at one or more of a variety of anatomical sites, some outside

the colon. To a large extent the genes responsible for these families have been identified (see Chapter 21). With knowledge of the genes involved, it is possible to determine precisely which relatives have inherited the predisposition, and those which can be removed from the burden of screening because they are not predisposed. The recognition of these families may be straightforward, although the confounding problems of limited family size may obscure the genetic susceptibility.

In some of the dominantly inherited bowel cancer syndromes, such as familial adenomatous polyposis (see below), the individuals at risk of developing colorectal cancer are revealed by clinical examination, looking for non-neoplastic colonic and extracolonic manifestations of the syndrome. For instance, in the polyposis patient, benign colonic adenomas develop around puberty, well ahead of the risk of colorectal cancer.

In other syndromes, such as hereditary non-polyposis colorectal cancer (HNPCC, see

Genetic Predisposition to Cancer. Edited by R.A. Eeles, B.A.J. Ponder, D.F. Easton and A. Horwich. Published in 1996 by Chapman & Hall, London.
0 412 56580 3

below), there may be no other phenotypic features other than the malignancies.

At the other extreme from these high-risk, clearly genetically-determined families, many individuals present with a family history consisting of one or two relatives with colorectal cancer. Clinically, the occurrence of such families does raise concerns about currently unaffected relatives. Could they be at high risk because in fact this is a syndromal family except that by chance only a few relatives have developed the cancer? Or, has there been a cluster of cancers in the families simply because they share an exposure to a medley of minor risk factors?

Definitive answers to these problems are not, in general, currently available. Epidemiological studies have suggested that relatives of colorectal cancer cases have a two- to three-fold increased risk of colorectal cancer themselves [1]. Although estimates vary widely, the mendelian dominant syndromes probably account for only a very small proportion of colorectal cancers in the population, possibly about 1–5% in all, so that by themselves, they cannot explain the family aggregation of colorectal cancer. It is possible, however, that lower penetrance genes may play a role in a much larger proportion of cases and be responsible for the majority of these other smaller familial clusters.

In this chapter, we discuss syndromes associated with colorectal cancer both in terms of identification and of clinical management. In a following chapter, our understanding of the genetic factors underlying these syndromes is presented although it is not possible to remove all such considerations from this discussion.

20.2 SYNDROMES ASSOCIATED WITH AN INCREASED RISK OF COLORECTAL CANCER

There are a number of rare, dominantly inherited syndromes which predispose to colorectal cancer. In each of these syndromes, the risk of colorectal cancer is high, being close to 100% over a lifetime. However, since these syndromes are so rare, together they explain only 1–5% of all colorectal cancer. The characteristics of each of these syndromes are distinct from each other and recently the genetic basis of a number of them has been elaborated (see Table 20.1). The best noted of these syndromes is familial adenomatous polyposis.

20.2.1 FAMILIAL ADENOMATOUS POLYPOSIS

Pathologists have appreciated for a long time that the majority of colorectal cancers develop in adenomatous polyps, and this was in part uncovered by the study of patients with familial adenomatous polyposis (FAP) [2,3]. FAP is a dominantly inherited cancer syndrome in which there is profuse covering of adenomas in the large bowel [4]. The adenomas start to develop in the second decade of life while the cancers in these individuals develop during the third and fourth decade, 20–30 years earlier than in the general population [5]. Without intervention, a number of these adenomas would progress to malignancy with the average age of colorectal cancer onset being 40 years [6]. The prevalence of polyposis is about one per 10 000 births [6].

FAP is not only a disease of the large bowel but also affects extracolonic sites. Upper gastrointestinal tract malignancy will develop in about 5% of patients [7] and 10% develop benign desmoid tumours; the latter, particularly when intra-abdominal, are also a cause of significant morbidity and mortality from local spread [8]. In addition, affected individuals may have other features which may help in diagnosis. Pigmented lesions of the fundus of the eye termed 'congenital hypertrophy of the retinal pigment epithelium' (CHRPE) are found in the majority of

Table 20.1 Characteristics of syndromes associated with increased risk of colorectal cancer

Syndrome	Gene	Chromosome	Usual clinical features	Other clinical features
Familial adenomatous polyposis/Gardner's/Flat adenoma syndrome	*APC*	5q21	Multiple colonic adenomas Classically >100; some families have fewer recorded	Congenital hypertrophy of retinal pigment epithelium (CHRPE) Epidermoid cysts, osteomas, desmoid tumours Malignancies Periampullary carcinoma/ polyps Papillary carcinoma of thyroid (females only) Hepatoblastoma
Hereditary non-polyposis colorectal cancer (HNPCC)	*hMSH2* *hMLH1* *hPMS2* *hPMS1*	2p 3p 7q 2q	Colorectal carcinoma	Lynch I: none Lynch II: other carcinoma Small bowel Endometrium Urinary tract Transitional cell Ovarian cancer Upper GI cancer Pancreatic cancer Muir–Torré: as Lynch II plus Sebaceous gland tumours Basal cell carcinomas Keratoacanthomas
Turcot	NK	NK	Colorectal adenomas; normally <100 Poor prognosis	Brain tumours Café au lait patches Syndactyly

FAP patients [9, 10], while osteomas, especially of the jaw, are also common [11]. Finally, epidermoid cysts, particularly if occurring prepubertally, are a useful diagnostic feature [12].

New mutations for FAP are not uncommon and the family history may therefore be unhelpful. For instance, Rustin *et al.* [13] found that 22% of their series of families did not have a previous family history and so were potentially new mutations. Even in the absence of a family history, however, the finding of profuse polyposis will be diagnostic and should be looked for, particularly in young colorectal cancer patients [14, 15].

The genetic basis of FAP has been unravelled in the last decade. First in 1987, Bodmer *et al.* [16] and Leppert *et al.* [17] showed that a gene for FAP was located on chromosome 5. Previously, FAP families were categorized separately as to whether the family members had extracolonic lesions such as epidermoid cysts or desmoid tumours in which case they were classified as 'Gardner's syndrome'. However, both types of family were found to be linked to 5q. In 1991, two groups cloned the gene for adenomatous polyposis coli (termed 'APC') [18, 19]. The gene is large, consisting of 15 exons, the last being the largest exon identified in any gene to date. Although a few FAP patients have been identified with deletions of the whole APC gene, the majority of patients have mutations that produce a truncated protein, most of which are found in the first half of the gene [20]. Subsequent analysis of mutations showed that the same mutation could be observed in either a family classified as Gardner's syndrome or simply as FAP [21], this evidence shows that other factors besides the APC gene determine the extent of expression and the number of complications. Families with CHRPEs have been found to have mutations in exons 9–15 while those with mutations in exons 1–8 only rarely have CHRPEs [22].

The mapping and cloning of the *APC* gene has provided evidence that mutations in the *APC* gene can cause widely varying differences in phenotype. For instance, it is now clear that there are some families with a later age of onset and less profuse polyposis as well as some families where the adenomas are predominantly sessile are also so attributed [23–25]. The finding of extracolonic features in these atypical individuals can be particularly helpful and be an indication for mutation analysis.

20.2.2 HEREDITARY NON-POLYPOSIS COLORECTAL CANCER (LYNCH SYNDROMES I AND II)

Hereditary non-polyposis colorectal cancer (HNPCC) is a dominantly inherited syndrome but the extracolonic features of FAP do not occur, there is no profuse polyposis and there appears to be a broader spectrum of cancers. Identification of these families usually relies on obtaining a recognizable family history of cancer. The sites of malignancies occurring in the family, as well as the number of affected relatives and the age at which they have been affected, are the accepted diagnostic features. The identification of three or more closely related individuals with bowel cancer, especially if the cases are young (<50 years) should arouse suspicion.

The families can be broadly classified according to the types of cancers occurring in the families. In Lynch syndrome I, the cancers are mainly gastrointestinal, while in Lynch syndrome II (also termed 'cancer family syndrome'), in addition to colorectal cancer, endometrial and ovarian cancer occur in women at a young age [26, 27]. In either condition, cancers occur at other sites, but with a much lower incidence. The majority of affected individuals will have adenomas, but usually only a few. The average age for developing colorectal cancer is 41 years and the anatomical distribution is predominantly right-sided as opposed to left-sided in the general population and indeed in FAP. Muir Torré is a related condition with additional skin manifestations, keratoacanthomas and sebaceous adenomas. The spectrum of malignancies is very similar but there is a tendency for affected individuals to develop multiple primaries, sometimes six or more. They also appear to develop metastases at unusual sites and anecdotal evidence suggests that they have improved survival.

Recently two genes involved in DNA mismatch repair have been identified, mutations in which produce HNPCC, one on chromosome 2p and the other on chromosome 3p. To date, there are few data to differentiate between the families with mutations in either gene. The majority of families with HNPCC are due to the 2p gene (perhaps 60% of all families), with the 3p gene responsible for perhaps another 30% [28]. Mutations in two other genes (*PMS1* and *PMS2*) involved in the repair pathway located on chromosomes 7 and 2 have been identified by one group but this remains to be confirmed.

The incidence of breast cancer is said not to be increased in cancer family syndrome; however, there appear to be dominant colorectal cancer families where breast cancer is occurring at an earlier age than in the general population and with an increased frequency. These families may represent a separate subgroup of HNPCC or could be breast cancer families which have been shown to be at an increased risk of bowel cancer [29].

20.2.3 OTHER SINGLE GENE DISORDERS WITH A HIGH RISK OF COLORECTAL CANCER

There are number of other rarer genetic disorders with a risk of colorectal cancer. The risk of bowel cancer in these conditions is variable. There are a number of other hamar-

tomatous polyposes, all of which can be associated with colorectal cancer, such as Peutz–Jeghers syndrome. The risk of large bowel malignancy is lower than in FAP and HNPCC.

(a) Turcot's syndrome

The name Turcot's syndrome has unfortunately been used to describe two different conditions. It has been applied to FAP patients with brain tumours (usually medulloblastomas); these patients have mutations in the *APC* gene. However, Turcot's syndrome was the name originally given to the condition associated with adenomatous polyposis; the adenomas are less profuse than in FAP and the phenotype quite different. The condition usually presents in childhood with brain tumours which are frequently astrocytomas. The children have scattered café au lait patches, occasionally syndactyly and appear to have a degree of radiosensitivity, often developing leukaemia after radiotherapy. The finding of this condition in sibs with healthy parents and the observation of consanguinity in a number of reported families makes it likely that this is recessive. Overall, the prognosis in affected children is poor. Genetic studies have shown that the *APC* gene does not appear to be involved.

However, recent studies in one patient have identified a mutation in one of the HNPCC genes. Perhaps Turcot is the recessive form of a mismatch repair defect [30].

(b) Juvenile polyposis

This is another autosomal dominant condition. It often presents in early childhood with anaemia and gastrointestinal symptoms. The polyps are hamartomatous but can undergo dysplastic change. They are less numerous than in FAP and are more evenly distributed throughout the gastrointestinal tract. Contrary to earlier belief there is an increased risk of colorectal cancer and the cumulative lifetime risk may be as high as 60–80%. The condition may be associated with developmental abnormalities such as congenital heart disease and some affected individuals are dysmorphic and have macrocephaly.

20.2.4 SPORADIC COLORECTAL CANCER

The majority of colorectal cancer arises outside the obvious context of the syndromes described above. Even then there is an increase in risk to family members of colorectal cancer cases. This observation has been made from a variety of epidemiological studies (see Chapter 1). Overall, these studies conclude that relatives of cases are at two- to three-fold increased risk of colorectal cancer over the general population. This risk, however, hides the fact that different family histories are associated with quite different levels of risk. St John *et al.* [31] in keeping with many other studies, showed convincingly that the highest risks are associated with the earliest ages of onset of colon cancer and having multiple affected relatives. For instance, while in summary, relatives of cases were found to have a 2 to 3-fold increased risk, the risk of colorectal cancer by age 70 years in a relative of a colorectal cancer case was estimated to be 6.5% (if the case was diagnosed before the age of 45 years), 4.5% (diagnosis between 45–54 years) and 2.2% (diagnosis after 55 years); all of these figures should be compared with the 1.2% risk to this age observed in the general population. Further, a 5 to 7-fold increased risk was found for relatives of two affected cases. Table 20.2 contains estimates of the importance of different family histories.

Table 20.2 Importance of family history for risk of colorectal cancer

Relative of	Risk
A case at any age	2–4 × population risk
A case diagnosed under the age of 45 years	5–7 × population risk
Two close relatives with colorectal cancer	5–7 × population risk

20.3 DIAGNOSIS AND MANAGEMENT

The finding of adenomatous polyposis or other unique phenotypic features may enable the diagnosis to be made of a recognizable genetic condition. However a genetic predisposition is indicated more frequently by the family history of malignancies or history of multiple primaries in an individual. Diagnoses of polyposes or polyps should be confirmed histopathologically and where there is doubt about the diagnosis of malignancy in relatives, confirmation should be sought.

The family history is important not only in diagnosis but also in management of the relatives of bowel cancer patients, since this also enables estimation of risk to relatives and provides a guide for who should be followed up by screening and the screening method that should be employed (also see Chapter 25).

20.3.1 SCREENING

Screening for those at high risk should aim at prevention of cancer and therefore at the detection of adenomas. This will necessitate the use of endoscopy as neither barium enema nor faecal occult bloods will have acceptable detection rates for people at increased risk. Compliance for screening from family cancer clinics tends to be very high.

(a) FAP

Screening for FAP can be adequately carried out by sigmoidoscopy, as the adenomas as a rule appear distally early. The age at which these examinations should begin is a matter of debate, but, even in FAP, colorectal cancer is rare before the age of 20. Most people usually start screening in their early teens. In addition the individual should have a thorough examination for any of the extracolonic manifestations and fundoscopy by an ophthalmologist may be useful. Most centres would proceed to colonoscopy if adenomas are found on sigmoidoscopy.

The finding of profuse polyposis is an indication for prophylactic colectomy, either with ileorectal anastomosis and careful follow-up for the rectum, or total colectomy and the creation of an ileal pouch.

(b) HNPCC

Screening in these conditions also requires endoscopy but as the distribution of cancers and adenomas is frequently right-sided, colonoscopy is the investigation of choice. Examinations should probably start around 25 years and should be repeated at least every 3–5 years, but this depends upon the findings. A high percentage of individuals from these families will have adenomas early compared with the general population and if an individual reaches 65–70 without problems then most of their risk from their family history is passed and examinations can probably be discontinued or at least made less frequent. Families who have a family of other cancers such as Cancer Family Syndrome should receive screening for the other malignancies that are common: annual pelvic ultrasound from 35 years for women with endometrial or ovarian cancer in the family, and breast screening from 35 where appropriate. In addition there are some families with a high incidence of renal tract cancers where annual urinary cytology and examination for microscopic haematuria may be useful.

(c) Familial clusters and young colorectal cancer patients

The finding of two relatives or a young relative with colorectal cancer confers a lifetime risk of colorectal cancer of 1 in 6 to 1 in 7. The consensus is that their relatives should also be offered screening. The relatives of a single young case who do go on to develop colorectal cancer appear to do so at a similar age as those patients without a family history and the distribution of the cancers is no different from that in the general population. This has implications for screening, suggesting that it does not need to be started until later as compared with those with more relatives affected. In addition, screening by flexible sigmoidoscopy in this group may be adequate particularly in those individuals whose affected relative is 55 and over.

20.4 DISCUSSION

In time, many of the genes causing susceptibility to bowel cancer will be identified and it will possible to test affected individuals to see if they have a mutation in a particular gene. Relatives may then be screened by a simple DNA test to see if they are also susceptible. This will of course greatly reduce the number of relatives who will need screening and concentrate resources on those at greatest risk. This is already possible in FAP, since there is an easily identified phenotype, very little genetic heterogeneity, and all the families appear to be due to the same gene on chromosome 5. In suitable families DNA linkage can be carried out before endoscopic screening to identify those who have not inherited the gene and therefore do not require endoscopy. If the family is not suitable for linked marker studies, mutation analysis can be carried out in an affected member of the family and if a defect is found this can be used for screening those at risk in the family.

Linkage has also been identified in HNPCC families, a significant proportion appearing to be due to a gene on chromosome 2. However, some families are definitely unlinked and others appear to be due to a gene on chromosome 3. Mutation analysis is still quite a laborious business because of locus heterogeneity in HNPCC, although hopefully, mutation analysis will ultimately become more routine and resolve this problem.

Finding susceptibility genes in families that show less evidence of a particular disorder or produce less obvious clustering is likely to take longer, but ultimately there will inevitably be an increase in those that have DNA screening and a decrease as a result in those that require clinical follow-up.

REFERENCES

1. Bishop, D. T. and Thomas, H. J. W. (1990) The genetics of colorectal cancer. *Cancer Surv.*, **9**, 585–604.
2. Morson, B.C., Bussey, H.J.R., Dawy, D.W. *et al.* (1983) Adenomas of the large bowel. *Cancer Surv.*, **2**, 451–77.
3. Tierney, R.P., Ballantyne, G.H., Modlin, I.M. *et al.* (1990) The adenoma of carcinoma sequence. *Surg. Gynecol. Obstet.*, **171**, 81–94.
4. Bussey, H.J.R. (1987) Historical developments in familial polyposis coli. *Semin. Surg. Oncol.*, **3**, 67–70.
5. Northover, J.M.A. and Murday, V. (1989) Familial colorectal cancer and familial adenomatous polyposis, in *Baillière's Clinical Gastroenterology: International Practice and Research*, Baillière Tindall, London, pp. 593–613.
6. Bülow, S. (1989) Familial adenomatous polyposis. *Ann. Med.*, **21**, 299–307.
7. Jagelman, D.G., DeCosse, J.J., Bussey, H.J.R. and The Leeds Castle Polyposis Group (1988) Upper gastrointestinal cancer in familial adenomatous polyposis. *Lancet*, **1**, 1149–51.
8. Klemmer, S., Pascoe, L.and DeCosse, J. (1987) Occurrence of desmoids in patients with familial adenomatous polyposis of the colon. *Am.J.Med.Genet.*, **28**, 385–92.
9. Burn, J., Chapman, P., Delhanty, J. *et al.* (1991) The UK Northern Region genetic register for familial adenomatous polyposis coli: use of age of onset, congenital hypertrophy of the retinal pigment epithelium and DNA markers in risk calculations. *J.Med.Genet.*, **28**, 289–96.
10. Hodgson, S.V., Bishop, D.T.and Jay, B. (1994) Genetic heterogeneity of congenital hypertrophy of the retinal pigment epithelium (CHRPE) in families with familial adenomatous polyposis. *J. Med. Genet.*, **31**, 55–8.
11. Northover, J.M.and Murday, V. (1989) Familial colorectal cancer and familial adenomatous polyposis. *Baillière's Clin. Gastroenterol.*, **3**(3), 593–613.
12. Leppard, B. and Bussey, H.J.R. (1975) Epidermoid cysts, polyposis coli and Gardner's syndrome. *Br. J. Surg.*, **62**, 387–93.
13. Rustin, R.B., Jagelman, D.G., McGannon, E. *et al.* (1990) Spontaneous mutation in familial adenomatous polyposis. *Dis. Colon Rectum*, **33**, 52–5.
14. Jagelamn, D.G. (1987) Extracolonic manifestations of familial polyposis coli. *Semin. Surg. Oncol.*, **3**, 88–91.
15. Bülow, S. (1989) Familial adenomatous polyposis. *Ann. Med.*, **21**, 299–307.
16. Bodmer, W.F., Bailey, C.J., Bodmer, J. *et al.* (1987) Localization of the gene for familial adenomatous polyposis on chromosome 5. *Nature*, **328**, 614–16.
17. Leppert, M., Dobbs, M., Scambler, P. *et al.* (1987) The gene for familial polyposis coli maps to the long arm of chromosome 5. *Science*, **238**, 1411–13.
18. Groden, J., Thliveris, A., Samowitz, W. *et al.* (1991) Identification and characterization of the familial adenomatous polyposis coli gene. *Cell*, **66**, 589–600.
19. Kinzler, K.W., Nilbert, M.C., Su, L.-K. *et al.* (1991) Identification of FAP locus genes from chromosome 5q21. *Science*, **253**, 661–5.
20. Cottrell, S., Bicknell, D., Kaklamandis, L. *et al.* (1992) Molecular analysis of *APC* mutations in familial adenomatous polyposis and sporadic colon carcinomas. *Lancet*, **340**, 626–30.

21. Nishisho, I., Nakamura, Y., Miyoshi, Y. *et al.* (1991) Mutations of chromosome 5q21 genes in FAP and colorectal cancer patients. *Science*, **253**, 665–9.

22. Olschwang, S., Tiret, A., Laurent-Puig, P. *et al.* (1993) Restriction of ocular fundus lesions to a specific subgroup of *APC* mutations in adenomatous polyposis coli patients. *Cell*, **75**, 959–68.

23. Leppert, M., Burt, R., Hughes, J.P. *et al.* (1990) Genetic analysis of an inherited predisposition to colon cancer in a family with a variable number of adenomatous polyps. *N. Engl. J. Med.*, **322**, 904–8.

24. Spirio, L., Otterud, B., Stauffer, D. *et al.* (1992) Linkage of a variant or attenuated form of adenomatous polyposis coli to the adenomatous polyposis coli (APC) locus. *Am. J. Hum. Genet.*, **51**, 92–100.

25. Spirio, L., Olschwang, S., Groden, J. *et al.* (1993) Alleles of the *APC* gene: an attenuated form of familial polyposis. *Cell*, **75**, 951–7.

26. Lynch, H.T., Lanspa, S., Smyrk, T. *et al.* (1991) Hereditary nonpolyposis colorectal cancer (Lynch syndromes I and II): genetics, pathology, natural history, and cancer control, Part 1. *Cancer Genet. Cytogenet.*, **53**, 143–60.

27. Watson, P.and Lynch, H.T. (1993) Extracolonic cancer in hereditary nonpolyposis colorectal cancer. *Cancer*, **71**, 677–85.

28. Sankiujl, M.A. and Bishop, T. (1994) Results of joint analysis of the EUROFAP Linkage Data, in *Genetic and Clinics of HNPCC: Proceedings of the 4th Copenhagen Workshop: EUROFAP* (ed. J. Mohr), P. 26.

29. Ford, D., Easton, D.F., Bishop, D.T., Narod, S.A. and Goldgar, D.E. (1994) Risks of cancer in BRCA1-mutation carriers. Breast Cancer Linkage Consortium. *Lancet*, **343**, 692–5.

30. Hamilton, S.R., Liu, B., Parsons, R.E. *et al.* (1995) The molecular basis of Turcot's syndrome. *N. Engl. J. Med.*, **332**, 839–47.

31. St John, D.J.B., McDermott, F.T. and Hopper, V.L. (1993) Cancer risk in relatives of patients with common colorectal cancer. *Ann. Intern. Med.*, **118**, 785–90.

Chapter 21

The genetics of familial colon cancer

SUSAN M. FARRINGTON and MALCOLM G. DUNLOP

21.1 INTRODUCTION

In developed countries, colorectal cancer is the second most common cause of death due to malignancy after lung cancer in males and third most common after lung and breast cancer in females. In the UK this manifests as a death rate due to colorectal cancer of more than 20 000 annually. Understanding the fundamental molecular genetic basis of colorectal carcinogenesis may allow the development of novel treatment approaches and may also lead to the identification of those who are at high risk of developing the disease when intensive screening combined with prophylactic surgery or drug therapy can be undertaken. In addition, colorectal carcinogenesis provides a model system in which to study the molecular events involved in the development of a number of epithelial cancers and may lead to an understanding of genetic predisposition to these common diseases.

Progress in understanding the molecular basis of colorectal cancer over the last 5 years has been breathtaking, particularly so with regard to understanding the genetic loci involved in predisposition to the disease. This chapter reviews and condenses some of the recent exciting work in this field.

For the majority of individuals, predisposition to bowel cancer is an ill-defined increased risk of the disease indicated by the history of having an affected relative. However, there are certain well-defined categories of patients characterized by a strong family history and an autosomal dominant genetic trait. There are several rare genetic predisposition syndromes which will not be discussed further in this review. We shall focus on familial adenomatous polyposis (FAP) and hereditary non-polyposis colorectal cancer (HNPCC). The prevalence of colorectal cancer due to FAP depends greatly on the assiduousness of screening programme of those at risk but is around 0.2% in most developed countries. HNPCC makes up a more substantial proportion (5–10% of all cases) [1] but since until recently there have been no biomarkers of HNPCC, diagnostic criteria have been purely pragmatic and are certainly not inclusive of all cases. Such criteria will only identify families where the

Genetic Predisposition to Cancer. Edited by R.A. Eeles, B.A.J. Ponder, D.F. Easton and A. Horwich. Published in 1996 by Chapman & Hall, London.
0 412 56580 3

gene defect is highly penetrant and the families are of sufficient size to allow the appropriate number of cases to arise and so it is certain that many small families are excluded inappropriately.

In the future, a reduction in the death rate from malignancy in genetically determined colorectal cancer seems likely. With improved awareness of patients and clinicians, the development of local FAP registries and colonic screening, FAP gene carriers should less frequently present with invasive cancer. Conversely, HNPCC kindreds are usually identified because several family members have already died from colorectal cancer before the familial nature of the problem is understood. Between these two defined syndromes, there are many patients who develop colorectal cancer as a result of genetic predisposition to the disease. However, because of small numbers of relatives, the genetic aspect is never apparent. Around 20–25% of all colorectal cancer cases are associated with a family history of the disease [2]. One screening study has shown that the predisposition is to the development of colorectal adenomas and the authors suggested that all cases of colorectal cancer occur on a background of genetic predisposition [3]. With the recent identification of a number of genes responsible for HNPCC (see below), it will be of great interest to elucidate the true prevalence of familial colorectal cancer.

21.2 FAMILIAL ADENOMATOUS POLYPOSIS (FAP)

FAP is an autosomal dominant disorder characterized by the development of more than 100, but frequently thousands of adenomatous polyps of the colon and rectum. The population frequency depends on the accuracy and completeness of the registration of cases, but the annual incidence is around 1/7000 live births (see Chapter 1). Malignancy is virtually inevitable if prophylactic colectomy is not undertaken. The syndrome is also associated with extracolonic features such as multiple craniofacial and long bone osteomata, epidermoid cysts, retinal pigmentation, gastroduodenal polyposis and malignancy and also desmoid tumours.

The discovery that a patient with FAP who also had multiple congenital abnormalities carried a constitutional deletion of the long arm of chromosome 5, indicated the location of the susceptibility gene responsible for FAP. Genetic linkage studies demonstrated that the gene lay in the region 5q21–22 [4, 5]. A number of positional cloning strategies were then employed involving genetic linkage, deletion mapping in sporadic colorectal cancers (which also exhibit loss of genetic material in 5q21–22) and mapping of constitutional microdeletions in FAP patients by pulse field gel electrophoresis. A number of candidate genes were cloned and eventually the gene was identified, sequenced and a number of FAP patients were shown to carry germline mutations [6–9]. The gene has been named adenomatous polyposis coli (*APC*) and was the first gene to be identified which confers germline susceptibility to colorectal neoplasia. Germline mutations have now been reported in around 250 FAP families [10–12] and all result in premature truncation of the *APC* product by either base substitution or deletion/insertion with a frameshift causing a downstream premature stop codon.

APC comprises an 8.5kb transcript encoding a 2843 amino acid polypeptide in 15 exons. The function of the *APC* gene product is not fully understood but antibodies to the APC protein have identified a 300KDa cytoplasmic protein expressed in colonic epithelial cells in the upper portions of the colonic crypts, suggesting involvement in colonocyte maturation [13]. Short repeat sequences within *APC* have been identified which are predicted to form coiled coil structures suggesting that normal *APC* product may be functional in dimeric configuration. Recently, interaction of APC with other proteins and subcellular structures has been investigated. APC has been shown to associate with alpha- and beta catenins. These proteins bind to the cell surface molecule, E-cadherin and are essential for its role in cellular adhesion. It is proposed that APC protein may affect the interaction between catenins and E-cadherin, thus influencing cellular adhesion and possibly intercellular communication [14, 15]. Further subcellular localization has demonstrated that wild-type APC is closely associated with microtubule formation [16, 17]. Indeed, *in vitro* studies indicate that wild-type APC not only binds to microtubules but also promotes their formation [16]. The organization and structure of microtubules are vital to cell division. Mutant APC product (missing the carboxy-terminal part of the molecule due to premature truncation) appears to be unable to bind microtubules. Once the underlying function of APC has been clearly determined it may be possible to restore or augment the effects of deleterious mutations by pharmacological means.

The wide spectrum of clinical presentation of FAP, even within a single family where affected individuals all carry the same *APC* mutation, indicates that there are factors other than the *APC* mutation which affect the phenotypic expression of the disease. A modifier locus has been identified in the Min mouse model of FAP. The Min (for *m*ultiple *i*ntestinal *n*eoplasia) mouse was generated by germline mutagenesis which fortuitously mutated the *APC* gene [18]. The resulting phenotype includes the development of multiple neoplastic lesions mainly affecting the foregut. This is somewhat at variance with the clinical presentation of FAP with almost universal neoplastic change in the hindgut, although upper gastro-intestinal polyposis is of course a problem. The Min mouse has been shown to carry a mutation in the murine *APC* gene [19] and hence represents a mouse

model of FAP. Phenotypic expression has been shown to be modulated by an unlinked locus [20]. Identification of the murine and homologous human modifier genes will be of great importance with regard to understanding and treating the human condition. A number of murine strains have recently been generated with germline *APC* mutations induced by targeted mutagenesis. These models and the Min mouse will allow the assessment of novel treatments for preventing the development of colorectal neoplasia in FAP and in particular for combatting the particularly capricious problems of desmoid disease and gastroduodenal cancer.

Around 80% of the *APC* mutations identified to date are in exon 15. Two specific exon 15 mutations occurring at codons 1061 and 1309 account for 15–20% of all *APC* mutations, but the remainder are spread throughout the gene with no particular 'hotspots' [9, 21–23]. The mutations detected to date are mainly deletions or insertions of short sequences [24], suggesting they are due to replication errors rather than to the action of environmental mutagens. All confirmed mutations generate a STOP codon, either directly or by a frame shift, and hence result in premature termination of transcription and resultant truncation of the protein. Truncated APC protein may interact with the normal APC product, resulting in a heterodimer which may impair the function of the normal protein in a dominant-negative manner [25].

Correlation of the specific location or type of *APC* mutation could in theory help clinicians predict the optimum timing for surgery or help predict whether extracolonic manifestations such as desmoid disease are likely. However, the number of reported mutations and quality of clinical data thus far have not allowed valid genotype–phenotype correlations. One study of 22 unrelated Japanese FAP patients predicted that the site of mutation may determine the number of colorectal polyps [24]. However, other groups have identified families with identical *APC* mutations but diverse phenotype in terms of both colorectal polyposis and extracolonic disease [26]. It may well be some time before valid correlations can be drawn, particularly in view of the likelihood of at least one modifier locus.

Identification of the mutation responsible for the FAP syndrome in a family has obvious advantages for presymptomatic diagnosis. Once the *APC* mutation has been identified in an affected individual (but preferably two or more), all at-risk offspring can be screened and prediction of carrier status based on mutation analysis can be made with 100% accuracy. However, the lack of a specific mutation or a small number of mutational 'hotspots' as the underlying genetic aetiology of FAP means that the entire gene must be screened laboriously for each different FAP family. Once the mutation has been identified mutation-specific PCR primers can be generated and used for each generation at risk. Due to the rapid introduction of mutation detection into the clinical sphere, it seems likely that the only FAP family members who are undergoing regular colon surveillance will be those who are known to carry a mutant *APC* gene and in whom the optimum timing for surgery is under assessment.

Future research into the molecular genetics of FAP will lead to better and more user-friendly methods of carrier status assessment such as *in vitro* transcription/translation with monoclonal antibody detection of truncated proteins. Greater understanding of the structure, function and interactions of the APC protein combined with the use of mouse models will undoubtedly lead to new treatment modalities of not only FAP but also sporadic colorectal cancer. Identification of the *APC* gene was only the start of what will be an exciting path for those in the field and particularly for those affected by the disorder.

21.3 HEREDITARY NON-POLYPOSIS COLORECTAL CANCER (HNPCC)

Hereditary non-polyposis colorectal cancer (HNPCC) is an autosomal dominant disorder with high penetrance in which colorectal cancer develops in gene carriers but without the myriads of adenomas seen in FAP [27]. Adenomatous polyps are found in HNPCC patients but these are in numbers comparable to that of the general population (usually <10). There is a propensity for both adenomas and carcinomas to develop in the proximal part of the colon. Expression of the HNPCC phenotype is diverse in terms of the age of onset and also the organs which develop malignancy. It can be inherited as a site-specific colorectal cancer susceptibility trait (Lynch type I) or can also be associated with uterine, gastric, ovarian, upper urinary tract, small intestinal and other malignancies (Lynch type II).

Large HNPCC families are fairly uncommon and so minimum criteria for the diagnosis of HNPCC have been drawn up. The effect of such criteria is to determine the prevalence which they set out to ascertain. Thus when diagnostic criteria are loosened, more cases of colorectal cancer will be attributed to HNPCC and vice versa. Conversely, simply because a family fulfils the minimum criteria for HNPCC does not unfailingly mean that the apparent familial aggregation is due to genetic predisposition. Colorectal cancer is a very common disease and so aggregation of cases in a family could occur by chance. The issue of diagnostic criteria has a major effect on the apparent prevalence of HNPCC and also considerably influences the apparent penetrance of the gene defect(s). Thus HNPCC is said to be a disorder with high penetrance, but it is the diagnostic criteria which demand a highly penetrant disease! Thus diagnostic criteria create considerable circularity in the assignment of penetrance and indeed the prevalence of

HNPCC. The criteria proposed by the International Collaborative Group on Hereditary Nonpolyposis Colorectal Cancer (ICG-HNPCC) require: (i) three or more relatives with histologically proven colorectal cancer, one being a first-degree relative of the other two; (ii) two or more generations affected; and (iii) at least one family member affected before age 50 years [28]. In addition to the predetermination of gene penetrance, such criteria will only identify families of sufficient size to allow the appropriate number of cases to arise and so many small families will be excluded inappropriately. With the recent identification of several causative genes, it will be of great interest to calculate the true penetrance of HNPCC.

As discussed above, around one-quarter of all cases of colorectal cancer are associated with a family history of the disease, which is significantly higher than in controls [2]. Abnormalities of colonic epithelial cell proliferation have been demonstrated in HNPCC [29] and have been shown to be more pronounced as the strength of family history increased [30]. This could be due to shared family environment but whereas the relatives of colorectal cancer patients are at increased risk of the disease, it has been shown that their spouses have the same risk as the general population [31]. Screening studies suggest the cancer susceptibility is due to predisposition to the development of colorectal adenomas [3]. Fortunately, not all adenomas become cancer since the population frequency of the 'adenoma-prone' allele was calculated as 19%. The effects of diet clearly must influence the expression of such an allele in terms of both adenoma and cancer but the trait could probably be thought of as a 'normal' variation of the human constitution. Perhaps most striking of all is the suggestion that colorectal neoplasms **only** occur in the presence of a genetic predisposition [3].

Since it is possible that genetic predisposition to colorectal cancer may be very preva-

lent indeed, identifying the gene or genes which might confer such susceptibility becomes of paramount importance. Four genes responsible for HNPCC have been identified and it will now be possible to assess the true prevalence of familial versus sporadic colorectal cancer.

21.3.1 THE GENES RESPONSIBLE FOR HNPCC

Several areas of research have recently come together to identify a number of genes responsible for HNPCC. These studies have also demonstrated a common functional deficit at the molecular level caused by mutation of such genes in humans, bacteria and yeast. Four human genes have been identified which are implicated in constitutional predisposition to colorectal cancer. These genes are human homologues of yeast and bacterial DNA repair genes and are known as *hMSH*2 on chromosome 2p [32, 33], *hMLH*1 on chromosome 3p [34, 35], *hPMS*1 on chromosome 2q [36] and *hPMS*2 on chromosome 7q [36].

*hMSH*2 was originally localized by linkage studies in two large unrelated HNPCC pedigrees [37]. A systematic linkage mapping strategy was embarked upon and a total of 345 RFLP and dinucleotide repeat markers spread evenly throughout the human genome were analysed for evidence of linkage to the disease phenotype. An anonymous marker, D2S123, mapping to the short arm of chromosome 2 was found to co-segregate with the disease in both families. Fourteen smaller families were also analysed and one-third showed no evidence of linkage to D2S123. A second locus was identified by a report of linkage to a marker on chromosome 3p shortly afterwards [38], clearly establishing genetic heterogeneity in HNPCC.

Around the same time, an apparently unrelated avenue of research on repeat sequences in genomic DNA from colorectal tumours identified widespread instability in short repetitive tracts which was very suggestive of a defect of DNA mismatch repair [39–41]. The most well-defined mismatch repair system is in *E. coli* (reviewed in [43]) and a number of gene products are required, namely MutL, MutH, MutS and MutU. Yeast also has a similar mismatch repair pathway which requires a homologue of MutS, MSH and two MutL homologues, MLH1 and PMS1 [43, 44]. With the finding that there was a dramatic increase in repetitive tract instability in yeast when mutations were included in MLH or PMS [45], such a group of genes became a strong candidate for the human condition of HNPCC with the characterstic change in repeat DNA.

A combination of positional cloning and candidate gene approaches to gene isolation was then employed by two groups to identify the human homologues of the yeast and bacterial DNA mismatch repair genes. The first to be isolated was *hMSH2* on chromosome 2p [32, 33]. Using degenerate PCR primers for the yeast MSH genes, Fishel *et al* [32] identified the human homologue *hMSH2* and localized it to the same region on chromosome 2p as the markers linked in HNPCC families. Vogelstein's group [33] employed a combination of positional cloning and candidate gene strategies, generating multiple markers within a 25 cM region defined by linkage studies. When analysed in HNPCC families which were linked to the 2p gene, recombination events were identified which designated a minimum region containing the gene of interest. After extensive screening of candidate genes mapping to this region, germline mutations were identified in HNPCC kindreds in a gene shown to be homologous to the bacterial MutS gene and so was named *hMSH2* (human Mut S Homologue). A 2802bp cDNA from *hMSH2* was found to contain a highly conserved region between codons 615–788 with considerable cross-species homology between human,

yeast and bacteria. Several mutations were identified within the highly conserved region including stop codons resulting in premature truncation of the protein product and a splice site alteration. Mutations were also shown to co-segregate with the disease in HNPCC families.

Once it became clear that human homologues of DNA mismatch repair genes were involved, the human homologues of other genes involved in the mismatch repair pathway were obvious candidates and these were quickly identified and mutations demonstrated to be responsible for the HNPCC syndrome [34, 35]. *hMLH1* was shown to be the gene segregating with chromosome 3p markers [38] and *hPMS1* and *hPMS2* lie on chromosomes 2q and 7q respectively [36].

At this early stage, the mutational spectrum in *hMSH*, *hMLH* and *hPMS* genes in HNPCC is very much affected by the selection of cases. However, reported mutations include base substitutions, short deletions, and deletions of a few hundred base pairs. The tendency for generation of stop codons as the underlying mechanism of inactivation has been exploited by Vogelstein's group to screen for mutations using the protein truncation test [35, 36, 46] used to such effect in *APC* mutation screening. The proportion of HNPCC families due to mutations in each of the genes remains to be elucidated but it would appear that around 40% of families fulfilling the ICG criteria for HNPCC carry mutations in *hMSH2* [46]. By extrapolating from published linkage and mutation data the proportion due to *hMLH1* appears to be around 20% while *hPMS1* and 2 appear to be rarely involved. Obviously there has been substantial selection of families for research purposes and with further work in this area, the proportion of colorectal cancer cases due to each gene will eventually become apparent.

Since, inactivation of either *MSH*, *MLH* or *PMS* in humans and in yeast results in a mutator phenotype [35, 36, 43–46] and the true penetrance of HNPCC gene mutations may well be relatively low and the population mutation frequency substantially higher than previously suspected, there are important implications for human population genetics. Lynch has calculated that the population gene frequency of an HNPCC allele may be around 0.005 [1]. Hence, it is perfectly reasonable to expect progeny from (say) an *hMLH*1- and *hMSH*2- pairing. This possibility has very substantial implications indeed for predictive testing in such offspring, particularly since very early-onset, highly penetrant disease has been selected for by most centres interested in the field. Since only 25% of offspring will be normal at both loci, it would seem wise to avoid any question of predictive testing until the true prevalence and penetrance of HNPCC gene mutations is clearly defined unless mutations in each of the other mismatch repair genes has been excluded by sequencing in an affected individual. While it is possible to be confident of the gene of major effect in large HNPCC families because linkage can be established with a high degree of certainty, the smaller families are of greater concern. It is possible that a causative mutation in (say) *hMSH*2 could be identified and non-carriers then reassured inappropriately while they **actually** carry a mutation in *hMLH*1. Such a possibility demands extreme caution before widespread introduction of genetic screening for HNPCC. It would seem wise to counsel at-risk individuals who are shown to be non-gene carriers in smaller families where the causative mutation has been identified in affected individuals but to recommend that colonoscopic and uterine screening continues.

The possibility of an *hMLH*1- and *hMSH*2-pairing also has intriguing implications for the DNA repair pathway of the progeny of such a pairing. It is possible that the *hMLH*1-/ *hMSH*2- genotype may be lethal, but all the evidence suggests that there is no effect of heterozygous inactivation of either gene and that homozygous inactivation is required for tumour formation [47]. In addition, MLH1/ PMS1 double mutants in yeast have very similar phenotypes to either MLH1 or PMS1 single mutant [43–45]. Clearly such individuals carrying such a genotype would be at risk of HNPCC-related cancers. It is also exciting to speculate that such a genotype may have a dramatic effect on repeat sequences in the germline on such double mutant gene carriers. Expansion of repeated sequences is known to cause disease such as Huntington's disease and Fragile X and perhaps it is passage through the germline of such a gene carrier, or even of the germline of a single mutant, that causes the expansion of triplet repeats characteristic of such genetic disorders.

21.3.2 MISMATCH REPAIR DEFECTS IN HUMANS AND DNA INSTABILITY IN TUMOURS

Tumours from HNPCC gene carriers exhibit a characteristic alteration in the stability of repetitive tract DNA [40, 48, 49]. There are dramatic variations in size of repeat sequences (predominantly poly CA and poly A) throughout the genome in the tumour DNA. However, such changes are also detectable in around one in six of apparently sporadic colorectal cancers [39–41, 50]. Such 'sporadic' tumours with microsatellite instability tend to be right-sided, diploid, with an inverse relationship with *TP*53 mutation and to be associated with a strong family history of colorectal cancer. Surprisingly, there is no age difference between patients with tumours exhibiting microsatellite instability and those that do not [39, 50]. The inverse relationship between microsatellite instability and aneuploidy and *TP*53 mutation is very suggestive that one of two mechanisms of genomic instability are required in colorectal cancer. One involves defects in mismatch repair in diploid cells while the other involves *TP*53 mutation and the development of aneuploidy [51].

Although it is possible that some tumours with microsatellite instability arise because of double somatic mutations of DNA repair genes, it seems likely that a substantial proportion of patients with such tumours will carry constitutional HNPCC gene mutations. Identification of microsatellite instability in tumours on a prospective basis from the general population may be a practical means of identification of HNPCC gene carriers. All tumours from patients with proven germline mismatch repair gene defects have microsatellite instability [49]. Hence by employing an initial screen of all colorectal cancers coming into pathology departments for microsatellite instability, screening of the entire population of colorectal cancer cases for mismatch repair gene defects may well become a practical possibility.

The detection of microsatellite instability in endometrial cancer [52] and in a number of cancers of different tissue origin in HNPCC gene carriers [49] is of great interest as it demonstrates that the underlying HNPCC gene mutation is indeed responsible for the mutator phenotype. In addition it has been shown that microsatellite instability occurs in tumours from patients with multiple different primary cancers [53], suggesting that such individuals may well carry DNA repair gene mutations, even without a family history of cancer.

The human mismatch repair system appears to be similar to that in yeast with MSH, MLH and PMS homologues. A human homologue of the *E. coli* MutH gene has not been detected in either humans or in yeast. Mismatch repair involves recognition and binding of mismatches by MSH2. The correct strand for excision is recognised by the fact that nascent DNA is transiently under-methylated. MLH and PMS then appear to work in concert to excise a segment of DNA some 1–2 kb in length which is then repaired by a DNA polymerase. There may well be further mismatch repair systems. One such candidate is a nucleotide-specific mismatch repair system which recognizes G·T mismatches [55]. Such a system is of great interest since G·T mismatches will result in a C→T transition if allowed to progress through mitosis. Such transitions are frequently seen in the *APC* gene in colorectal tumours in addition to short deletions or insertions at repetitive sequences. Hence this opens the intriguing possibility that many of the somatic changes that are involved in the very genesis of colorectal cancer and indeed of FAP are caused by defects in mismatch repair.

The possibility that mismatch repair defects are causal in colorectal carcinogenesis is also supported by the finding that microsatellite instability is detectable in early adenomas in patients carrying HNPCC gene mutations [49]. In addition, colorectal cancer cell lines which exhibit microsatellite instability (and hence are assumed to have a defect in mismatch repair) have been shown to have a continuing defect in mismatch repair with progressive alterations in repetitive tracts [47, 55, 56]. The data also strongly support the notion that the change occurs early in the neoplastic process [55]. Although loss of heterozygosity at the *hMSH*2 or chromosome 3p locus is rare [40], second somatic inactivating mutations have been identified in tumours from patients with germline mutations in *hMSH*2 and *hMLH*1 [33, 35].

The finding that a lymphoblastoid cell line from a patient with HNPCC was repair-proficient [47] is suggestive that homozygous inactivation of a DNA repair gene is required for tumour formation. However, as discussed above there is a phenotype for heterozygous carriers since abnormal colonic crypt cell production rate and DNA repair has been reported in the apparently normal colorectal mucosa of affected and at-risk HNPCC family members [29, 30]. Only one HNPCC lymphoblastoid cell line has been examined for DNA repair proficiency and so it remains an interesting possibility that HNPCC gene carriers do have a low level of instability in the normal colorectal mucosa and in other tissues which is manifest in subtle ways such as alteration in cell turnover.

Much work remains to be done in understanding the effects of HNPCC gene mutations in carcinogenesis, their effect on mutation rate in the homozygous and heterozygous state, on population gene frequency, penetrance and the question of other DNA repair systems which may be involved in heritable predisposition to colorectal cancer. With the rapid technical advances in molecular biology and the availability of commercial sequence databases, it seems likely that much progress will be made in HNPCC in the foreseeable future.

21.3.3 THE *DCC* (DELETED IN COLON CANCER) GENE

The location of a tumour suppressor gene on chromosome 18q was first indicated by the demonstration of frequent deletions involving that region in colorectal cancer tissue by tumour cytogenetic studies. Further molecular genetic studies detected frequent allele loss on 18q, occurring in approximately 80% of colorectal cancers and 50% of large adenomas [57]. The region 18q21-qter was identified as the common area of allele loss. A rearrangement involving a relatively small deletion in a single cancer indicated the position of the gene from which point chromosomal walking resulted in the isolation of a 1.2Mb gene which was named the *DCC* gene (for deleted in colon cancer) [59]. *DCC* comprises a 12.5 kb transcript which is expressed at low level in many tissues including normal colonic mucosa, but it is reduced or absent in colorectal cancer tissue. This strongly suggests that the *DCC* gene is indeed a tumour suppressor gene involved in colorectal tumourigenesis. Further evidence for tumour suppressor activity of *DCC* was demonstrated by the introduction of normal chromosome 18 into a human colon cancer cell line with resultant suppression of tumourigenicity [59].

Inactivating *DCC* mutations or loss of one gene copy by allele loss occurs frequently in colorectal cancer tissue and, given the paradigm of the *APC* gene, it is also possible that constitutional *DCC* mutations may predispose to colorectal cancer. There is some evidence to suggest *DCC* may be involved in colorectal cancer predisposition. One large pedigree exhibited genetic linkage of the Kidd blood group with a dominant non-polyposis trait manifest as colorectal cancer at a young age of onset [60]. The Kidd blood group has been shown to map to a region very close to *DCC* on chromosme 18q. However, published data [62] and our own unpublished findings have not detected any evidence for linkage of intragenic *DCC* markers in a number of HNPCC kindreds. However, it is possible that *DCC* is a colorectal cancer susceptibility locus in a minority of families. It will be of great interest to carry out further analysis of *DCC* in HNPCC families who are shown not to be linked to the mismatch repair loci on chromosomes 2, 3 and 7.

The involvement of *DCC* in colorectal cancer susceptibility remains to be clarified but it seems certain that if this gene is involved at all in genetic predisposition to colorectal cancer, only a minority of families carry a constitutional *DCC* mutation. Due to its large size, the impracticalities of screening the entire *DCC* gene for mutations have mitigated against direct mutation analysis but as more efficient mutation detection methods become available, this may become a realistic proposition for those families who do not carry mismatch repair gene mutations.

21.3.4 THE *TP*53 GENE

The involvement of the *TP*53 gene in colorectal carcinogenesis is now becoming well understood. Normal *TP*53 is a nuclear phosphoprotein which functions as a transcription regulator with sequence specific DNA binding sites. Alterations to *TP*53 function by loss of heterozygosity involving the region of chromosome 17p where *TP*53 is located occurs in around 75% of colonic carcinomas while 17p allele loss is rare in even relatively advanced adenomas [58]. Many colorectal carcinomas contain *TP*53 missense mutations in addition to *TP*53 allele loss and it is clear that expression of both wild-type and mutant *TP*53 mRNA can occur [63]. The data suggest that mutated *TP*53 alleles may act in a dominant-negative fashion. This could occur either by binding of mutated protein to wild-type protein, therefore preventing access to its receptor molecules or by altering its overall conformation. Clearly, because of its well established role in carcinogenesis, *TP*53 is a candidate colorectal cancer susceptibility gene. *TP*53 mutations have been shown to be responsible for the rare, autosomal dominant Li–Fraumeni syndrome [63 see Chapter 8] which is characterized by predisposition to a variety of cancers including brain tumours, breast carcinomas, soft tissue sarcomas, leukaemia, osteosarcomas and adrenocortical carcinomas. However, colorectal cancer is very rare in Li–Fraumeni gene carriers. We have studied the role of *TP*53 in colorectal cancer susceptibility in a group of 35 unrelated patients who developed colorectal cancer at a very young age, many of whom are part of HNPCC kindreds [63]. Despite screening *TP*53 for mutations using a highly sensitive mutation detection technique, we did not detect any constitutional *TP*53 mutations.

Hence, it seems highly unlikely that *TP*53 mutations confer susceptibility to colorectal cancer despite frequent abnormalities of *TP*53 in somatic colorectal cancer tissue.

21.3.5 THE *RAS* GENES

Activated proto-oncogenes have been shown to play a major role in many human cancers. The *RAS* family gene family are cytoplasmic proto-oncogenes with signal transduction functions and have been shown to be commonly activated in colorectal neoplasms. *ras* mutations, particularly Kirsten *RAS*, have been demonstrated in 50% of colorectal carcinomas and in a similar proportion of sporadic adenomas over 1 cm [57]. The frequency of *RAS* mutations is much lower in adenomas <1 cm while recent evidence has associated k-*RAS* mutations with histologic dysplasia but does not appear to precede the formation of adenomas, being involved in the progression of adenoma to carcinoma [64]. It also appears that *RAS* expression, although high in primary carcinomas, tends to be lower in the more pathologically advanced cases, indicating that when the tumour progresses to a certain stage, then *RAS* activation is no longer required.

Clearly the *RAS* family of genes are candidate colorectal cancer susceptibility genes. There have been a number of studies which have examined the apparent association of rare Harvey *RAS* alleles with various cancers. However, the association was not upheld until a recent study examined a *H-RAS* minisatellite locus and also carried out a metanalysis of all published literature on the association of rare H-*RAS* alleles with cancer [65]. The authors propose from their findings that 1 in 11 colorectal cancers occur as a result of inheritance of a predisposing *RAS* allele. These data clearly require confirmation, but *RAS* alleles may indeed represent one of a number of genetic factors involved in polygenic inherited colorectal cancer susceptibility which does not involve the mismatch repair loci.

21.4 PRACTICAL IMPLICATIONS FOR THE DISCOVERY OF COLORECTAL CANCER SUSCEPTIBILITY GENES

All available data suggest that colorectal cancer is preventable by removal of premalignant polyps. Survival is undoubtedly related to the time of clinical presentation with respect to the natural history of the tumour. Both of these factors indicate that if individuals who carry a colorectal cancer susceptibility allele could be identified and were to undergo colonoscopic screening, mortality from cancer death in families with familial large bowel cancer would be dramatically reduced. The risk may be so high in some patients that prophylactic colectomy is offered to some family members. Molecular genetic screening is already underway in FAP kindreds [66, 67] and has already influenced clincal screening protocols. Now that a number of HNPCC genes have been identified, and causative mutations characterized, a similar effect on clinical screening in these families can be expected.

With the advent of transgenic technology it has already been possible to generate animal models of FAP and similar techniques will undoubtedly be employed to create transgenic animals with mutator gene defects. These animals will allow study of gene function, of regulatory elements and of the influence of modifier genes on colorectal cancer susceptibility. It will be possible to develop novel preventive treatment regimes with the use of transgenic animals. Already such studies are underway in the Min 1 mouse using non-steroidal anti-inflammatory agents in view of the known effect of such agents on reducing colorectal cancer risk [68] and in causing polyp regression in FAP patients [69]. Given the enormity of the problem of colorectal cancer throughout the industrialized world, there will no doubt be intense commercial interest in the development of chemopreventive agents using transgenic animals as the test system.

The rapid progress in understanding of colorectal carcinogenesis seems set to continue. Molecular genetic studies seem set to radically alter our approach by targetting screening to those at high risk of the disease and allowing the development of agents that will prevent the disease which for so long has resisted the best efforts of medical research.

Within recent months, further advances have been made in understanding the role of DNA mismatch repair in colorectal carcinogenesis. A new component of mismatch repair has been identified as a GT binding protein (GTBP) [70–72] and it has become clear that some patients with germline mismatch repair gene mutations are prone to develop mutations in normal tissues [73].

REFERENCES

1. Lynch, H.T., Smryk, T.C., Watson, P. *et al.* (1993) Genetics, natural history, tumor spectrum, and pathology of hereditary nonpolyposis colorectal cancer: an updated review. *Gastroenterology*, **104**, 1535–49.
2. Bonelli, L., Martines, H., Conio, M. *et al.* (1988) Family history of colorectal cancer as a risk factor for benign and malignant tumours of the large bowel. A case control study. *Int. J. Cancer*, **41**, 513–17.
3. Cannon-Albright, L.A., Solnick, M.H., Bishop, D.T. *et al.* (1988) Common inheritance of susceptibility to colonic adenomatous polyps and associated colorectal cancers. *N. Engl. J. Med.*, **319**, 533–7.
4. Bodmer, W.F., Bailey, C.J., Bodmer, J. *et al.* (1987) Localisation of the gene for familial adenomatous polyposis on chromosome 5. *Nature*, **328**, 614–6.
5. Leppert, M., Dobbs, M., Scambler, P. *et al.* (1987) The gene for familial polyposis maps to the long arm of chromosome 5. *Science*, **238**, 1411–13.
6. Kinzler, K.W., Nilbert, M.C., Su, L-K. *et al.*

(1991) Identification of FAP locus genes from chomosome 5q21. *Science*, **253**, 661–4.

7. Joslyn, L., Carlson, M., Thliveris, A. *et al.* (1991) Identification of deletion mutations and three new genes at the Familial Polyposis locus. *Cell*, **66**, 601–13.

8. Groden, J., Thliveris, A., Samowitz, W. *et al.* (1991) Identification and characterization of the Familial Adenomatous Polyposis Coli gene. *Cell*, **66**, 589–600.

9. Miyoshi, Y., Ando, H., Nagase, H. *et al.* (1992) Germ-line mutations of the *APC* gene in 53 familial adenomatous polyposis patients. *Proc. Natl. Acad. Sci. USA*, **89**, 4452–6.

10. Nagase, H., Miyoshi, Y., Horii, A. *et al.* (1992) Screening for germ-line mutations in familial adenomatous polyposis patients: 61 new patients and a summary of 150 unrelated patients. *Hum. Mutat.*, **1**, 467–73.

11. Nagase, H. and Nakamura, Y. (1993) Mutations of the *APC* (adenomatous polyposis coli) gene. *Hum. Mutat.*, **2**, 425–34.

12. Mandl, M., Paffenholz, R., Friedl, W. *et al.* (1994) Frequency of common and novel inactivating *APC* mutations in 202 families with familial adenomatous polyposis. *Hum. Mol. Genet.*, **3**, 181–4.

13. Smith, K.J., Johnson, K.A., Bryan, T.M. *et al.* (1993) The *APC* gene product in normal and tumour cells. *Proc. Natl. Acad. Sci. USA*, **90**, 2846–50.

14. Rubinfeld, B., Souza, B., Albert, I. *et al.* (1993) Association of the *APC* gene product with b-catenin. *Science*, **262**, 1731–4.

15. Su, L.-K., Vogelstein, B. and Kinzler, K. (1993) Association of the APC tumour suppressor protein with catenins. *Science*, **262**, 1734–7.

16. Munemitsu, S., Souza, B., Muller, O. *et al.* (1994) The *APC* gene product associates with microtubules *in vivo* and promotes their assembly *in vitro*. *Cancer Res.*, **54**, 3676–81.

17. Smith, K.J., Levy, D.B., Maupin, P. *et al.* (1994) Wild-type but not mutant APC associates with microtubule cytoskeleton. *Cancer Res.*, **54**, 3672–5.

18. Moser, A.R., Pitot, H.C. and Dove, W.F. (1990) A dominant mutation that predisposes to multiple intestinal neoplasia in the mouse. *Science*, **247**, 322–4.

19. Su, L.-K., Kinzler, K.W., Vogelstein, B *et al.*

(1992) Multiple intestinal neoplasia caused by a mutation in the murine homolog of the *APC* gene. *Science*, **256**, 668–70.

20. Moser, A.R., Dove, W.F., Roth, K.A., *et al.* (1992) The *Min* (Multiple Intestinal Neoplasia) Mutation: its effect on gut epithelial cell differentiation and interaction with a modifier system. *J. Cell Biol.*, **116** (6) 1517–26.

21. Cottrell, S., Bicknell, D., Kaklamanis, L. *et al.* (1992) Molecular analysis of *APC* mutations in familial adenomatous polyposis and sporadic colon carcinomas. *Lancet*, **340**, 626–30.

22. Olschang, S., Laurent-Puig, P., Groden, J. *et al.* (1993) Germ-line mutations in the first 14 exons of the adenomatous polyposis coli (*APC*) gene. *Am. J. Hum. Genet.*, **52**, 273–9.

23. Groden, J., Gelbert, L., Thliveris, A. *et al.* (1993) Mutational analysis of patients with adenomatous polyposis: identical inactivating mutations in unrelated individuals. *Am. J. Hum. Genet.*, **52**, 263–72.

24. Nagase, H., Miyoshi, Y., Horii, A. *et al.* (1992) Correlation between the location of germ-line mutations in the *APC* gene and the number of colorectal polyps in familial adenomatous polyposis patients. *Cancer Res.*, **52**, 4055–7.

25. Su, L-K., Johnson, K.A., Smith, K.J. *et al.* (1993). Association between wild-type and mutant *APC* gene products. *Cancer Res.* **53**, 2728–31.

26. Paul, P., Letteboer, T., Gelbert, L. *et al.* (1993) Identical *APC* exon 15 mutations result in a variable phenotype in familial adenomatous polyposis. *Hum. Mol. Genet.* **2**, 925–31.

27. Lynch, H.T., Kimberling, W.J., Albano, W.A. *et al.* (1985) Hereditary nonpolyposis colorectal cancer (Lynch Syndromes 1 and 2).1.Clinical description of resource. *Cancer*, **56**, 934–8.

28. Vasen, H.F.A., Mecklin, J-P., Meera–Khan, P. *et al.* (1991). The International Collaborative Group on Hereditary Non-Polyposis Colorectal Cancer (ICG–HNPCC). *Dis. Colon Rectum*, **34**, 424–25.

29. Lipkin, N., Blattner, W.E., Fraumeni, J.F. *et al.* (1983) Tritiated thymidine labelling distribution as a marker for hereditary predisposition to colon cancer. *Cancer Res.* **43**, 1899–904.

30. Gerdes, H., Gillin, J.S., Zimbalist, E. *et al.* (1993) Expansion of the epithlial cell proliferative compartment and frequency of adenoma-

tous polyps in the colon correlate with the strength of family history of colorectal cancer. *Cancer Res.*, **53**, 279–82.

31. Jenson, O.M., Bolander, A.M., Sigtryggsson, P. *et al.* (1980) Large-bowel cancer in married couples in Sweden. A follow-up study. *Lancet*, **1**, 1161–3.

32. Fishel, R., Lescoe, M.K., Rao, M.R.S. *et al.* (1993) The human mutator gene homolog *MSH2* and its association with hereditary nonpolyposis colon cancer. *Cell*, **75**, 1027–38.

33. Leach, F.S., Nicolaides, N.C., Papadopolous, N. *et al.* (1993) Mutations of a *MutS* homolog in hereditary non-polyposis colorectal cancer. *Cell*, **75**, 1215–25.

34. Bronner, C.E., Baker, S.M., Morrison, P.T. *et al.* (1994) Mutation in the DNA mismatch repair gene homologue *hMLH1* is associated with hereditary non-polyposis colon cancer. *Nature*, **368**, 258–61.

35. Papadopolous, N., Nicolaides, N.C., Wei, Y-F. *et al.* (1994) Mutation of a *mutL* homolog in hereditary colon cancer. *Science*, **263**, 1625–9.

36. Nicolaides, N.C., Papadopoulos, N., Wei, Y.F., *et al.* (1994) Mutations of two *PMS* homologues in hereditary nonpolyposis colon cancer. *Nature*, **371**, 75–80.

37. Peltomaki, L., Aaltonen, L.A., Sistonen, P. *et al.* (1993) Genetic mapping of a locus predisposing to human colorectal cancer. *Science*, **260**, 810–12.

38. Lindblom, A., Tannergard, P., Werelius, B. and Nordenskjold, M. (1993) Genetic mapping of a second locus predisposing to hereditary non-polyposis colon cancer. *Nature Genet.*, **5**, 279–82.

39. Ionov, Y., Peinado, M.A., Malkhosyan, S. *et al.* (1993) Ubiquitous somatic mutations in simple repeated sequences reveal a new mechanism for colonic carcinogenesis. *Nature*, **363**, 558–61.

40. Aaltonen, L.A., Peltomaki, P., Leach, F.S. *et al.* (1993) Clues to the pathogenesis of familial colorectal cancer. *Science*, **260**, 812–16.

41. Thibodeau, S.N., Bren, G. and Schaid, D. (1993) Microsatellite instability in cancer of the proximal colon. *Science*, **260**, 816–19.

42. Grilley, M., Holmes, J., Yashar, B. and Modrich, P. (1990) Mechanisms of DNA-mismatch correction. *Mutat. Res.*, **26**, 253–67.

43. Prolla, T.A., Christie, D-M. and Liskay, R.M. (1994) Dual requirement in yeast DNA mismatch repair for MLH1 and PMS1, two homologs of bacterial *MutL* gene. *Mol. Cell. Biol.*, **14**, 407–15.

44. Prolla, T.A., Pang, Q., Alani, E. *et al.* (1994) MLH1, PMS1 and MSH2 interactions during the initiation of DNA mismatch repair in yeast. *Nature*, **365**, 1091–3.

45. Strand, M., Prolla, T.A., Liskay, R.M. *et al.* (1993) Destabilization of tracts of simple repetitive DNA in yeasts by mutations affecting DNA mismatch repair. *Nature*, **365**, 274–6.

46. Liu, B., Parsons, R.E., Hamilton, S.R. *et al.* (1994) h*MSH*2 mutations in hereditary nonpolyposis colorectal cancer kindreds. *Cancer Res.*, **54**, 4590–4.

47. Parsons, R.E., Li, G.-M., Longley, M.J. *et al.* (1993) Hypermutability and mismatch repair deficiency in RER+ tumour cells. *Cell*, **75**, 1227–36.

48. Peltomaki, P., Lothe, R.A., Aaltonen, L.A. *et al.* (1993) Microsatellite instability is associated with tumours that characterize the hereditary non-polyposis colorectal carcinoma syndrome. *Cancer Res.* **53**, 5853–5.

49. Aaltonen, L.A., Peltomaki, P. and Mecklin, J.-P. (1994) Replication errors in benign and malignant tumours from hereditary non-polyposis colorectal cancer patients. *Cancer Res.*, **54**, 1645–8.

50. Lothe, R.A., Peltomaki, P., Meling, G.I. *et al.* (1993) Genomic instability in colorectal cancer: relationship to clinicopathological variables and family history. *Cancer Res.*, **53**, 5849–52.

51. Carder, P., Wyllie, A.H., Purdie, C.A. *et al.* (1993) Stabilised p53 facilitates aneuploid clonal divergence in colorectal cancer. *Oncogene*, **8**, 1397–401.

52. Risinger J.I., Berchuck, A., Kohler, M.F. *et al.* (1993) Genetic instability of microsatellites in endometrial carcinoma. *Cancer Res.*, **53**, 5100–3.

53. Horii, A., Han, H.-J., Shimada, M. *et al.* (1994) Frequent replication errors at microsatellite loci in tumrs of patients with multiple primary cancers. *Cancer Res.*, **54**, 3373–82.

54. Wiebauer, K.M. and Jiricny, J. (1990) Mismatch-specific thymine DNA glysosylase and DNA polymerase B mediate the correction of G.T mispairs in nuclear extracts from

human cells. *Proc. Natl. Acad. Sci. USA*, **87**, 5842–5.

55. Shibata, D., Peinado, M.A., Ionov, Y. *et al.* (1994) Genomic instability in repeated sequences is an early somatic event in colorectal tumorigenesis that persists after transformation. *Nature Genet.*, **6**, 273–81.

56. Bhattacharyya, N.P., Skandalis, A., Groden, J. and Meuth, M. (1994) Mutator phenotypes in human colorectal carcinoma cell lines. *Proc. Natl Acad. Sci. USA*, **91**, 6319–23.

57. Vogelstein, B., Fearon, E.R., Hamilton, S.R. *et al.* (1988) Genetic alterations during colorectal tumour development. *N. Engl. J. Med.*, **319**, 525–32.

58. Fearon, E.R., Cho, K.R., Nigro, J.M. *et al.* (1990) Identification of a chromosome 18q gene that is altered in colorectal cancers. *Science*, **247**, 49–56.

59. Tanaka, K., Oshimura, M., Kikuchi, R. *et al.* (1991) Suppression of tumourigenicity in human colon carcinoma cells by introduction of normal chromosome 5 or 18. *Nature*, **349**, 340–2.

60. Lynch, H.T., Schuelke, G.S., Kimberling, W.J. *et al.* (1985) Hereditary non-polyposis colorectal cancer (Lynch Syndromes 1 and 2): 2. Biomarker studies. *Cancer*, **56**, 939–51.

61. Peltomaki, P., Sistonen, P., Mecklin, J.-P., *et al.* (1991) Evidence supporting exclusion of the *DCC* gene and a portion of chromosome 18q as the locus for susceptibility to hereditary non-polyposis colorectal carcinomas in five kindreds. *Cancer Res.*, **51**, 4135–40.

62. Nigro, J.M., Baker, S.J., Preisinger, A.C. *et al.* (1989) Mutations in the p53 gene occur in diverse human tumour types. *Nature*, **342**, 705–8.

63. Bhagirath, T.H., Condie, A., Dunlop, M.G. *et al.* (1993) Exclusion of constitutional p53 mutations as a cause of genetic susceptibility to colorectal cancer. *Br. J. Cancer*, **68**, 712–14.

64. Shibata, O., Schaeffer, J., Li, Z.-H. *et al.* (1993) Genetic heterogeneity of c-K-*ras* locus in colorectal adenomas but not adenocarcinomas. *J. Natl Cancer Inst.*, **85**, 1058–63.

65. Krontiris, T.G., Devlin, B., Karp, D.D. *et al.* (1989) An association between the risk of cancer and mutations in the HRAS1 minisatellite locus. *N. Engl. J. Med.*, **329**, 517–23.

66. Petersen, G.M., Francomano, C., Kinzler, K. *et al.* (1993) Presymptomatic direct detection of adenomatous polyposis coli (*APC*) gene mutations in familial adenomatous polyposis. *Hum. Genet.*, **91**, 307–11.

67. Maher, E.R., Barton, D.E., Slatter, R. *et al.* (1993) Evaluation of molecular genetic diagnosis in the management of familial adenomatous polyposis coli: a population based study. *J. Med. Genet.*, **30**, 675–8.

68. Thun, M.J., Namboodiri, M.M. and Heath, C.W. (1991) Aspirin use and reduced risk of fatal colon cancer. *N. Engl. J. Med.*, **325**, 1593–6.

69. Giardiello, F.M., Hamilton, S.R., Krush, A.J., *et al.* (1993) Treatment of colonic and rectal adenomas with sulindac in familial adenomatous polyposis. *N. Engl. J. Med.*, **328**, 1313–16.

70. Drummond, J.T., Li, G-M., Longley, M.J. *et al.* (1995) Isolation of an hMSH2-p160 heterodimer that restores DNA mismatch repair to tumor cells. *Science*, **268**, 1909–12.

71. Palombo, F., Galtiari, P., Laccarino, I. *et al.* (1995) GTBP, a 160 kilodalton protein essential for mismatch-binding activity in human cells. *Science*, **268**, 1912–15.

72. Papadopoulos, N., Nicolaides, N.C., Liu, B. *et al.* (1995) Mutations of GTBP in genetically unstable cells. *Science*, **268**, 1915–17.

73. Parsons, R., Li, G-M., Longley, M.J. *et al.* (1995) Mismatch repair deficiency in phenotypically normal human cells. *Science*, **268**, 738–40.

Chapter 22

Familial prostate cancer and its management

ROSALIND A. EELES and LISA CANNON-ALBRIGHT

22.1 INTRODUCTION

Prostate cancer is a significant public health problem. There are 10 180 cases per year in England and Wales, and 8098 deaths [1]. In the US, it is the most common malignancy and the second most common cause of cancer deaths, with 200 000 cases per year and 44 000 deaths [2]. It has been estimated that 5–10% of breast cancer is due to an autosomal dominant gene [3]; if the same applied for prostate cancer, at least 500 prostate cases per year in England and Wales, and 10 000 in the US would be gene carriers. Furthermore, the incidence of the disease is increasing by 10–20% every 5 years [4].

The disease is usually asymptomatic until it is advanced. In the UK, where there is no widespread screening programme, the disease has often metastasized at presentation. Only 13% of cases localized to the pelvis, treated at The Royal Marsden Hospital, UK from 1970–89 presented with stage T1 disease confined to the prostate. Even in the US, where there has been a greater emphasis on earlier detection in the past few years, at least 40% of cases currently have metastases at presentation. This proportion may decrease as screening becomes more widespread. The 5-year survival rate for all stages is 55–78% depending on the series reported, but for T1 overall is 74–95% [5], the higher grade tumours having the lower survival rate. The improved survival in earlier stage disease provides a rationale for early detection. However, the argument against screening the general population is that large numbers of men would have to be screened to detect a few cancers, for example, male general population prostate-specific antigen screening detects cancer in about 2–4% of those screened [6]. If a predisposition gene or genes could be characterized, then men at increased risk of prostate cancer could be identified and offered targetted screening and prevention.

22.2 EVIDENCE FOR A GENETIC PREDISPOSITION TO PROSTATE CANCER

The first piece of evidence that prostate cancer may be familial in some instances is the observed clustering of cases, the best examples being the large high-risk Utah

Genetic Predisposition to Cancer. Edited by R.A. Eeles, B.A.J. Ponder, D.F. Easton and A. Horwich. Published in 1996 by Chapman & Hall, London.
0 412 56580 3

kindreds (Figure 22.1) [7]. Woolf [8] first described an increased incidence of prostate cancer in the relatives of cases. He studied the incidence of prostate cancer in the first-degree relatives (fathers and brothers) of 228 individuals with prostate cancer in the Utah population and age-matched controls. Using death certificate data, he found that first-degree relatives of prostate cancer cases had a relative risk of 3 of developing prostate cancer. This is similar to the relative risks seen in the other common cancers where there is a recognized genetic component.

There have been two types of study to demonstrate an increased risk of prostate cancer in relatives of cases. The relative risk values in first-degree relatives of cases range from 3–11 when rates of first-degree relatives are compared between cases and controls. When family history of cases is compared with family history of controls, the relative risk estimates range from 0.64–7.5. Only one study [13] reported to date shows a reduced relative risk in relatives, and it only consisted of 39 cases. These studies are summarized in Table 22.1.

22.3 STUDIES OF FAMILIAL PROSTATE CANCER IN THE UTAH POPULATION

Utah has a 1.2-times increased rate of prostate cancer when compared with the rest of the US [18]. Studies of familial cancer in Utah have been revolutionized by three data sources: the genealogy records of the church of Jesus Christ of Latter Day Saints (LDS, or Mormon) computerized by Skolnick, the Utah SEER Cancer Registry, and the Utah Death Certificates. Together, these data comprise the Utah Population Data Base or UPDB [19].

Genealogical work is central to membership in the LDS church. Pioneers from much of Northern Europe emigrated to the US in the 19th century, and persecution drove them West in the US, until they came to the Salt Lake valley in Utah, and built Salt Lake City. This is now the centre for the LDS church, and houses the Family History Library, which was started in 1894. Each family compiles family group sheets and the library contains 8 million of these. All those family group sheets containing at least one birth or death date in Utah or along the pioneer Western trail were obtained from the society and formed the basis of the Utah Genealogical Database [19] in the 1970s. The data containing 185 000 families (1.5 million individuals) have been computerized and all individuals linked into a genealogy representing the Utah descendants of the Mormon pioneers. The relatives of a given individual in this population can therefore be traced.

The Utah Cancer Registry was made statewide in 1966, and in 1973 became one of eleven population-based registries of the Surveillance, Epidemiology and End Results (SEER) Program of the National Cancer Institute in America. The registry maintains abstracts of clinical records and follow-up data on all cancer cases in the state. The Utah death certificates have been computerized for all individuals who have died since 1955. The computerized genealogy, death records and Cancer Registry have been linked to create the Utah Population Database (UPDB).

The advantage of this population for genetic studies is that early polygamy (occurring in 10–20% of the male pioneers until 1890), high fertility, low non-paternity and a high degree of cooperation, has resulted in very large, well-documented, extended families. The gene pool is large because the original Mormon pioneers were unrelated and numerous. Many Mormons have remained in Utah, and those that have migrated are still often traceable through family reunions, a Mormon custom. The genetic make-up is

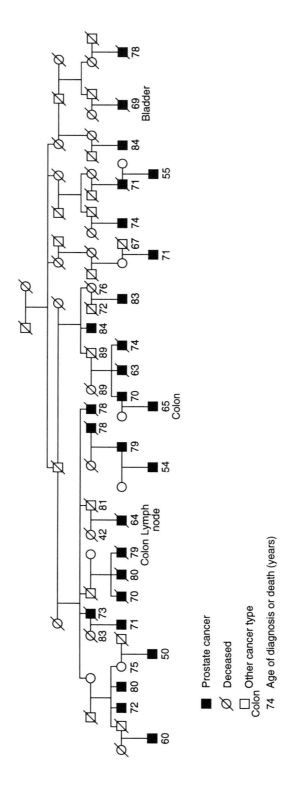

Fig. 22.1 Example of one of the large Utah pedigrees. (Courtesy of Dr Cannon-Albright.)

■ Prostate cancer

⊘ Deceased

□ Other cancer type

74 Age of diagnosis or death (years)

Table 22.1 Evidence for genetic predisposition to prostate cancer

Reference	No. of cases	No. of cases in first-degree relatives of cases	No. of cases in first-degree relatives of controls	Relative risk
[9][1]	183	11	1	11
[8][2]	228	15	5	3
[10][1]	221	12	2	6
[11][1]	382	58	31	3.2
[7][2]	2824	GI	GI	2.4
[12][2]	150	11	1	4 (at age 80)
		(brothers only)		16.6 (at age <49)

Reference	No. of cases	Cases with positive family history (%)	Controls with positive family history (%)	
[13][1]	39	12.8	20.0	0.64
[14][1]	40	16.7	7.3	2.3
[15][1]	691	15.0	8.0	1.9
[16][1]	378	13.0	5.7	2.3
[17][1]	140	15.0	2.0	7.5

[1] Information from patient/control questionnaire only.
[2] Diagnosis verified by hospital records, cancer registration or death certificate.
GI, genealogical index measured – see text for details.

very similar to that of Northern Europeans, as has been shown from gene frequency studies [20] and due to a continued influx of immigrants, there are normal levels of inbreeding [21].

22.3.1 GENEALOGICAL INDEX

The genealogical index (GI) measure of familiality has been used on the UPDB data to assess the relationship between a pair of individuals. All cases of a particular cancer are considered and the degree of relatedness between the affected individuals is measured. The degree of relatedness is quantified by the Malecot coefficient of kinship [22]. This expresses the probability that randomly selected homologous genes from two individuals are identical by descent from a common ancestor. In the absence of inbreeding, it is calculated in integral powers of 1/2 (the power of 1/2 is the kinship exponent). For example, for siblings, since there are two genetic steps between them, the coefficient is $(1/2)^2$; for uncle–nephew, it is $(1/2)^3$, with kinship exponents 2 and 3 respectively. Tens of thousands of pairs of cases are analysed to assess the kinship components, and these are then averaged to obtain a figure for the disease site. This figure is called the genealogical index (GI) and is expressed as a figure ($\times 10^{-5}$). In 1982, Cannon *et al.* [7] measured the GI in prostate cancer cases traceable back to a common ancestor in the UPDB. The GI was 2.57 for prostate cancer cases and only 1.45 for controls. This excess familiality extended out to seventh-degree relatives,

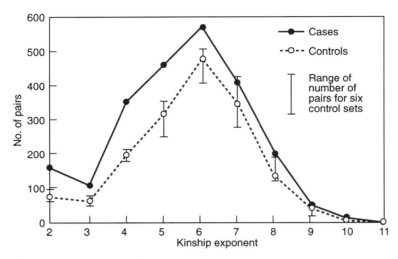

Fig. 22.2 Kinship distribution of prostate cancer showing statistically significant excess familiality in cases extending to seventh-degree relatives.

many of whom will not even know each other, indicating that it is likely that a common gene has predisposed to these cancers in distantly related relatives (Figure 22.2). A potential bias that cases within the UPDB have more complete information than controls was excluded by studying internal controls.

This analysis has recently been updated using 41 940 Cancer Registry records linked to the UPDB genealogy [23]. The GI is more recently termed the GIF for genealogical index of familiality. Of the common cancers, prostate cancer is one of the most familial (case GIF of 3.70 versus 2.76 in controls, $P=0.00$). It is surpassed by melanoma (4.06 versus 2.64) and is followed by colon cancer (3.53 versus 2.76) and breast cancer (3.23 versus 2.73), all these latter case GIFs being statistically in excess of controls. Both breast and colon cancer, which have lower GIFs, are recognized to have a genetic component. Younger prostate cases had a higher GIF than older cases (≤69 years: GIF 3.89 versus 3.76 for older cases, $P=0.00$).

22.4 EPIDEMIOLOGICAL EVIDENCE THAT THE INCREASED RISK TO RELATIVES IS A GENETIC EFFECT

The magnitude of the relative risks from most of the case-control studies suggest a genetic effect. The relative risk of prostate cancer due to other factors such as age at first marriage are all about 1.5, which is the level of risk from hormonal factors in breast cancer aetiology. All but one of the relative risk figures in the familial studies are higher than this, and all but two are higher than 2.0. The fact that an increased level of relatedness is present in the UPDB data even as distant as sixth- or seventh-degree relatives may suggest this, since such distant relatives would not even know each other. However, common environmental factors cannot be excluded.

The best evidence that there is a genetic effect is the fact that the relative risk markedly increases as the age of the proband decreases (Table 22.2), as the number of affecteds increases (Tables 22.3 and 22.4), or both (Table 22.5). The degree of this rise in risk cannot be explained solely by an environ-

Table 22.2 Relative odds for prostate cancer in brothers of prostate cancer cases by age. (From [7].)

Age of affected (years)	Age of brother (years)		
	<65	65–79	80+
<65	5.97**	2.77*	2.29
65–79	2.77*	2.04**	2.52*
80+	2.29	2.52*	1.14

*P<0.01; **P<0.001.

Table 22.3 Relative risks for prostate cancer in relatives of prostate cancer cases by degree of relationship. (From [15].)

Affected relatives	Relative risk (95% C.I.)
First-degree	2.0 (1.2–3.3)
Second-degree	1.7 (1.0–2.9)
First- and second-degree	8.8 (2.8–28.1)

Table 22.4 Age-adjusted relative risk estimates for prostate cancer by number of additional affected family members. (From [15].)

Affected relatives (besides proband)	Odds ratio (95% C.I.)
1	2.2 (1.4–3.5)
2	4.9 (2.0–12.3)
3	10.9 (2.7–43.1)

mental effect. The relative risk of prostate cancer if a first-degree relative is affected at less than 50 years of age is estimated to be 16.6 versus 4.0 if the affected relative is 80 at diagnosis, although the former estimate is based on very small numbers [12].

22.5 THE GENETIC MODEL

Segregation analysis has only been performed in one data set using nuclear families,

Table 22.5 Estimated risk ratios for prostate cancer in first-degree relatives of probands, by age at onset in proband and additional affected family members. (From [24].)

Age at onset of proband (years)	Risk ratio	
	No additional relatives affected	One or more additional first-degree relatives affected
50	1.9 (1.2–2.8)	7.1 (3.7–13.6)
60	1.4 (1.1–1.7)	5.2 (3.1–8.7)
70	1.0[1]	3.8 (2.4–6.0)

[1] Reference group. Hazard ratio is shown with 95% C.I. in brackets.

and suggests that familial prostate cancer is due to a rare highly penetrant dominant gene (gene frequency of 0.003) which causes 43% of cases by age 55, and 9% by age 80. The penetrance in carriers would be 88% by age 85 [24]. Until recently, all familial cancers were thought to be caused by tumour suppressor genes. Carcinogenesis in such cases arises following the Knudson two-hit hypothesis, where the first hit is inherited, and loss of the remaining normal or wild-type allele results in tumour development [25]. However, it is now thought that at least one familial syndrome (MEN 2) is caused by mutations in a dominant oncogene since loss of the normal allele does not occur at the predisposition locus in tumours (see Chapter 6). The mechanism of action of the prostate cancer-predisposition gene is unknown.

22.6 COAGGREGATION OF PROSTATE CANCER WITH OTHER CANCERS

A higher incidence of prostate cancer among male relatives of breast cancer patients has been reported [26]. Anderson and Badzioch [27] reported a doubling of familial breast cancer risk when prostate cancer was present in the family history. Male carriers of the *BRCA*1 gene also have a three-fold increased risk of prostate cancer [28]. Carter *et al.* [29] showed a significant association of prostate cancer with brain tumours.

Prostate cancer is also now considered to be part of the extended definition of the Li–Fraumeni syndrome. A study of relatives of cases of soft tissue sarcoma has shown that there is a 1.9 increased risk of prostate cancer in these relatives (95% C.I. 0.7–5.1) [30]. In Li–Fraumeni-like families, the incidence of germline mutations in the oncogene *TP*53 is about 10% [31], and although families with *TP*53 germline mutations which contain cases of prostate cancer have been described [32], this gene still has to be studied as a candidate for the cause of large familial prostate cancer kindreds.

22.7 THE SEARCH FOR GENE(S) PREDISPOSING TO FAMILIAL PROSTATE CANCER

The study of familial prostate cancer is complicated by the fact that there may be a high number of sporadic cases in families since prostate cancer is common. In addition, screen-detected prostate cancer may behave differently from symptomatic disease since 15–30% of men will have histological evidence of prostate cancer by the age of 50 as has been ascertained from post-mortem studies [33], but not all these progress to clinical disease. Men with a positive family history may be more likely to undergo screening, which may detect histological disease which would not progress.

To perform linkage analyses, several groups have been collecting nuclear families and have been trying to extend them to find further cases. Some of the most dramatic families are those from Utah. An ideal candidate gene would be the androgen receptor gene which is on Xq. From the Utah family

shown in Figure 22.1, however, it appears that male/male transmission of the disease can occur, so unless there are a high number of sporadics in this family, it is unlikely that the susceptibility gene in this family is on the X chromosome. Carter *et al.* [29] have shown the same phenomenon in some nuclear families. In other kindreds, maternal transmission excludes the Y chromosome as a site for the predisposition gene. To date, the susceptibility gene for prostate cancer has not been located.

22.7.1 PUTATIVE LOCATION OF THE PROSTATE CANCER SUSCEPTIBILITY LOCUS FROM TUMOUR STUDIES

Although its location is unknown, the prostate cancer susceptibility locus has been named *PRCA*1 by the genome nomenclature committee. A definitive multistep genetic pathway has not been determined as yet for prostate cancer. Such a pathway would be useful in providing clues for the identity of the prostate susceptibility locus since this would be expected to be the earliest event. As discussed under the genetic model section, the susceptibility locus does not necessarily have to be a tumour suppressor gene. However, in prostate tumour studies, all the reported mutations in dominant oncogenes seem to be associated with disease progression rather than early stages of prostate cancer development. It is also unclear at present whether prostatic hypertrophy predisposes to carcinoma. These both argue against a dominant oncogene model for prostate cancer predisposition. However, once the gene(s) is located, loss of heterozygosity studies will confirm this.

Candidate locations and genes for *PRCA*1 come from several study types: cytogenetics, allele loss studies which indicate sites of tumour suppressor genes and dominant oncogene studies.

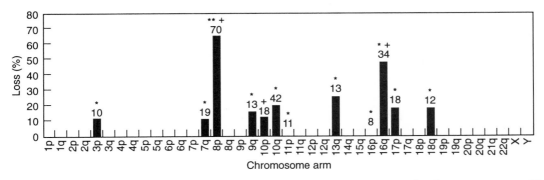

Fig. 22.3 Results of loss of heterozygosity (LOH) studies in prostate tumours by chromosome arm. The numbers at the top of each bar are the numbers of informative tumours studied; symbols refer to reference sources *[38]; **[40]; +[41].

22.7.2 CYTOGENETICS

The amount of cytogenetic information on prostate cancer is sparse in comparison with other carcinomas, possibly due to overgrowth in culture of normal cells [34]. All studies have been performed in sporadic tumours. Cytogenetics of prostate tumours are difficult to perform, but the reported studies to date show loss of the long arms of chromosome 10 (e.g. [35]), and 7 [36] and loss of chromosomes 1, 2, 5 and Y [37]. Some studies have reported trisomy 7, 14, 20 and 22, one patient with trisomy 4 has been reported, and one with a translocation from 5q to 7q [37]. Rearrangements involving chromosomes 2p, 7q and 10q are the most commonly observed [37].

22.7.3 ALLELE LOSS STUDIES AND TUMOUR SUPPRESSOR GENES

Allele loss or loss of heterozygosity (LOH) studies indicate the sites of tumour suppressor genes since, in the tumour, the wild-type allele is lost. This results in the tumour suppressor gene exerting an unopposed effect. Individuals heterozygous for markers in the area of loss have their heterozygous state reduced to homozygosity, hence the term LOH. The most favoured candidates for locations of a tumour suppressor gene from LOH studies in prostate cancer are 8p, 10q and 16q because the highest percentage of loss (30–50% of tumours) is in these regions [38, 39]. LOH has also been seen in other regions (see Figure 22.3). In one study of 52 tumours, the loss at 8p was in 63% of those studied [40] and in a metastasis, a homozygous deletion of part of 8p (8p22) has been found. This deletion narrowed down the area of loss to a 14 cM interval [40] and is strongly suggestive of a tumour suppressor gene in this region. *TP53* mutations are the most common genetic changes in many cancer types [42]; however, in prostate cancer, *TP53* mutation is not very common in primary tumours. Mutations of *TP53* were seen in 25% of 92 tumours in one study [43], but all the mutations were seen in metastatic disease, and were a late event. Similar results have been obtained for the retinoblastoma gene [44] and the DNA polymerase β genes [45] where changes are more common in metastatic disease than in earlier disease.

Chromosome transfer studies using microcell-mediated chromosome transfer have shown that introduction of chromosome 8 or 11 suppresses metastatic ability, but not tumourigenicity in the highly metastatic Dunning rat AT3.1 prostatic cancer cell line [46, 47]. Loss of chromosome 2 has also been associated with the development of metastasis [48]. Suppression of tumourigenicity of the human prostate cancer cell line, DU 145 in nude mice [49] can be achieved by transfer of a portion of chromosome 12 (12pter-12q13). These would therefore be candidate areas for the sites of tumour suppressor genes.

22.7.4 DOMINANT ONCOGENES

(a) *RAS*

Mutations in the *RAS* oncogene are infrequent and are usually a late event in prostate cancer [50]. Treiger and Isaacs [51] have shown that expression of a mutated v-H-*RAS* oncogene can convert a tumourigenic non-metastatic Dunning rat prostatic cell line into a highly metastatic state. The acquisition of metastatic potential is accompanied by genomic instability, in particular, loss of chromosome 10 occurred in all of the transfectants, which would correlate with LOH studies which suggest that there is a tumour suppressor gene on chromosome 10.

Increased levels of *MYC* transcripts have been found in high-grade prostate cancers [52] and *BCL*-2 overexpression, associated with the overriding of apoptosis, has been shown to occur when prostate cancer progresses from androgen-dependence to independence [53]. All these genetic alterations are associated with advanced disease and would therefore not be prime candidates for *PRCA*1.

22.8 CLINICAL CONSIDERATIONS

22.8.1 GENE–ENVIRONMENT INTERACTIONS

Epidemiological studies of the aetiology of prostate cancer suggest many causal factors (reviewed in [7, 54]), of which genetic predisposition is a component. The incidence of the disease is very high in certain racial groups, particularly negroes, where the prognosis is also worse. It is a relatively uncommon disease in Japan, but there is a higher mortality in Japanese immigrants to the US, suggesting an environmental component. Some studies suggest this is dietary fat, and this is effected via hormonal changes.

Hormonal factors have been studied, with conflicting results. Testosterone and derivative hormone levels are not consistently different between cases and controls in different studies; however, it has been shown from a study in twins that the production of testosterone and dihydrotestosterone is under genetic influence [55]. Prostate cancer is also associated with a higher fertility rate and marital status. Other sexual factors such as age at puberty and at first sexual intercourse vary in their effects on risk between studies. The effect of vasectomy is controversial, some studies suggesting an associated increased risk of prostate cancer, and others refuting this [56].

It has been suggested that an infectious agent may be responsible, since higher rates are correlated with crude measures of increased sexual activity, namely ever-married men versus single men, lower age at first sexual intercourse and at first marriage than controls [13], and correlate with the frequency of venereal disease [12]. Virus-like particles have been found in prostatic cancer tissue and higher antibody titres are present in such cases [57].

The disease is more common in urban than rural areas, but socioeconomic factors are unrelated and there is no significant relationship to previous diseases, height, circumcision, smoking or alcohol consumption. Some occupations carry an increased risk, namely cadmium workers and rubber workers.

The interactions of all these factors upon a

genetic effect will be able to be studied once the predisposition genes have been located.

22.8.2 MANAGEMENT OF FAMILIAL PROSTATE CANCER

When advising individuals in prostate cancer families about their risk, there are a few epidemiological studies which provide data on the relative risks of developing prostate cancer according to the number of relatives affected in the family. Tables 22.4 and 22.5 show the relative risks according to the number of relatives affected and the age at diagnosis. For example, if there are two first-degree relatives affected with prostate cancer aged about 60 years, the relative risk in the unaffected, related individual is about 5. The normal population risk is 0.5% by age 64 and 2% by age 74 [58].

Since relatives of prostate cancer patients are at increased risk of the disease, the question arises whether they should be offered targeted screening. It has been shown that earlier diagnosis results in a better survival [5], but improved survival as a result of screening for prostate cancer remains to be proven.

Population studies worldwide have reported a prostate-specific antigen (PSA) screening:cancer-detection ratio of 13–83 to 1 (e.g. [6]). If a higher risk population could be identified, in theory, PSA screening should result in a higher yield of cancer cases detected per number screened. McWhorter *et al.,* [59] have studied first-degree relatives of 17 sets of two brothers with prostate cancer. A total of 34 relatives were studied (sons and brothers, aged 55–80). They underwent intensive screening with PSA, digital rectal examination (DRE), transrectal ultrasound (TRUS) and systematic as well as clinically directed core biopsies. Six had a positive PSA (18%), but only three of these had cancer. Both PSA and DRE were abnormal in four, and TRUS showed a lesion in seven.

Although eight cancers were detected in the study, in only seven was there a detectable lesion on ultrasound. The problem with such screening is that it may detect cancer which will not become clinically relevant in terms of causing morbidity to the patient within their lifetime. However, this was not the case in this study. One of these eight cancers was stage C and so the other seven underwent prostatectomy and lymph node dissection. Pathologically, the stages were three-stage B and four-stage C. The overall cancer detection percentage was therefore 8/36, or 9%, and all had clinically significant disease. Using a similar screening protocol in the general population, with the difference that biopsy was only performed if indicated, Catalona *et al.* [6] found only 36 cancers (2.2%) in a population of 1630 men aged 50–79. From these limited data, there would be supporting evidence for targeted prostatic cancer screening in relatives of cases, at least if two brothers have both been affected with the disease.

Chemoprevention of prostate cancer in those at increased risk due to a genetic predisposition is an exciting new area in cancer prevention. Finasteride, a 5-alpha reductase inhibitor previously used to treat benign prostatic hypertrophy, is being piloted in a randomized controlled trial in the US to assess if it will reduce mortality from prostate cancer. Men at increased risk of the disease due to older age, and also those with a positive family history are randomized to finasteride or placebo [60].

22.9 SUMMARY

Although there is compelling evidence for genetic predisposition to prostate cancer, the susceptibility locus is not yet known. The characterization of genetic changes which predispose to prostate cancer will enable the identification of individuals at risk of developing the disease, so that they can be offered early treatment or prevention.

REFERENCES

1. *Office of Population Censuses and Surveys*, UK. (1992).
2. Cancer facts and figures (1994) *American Cancer Society*, USA.
3. Claus E.B., Risch, N.J. and Thompson, W.D. (1991) Genetic analysis of breast cancer in the Cancer and Steroid Hormone Study. *Am. J. Hum. Genet.*, **48**, 232–42.
4. Coleman, M.P., Esteve J., Damiecki, P. *et al.* (1993) Trends in cancer incidence and mortality. *IARC.*, **21**, Chapter 21.
5. Hanks, G.E., Diamond, J.J., Krall, J.M. *et al.* (1987) A ten year follow-up of 682 patients treated for prostate cancer with radiation therapy in the United States. *Int. J. Radiat. Oncol. Biol. Phys.*, **13**, 449–505.
6. Catalona, W.J., Smith, D.S., Ratliff, T.L. *et al.* (1991) Measurement of prostate-specific antigen in serum as a screening test for prostate cancer. *N. Engl. J. Med.*, **324**, 1156–61.
7. Cannon, L.A., Bishop, D.T., Skolnick, M. *et al.* (1982) Genetic epidemiology of prostate cancer in the Utah Mormon Genealogy. *Cancer Surv.*, **1**, 47–69.
8. Woolf, C.M. (1960) An investigation of the familial aspects of carcinoma of the prostate. *Cancer*, **13**, 739–44.
9. Morganti, G., Gianferrari, L., Cresseri, A. *et al.* (1956) Recherches clinico-statistiques et genetiques sur les neoplasies de la prostate. *Acta Genetica Statistica*, **6**, 304–5.
10. Krain, L.S. (1974) Some epidemiologic variables in prostatic carcinoma in California. *Preventive Medicine*, **3**, 154–9.
11. Fincham, S.M., Hill, G.B., Hanson, J. *et al.* (1990) Epidemiology of prostate cancer: a case control study. *Prostate*, **17**, 189–206.
12. Meikle, A.W., Smith, J.A. and West, D.W. (1985) Familial factors affecting prostatic cancer risk and plasma sex-steroid levels. *Prostate*, **6**, 121–8.
13. Steele, R., Lees, R.E.M., Kraus, A.S. *et al.* (1971) Sexual factors in the epidemiology of cancer of the prostate. *J. Chron. Dis.*, **24**, 29–37.
14. Schuman, T., Mandel, J., Blackard, C. *et al.* (1977) Epidemiologic study of prostatic cancer: preliminary report. *Cancer Treat. Rep.*, **61**, 181–6.
15. Steinberg, G.D., Carter, B.S., Beaty, T.H. *et al.* (1990) Family history and the risk of prostate cancer. *Prostate*, **17**, 337–47.
16. Spitz, M.R., Currier, R.D., Fueger, J.J. *et al.* (1991) Familial patterns of prostate cancer: a case-control analysis. *J. Urol.*, **146**, 1305–7.
17. Ghadirian, P., Cadotte, M., Lacroix, A. *et al.* (1991) Family aggregation of cancer of the prostate in Quebec: the tip of the iceberg. *Prostate*, **19**, 43–52.
18. *Cancer in Utah, Report No. 3*, 1967–77. Utah Cancer Registry, Salt Lake City.
19. Skolnick, M.H. (1980) The Utah genealogical data base: a resource for genetic epidemiology, in *Banbury Report No.4: Cancer Incidence in Defined Populations*, (eds J. Cairns, J.L. Lyon and M.H. Skolnick), Cold Spring Harbor Laboratory Press, New York, pp. 285–97.
20. McLellan, T., Jorde, L.B. and Skolnick, M.H.(1984) Genetic distances between the Utah Mormons and related populations. *Am. J. Hum. Genet.*, **36**, 836–7.
21. Jorde, L.B., and Skolnick, M.H. (1981) Demographic and genetic application of computerized record linking: the Utah Mormon genealogy. *Information et Sciences Humaines*, **56–57**, 105–17.
22. Malecot, G. (1948) Les mathematiques de l'heredite. *Masson et Cie*, Paris.
23. Cannon–Albright, L.A., Thomas, A., Goldgar, D.E. *et al.* (1994) Familiality of cancer in Utah. *Cancer Res.*, **54**, 2378–85.
24. Carter, B.S., Beaty, T.H., Steinberg, G.D. *et al.* (1992) Mendelian inheritance of familial prostate cancer. *Proc. Natl Acad. Sci. USA*, **89**, 3367–71.
25. Knudson, A.G. (1985) Hereditary cancer, oncogenes and antioncogenes. *Cancer Res.*, **45**, 1437–43.
26. Tulinius, H., Egilsson, V., Olafsdottir, G.H., *et al.* (1992) Risk of prostate, ovarian, and endometrial cancer among relatives of women with breast cancer. *Br. Med. J.*, **305**, 855–7.
27. Anderson, D.E. and Badzioch, M.D. (1992) Breast cancer risks in relatives of male breast cancer patients. *J. Natl Cancer Inst.*, **84**, 1114–7.

28. Ford, D., Easton, D.F., Bishop, D.T., Narod, S.A., Goldgar, D.E. and the Breast Cancer Linkage Consortium (1994) Risks of cancer in BRCA1-mutation carriers. *Lancet*, **343**, 692–5.

29. Carter, B.S., Bova, G.S., Beaty, T.H. *et al.* (1993) Hereditary prostate cancer: epidemiologic and clinical features. *J. Urol.*, **150**, 797–802.

30. Zahm, S.H., Blair, A., Holmes, F.F. *et al.* (1989) A case-control study of soft tissue sarcoma. *Am. J. Epidemiol.*, **130**, 665–74.

31. Birch, J.M., Hartley, A.T., Tricker, K.J. *et al.* (1994) Prevalence and diversity of constitutional mutations in the p53 gene among 21 Li–Fraumeni families. *Cancer Res.*, **54**, 1298–304.

32. Eeles, R.A., Warren, W., Knee, G. *et al.* (1993) Constitutional mutation in exon 8 of the p53 gene in a patient with multiple independent primary tumours: molecular and immunohistochemical findings. *Oncogene*, **8**, 1269–76.

33. Haas, G.P., Sakr, W., Cassin, B. *et al.* (1992) The prevalence of prostate cancer in young black and white males. *J. Urol.*, **147**: 290A.

34. Sandberg, A.A. (1992) Chromosomal abnormalities and related events in prostate cancer. *Hum. Pathol.*, **23**, 368–80.

35. Lundgren, R., Mandahl, N., Heim, S. *et al.* (1992) Cytogenetic analysis of 57 primary prostatic adenocarcinomas. *Genes Chromosomes Cancer*, **4**, 16–24.

36. Atkin, N.B. and Baker, M.C. (1993) Chromosome 7q deletions: observations on 13 malignant tumors. *Cancer Genet. Cytogenet.*, **67**, 123–5.

37. Brothman, A.R., Peehl, D.M., Patel, A.M. *et al.* (1990) Frequency and pattern of karyotypic abnormalities in human prostate cancer. *Cancer Res.*, **50**, 3795–803.

38. Carter, B.S., Ewing, C.M., Ward, W.S. *et al.* (1990) Allelic loss of chromosomes 16q and 10q in human prostate cancer. *Proc. Natl Acad. Sci. USA*, **87**, 8751–5.

39. Collins, V.P., Kunimi, K., Bergerheim, U. *et al.* (1991) Molecular genetics and human prostatic carcinoma. *Acta Oncologica*, **31**, 181–5.

40. Bova, G.S., Carter, B.S., Bussemakers, M.J.G. *et al.* (1993) Homozygous deletion and frequent allele loss of chromosome 8p22 loci in human prostate cancer. *Cancer Res.*, **53**, 3869–73.

41. Bergerheim, U.S.R., Kunimi, K., Collins, V.P. *et al.* (1991) Deletion mapping of chromosomes 8, 10 and 16 in human prostate carcinoma. *Genes Chromosomes Cancer*, **3**, 215–20.

42. Hollstein, M.C., Sidransky, D., Vogelstein, B. *et al.* (1991) p53 mutations in human cancers. *Science*, **253**, 49–53.

43. Navone, N.M., Troncosco, P., Pisters, L.L. *et al.* (1993) p53 protein accumulation and gene mutation in the progression of human prostate carcinoma. *J. Natl Cancer Inst.*, **85**, 1657–69.

44. Bookstein, R., Rio, P., Madreperla, S.A. *et al.* (1990) Promoter deletion and loss of retinoblastoma gene expression in human prostate cancer. *Proc. Natl Acad. Sci. USA*, **87**, 7762–6.

45. Dobashi, Y., Shuin, T., Tsuruga, H. *et al.* (1994) DNA polymerase β gene mutation in human prostate cancer. *Cancer Res.*, **54**, 2827–9.

46. Ichikawa, T., Niheii, N., Suzuki, H. *et al.* (1994) Suppression of metastasis of rat prostatic cancer by introducing human chromosome 8. *Cancer Res.*, **54**, 2299–302.

47. Ichikawa, T., Ichikawa, Y., Dong, J. *et al.* (1992) Localization of metastasis suppressor gene(s) for prostatic cancer to the short arm of human chromosome 11. *Cancer Res.*, **52**, 3486–90.

48. Ichikawa, T., Ichikawa, Y. and Isaacs, J.T. (1991) Genetic factors and suppression of metastatic ability of prostatic cancer. *Cancer Res.*, **51**, 3788–92.

49. Berube, N.G., Speevak, M.D. and Chevrette, M. (1994) Suppression of tumourigenicity of human prostate cancer cells by introduction of human chromosome del(12)(q13). *Cancer Res.*, **54**, 3077–81.

50. Carter, B.S., Epstein, J.L. and Isaacs, W.B. (1992) *ras* gene mutations in human prostate cancer. *Cancer Res.*, **50**, 6830–2.

51. Treiger, B. and Isaacs, J. (1988) Expression of a transfected v-H-ras oncogene in a Dunning rat prostate adenocarcinoma and the development of high metastatic ability. *J. Urol.*, **140**, 1580–6.

52. Buttyan, R., Sawczuk, I.S., Benson, M.C. *et al.* (1987) Enhanced expression of the c-myc proto-oncogene in high grade human prostate cancers. *Prostate*, **67**, 327–37.

53. McDonnell, T.J., Troncoso, P., Brisbay, S.M. *et al.* (1992) Expression of the protooncogene *bcl*-2 in the prostate and its association with emergence of androgen-independent prostate cancer. *Cancer Res.*, **52**, 6940–4.

54. Zaridze, D.G. and Boyle, P. (1987) Cancer of the prostate: epidemiology and aetiology. *Br. J. Urol.*, **59**, 493–502.

55. Meikle, A.W., Stringham, J.D., Bishop, D.T. *et al.* (1988) Quantitating genetic and nongenetic factors influencing androgen production and clearance in men. *J. Clin. Endocrinol. Metab.*, **67**, 104–9.

56. Skegg, D.C.G. (1993) Vasectomy and risk of cancers of prostate and testis. *Eur. J. Cancer*, **29A**(7), 935–6.

57. Ablin, R.J. (1976) Serum antibody in patients with prostatic cancer. *Br. J. Urol.*, **48**, 355–61.

58. Parkin, D.M., Muir, C.S., Whelan, S.L. *et al.* (1993) Cancer incidence in five continents. *IARC.*, **6**, 971.

59. McWhorter, W.P., Hernandez, A.D., Meikle, A.W. *et al.* (1992) A screening study of prostate cancer in high risk families. *J. Urol.*, **148**, 826–8.

60. Donodeo, F. (1994) Prevention trial for prostate cancer piques public interest. *J. Natl Cancer Inst.*, **85**, 1801–2.

Chapter 23

Familial melanoma and its management

ALISA M. GOLDSTEIN and MARGARET A. TUCKER

23.1 INCIDENCE

Cutaneous malignant melanoma (CMM) is a potentially fatal form of skin cancer whose incidence is rising in many regions of the world [1–4]. Data from the Scottish Melanoma Group showed that in Scotland the incidence of CMM increased 82% over an 11-year period from 3.4 per 100 000 in 1979 to 7.1 per 100 000 in 1989 for men and from 6.6 per 100 000 to 10.4 per 100 000 for women [4]. In Queensland, Australia, which has the highest incidence of cutaneous melanoma in both men and women, the cumulative risks of invasive melanoma have increased to 1 in 19 for men and to 1 in 25 for women. The incidence of CMM increased from 25.3 per 100 000 in 1979–1980 to 55.8 per 100 000 in 1987 for men and from 27.1 per 100 000 to 42.9 per 100 000 in women [1]. In the US, over the period 1973–1990, the incidence of malignant melanoma among whites increased nearly 95%, more than that of any other cancer. The overall age-adjusted incidence rate of invasive melanoma for 1986–1990 was 10.9 per 100 000, 12.1 per 100 000 in whites and 0.8 per 100 000 in blacks. For white men,

the overall age-adjusted incidence was 14.1 per 100 000, and for white women, 10.6 per 100 000 [3].

Approximately 8–12% of cases of malignant melanoma occur in individuals with a familial predisposition [5], often in association with clinically dysplastic naevi, a major precursor lesion of melanoma [6].

23.2 RISK FACTORS

Several environmental and host variables have been identified as risk factors for malignant melanoma. The major environmental risk factor for CMM is ultraviolet radiation. For melanoma, early intermittent sun exposure (i.e. childhood sunburns) appears to be the major risk determinant [7, 8].

In addition to ultraviolet radiation, there is a strong association between melanoma and melanocytic naevi, both clinical benign [9, 10] and clinically atypical (clinically dysplastic) (Figures 23.1 and 23.2, colour plate section). The characteristics of a clinically atypical or clinically dysplastic naevus (CAN or DN)

Genetic Predisposition to Cancer. Edited by R.A. Eeles, B.A.J. Ponder, D.F. Easton and A. Horwich. Published in 1996 by Chapman & Hall, London.
0 412 56580 3

include a macular component, irregular and indistinct borders, variable colour (including tan, brown, dark brown and pink), size >5 mm, and distribution similar to normal naevi but also occurring in areas unusual for common acquired naevi, such as the scalp, buttocks and, in women, the breasts [11–13]. Clinically dysplastic naevi have been shown to be an independent predictor of melanoma risk in both non-familial and familial melanoma [13–15].

In a study of 23 US melanoma-prone families, the strongest risk factor for melanoma was the presence of clinically dysplastic naevi. The cumulative risk of melanoma by age 50 years among people with dysplastic naevi was 48.9% ± 4.2% [13]. In addition to DN, categorical number of naevi, number of sunburns (particularly at an early age) and skin type (i.e. the skin's response to exposure to the sun) were also associated with an increased risk of melanoma [16].

Other host factors implicated in both familial and non-familial melanoma include hair colour, eye colour, extent of freckling, and skin type [17, 18]. Individuals with blonde/fair hair, blue eyes, many freckles, and an inability to tan are at increased risk of melanoma.

23.3 FAMILIAL MELANOMA

Hereditary cutaneous malignant melanoma has been defined as the presence of at least 2 cases of cutaneous melanoma in a kindred [19]. An example of a hereditary CMM pedigree is shown in Figure 23.3. It is possible, however, especially in heavily insolated regions such as Australia, that familial clustering of melanoma may occur because family members share the same risk factors such as hair colour, eye colour, freckling, and skin type.

23.3.1 COMPARISON OF FAMILIAL AND NON-FAMILIAL MELANOMA

(a) Similarities

In general, familial melanoma is clinically and histologically indistinguishable from non-familial melanoma. Barnhill *et al.* [19] directly compared the characteristics of 145 non-familial CMM patients and six patients with familial melanoma, all ascertained in the Yale Melanoma Unit. Eligibility criteria included diagnosis of malignant melanoma between 1st January, 1983 and 1st July, 1987, non-Hispanic Caucasian, and age >20 but <70 years. No striking differences were observed between the patients with familial and non-familial melanoma with respect to hair colour, skin type, sunburn history, numbers of naevi per person, and histological features of naevi [19]. These results were similar to an earlier larger study [20] that compared 69 patients with familial melanoma to 1099 melanoma patients without a positive family history. Kopf *et al.* [20] found no differences between the two groups with respect to hair colour, skin type, skin reaction to sunlight and previous history of sun exposure, estimate of melanocytic naevi on the body, and freckling.

(b) Differences

However, differences in age at diagnosis, lesion thickness, and frequency of multiple lesions were observed [20]. As has been observed in most studies comparing hereditary melanoma and unselected or non-familial melanoma [13, 16, 19–21], younger ages at diagnosis of CMM, relatively thinner lesions, and greater frequencies of multiple primary melanomas were observed in familial melanoma cases versus non-familial melanoma cases.

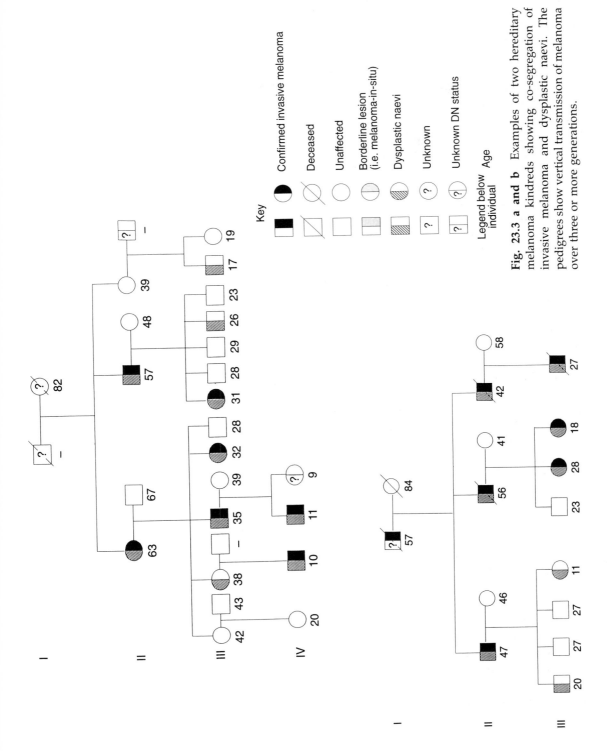

Fig. 23.3 a and b Examples of two hereditary melanoma kindreds showing co-segregation of invasive melanoma and dysplastic naevi. The pedigrees show vertical transmission of melanoma over three or more generations.

23.4 PREDISPOSITION TO OTHER CANCERS

Several researchers have investigated whether a familial susceptibility to melanoma also predisposes individuals to an increased risk of other cancers independent of other known family cancer syndromes (e.g. Li–Fraumeni syndrome) [22]. Prospective follow-up of 23 US melanoma-prone families revealed no significant excess of cancers other than melanoma. The relative risk of a prospective melanoma among family members with previous melanoma was 229 (95% C.I. 110–422). This risk decreased over time from 362 (95% C.I. 147–759) in the first 5 years to 120 (95% C.I. 24–351) after 5 years [13]. In addition, Kopf *et al.* [20] observed that individuals with familial melanoma had fewer other cancers than individuals with sporadic melanoma.

In contrast, Lynch *et al.* [23] reported several melanoma-prone families with an increased risk of several other cancers in addition to melanoma. Since this research group is well known for studying families with unusual numbers or types of cancer, it is possible that the reported excess may represent chance co-segregation of rare cancers rather than an increased risk of other cancers in typical melanoma-prone families. However, Bergman *et al.* [24] studied several Dutch melanoma-prone kindreds and observed an increased frequency of gastro-intestinal tract neoplasms, particularly carcinoma of the pancreas, in a subset of the kindreds similar to those observed by Lynch *et al.* [23].

Recently, Goldstein *et al.* [24a] reported an increased risk of pancreatic cancer in 10 melanoma-prone kindreds with *p*16 (a melanoma tumour-suppressor gene) mutations but not in 9 kindreds without *p*16 mutations. Genetic factors, such as *p*16 mutations, may help explain the inconsistent occurrence of other cancers in melanoma-prone kindreds.

More research needs to be done to determine whether subsets of melanoma-prone families may have excesses of non-melanoma tumors. If excesses are confirmed, this information may help to unravel the genetics and epidemiology of subtypes of familial melanoma.

23.5 MANAGEMENT OF FAMILIAL MELANOMA

23.5.1 SURVIVAL

Survival after early melanoma is very high. Patients diagnosed with melanoma *in-situ* have a greater than 99% long-term, disease-free survival. Patients with early melanoma, defined as lesions <1 mm in depth, have a greater than 90% long-term overall survival [25]. In fact, the single most predictive factor for recurrence and long-term prognosis of melanoma is the depth of invasion of the original lesion. Other prognostic factors include regression, level of invasion (Clark), ulceration, anatomic location, radial versus vertical growth phase, and sex of the patient [25]. If thin melanomas (<1 mm in depth) are subdivided between radial and vertical growth phases, only those tumours with vertical growth phase progress to metastatic disease [26]. In contrast, the 5-year survival rate for thick tumours (>3.5 mm) is only about 50% [4].

23.5.2 AIMS OF MANAGEMENT

Because early diagnosis of thin lesions is essential to survival following melanoma, it is important to identify individuals at increased risk for melanoma and appropriately screen and manage this high-risk population. There should be two aims in the management of individuals at high risk for melanoma and individuals in melanoma-prone families: (i) prevention of melanoma by reducing risk factors that promote tumourigenesis; and (ii) early detection of melanoma by recognizing and biopsying naevi suspicious for melanoma [27]. Clinical follow-up of high-risk patients can lead to the detection of early thin melanomas [13, 28, 29] and ultimately increased survival.

23.5.3 WHO SHOULD BE SCREENED?

Since familial melanoma is clinically indistinguishable from non-familial melanoma, it is essential for the clinician to obtain a detailed family history from all individuals with melanoma. All first-degree relatives (parents, siblings and children) of individuals with invasive melanoma (or clinically atypical naevi) should be screened. Although the inheritance of familial melanoma is not completely understood, first-degree relatives of melanoma patients are at increased risk of developing melanoma and members of melanoma-prone families are at very high risk of melanoma [13]. In addition, since individuals with familial melanoma tend to develop multiple primary lesions, they need to be followed closely.

23.5.4 MANAGEMENT OF HIGH-RISK PATIENTS

Individuals with melanoma or clinically dysplastic naevi from melanoma-prone families should be examined by a skilled physician or nurse every 3–6 months. The examination should be conducted in a brightly lit room with adequate accessory lighting to allow bright-field illumination of the area being examined. A halogen light source is very effective, because it emits a continuous-spectrum white light, fluorescent light should be avoided because its discontinuous emission spectrum turns the pink hues of clinically dysplastic naevi to a dull grey [30]. The entire skin surface should be examined, including the scalp, breasts, buttocks, genital area, and soles of feet. Baseline colour photographs, including body overviews, segmental overviews, and 1-to-1 close-ups (with a ruler next to the naevi) of the most atypical naevi should be taken. Close-up photography of selected naevi is an important tool in following such lesions over time.

Lesions suspicious for melanoma should be removed by excisional biopsy [31]. In addition, changing naevi that are becoming more abnormal should also be biopsied. Routine or 'prophylactic' removal of non-changing, clinically dysplastic naevi is not recommended. The chances of any one naevus becoming melanoma are slight: biopsying only changing naevi minimizes the amount of surgery. Over time, most dysplastic naevi will involute, differentiate, or disappear [32].

23.5.5 MANAGEMENT OF CHILDREN

It is very important to protect young children in these families. Complete avoidance of sunburn from the time of birth and use of sunscreens and protective clothing are strongly recommended. Since it is frequently difficult to detect clinically dysplastic naevi on children until puberty, it should be assumed that everyone is at risk, and should be protected from the sun. Children should have their first skin examination by age 10 but should be seen by a skilled clinician earlier if they have suspicious lesions. In a study of 23 US high-risk CMM/DN families, 10% of the melanoma cases developed melanoma before 20 years of age [13] compared with 2% in the general population [33].

23.5.6 EDUCATION

Family members need to be taught self-examination of the skin, including the scalp, so that they can examine their naevi monthly. Individuals should look for changes in the size, shape, colour, elevation, consistency (softening or hardening), and sensation of the naevus itself and the skin surrounding a naevus [34]. This task is greatly aided if

Table 23.1 Melanoma warning signs: changes in moles that may signal melanoma

Large size: usually >5 mm
Shape: irregular border, asymmetric shape
Surface: scaly, flaky, oozing, bleeding, ulceration, non-healing sore
Colour: multiple colours including tan, brown, white, pink and black. Rapid darkening, especially of new areas of black or dark brown
Elevation: development of raised areas on a previously flat lesion
Consistency: softening or hardening
Sensation in naevus: unusual sensation in naevus including itchy, painful and tenderness
Sensation in surrounding skin: redness, inflammation, loss of pigmentation (become white or grey), or bleeding of pigment from mole into surrounding skin

family members have a copy of their clinical photographs. Patients can observe changes in individual naevi relative to the clinical close-up, as well as identify variation in their naevi from comparison with the segmental overviews. Patients should be taught melanoma warning signs and recognition of clinically atypical naevi and melanoma [34] (Table 23.1).

Family members should be taught to avoid sun exposure between 10 a.m. and 3 p.m., to wear protective clothing including hats, long-sleeve shirts, and long trousers, and to use sunscreens with a sun protection factor (SPF) of at least 15 when exposed to the sun for prolonged periods of time. Family members should also be taught to avoid overexposure to the sun, to never sunburn again, and to avoid sunbathing, sunlamps, and tanning parlours [34]. Patients should be taught that changes in the hormonal milieu (e.g. during pregnancy and puberty) may cause moles to change and that these changes should be carefully watched [34].

These guidelines may undergo modifications as more data are gathered and more information is learned about the aetiology of melanoma. At present, these guidelines are effective and careful follow-up of family members from 23 high-risk, melanoma-prone families has led to a substantial decrease in the thickness of melanomas over time. In addition, intense educational efforts have contributed to positive changes in many family members' sun habits over time [13].

23.5.7 MANAGEMENT OF FAMILIAL CMM IN NON-HEREDITARY CMM KINDREDS

Again, since familial melanoma is indistinguishable from both hereditary and non-familial melanoma, it is essential for the clinician to obtain a good family history. All first-degree relatives of patients with invasive melanoma should be screened. These individuals should receive the same initial screening as members of melanoma-prone families, but then less frequent follow-up unless their moles are rapidly changing, they have had multiple primary melanomas, or they have other identified risk factors for melanoma.

23.6 GENETICS OF FAMILIAL MELANOMA

The genetics of familial melanoma appear to be complex and heterogeneous. Although evidence exists for autosomal dominant transmission of CMM (see [35]), the inheritance pattern has not been firmly established. Debate continues about the existence of a major susceptibility locus (or loci) and the localization of such a locus (or loci).

23.6.1 CHROMOSOME 1p

In 1989, a susceptibility locus for CMM/DN was provisionally mapped to chromosome 1p [36]. This mapping assignment remained controversial, with several laboratories reporting evidence against linkage to the chromosome 1p region [21, 37–39] and no confirmation of the positive linkage results. Recently, Goldstein *et al.* [40] examined the relationship between CMM/DN and chromosome 1p in seven new families plus updated versions of six previously reported families [36]. The results showed significant evidence for a CMM locus linked to chromosome 1p marker D1S47, as well as significant evidence for genetic heterogeneity with only a subset of the families appearing linked to chromosome 1p [40].

23.6.2 CHROMOSOME 6p

One of the first genomic regions implicated in familial melanoma was the HLA region on chromosome 6p. Several linkage and co-segregation studies of CMM and HLA found suggestive evidence for linkage of a CMM locus to HLA [41–44] but no significant results were obtained. In 1985 Bale *et al.* [45] conducted linkage analysis on all previously reported pedigrees plus 11 new CMM/DN families. No evidence for linkage of a CMM locus or a CMM/DN locus to HLA was observed in all 30 pedigrees combined. In fact strong evidence against linkage was obtained for both phenotypes examined. There was however, significant evidence for heterogeneity between the 11 new CMM/DN families and the previously reported pedigrees [45]. Although there is little evidence for a CMM locus linked to HLA across all families tested it is possible that families with other immune-related tumors such as Hodgkin's disease, non-Hodgkin's lymphoma, leukaemia, and sarcoma may be genetically and aetiologically different from families without an underlying immune dysfunction. Families with other immune-related tumours may have a relationship with HLA independent of typical melanoma-prone families.

23.6.3 CHROMOSOME 9p

Recent research on the genetics of familial melanoma has focused on chromosome 9p. This region had been proposed as a candidate region for melanoma based on positive results from cytogenetic, loss of heterozygosity, and tumour-progression studies [46–50]. Fountain *et al.* [50] performed loss-of-heterozygosity studies using eight genetic markers on chromosome 9p. Loss-of-heterozygosity for two or more of the loci were observed in 86% (12/14) of the informative metastatic melanoma tumour and cell-line DNAs. In addition, homozygous deletions of the anonymous DNA marker D9S126 were observed in 10% (2/20) of melanoma cell lines. These results identified a 2–3 Mb region of chromosome 9p21 in which a putative tumour suppressor gene appears likely to reside. The critical region on chromosome 9p21 appears to reside proximal to the interferon-α and -β loci and is defined by the two homozygous deletions of D9S126 [50].

Cannon-Albright *et al.* [51] conducted linkage analysis on 10 Utah kindreds and one Texas kindred with multiple cases of invasive melanoma. The results provided strong evidence for linkage of a familial melanoma locus (MLM) to the chromosomal region 9p13–9p22 near interferon-α and D9S126. The authors reported no evidence for heterogeneity in the 11 kindreds and did not examine a combined CMM/DN trait [51]. A second study of invasive melanoma in 26 Australian kindreds confirmed the chromosome 9p linkage [52]. Nancarrow *et al.* [52] showed significant evidence for linkage to chromosome 9p based on multipoint linkage analysis. Again, there was no significant evidence for heterogeneity and a combined CMM/DN trait was not investigated. Finally, examination of the relationship between CMM/DN and chromosome 9p in 13 pedigrees previously examined for linkage to chromosome 1p [40] showed significant evidence for linkage of both CMM alone and CMM/DN to chromosome 9p marker IFNA (interferon-α). In addition, there was significant evidence for heterogeneity when a homogeneity test allowing for linkage to chromosome 9p, chromosome 1p, or neither region was used [53].

Recently, Serrano *et al.* [54] isolated a human p16 complementary DNA and demonstrated that p16 binds to cyclin-dependent kinase 4 (CDK4), and inhibits the catalytic activity of the CDK4/cyclin D enzymes. Deletions or mutations in the *p*16 gene may affect the relative balance of functional *p*16 and cyclin D, resulting in abnormal cell growth. The *p*16 gene has been localized to the chromosome 9p21 region [55, 56] implicated in melanoma from linkage, cytogenetic and loss of heterozygosity studies [46–51]. In addition, *p*16 has been shown to be frequently deleted or rearranged in cell lines derived from melanoma tumours [55, 56], thus making it a strong candidate for a chromosome 9p21 melanoma tumour suppressor gene.

Familial melanoma kindreds from the USA, Europe, and Australia have been examined for *p*16 germline mutations. To date, mutations have been identified in ⅓–½ of these kindreds [57–63]. In one study [57], eight germline mutations (one nonsense, one splice donor site and six missense) were observed in 13/18 kindreds. Functional studies showed that 3 of the missense mutations were unable to bind to CDK4 or CDK6 [64]. Thus, $^9/_{18}$ kindreds had melanoma-specific mutations that impaired *p*16 function. The putative melanoma-specific mutations were detected in 9p21-linked, but not in non-9p-linked, families, thereby confirming previous reports of genetic heterogeneity. A second study [58] evaluated 13 American or Dutch putative 9p-linked familial melanoma kindreds, plus 38 other Utah or Australian melanoma-prone families not previously examined for chromosome 9p linkage. In

only two families were potential predisposing mutations identified. Further examination of the 5 Dutch kindreds plus 10 additional ones, however, revealed a 19 basepair deletion in 13 of them [60]. Nevertheless, in a small number of putative 9p-linked kindreds, no p16 mutations have been detected to date [57–63]. These kindreds may have *p*16 mutations outside the coding region or there may be another gene relevant to melanoma in this chromosomal region.

23.6.4 FUTURE RESEARCH

Although there is strong evidence for a susceptibility locus for familial melanoma (MLM) on chromosome 9p, it appears likely that familial melanoma is heterogeneous and not all families are linked to a locus in this region. Studies on non-familial melanoma continue to implicate other regions of the genome [35, 50, 65, 66]. Further research will be required to resolve the genetic and molecular bases of familial melanoma.

REFERENCES

1. MacLennan, R., Green, A.C., McLeod, G.R.C. and Martin, N.G. (1992) Increasing incidence of cutaneous melanoma in Queensland. Australia. *J. Natl Cancer Inst.*, **84**, 1427–32.
2. Osterlind, A., Hou-Jensen, K. and Moller Jensen, O. (1988) Incidence of cutaneous malignant melanoma in Denmark 1978–1982. Anatomic site distribution. histologic types, and comparison with non-melanoma skin cancer. *Br. J. Cancer*, **58**, 385–91.
3. Miller, B.A., Gloeckler Ries, L.A., Hankey, B.F. *et al.* (eds) (1993) Cancer Statistics Review 1973–1990. US Department of Health and Human Services, NIH Publication No. 93–2789.
4. MacKie, R., Hunter, J.A.A., Aitchison, T.C. *et al.* (1992) Cutaneous malignant melanoma, Scotland, 1979–89. *Lancet*, **339**, 971–5.
5. Greene, M.H. and Fraumeni, J.F. Jr (1979) *The*

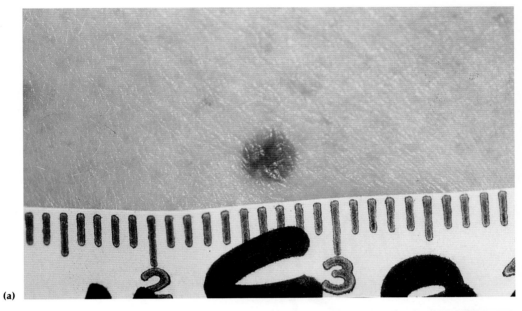

(a)

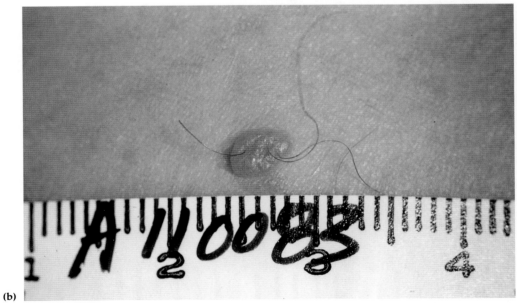

(b)

Figure 23.1 a and b Features of normal moles include uniformly tan or brown colour, round or oval shape with clearly-defined borders, and size usually <5 mm. Clinically, typical moles usually start as flat, smooth spots which progress to smooth papules. They are usually located above the waist and are rarely found on the scalp, breasts or buttocks.

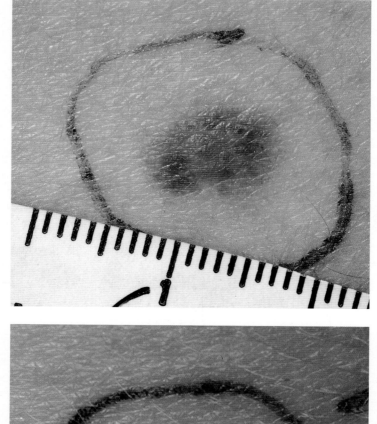

(a)

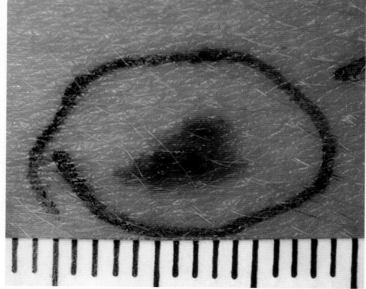

(b)

Figure 23.2 a and b Features of dysplastic moles include a macular component, irregular or indistinct borders, variable colour including tan, brown, dark brown and pink. Frequently size is >5 mm, and the distribution is similar to normal naevi but lesions also occur on the scalp, breasts and buttocks.

Hereditary Variant of Malignant Melanoma, Grune and Stratton, New York.

6. Tucker, M.A. (1988) Individuals at high risk of melanoma. *Pigment Cell.*, **9**, 95–109.

7. Osterlind, A., Tucker, M.A., Stone, B.J. and Jensen, O.M. (1988) The Danish case-control study of cutaneous malignant melanoma II. Importance of UV-light exposure. *Int. J. Cancer*, **42**, 319–24.

8. Zanetti, R., Franceschi, S., Rosso, S. *et al.* (1992) Cutaneous melanoma and sunburns in childhood in a Southern European population. *Eur. J. Cancer*, **28A**, 1172–6.

9. Holly, E.A., Kelly, J.W., Shpall, S.N. and Chiu, S.-H. (1987) Number of melanocytic nevi as a major risk factor for malignant melanoma. *J. Am. Acad. Dermatol.*, **17**, 459–68.

10. Swerdlow, A.J., English, J., MacKie, R.M. *et al.* (1986) Benign melanocytic naevi as a risk factor for malignant melanoma. *Br. Med. J.*, **292**, 1555–9.

11. Reimer, R.R., Clark, W.H. Jr, Greene, M.H. *et al.* (1978) Precursor lesions in familial melanoma: a new genetic preneoplastic syndrome. *JAMA*, **239**, 744–6.

12. Greene, M.H., Clark, W.H. Jr, Tucker, M.A. *et al.* (1985) Acquired precursors of cutaneous malignant melanoma: the familial dysplastic nevus syndrome. *N. Engl. J. Med.*, **312**, 91–7.

13. Tucker, M.A., Fraser, M.C., Goldstein, A.M. *et al.* (1993) The risk of melanoma and other cancers in melanoma-prone families. *J. Invest. Dermatol.*, **100**, S350–5.

14. Halpern, A.C., Guerry, D. IV, Elder, D.E. *et al.* (1991) Dysplastic nevi as risk markers of sporadic (nonfamilial) melanoma. *Arch. Dermatol.*, **127**, 995–9.

15. Rousch, G.C., Nordlund, J.J., Forget, B., *et al.* (1988) Independence of dysplastic nevi from total nevi in determining risk for nonfamilial melanoma. *Prev. Med.*, **17**, 273–9.

16. Goldstein, A.M., Fraser, M.C. and Tucker, M.A. (1993) Risk factors for familial melanoma. *Am. J. Hum. Genet.*, **53** (Suppl.), 808.

17. Elwood, J.M., Whitehead, S.M., Davison, J. *et al.* (1990) Malignant melanoma in England: risks associated with naevi, freckles, social class, hair colour, and sunburn. *Int. J. Epidemiol.* **19**, 801–10.

18. Osterlind, A., Tucker, M.A., Hou-Jensen, K. *et al.* (1988) The Danish case-control study of cutaneous melanoma. I. Importance of host factors. *Int. J. Cancer*, **42**, 200–6.

19. Barnhill, R.L., Rousch, G.C. and Titus-Ernstoff, L. (1992) Comparison of nonfamilial and familial melanoma. *Dermatology*, **184**, 2–7.

20. Kopf, A.W., Hellman, L.J., Rogers, G.S. *et al.* (1986) Familial malignant melanoma. *JAMA*, **256**, 1951–9.

21. Kefford, R.F., Salmon, J., Shaw, H.M. *et al* (1991) Hereditary melanoma in Australia. Variable association with dysplastic nevi and absence of genetic linkage to chromosome 1p. *Cancer Genet. Cytogenet.*, **51**, 45–55.

22. Li, F.P., Fraumeni, J.F.-Jr, Mulvihill, J.J. *et al.* (1988) A cancer family syndrome in twenty-four kindreds. *Cancer Res.*, **48**, 5358–61.

23. Lynch, H.T., Fusaro, R.M., Kimberling, K.J. *et al.* (1983) Familial atypical multiple mole melanoma (FAMMM) syndrome: segregation analysis. *J. Med. Genet.*, **20**, 342–4.

24. Bergman, W., Watson, P., deJong, J. *et al.* (1990) Systemic cancer and the FAMMM syndrome. *Br. J. Cancer*, **61**, 932–6.

24a Goldstein, A.M., Fraser, M.C., Struewing, J.P. *et al.* (1995) Increased risk of pancreatic cancer in melanoma-prone kindreds with p16^{INK4} mutations. *N. Engl. J. Med.*, **333**, 970–4.

25. NIH Consensus Statement: Diagnosis and treatment of early melanoma. NIH Consensus Development Conference, January 27–29, 1992, Vol.10, no. 1.

26. Clark, W.H. Jr, Elder, D.E., Guerry, D. IV *et al.* (1989) Model predicting survival in stage I melanoma based on tumor progression. *J. Natl Cancer Inst.*, **81**, 1893–904.

27. Tokar, I.P., Fraser, M.C. and Bale, S.J. (1992) Genodermatoses with profound malignant potential. *Semin. Oncol. Nursing*, **8**, 272–80.

28. Mackie, R.M., McHenry, P. and Hole, D. (1993) Accelerated detection with prospective surveillance for cutaneous malignant melanoma in high-risk groups. *Lancet*, **341**, 1618–20.

29. Masri, G.D., Clark, W.H. Jr, Guerry, D. IV *et al.* (1990) Screening and surveillance of patients at high risk for malignant melanoma result in detection of earlier disease. *J. Am. Acad. Dermatol.*, **22**, 1042–8.

30. Crutcher, W.A. and Cohen, P.J. (1990) Dysplastic nevi and malignant melanoma. *Am. Family Physician*, **42**, 372–85.

31. Friedman, R.J., Rigel, D.S., Silverman, M.K. *et al.* (1991) Malignant melanoma in the 1990's: the continued importance of early detection and the role of physician and self-examination of the skin. *Cancer J. Clin.*, **41**, 201–26.

32. Halpern, A.C., Guerry, D. IV, Elder, D.E. *et al.* (1993) Natural history of dysplastic nevi. *J. Am. Acad. Dermatol.*, **29**, 51–7.

33. Young, J.L., Percy, C.L. and Asire, A.J. (eds) (1981) *Surveillance, Epidemiology, and End Results: Incidence and Mortality Data 1973–77*. NIH Publication 81–2330, Department of Health and Human Services, Bethesda, MD.

34. National Cancer Institute. NIH. US Department of Health and Human Services. (1990) *What you need to know about dysplastic nevi*. NIH Publication No. 91–3133.

35. Fountain, J.W., Bale, S.J., Housman, D.E. and Dracopoli, N.C. (1990) Genetics of melanoma. *Cancer Surv.*, **9**, 645–71.

36. Bale, S.J., Dracopoli, N.C., Tucker, M.A. *et al.* (1989) Mapping the gene for hereditary cutaneous malignant melanoma-dysplastic nevus to chromosome 1p. *N. Engl. J. Med.*, **320**, 1367–72.

37. van Haeringen, A., Bergman, W., Nelen, M.R. *et al.* (1989) Exclusion of the dysplastic nevus syndrome (DNS) locus from the short arm of chromosome 1 by linkage studies in Dutch families. *Genomics*, **5**, 61–4.

38. Cannon-Albright, L.A., Goldgar, D.E., Wright, E.C. *et al.* (1990) Evidence against the reported linkage of the cutaneous melanoma-dysplastic nevus syndrome locus to chromosome 1p36. *Am. J. Hum. Genet.*, **46**, 912–8.

39. Nancarrow, D.J., Palmer, J.M., Walters, N.K. *et al.* (1992) Exclusion of the familial melanoma locus (MLM) from the PND/D1S47 and MYCL1 regions of chromosome arm 1p in 7 Australian pedigrees. *Genomics*, **12**, 18–25.

40. Goldstein, A.M., Dracopoli, N.C., Ho, E.C. *et al.* (1993) Further evidence for a locus for cutaneous malignant melanoma-dysplastic nevus (CMM/DN) on chromosome 1p and evidence for genetic heterogeneity. *Am. J. Hum. Genet.*, **52**, 537–50.

41. Hawkins, B.R., Dawkins, R.L., Hockey, A. *et al.* (1981) Evidence for linkage between HLA and malignant melanoma. *Tissue Antigens*, **17**, 540–1.

42. Pellegris, G., Illeni, M.T., Rovini, D. *et al.* (1982) HLA complex and familial malignant melanoma. *Int. J. Cancer*, **29**, 621–3.

43. Demenais, F., Cesarini, J.P., Daveau, M. *et al.* (1984) A linkage study between HLA and cutaneous malignant melanoma or precursor lesions or both. *J. Med. Genet.*, **21**, 429–35.

44. Mueller-Eckhardt, G., Schendel, D.J., Hundeiker, M. *et al.* (1984) Possible association between HLA-DR5 and superficial spreading melanoma (SSM). *Int. J. Cancer*, **34**, 751–5.

45. Bale, S.J., Greene, M.H., Murray, C. *et al.* (1985) Hereditary malignant melanoma is not linked to the HLA complex on chromosome 6. *Int. J. Cancer*, **36**, 439–43.

46. Cowan, J.M., Halaban, R. and Francke, U. (1988) Cytogenetic analysis of melanocytes from premalignant nevi and melanomas. *J. Natl Cancer Inst.*, **80**, 1159–64.

47. Dracopoli, N.C., Alhadeff, B., Houghton, A.N. and Old, L.J. (1987) Loss of heterozygosity at autosomal and X-linked loci during tumor progression in a patient with melanoma. *Cancer Res.*, **47**, 3995–4000.

48. Petty, E.M., Gibson, L.H., Fountain, J.W. *et al.* (1993) Molecular definition of a chromosome 9p21 germ-line deletion in a woman with multiple melanomas and a plexiform neurofibroma: implications for 9p tumor suppressor gene(s). *Am. J. Hum. Genet.*, **53**, 96–104.

49. Pedersen, M.I. and Wang, N. (1989) Chromosomal evolution in the progression and metastasis of human malignant melanoma. *Cancer Genet. Cytogenet.*, **41**, 185–201.

50. Fountain, J.W., Karayiorgou, M., Ernstoff, M.S. *et al.* (1992) Homozygous deletions within human chromosome band 9p21 in melanoma. *Proc. Natl Acad. Sci. USA*, **89**, 10557–61.

51. Cannon-Albright, L.A., Goldgar, D.E., Meyer, L.J. *et al.* (1992) Assignment of a locus for familial melanoma, MLM, to chromosome 9p13-p22. *Science*, **258**, 1148–52.

52. Nancarrow, D.J., Mann, G.J., Holland, E.A. *et*

al. (1993) Confirmation of chromosome 9p linkage in familial melanoma. *Am. J. Hum. Genet.*, **53**, 936–42.

53. Goldstein, A.M., Dracopoli, N.C., Engelstein, M. *et al.* (1994) Linkage of cutaneous malignant melanoma/dysplastic nevus (CMM/DN) to chromosome 9p and evidence for genetic heterogeneity. *Am. J. Hum. Genet.*, **54**, 489–96.

54. Serrano, M., Hannon, G.J. and Beach, D. (1993) A new regulatory motif in cell-cycle control causing specific inhibition of cyclin D/CDK4. *Nature*, **366**, 704–7.

55. Kamb, A., Gruis, N.A., Weaver-Feldhaus, J. *et al.* (1994) A cell cycle regulator potentially involved in genesis of many tumor types. *Science*, **264**, 436–40.

56. Nobori, T., Miura, K., Wu, D.J. *et al.* (1994) Deletions of the cyclin-dependent kinase-4 inhibitor gene in multiple human cancers. *Nature*, **368**, 753–6.

57. Hussussian, C.J., Struewing, J.P., Goldstein, A.M. *et al.* (1994) Germline p16 mutations in familial melanoma. *Nature Genet.*, **8**, 15–21.

58. Kamb, A., Shattuck-Eidens, D., Eeles, R. *et al.* (1994) Analysis of the p16 gene (CDKN2) as a candidate for the chromosome 9p melanoma susceptibility locus. *Nature Genet.*, **8**, 22–6.

59. MacGeoch, C., Newton Bishop, J.A., Bataille, V. *et al.* (1994) Genetic heterogeneity in familial malignant melanoma. *Hum. Mol. Genet.*, **3**, 2195–200.

60. Gruis, N.A., van der Velden, P.A., Sandkuijl, L.A., *et al.* (1995) Homozygotes for CDKN2 (p16) germline mutation in Dutch familial melanoma kindreds. *Nature Genet.*, **10**, 351–3.

61. Ohta, M., Nagai, H., Shimizu, M. *et al.* (1994) Rarity of somatic and germline mutations of the cyclin-dependent kinase 4 inhibitor gene, CDK4I, in melanoma. *Cancer Res.*, **54**, 5269–272.

62. Liu, L., Lassam, N.J., Slingerland, J.M. *et al.* (1995) Germline p16INK4A mutation and protein dysfunction in a family with inherited melanoma. *Oncogene*, **11**, 405–12.

63. Walker, G.J., Hussussian, C.J., Flores, J.F. *et al.* (1995) Mutations of the CDKN2/p16INK4 gene in Australian melanoma kindreds. *Hum. Mol. Genet.*, **4**, 1845–52.

64. Ranadi, K., Hussussian, C.J., Sikorski, R.S. *et al.* (1995) Mutations associated with familial melanoma impair p16INK4 function. *Nature Genet.*, **10**, 114–16.

65. Millikin, O., Meese, E. and Vogelstein, B. (1991) Loss of heterozygosity for loci on the long arm of chromosome 6 in human malignant melanoma. *Cancer Res.*, **51**, 5449–53.

66. Parmiter, A.H. and Nowell, P.C. (1993) Cytogenetics of melanocytic tumors. *J. Invest. Dermatol.*, **100**, S254–8.

Chapter 24

Familial predisposition to lung cancer

THOMAS A. SELLERS

24.1 INTRODUCTION

There can be little doubt that lung cancer is the product of environmental exposures, primarily tobacco but also radioactive ores, heavy metals and petrochemicals. However, the idea that individuals differ in their response to these environmental exposures is at least 30 years old. Recognizing that cigarette smoking was the principal cause of lung cancer, Goodhart [1] noted: '. . . different individuals show wide variation in the type and strength of stimulus needed for a neoplastic reaction so that, although even quite light smokers run a significantly higher risk of lung cancer than non-smokers, nine out of ten of the heaviest smokers never get it at all. Personal idiosyncrasy seems to be an important factor in carcinogenesis and this suggests the hypothesis that the population may be genetically heterogeneous for susceptibility to cancer, some individuals being more 'cancer-prone' than others.

This chapter will review the evidence that a familial predisposition, be it genetic, common transmissible environment, or both, is involved in the pathogenesis of lung cancer.

24.2 CASE REPORTS OF FAMILIAL AGGREGATIONS OF LUNG CANCER

Published case reports on the familial aggregation of lung cancer are rare: Brisman *et al.* [2] reported a family in which four of eight sibs had lung cancer; Nagy [3] described a family in which three of 15 sibs were affected and Jones [4] reported the clustering of bronchogenic carcinoma in three of five sibs. Goffman *et al.* [5] studied two families with over 40% of sibs affected with lung cancer, Joishy *et al.* [6] reported 58-year-old identical twins who developed alveolar cell carcinoma with nearly synchronous onset and Paul *et al.* [7] observed three sibs affected with the same histological cell type. While dramatic case reports such as these may offer a striking clinical impression, they are insufficient evidence for the role of a genetic effect. In particular, rare familial clusters of a disease with such strong environmental influences may simply represent a chance occurrence.

Genetic Predisposition to Cancer. Edited by R.A. Eeles, B.A.J. Ponder, D.F. Easton and A. Horwich. Published in 1996 by Chapman & Hall, London.
0 412 56580 3

Table 24.1 Studies of family history and lung cancer

Reference	Lung cancer		Any cancer	
	Family history (%)	Odds ratio	Family history (%)	Odds ratio
Ooi *et al.*, 1986 [9]	25.6	3.2	58.3	1.5
Samet *et al.*, 1986 [10]	6.9	5.3	31.3	1.6
McDuffie *et al.*, 1988 [11]	9.3	2.0	24.4	1.3
Shaw *et al.*, 1991 [12]	26.1	1.8	58.1	1.3
McDuffie, 1991 [13]	2.6	2.0	13.2	1.2

24.3 EPIDEMIOLOGICAL STUDIES OF FAMILY HISTORY

The question of whether or not lung cancer clusters in families more often than could be expected by chance alone requires proper epidemiological evaluation. One approach is to select a group of patients with lung cancer and a group of cancer-free controls and compare the frequency with which each group reports a positive family history of the disease. The first landmark study of this type was conducted by Tokuhata and Lilienfeld in 1963 [8]. They showed that the occurrence of lung cancer among the parents and siblings of 270 lung cancer patients was three times greater than the frequency among relatives of the patients' spouse. This report remained uncorroborated for over 20 years until the study by Ooi and colleagues [9] in a 10-county geographic area referred to as the 'lung cancer belt' of southern Lousiana. Studies conducted since these early reports [10–13] demonstrate a wide range in the reported frequency of a family history of lung cancer (Table 24.1). However, the finding of a statistically significant excess occurrence of lung cancer among relatives of lung cancer cases is, with few exceptions [14, 15], quite consistent. Similar findings have been observed when investigators considered the occurrence of cancer at all sites, although the magnitude of the risk elevation is generally lower [12, 16]. When examined on a site-specific basis, the malignancies observed to be most frequent were usually smoking-associated.

24.4 STUDIES OF FAMILY HISTORY BY HISTOLOGICAL CELL TYPE

Adenocarcinoma of the lung demonstrates a weaker association with the use of tobacco products than does lung cancer of small-cell, squamous or large-cell histologies. One might therefore expect to observe stronger evidence for familial factors in adenocarcinoma of the lung; most of the studies that have examined familial risk by histological categories seem to support this hypothesis. Wu *et al.* [17] studied 336 females with adenocarcinoma of the lung and found that, after adjusting for personal smoking habits, cases were 3.9 times as likely to report a family history of lung cancer than neighbourhood controls. Osann [18] reported another study of females with lung cancer and noted a stronger association of family history of lung cancer with adenocarcinoma (odds ratio 3.0) than with smoking-associated histologies (odds ratio 1.4). Although Lynch *et al.* [14] observed no association of histology with a family history of lung cancer, they did find that the greatest familial risk of smoking-associated cancers occurred among relatives of patients with adenocarcinoma. When Shaw *et al.* [12] stratified their cases according to histology, the greatest familial risk was noted for the cases with adenocarcinoma (odds ratio = 2.1), but significantly elevated risks were observed for other histologies: squamous (1.9), small cell (1.7). In contrast to these studies is the report by Sellers *et al.* [19] of 300 lung cancer patients that found the lowest familial risk among those with adeno-carcinoma and the highest among those with small-cell carcinoma. Ambrosone and colleagues [20] examined family history of cancer at all sites in a much larger sample and observed the greatest familial risks among patients with small-cell and squamous cell histologies. Clearly, additional work needs to be done in this area.

24.5 EPIDEMIOLOGICAL STUDIES OF FAMILIES

It is well known that cigarette smoking habits are familial in nature [21, 22]. That is, children are more likely to smoke if their parents also smoke. Therefore, when making comparisons of the prevalence of lung cancer among relatives of lung cancer cases and controls, one must take into consideration the distinct possibility that, unless cases and controls are matched on smoking behaviour, relatives of cases would be more likely to smoke than relatives of controls. The clustering of such behaviours might well explain why lung cancer cases are more likely to have a positive family history of the disease than controls. To date, only three studies have been conducted in which smoking data on the majority of family members were collected.

In the study by Tokuhata and Lilienfeld [8], the expected number of lung cancer deaths was determined separately by sex, smoking status, age and category of relative (father, mother, brother, sister). The observed number of lung cancer deaths among men who smoked was two-fold greater than expected ($P = 0.01$) and four-fold greater than expected among men who did not smoke ($P = 0.02$). There were no cases of lung cancer among smoking female relatives of the index cases. However, among non-smoking female relatives there was a 2.4-fold excess prevalence of lung cancer.

The study by Ooi *et al.* [9] in southern Louisiana also obtained specific exposure data on relatives. Similar to the Tokuhata and Lilienfeld [8] study, the excess risk was evident among non-smokers as well as smokers. The risk to smoking fathers of the cases was increased five-fold, while the risk of lung cancer to non-smoking female relatives of the cases was elevated nine-fold. This excess risk could not be explained by age, sex, smoking status, pack-years of tobacco exposure, or a cumulative index of occupational/industrial exposures.

The third study that considered specific environmental measures in family members was not restricted to patients with lung cancer. Since a number of studies had noted a greater-than-normal likelihood of cancer among relatives of lung cancer patients, Sellers and co-workers [23] in southern Louisiana undertook a study to evaluate the familial risk of lung and other cancers among a randomly selected sample of cases with malignancy at any site. An excess of lung cancer was observed among relatives of lung cancer probands (odds ratio = 2.5) as well as among relatives of probands with cancers other than lung or breast (odds ratio = 1.6). This excess risk was evident even after allowing for each family member's age, sex, frequency of alcohol consumption (<1 versus ≥1 drink per day), pack-years of tobacco consumption and a cumulative index of occupational/industrial exposures.

In summary, those studies in which specific environmental and lifestyle exposures were determined on individual family members suggest that, even after allowing for the effects of age, sex and smoking, close relatives of lung cancer patients are still at an increased risk for the disease.

Table 24.2 Distribution of smoking and cancer sites among relatives of 337 lung cancer probands ascertained in southern Louisiana, 1976–1979

Characteristic		Relative				
	Proband	Father	Mother	Brother	Sister	Spouse
Number[1,2]	337	337	337	940	896	304
Average age (years)	64.4	66.9	70.9	58.1	61.4	61.5
Smokers (%)	91.7	63.5	11.8	73.6	31.7	47.6
Average pack-years	62.2	23.3	6.6	28.3	12.1	18.0
No. with cancer						
Lung	337	29	7	42	20	1
Larynx	0	12	0	9	5	1
Bladder	0	3	1	5	2	0
Oral cavity	0	2	0	5	0	1
Pancreas	0	3	1	2	1	1
Kidney	0	1	1	2	2	1
Cervix	0	–	2	–	4	0
Oesophagus	0	0	1	1	1	0
Total	337	50	13	66	35	5

[1] Numbers with information on age and smoking status are: fathers (222), mothers (263], brothers (745), sisters (732) and spouses (252).
[2] Table does not include sons (one with cancer of larynx, one with lung cancer), daughters, and half-siblings (two with lung cancer).

24.6 MAJOR GENE HYPOTHESES FOR LUNG CANCER

To address the issue of whether the familial aggregation of lung cancer is consistent with an inherited predisposition, one requires a data set in which several family members have been affected and specific risk factor (level and type of environmental exposures, etc.) and disease information (including age of onset), are available on individual family members. The statistical determination of whether a major gene may be operative in the pathogenesis of the disease is achieved, in essence, by asking the question: 'Given the pattern of disease observed in these families, the ages of onset and the level of environmental exposure of the affected relatives, what is the most likely explanation?'

To date, only one attempt to answer this question has been published [24]. The analysis was based on the 337 lung cancer families collected by Ooi *et al.* [9]. Families included the index cases (probands), their parents, sibs, offspring and spouses. A total of 4357 family members were studied but, because of missing values on tobacco consumption, only 3276 individuals were included in the analysis (Table 24.2). Excluding the probands, there were 86 families (35.6%) with at least one other family member affected with lung cancer (total *n*=106 lung cancers).

Maximum likelihood segregation analyses were performed using the S.A.G.E. package of computer programs that are based on the regressive models of Bonney [25]. Mendelian inheritance, if present, was assumed to be through a single autosomal locus with two alleles (A and B), with allele A associated with the affected state. Under these models, the concept of susceptibility refers to the cumulative probability of being affected if one both lives to the oldest possible age and has the highest possible levels of measured

Table 24.3 Results of segregation analysis of lung cancer in 337 families from southern Louisiana ascertained between 1976 and 1979

Hypothesis	Significance of goodness-of-fit	Allele frequency	Percentage of population susceptible	Mean age of onset (years)		
				AA	AB	BB
No major gene	0.004	–	28	80	80	80
Environmental	0.006	0.037	23	33	53	78
Mendelian						
Dominant	0.075	0.045	60	76	76	101
Recessive	0.04	0.20	26	56	81	81
Codominant	0.90	0.052	28	36	67	82

environmental risk factors (covariates). In other words, susceptibility is not a surrogate measure of genetic predisposition, but rather the proportion of the population at risk because of the (unmeasured) environment in which they live. The models are constructed so that any effect of the high-risk allele would be reflected as an earlier age of onset among susceptible individuals.

The likelihood of each pedigree was conditioned on each person's smoking history and on the age at which the proband became affected. Five hypothetical modes of transmission were considered:

1. No major gene effect can be discerned and lung cancer is independent of genetic factors, but rather is due to known environmental influences (e.g. cigarette smoking) and unmeasured environmental factors.
2. Environmental factors – like the no major gene hypothesis, only random environmental factors contribute to cancer risk, but differences in exposure to unmeasured environmental factors can result in two or three distributions of age-of-onset in the population.
3. Mendelian dominant implies that, given equal environmental exposures, a single copy of the putative high-risk allele is sufficient for an earlier age of onset.
4. Mendelian recessive states that, given equal

environmental exposures, inheritance of two copies of the high-risk allele is necessary for an earlier age of onset.
5. Mendelian codominant, a more general model that includes the preceding two hypotheses as special cases, allows for each of the three genotypes to have a different (not necessarily additive) mean age of onset, again assuming equal environmental exposures.

These hypotheses were tested under the likelihood of an unrestricted (general) model in which all parameters were adjusted to the empirical data, without restrictions, thereby providing the best fit to the data. Twice the difference in the $\log_e$ likelihood (lnL) for the data under the hypothesis of interest (dominant, environmental, etc.) and that under the unrestricted model was compared to the χ^2 distribution to assess departure. The degrees of freedom for the χ^2 statistic are given by the difference in the number of parameters estimated between the hypotheses and the model. A significant χ^2 indicates that the genetic or environmental hypothesis considered can be rejected.

Results of the segregation analyses are presented in Table 24.3 Three hypotheses could be rejected; environmental ($P < 0.01$), no-major-gene ($P < 0.01$) and mendelian recessive ($P < 0.05$). Although the mendelian dominant hypothesis could not be rejected

($P=0.075$), mendelian codominant inheritance provided a significantly better fit to the data ($P >0.90$). The estimated gene frequency of 0.052 implies that approximately 10% of the population can be expected to carry the putative gene. The model further estimates that 28% of the population, regardless of genotype, would develop lung cancer. Based on parameters of the model it was determined that the gene and its interaction with smoking contributed to 69%, 47% and 22% of lung cancers through ages of 50, 60 and 70, respectively. While these percentages are quite high, it is important to consider that only 6% of lung cancer is diagnosed before the age of 50 and approximately 22% occur before the age of 60. Therefore, based on these results, the actual number of lung cancers due to inheritance of a major susceptibility gene is low.

24.7 EFFECT OF COHORT DIFFERENCES IN SMOKING PREVALENCE

Lung cancer rarely occurs in the absence of environmental exposure; approximately 95% of the attributable risk is due to tobacco consumption [26]. Therefore, if lung cancer is the result of a gene–environment interaction, then in the absence of environmental exposure (i.e. cigarette consumption), an inherited susceptibility to the disease is less likely to be expressed. Therefore, intergenerational differences in the prevalence of the relevant environmental exposures, particularly tobacco, may obscure the true pattern of inheritance of a genetic factor.

The probands (index cases) selected for the Louisiana studies on lung cancer were ascertained over a 4-year period (1976–1979) and ranged in age at onset from 32 to 91 years. A potential complicating factor in these analyses is the temporal trend in smoking. In the US, smoking was uncommon before World War I, after which time there was a dramatic increase in tobacco use. Because of this cohort phenomenon and the wide range in the age of the probands, there was little uniformity in the exposure of the parental generations to the use of tobacco products. In particular, the parents of probands born before World War I (and hence with an age of onset greater than 60 years) would be less likely to smoke than the parents of probands born subsequent to World War I (and hence with an age of onset less than 60 years). If the previous segregation analyses are correct, one would assume that, at least for some families, one of the proband's parents carries a lung cancer susceptibility gene. If the genetically predisposed parent smokes, they are at significantly increased risk of developing lung cancer. Therefore, from a genetic modelling standpoint, one is analysing pedigrees in which there is at least one affected parent and at least one affected offspring – giving the appearance of mendelian dominant transmission. Conversely, if the genetically predisposed parent does not smoke, he or she would be less likely to develop lung cancer. Consequently, the pattern of disease in these families might appear to be inherited in a recessive or sporadic manner (i.e. no affected parents but lung cancer among their offspring). To address this possible scenario, additional analyses were performed in which the lung cancer families were partitioned into two groups: (i) probands older than age 60 at the time of ascertainment (born before World War I and unlikely to have parents who smoke); and (ii) probands younger than age 60 at the time of ascertainment (higher probability of smoking among parents) [27].

Of the 337 lung cancer families studied, 106 were ascertained through a proband whose age at death was less than 60 years and 231 through a proband whose age at death was 60 years or greater. Results of the segregation analyses on the early-onset proband families (higher probability of smoking parents) suggested that the pattern of disease was

Table 24.4 Results of segregation analysis of lung cancer in 337 families from southern Louisiana stratified by age of onset of proband

Hypothesis	Significance of goodness-of-fit*	Allele frequency	Percentage of population susceptible	Mean age of onset (years)		
				AA	AB	BB
Early onset (n = 106 families)						
No major gene	0.05	–	43	78	78	78
Environmental	0.025	0.035	40	273	58	79
Mendelian						
Dominant	0.025	0.090	86	79	79	295
Recessive	0.05	0.16	42	62	79	79
Codominant	0.25	0.062	60	61	79	279
Late onset (n = 231 families)						
No major gene	0.001	–	25	82	82	82
Environmental	0.05	0.25	19	48	77	77
Mendelian						
Dominant	0.95	0.025	22	50	50	82
Recessive	0.50	0.23	20	49	78	78
Codominant	0.90	0.17	22	47	73	84

*Compared with best fitting model.

explained only by mendelian codominant inheritance; all other hypotheses could be rejected (Table 24.4). Compared with the results obtained for all families, the estimated gene frequency was little changed, but the proportion of the population susceptible to the affected state doubled (from 28% to 60%). For the late-onset proband families (lower probability of smoking parents), the hypotheses of no major gene and random environment were still rejected, but the models of mendelian transmission considered could not be distinguished. Compared with the results obtained for all families, the estimated proportion of susceptibles under the codominant hypothesis was little changed (from 28% to 22%). The estimated gene frequency was considerably increased (0.052 to 0.17), but the estimates of gene frequencies in the two subsets were not significantly different from each other ($P = 0.1$).

As expected, the prevalence of smoking was greater among the fathers ($P < 0.05$) and mothers ($P < 0.01$) of early-onset probands than among the parental generation of late-onset probands. Age of onset of affected relatives, however, was not significantly different for the two subsets. These results suggest that the observed heterogeneity is more likely to be environmentally-related rather than mere isolation of a high-risk, early-onset subset of families.

24.8 POTENTIAL SOURCES OF HETEROGENEITY BETWEEN EARLY- AND LATE-ONSET FAMILIES

Although apparently different results were obtained when the families were stratified according to the age of onset of the proband, a statistical test was performed to evaluate whether the difference was significant. The test compares how well the various hypotheses fit the two subsets of the data versus how well the hypotheses fit the data on all families analysed together. The heterogeneity test confirmed that the stratification of the families into two groups was important ($P < 0.001$). Several possible sources of this heterogeneity were then examined [28], including sex differences in smoking prevalence, sex differences in age of onset, sex differences in susceptibility and a linear effect of the age of onset of the proband. None of these changes in the model could account for the observed heterogeneity.

24.9 IMPLICATIONS OF THE SEGREGATION ANALYSIS RESULTS

Because lung cancer rarely occurs in the absence of tobacco exposure, the results observed for the subset of early-onset families (where exposures were more uniform across generations) may be more likely to reflect the true underlying biology. If so, the results suggest a much greater influence of genetic factors in lung cancer pathogenesis than the results obtained when all families were analysed together: the cumulative probability of lung cancer at age 80 for a non-carrier of the gene, at the average level of tobacco consumption, was 2.8×10^{-27}, implying that virtually all lung cancer occurs among gene carriers. However, the results do not suggest that lung cancer is primarily a genetic disease. The cumulative probability that a non-smoking gene carrier develops lung cancer by age 80 was estimated to be only 52 per 100 000 (compared with 2175 per 100 000 for gene carriers who smoked). Thus, the data are more consistent with the hypothesis that a genetic predisposition to lung (and perhaps other smoking-associated cancers) is inherited and that the trait is expressed only in the presence of the major environmental insult: tobacco smoke.

Given the observational nature of the study design and analysis, it is premature to suggest screening, counselling or education for individuals with a positive family history of lung cancer; the results need to be corroborated by linkage studies. It is also imperative that the results be replicated in other populations, allowing for potentially important risk

factors that were not measured in the Louisiana study (e.g. carotenoid intake, alcohol use, physical activity, passive smoking, radon exposure, occupation). If shown to be correct, however, these findings would have tremendous public health implications: for the lung cancer-susceptible, smoking would appear to be universally lethal. Moreover, individuals without a family history of lung cancer should not be lulled into a false sense of security; (i) if parents and siblings have not been challenged by environmental (tobacco) exposure, susceptibility may not have been 'unmasked'; and (ii) given the variable age of onset of lung cancer, whether or not a person has a positive family history is a dynamic rather than a static characteristic. Furthermore, for the lung cancer non-susceptible, a variety of other disorders are highly likely, especially cardiovascular disease, which accounts for the greatest smoking-related morbidity and mortality [26].

24.10 CANDIDATE GENES FOR LUNG CANCER PREDISPOSITION

It is beyond the purpose of this chapter to review the results of laboratory studies designed to identify the molecular genetic changes associated with lung cancer progression, any of which might be inherited rather than acquired mutations in some families. The reader is referred to one of several excellent reviews on the topic [29, 30]. Briefly, while there are a number of candidate genes that may prove to be important in the pathogenesis of lung cancer, no definitive answer as to the molecular/genetic basis for an inherited predisposition to lung cancer is available. The prevailing hypothesis for susceptibility to chemically induced carcinogenesis is variation in metabolic activation of procarcinogens, primarily by the *CYP*2 genes [3, 32]. Related factors include variation in the formation of DNA adducts [33] and DNA repair [34]; both are important steps in the carcinogenic process that may determine susceptibility. While inherited *TP*53 mutations are associated with a variety of malignancies, the low frequency of inherited *TP*53 mutations in the general population make this an unlikely candidate.

24.11 SUMMARY AND CONCLUSION

The published studies of lung cancer to date suggest that the disease does aggregate in some families, that the clustering does not appear to be entirely the result of shared environmental factors and that the pattern of disease among relatives is consistent with the hypothesis of major gene segregation. Investigations to confirm these findings and isolate a putative susceptibility gene(s) for lung cancer are being actively pursued.

REFERENCES

1. Goodhart, C.B. (1959) Cancer-proneness and lung cancer. *Practitioner*, **182**, 578–84.
2. Brisman, R., Baker, R.R., Elkins, R. and Hartmann, W.H. (1967) Carcinoma of the lung in four siblings. *Cancer*, **20**, 2048–53.
3. Nagy, I. (1968) Zur Beobachtung von Bronchialkarzinomen bei drei Brudern. *Prax. Pneumol.*, **22**, 718–23.
4. Jones, F.L. Jr (1977) Bronchogenic carcinoma in three siblings. *Bull. Geisinger. Med. Cen.*, **29**, 23–5.
5. Goffman, T.E., Hassinger, D.D. and Mulvihill, J.J. (1982) Familial respiratory tract cancer: opportunities for research and prevention. *JAMA*, **247**, 1020–3.
6. Joishy, S.K., Cooper, R.A. and Rowley, P.T. (1977) Alveolar cell carcinoma in identical twins: Similarity in time of onset, histochemistry and site of metastases. *Ann. Intern. Med.*, **87**, 447–50.
7. Paul, S.M., Bacharach, B. and Goepp, C. (1987) A genetic influence on alveolar cell carcinoma. *J. Surg. Oncol.*, **36**, 249–53.
8. Tokuhata, G.K. and Lilienfeld, A.M. (1963) Familial aggregation of lung cancer in humans. *J. Natl Cancer Inst.*, **30**, 289–312.
9. Ooi, W.L., Elston, R.C., Chen, V.W., Bailey-Wilson, J.E. and Rothschild, H. (1986) Increased familial risk for lung cancer. *J. Natl Cancer Inst.*, **76**, 217–22.
10. Samet, J.M., Humble, C.G. and Pathak, D.R. (1986) Personal and family history of respiratory disease and lung cancer risk. *Annu. Rev. Respir. Dis.*, **134**, 466–70.
11. McDuffie, H.H., Klaassen, D.J. and Dosman, J.A. (1988) Cancer, genes and agriculture, in *Principles of Health and Safety in Agriculture*, (eds J.A. Dosman and D.W. Cockroft), CRC Press, Boca Raton, FL, pp. 258–61.
12. Shaw, G.L., Falk, R.T., Pickle, L.W., Mason, T.J. and Buffler, P.A. (1991) Lung cancer risk associated with cancer in relatives. *J. Clin. Epidemiol.*, **44**, 429–37.
13. McDuffie, H.H. (1991) Clustering of cancer in families of patients with primary lung cancer. *J. Clin. Epidemiol.*, **44**, 69–76.
14. Lynch, H.T., Kimberling, W.J., Markvicka, S.E. *et al.*. (1986) Genetics and smoking-associated cancers: a study of 485 families. *Cancer*, **57**, 1640–6.
15. Pierce, R.J., Kune, G.A., Kune, S. *et al.* (1989) Dietary and alcohol intake, smoking pattern, occupational risk, and family history in lung cancer patients: results of a case-control study in males. *Nutr. Cancer*, **12**, 237–48.
16. Sellers, T.A., Ooi, W.L., Elston, R.C., Chen, V.W., Bailey-Wilson, J.E. and Rothschild, H. (1987) Increased familial risk for non-lung cancer among relatives of lung cancer patients. *Am. J. Epidemiol*, **126**, 237–46.
17. Wu, A.H., Yu, M.C., Thomas, D.C., Pike, M.C. and Henderson, B.E. (1988) Personal and family history of lung disease as risk factors for adenocarcinoma of the lung. *Cancer Res.*, **48**, 7279–84.
18. Osann, K.E. (1991) Lung cancer in women: the importance of smoking, family history of cancer and medical history of respiratory disease. *Cancer Res.*, **51**, 4893–7.
19. Sellers, T.A., Elston, R.C., Atwood, L.D. and Rothschild, H. (1992) Lung cancer histologic type and family history of cancer. *Cancer*, **69**, 86–91.
20. Ambrosone, C.B., Rao, U., Michalek, A.M., Cummings, K.M. and Mettlin, C.J. (1993) Lung cancer histologic types and family

history of cancer. Analysis of histologic sub-types of 872 patients with primary lung cancer. *Cancer*, **72**, 1192–8.

21. Horn, D., Courts, F.A., Taylor, R.M. and Solomon, E.S. (1959) Cigarette smoking among high school students. *Am. J. Public Health*, **49**, 1497–511.

22. Salber, E.J. and MacMahon, B. (1961) Cigarette smoking among high school students related to social class and parental smoking habits. *Am. J. Public Health*, **51**, 1780–9.

23. Sellers, T.A., Elston, R.C., Stewart, C. and Rothschild, H. (1988) Familial risk of cancer among randomly selected cancer probands. *Genet. Epidemiol.*, **5**, 381–91.

24. Sellers, T.A., Bailey-Wilson, J.E., Elston, R.C. *et al.* (1990) Evidence for mendelian inheritance in the pathogenesis of lung cancer. *J. Natl Cancer Inst.*, **82**, 1272–9.

25. Bonney, G.E. (1986) Regressive logistic models for familial disease and other binary traits. *Biometrics*, **42**, 611–25.

26. Doll, R. and Hill, A.B. (1956) Lung cancer and other causes of death in relation to smoking. A second report on the mortality of British doctors. *Br. Med. J. (Clin. Res.)*, **57**, 1071–5.

27. Sellers, T.A., Potter, J.D., Bailey-Wilson, J.E., Rich, S.S., Rothschild, H. and Elston, R.C. (1992) Lung cancer detection and prevention: evidence for an interaction between smoking and genetic predisposition. *Cancer Res.*, **52**. S2694–7.

28. Sellers, T.A., Bailey-Wilson, J.E., Potter, J.D., Rich, S.S., Rothschild, H. and Elston, R.C. (1992) Effect of cohort differences in smoking prevalence on models of lung cancer susceptibility. *Genet. Epidemiol.*, **9**, 261–71.

29. Amos, C.I., Caporaso, N.E. and Weston, A. (1992) Host factors in lung cancer risk: a review of interdisciplinary studies. *Cancer Epidemiol. Biomarkers Prev.*, **1**, 505–13.

30. Shields, P.G. and Harris, C.C. (1993) Genetic predisposition to lung cancer, in *Lung Cancer*, 1st edn, (eds J.A. Roth, J.D. Cox and W.K. Hong), Blackwell Scientific Publications, Boston, pp. 3–19.

31. Guengerich, F.P. and Shimada, T. (1991) Oxidation of toxic and carcinogenic chemicals by human cytochrome P-450 enzymes. *Chem. Res. Toxicol.*, **4**, 391–407.

32. Uematsu, F., Kikuchi, H., Motomiya, M. *et al.* (1991) Association between restriction fragment polymorphism of the human cytochrome p450IIE1 gene and susceptibility to lung cancer. *Jpn J. Cancer Res.*, **82** 254–6.

33. Foiles, P.G., Murphy, S.E., Peterson, L.A., Carmella, S.G. and Hecht, S.S. (1992) DNA and hemoglobin adducts as markers of metabolic activation of tobacco-specific carcinogens. *Cancer Res.*, **52**, S2698–701.

34. Harris, C.C. (1989) Interindividual variation among humans in carcinogen metabolism, DNA adduct formation and DNA repair. *Carcinogenesis*, **10**, 1563–6.

353

Part Five

Health Care Aspects

Chapter 25

The cancer family clinic

ROSALIND A. EELES and VICTORIA A. MURDAY

25.1 WHAT IS THE CANCER FAMILY CLINIC AND WHY IS IT NEEDED?

Until recently, the study of the genetics of cancer was confined to the rarer familial cancer syndromes such as multiple endocrine neoplasia type 2 and familial polyposis coli. This was restricted to a relatively small number of families which were managed by clinicians with a specialized research interest in these conditions. With the advent of the knowledge that at least a proportion of many of the common cancers is due to an inherited genetic predisposition, although the percentage within each site may be low, the overall numbers of individuals at risk will be large because the cancers are more common. For example, it has been estimated that about 5% of breast cancers may occur as a result of the inheritance of a dominant gene [1]. This would equate to 1250 cases per year in the UK. This has led to the development of cancer family clinics, specializing in the management of hereditary cancers.

The functions of the cancer family clinic are to detect whether a family pattern of common cancers is likely to be genetic, diagnose rarer cancer family syndromes, provide cancer risk assessment, keep accurate records according to the Data Protection Act (1984), link familial data via confidential family registers, provide genetic counselling and genetic testing if appropriate, give advice on early detection and preventative options, and participate in clinical trials of these options, train other health care professionals so that the appropriate individuals are referred, guide and support voluntary bodies, monitor the effectiveness and quality of services, provide a resource for research and development, and provide a source of expert advice for purchasers and providers of these services.

25.2 NATIONWIDE ORGANIZATION OF CANCER FAMILY CLINICS

In the UK, the first clinical genetics service was established in 1946, and currently, the genetics service is organized on a regional basis. The ideal cancer family clinic would be the provision of a specialist clinic with access not only to personnel with experience in genetics, but also to oncological experience, counsellors and psychologists. It is therefore likely that these clinics will develop as joint clinics serving a regional area. National registers have been proposed in several countries for recording familial cancers. In France, the French Cooperative Group Network has been

Genetic Predisposition to Cancer. Edited by R.A. Eeles, B.A.J. Ponder, D.F. Easton and A. Horwich. Published in 1996 by Chapman & Hall, London.
0 412 56580 3

formed to coordinate the data collected from such clinics, and has already proved highly effective in identifying families with certain cancer phenotypes for collaborative international research (Y. Bignon and H. Sobol, personal communication).

It is likely that centres with an interest in certain inherited cancer syndromes which are rare (e.g. Li–Fraumeni syndrome), will become the national centre(s) for these diseases and other cancer family clinics will refer to them as tertiary referrals. However, personnel staffing all clinics have to have a working knowledge of the entire area of cancer genetics to be able to recognize these rare syndromes and know the correct channel of referral. The majority of the work in the cancer family clinic will be with families with inherited forms of the common cancer types, especially breast and colon cancer.

25.3 WHAT IS THE OPTIMAL STAFFING ORGANIZATION OF THE CLINIC?

The individuals at increased risk of cancer due to a genetic predisposition need both genetic and oncological advice. The ideal staffing of such a clinic therefore includes a geneticist, oncological specialist, and counselling and psychological support from trained nurses and clinical psychologists. Data management is important, for research and audit. A mechanism is needed for confirming diagnoses from medical records and retrieving death certificates. Such clinics are therefore labour intensive.

Another model is the attendance of a geneticist with a special interest in cancer genetics (or oncologist with experience of genetics) at joint clinics for the common cancers. This avoids a separate appointment in the cancer family clinic in some cases; however, the extensive cancer families would still have to be referred as these families require the back-up of the personnel listed above.

Liaison with a laboratory (preferably within the regional genetics service) is essential for the storage of blood and tumour samples.

25.4 REFERRAL PATTERNS

General practitioners are increasingly being consulted about genetic risk for cancer. The numbers involved with respect to the common cancers will make it very difficult for all the concerned individuals to be seen in a specialized cancer family clinic, nor indeed do all these people require the specialized services of such a clinic. A key role of the personnel in these clinics in the next few years will be education of both the primary care sector, other oncologists, and the general public. Research in the area of cancer genetics is urgently needed to identify the current knowledge and educational needs of the public and their care providers.

Ideally, one would refer potential gene carriers to the clinic, but the problem is identifying these individuals. The chance of being a gene carrier rises as the age of cancer diagnosis falls, for example, if female relatives of all cases of breast cancer diagnosed below 50 years were referred to cancer family clinics, this would involve 10 000 new women at risk each year in the UK. This is estimated from the figures that 20% of breast cancer arises in the under 50s (5000 cases/year in the UK), and on average, each woman has a mother and one sister at risk (A. Howell, personal communication). According to the Claus model [1], only up to 36% of isolated breast cancers diagnosed under the age of 40 are due to dominant high-risk predisposition genes, and so the remaining 64% are sporadic and would have no implications for the patient's relatives. The problem is the lack of markers which can identify gene carriers from sporadic cases.

Table 25.1 Referral guidelines for a cancer family clinic.[1] (Modified from [2].)

The cancers should be through the same genetic lineage, but can be through either the mother or father's side

1. Two or more unusual cancers in the same individual or in close relatives (e.g. brain tumour and sarcoma)
2. Cancer in the context of an associated syndrome (e.g. glioma in neurofibromatosis, type I; melanoma in dysplastic naevus syndrome)
3. Clustering of common cancers
   (a) Three or more cancers or the same type or related types in close relatives (e.g. breast/ovary/endometrium/colon/prostate)
   (b) Two cancers of the same type or related types in close relatives where one is diagnosed before age 50
   (c) A first-degree relative with one of the common cancers diagnosed before age 40 (in the case of prostate, before age 55)

[1] These guidelines are for referral only. Not all cases where there is a significant predisposition will fall within these groups; conversely, many individuals or families which meet these criteria will not in fact have a cancer-predisposition. The aim is to provide a simple scheme for ease of referal from GPs and oncology clinics.

The ideal situation would be computer-generated packages which would provide risk estimates for general practitioners when the family history is entered into a desktop computer. This would then advise when an individual should be referred to a cancer family clinic. Some groups are trying to produce such programs. The problem is designing a program which will cater for every possible familial cancer pattern.

Instead, guidelines can be followed and Ponder [2] has provided some easy guidelines for referral (see Table 25.1).

25.5 GENETIC COUNSELLING

Genetic counselling is the term which describes the interview which occurs when an individual attends a genetic clinic, although this is only part of what actually happens when a patient visits the clinic. Counselling is important in genetics, and its non-directive nature, offering choices to patients, has been the basis of the practice. This situation is likely to remain until proven preventive options are available for the common cancers. This is likely only to be a matter of time, and then it is possible that this traditional approach will cease and preventive options will be offered in the same way as treatments are offered for clinical disease. Currently, much of the consultation, like any other outpatient appointment, is for diagnosis and management of disease, and this is carried out ordinarily using the history and examination of an affected individual. With genetic disease, it may be the family history that holds the clue to diagnosis, and in a family cancer clinic, diagnosis of a genetic susceptibility to cancer may be largely determined by the family history.

25.6 THE FAMILY HISTORY

Establishing the pedigree is an important part of the interview. This is standardized to include the family history of cancer, other diseases, developmental and congential abnormalities, and a history of miscarriages. The diagnosis of a particular cancer-syndrome may be possible from the familial pattern of cancers or associated non-malignant problems. Information about at least first- (parents/siblings) and second- (grandparents) degree relatives should be requested (preferably also third-degree such as cousins) and, where appropriate, the family history sould be extended as far as possible [3].

The age at which cancer was diagnosed, the site(s), and the name of the treatment/hospital involved should be ascertained. This will allow assessment of risks to relatives, and confirmation of diagnosis from hospital records. For example, a common inaccuracy is the diagnosis of ovarian cancer which can be reported as stomach or uterine cancer. The presence of ovarian cancer in a breast cancer family raises the possibility that *BRCA1* is present and is therefore important.

25.7 PEDIGREE CONSTRUCTION

Many cancer family clinics send the client a questionnaire and have the family history available and reviewed before the client is seen in the clinic, where the doctor then simply comments on the pedigree. This saves about 20–30 minutes and can increase the throughput of the clinic. There are advantages and disadvantages of this approach. The family dynamics which are detected when taking a family history, can be missed and details of the pedigree should be confirmed since inaccuracies can occur when a client fills out a family history from a questionnaire, or further details may have been ascertained since the questionnaire was completed. However, the advantages are that the information will be more comprehensive since clients will ask family members about pieces of missing information before the consultation. In addition, diagnoses such as 'womb/ovarian cancer' can be confirmed from medical records or death certificates before the consultation.

One example of the expediency of this approach was the case of an individual referred for ovarian cancer screening and cancer risk assessment because of a family history of ovarian cancer in two relatives. The client reported in her questionnaire that one relative had 'stomach cancer' and the other ovarian cancer. Confirmation of the diagnoses by medical records in one case and death certification in the other revealed that only one relative had had ovarian cancer. The client was therefore at a lower ovarian cancer risk than she had feared and did not need

screening. All this was possible in one consultation, saving time and resources for the client and clinic staff.

For formal computation of pedigrees there are several computer packages which are PC-based (Cyrillic or Ped-Draw). There is an attempt to standardize pedigree symbols internationally [4], but until this occurs, the symbols unique to each centre should be explained in a legend accompanying the pedigree.

25.8 RISK ASSESSMENT

Genetic risks have two components: (i) the probability that a particular disorder will occur; and (ii) the damage and burden that it will inflict, both on the person that suffers the disease, and their family. The risk of cancer to the individual undergoing counselling is assessed from the family history. This is used to determine the likelihood that there is a cancer-predisposition gene in the family. If the gene involved has been identified, the cancer risks are determined from the genetic epidemiological studies of that gene. If the particular gene has not yet been identified, as is the case in many instances of the common cancers, risk estimates are calculated using the epidemiological studies of risks to relatives of cases with those cancers. There is also an additional component from environment–gene interactions, a relatively unstudied area at present. These will be more clearly defined as further cancer-predisposition genes are cloned and genetic epidemiological studies are performed.

As a general rule, the occurrence of the same cancer in three close blood relatives of a family is suggestive that there is a genetic susceptibility, particularly if they were affected at an early age.

If there are two close relatives with the same cancer, then the population risk of that cancer is an important guide as to the chance of a genetic susceptibility, i.e. if a cancer is

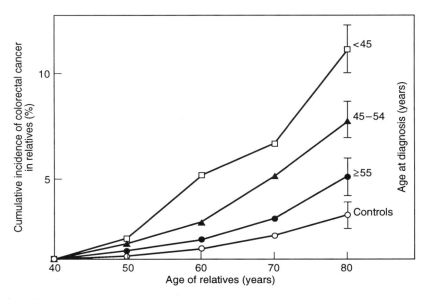

Fig. 25.1 Cumulative risk of colorectal cancer in relatives of a patient diagnosed at various ages from [5].

rare, then two cases in a family are less likely to have occurred by chance.

Having a single relative with a particular cancer often does not greatly increase the risk to relatives. The exception to this is if the relative is young or has had multiple primaries or a recognizable cancer syndrome. The risk of bowel cancer in the relatives of a single case illustrates the importance of age at diagnosis (Figure 25.1, from [5]).

Some cancer syndromes have phenotypes that can be diagnosed in an individual. Frequently, it is the premalignant phenotype, such as numerous adenomatous polyps in familial adenomatous polyposis (FAP; see Chapter 20).

There is now published information on the risks for relatives of cancer patients, particularly for common cancers such as breast cancer and colorectal cancer [1,5,6] and these are particularly useful for genetic counselling, permitting visual demonstration of risk assessment to the patient. The likelihood of a genetic susceptibility can be calculated, by combining information on the number and age of affected individuals. The risk to the patient will depend upon their relationship to the affected family members, and their own age since the risk will decrease the longer they remain free of disease. An example of such a risk assessment for the kindred is illustrated in Figure 25.2. Table 25.2 shows the method of combining the information by an approximate Bayesian calculation to determine the residual risk for the patient. The prior probability is the chance that the individual at risk has the predisposition gene. As II.1 is a daughter of I.2 who is assumed to be a gene carrier, the probability of II.1 having the gene is half of the chance that the cases in the family have a breast cancer predisposition gene (60%/2 = 30% or 0.3). The posterior probability is the probability that the person will have the predisposition gene given all the information available, such as age of the individual.

When a specific diagnosis of cancer susceptibility is possible in a family, then there may be more information available to impart, both in terms of the chances of developing cancer and possible non-malignant problems. For

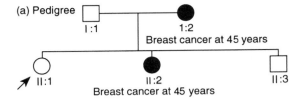

(a) Pedigree

I:1   1:2
Breast cancer at 45 years

II:1   II:2   II:3
Breast cancer at 45 years

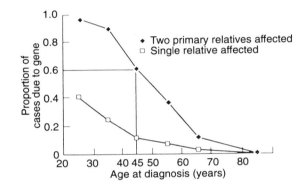

(b) Probability curve for breast cancer

• Two primary relatives affected
□ Single relative affected

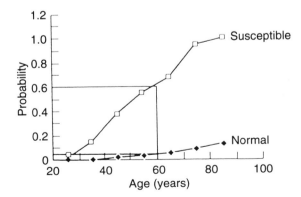

(c) Penetrance of breast allele

Fig. 25.2

instance, if a *BRCA*1 mutation is the likely cause of breast cancer in a family, then detailed information is available on the cumulative risk of both ovarian and breast cancer as well as the possibility of other cancers, such as bowel and prostate, for which there is an increased relative risk in affected individuals (see Chapter 15). A *BRCA*1 mutation may be suspected either from the family structure, a dominant susceptibility to early breast cancer associated with ovarian cancer, or by demonstration of linkage to the *BRCA*1 region on chromosome 17, or, best of all, by the demonstration by direct mutation analysis of a cancer-causing mutation in the gene.

25.9 RISK PERCEPTION

One of the primary reasons for identifying hereditary cancer is to enable family members to be targetted for advice on risk. This raises the important issue of the process of giving risk information. The uptake of preventive strategies may depend on the individual's perception of risk; for example, Croyle *et al.* [7] have shown that individuals at a perceived increased risk of heart disease were more likely to express their intentions to modify their lifestyle than those at population risk. The understanding and retention of

Fig. 25.2 (a) The patient (II:1 arrowed) has a mother (I:2) diagnosed with breast cancer at 45 years of age and a sister (II:2) with breast cancer diagnosed at the age of 45 years. (b) The probability of a dominant gene giving rise to the breast cancer in two primary relatives affected is 60%. (c) Since the woman at risk is a sister or daughter of an affected individual her risk of having the 'gene' is 30%, i.e. 1/2 that of the affected relatives. She is 60 years of age, by which age 60% of individuals with the genetic susceptibility will have developed breast cancer. (Actually the true prior probability that II:1 is a gene carrier is very slightly lower than this since the fact that she is unaffected at age 60 slightly reduces the figure from 25.2(b).)

Table 25.2 Determination of residual risk for patients

	Susceptible	Non-susceptible
Prior probability (from Figure 25.2(b))	0.30	0.70
Disease-free at 60 years (from Figure 25.2(c))	0.40	0.96
Posterior probability	$\dfrac{0.30 \times 0.4}{0.3 \times 0.4 + 0.7 \times 0.96} = 0.15$	0.85

this information may depend on the format in which it is presented and the individual's attitudes to risk. Even with the recent advances in the cloning of several cancer-predisposition genes, incomplete penetrance (i.e. not all gene carriers develop cancer, they are however at increased risk) means that even known gene carriers still have to comprehend that thay are at a certain level of **risk** and the development of cancer still has an element of uncertainty. Geneticists are still trying to determine the best method for providing information to those at increased risk due to a genetic predisposition.

Risk information is often complex and can be expressed in various ways. It is current practice in genetic counselling clinics and the more recent specialized cancer family clinics, to convey risk information numerically, either as a risk of developing disease per year, or risk by a certain age [8]. The risk value is either given as a percentage risk or a '1 in x' value. However, the optimal format for conveying risk information is unknown. Studies have examined whether women correctly assess their level of risk [9], but few examine the best way to present genetic information to those who may be at increased risk of familial cancer, and it is not clear whether clients understand the rather complex explanations or what they remember of this information. We have preliminary data which suggest that women do not wish to have or remember numerical information. For example, 98% of women attending because of a family history of breast cancer

could not remember their percentage annual risk, even when this was given both verbally in the clinic, and by follow-up letter. They were somewhat better at providing feedback on their lifetime risk, but 35% gave an incorrect figure. More importantly though, they were able to report the category of their risk (low, medium, high) with reasonable accuracy, but this did not relate to their perception that they were more or less likely to get cancer. This suggests that clients have a poor understanding of the risk information being given. In general, this sample was also unclear about what action to take as a result of this consultation, despite the options being reiterated in a follow-up letter. Some women in this study reported that they did not actually find numerical risk information useful, despite wishing to know their risk status, and being able to report that a risk category, such as high risk, was helpful.

Green and Brown [10] have suggested that the **qualitative** aspect of risk is more important than the **quantitative** aspect, and Sorensen *et al.* [11] suggested that many patients do not remember or understand the genetic information given. Leonard *et al.* [12] claim that 'clients are bad at probabilistic reasoning and find quantitative risk estimates difficult to understand'. However, this finding contrasts with that of Josten *et al.* [13], who report from a cancer family clinic in Wisconsin, US that 'clients say that a number gives them boundaries rather than having an ambiguous sense of being high risk'. Interestingly, however, even 5–10% of individuals in this American study did not wish to have numerical risk information.

The individual's background information, sociodemographic factors (e.g. educational level) and psychological profile could conceivably alter the optimal method of risk presentation since these can act as barriers to adequate informed consent [14, 15].

Much of the research on risk perception has been done in industrial contexts. Familiarity with the risk has been shown to lower the perception of the risk level. For example, the perception of radiation risk by people living near nuclear power plants is lower than in those not living near to such installations [16]. However, in cancer families, it is possible that a larger cancer burden (the number and age at diagnosis of the cancer cases) may distort the risk above the true level, as is the case in families with cystic fibrosis [12]. Many people in cancer families think erroneously that their risk of developing cancer is 100%, and the only uncertainty is the point in time when the disease will occur. Lerman *et al.* [15] have reported that members of cancer families distort their risk, even when their family history consists of only one affected relative. There is evidence that overestimation of rare events can occur if the event concerned is salient, for example, a recent cancer diagnosis in a young family member.

The definitions of risk are multidimensional. They consist of the probability of a negatively valued event occurring, the consequences of that event, and the possible consequences of a person's behaviour (e.g. preventive actions) upon both these factors [17].

Vlek [18] claims that there are five factors underlying perception of risk. These are: (i) the potential degree of harm or lethality associated with the risk; (ii) the controllability through safety/rescue measures (i.e. prevention/early detection); (iii) the number of people exposed (this would equate to the cancer burden in the family); (iv) the familiarity with the effects of the risk; and (v) the degree of voluntariness of exposure to the risk.

Some individuals in our study expressed a wish only to know if they fall into a high, moderate or low risk category (S. Lloyd, in preparation); however, it is unclear what these categories mean to patients. Wilkie [19] assessed the perceived risk of inheriting adult polycystic kidney disease in children of an affected parent, who are at a 1 in 2 risk. Although in the same risk category, the perceived risk category was variable, 26% describing a high risk and 53% a medium risk. However, descriptive rather than numerical risk levels may be more easily retained, as has been shown in a study of AFP screening in pregnancy [20].

There are several reports regarding the perception of risk and the resultant effects on health monitoring behaviours [10, 21, 22], some suggesting that those at highest risk have a lower uptake of health preventive measures.

25.9.1 THE FORMAT OF GENETIC RISK INFORMATION

There are several options for the form of presentation of risk information for the risk of developing cancer:

1. Numerical
   Risk per year
   Risk by a certain age
   1 in X value or percentage format
   Relative risk corrected for age
2. General categorization
   High/moderate/low risk
   The problem with this concept is that different individuals and doctors assign the same risk levels to different categories
3. Situation analogy
   A situation carrying an equivalent risk without any numerical information, e.g.

the chances of picking an ace if one card is chosen blind from a card pack
4. The risk figure measure
   Risk of developing cancer
   Risk of **not** developing cancer
   Risk of death from cancer (this is very rarely given in clinics as it is perceived as too distressing)

From studies of lung cancer, there is some evidence that the perceived risk of **not** developing cancer is different from that of **developing** the disease [23]. For example, a *BRCA*1 carrier has a lifetime risk (by age 80) of developing breast cancer of 85%, and therefore has a 15% chance of **not** developing the disease. However, many women still believe that this risk level means they will inevitably develop breast cancer by age 80.

Clearly, if cancer family clinics are to provide a useful service it would be important to ensure that counsellees understand the risk information and advice they are given. Lack of understanding of their risk could impact on their ability to use this information when making decisions about the future management of their health and may also affect their mental health if cancer-related worries are increased through misunderstanding of information given in the clinic.

25.10 MEDICAL HISTORY AND EXAMINATION

It must be established from the history and examination whether the patient is an affected or an at-risk member of the family, and the patient should be questioned on any symptoms indicative of cancer or congenital abnormalities. Initial clinical examination involves looking for any dysmorphic features and congenital anomalies. The skin should be carefully examined, as many cancer syndromes are associated with dermatological features, such as pigmentary abnormalities, e.g. freckles are seen in Peutz–Jeghers syn-

drome, café au lait patches in neurofibromatosis or Turcot's syndrome, basal cell naevi in Gorlin's syndrome, etc. Skin tumours, like the epidermoid cysts seen in FAP or keratoacanthomas seen in Muir–Torré or tricholemmas of Cowden's syndrome, can be indicators that the individual is in fact a gene carrier without the need for formal DNA genetic testing.

25.11 DISCUSSION OF CANCER SUSCEPTIBILITY AND RISKS

The following part of the interview involves communicating to the patient the results of the pedigree assessment, risk assessment and clinical examination. If a particular diagnosis is made, then information about that disease is given.

Those attending genetic clinics may have a very rudimentary knowledge of genetics, and it is important that they have a simple explanation of mendelian genetics and how their risk has been assessed. A simple explanation of how cancer develops as a result of somatic genetic events is also sometimes helpful. In this way patients can understand the information they are given. If they are being given empiric risks then the method by which these figures are derived must be explained. If there are no data, then this must also be discussed, and if the geneticist has a clinical impression that there may be something unusual occurring, but it is no more than a clinical judgement, then this must be made clear. Having a risk figure is useful for the clinician as this will dictate what options for management are available, but may only be useful to patients if they are put into context, i.e. in relation to the population risk of that and other cancers (see above). In particular, the age at which they are at greatest risk must be discussed, to enable management choices to be made, as they may affect the timing of prophylactic surgery or screening programmes.

Discussion of possibilities for screening and prevention should follow. Suggested screening protocols are shown in Table 25.3. What is known about the value of any particular strategy, including its rationale, is explored. Since some individuals may wish to do nothing, it is important that this is also discussed as an acceptable option, and may be the right decision for some people. In some instances prophylactic surgery needs to be discussed, but this must be approached with caution as some patients are frightened or even horrified at the suggestion. They may feel that this is confirmation from the doctor that their risk of cancer is unacceptably high, and may accentuate any fears they may have of the disease and its treatment.

Throughout the interview, it is important to be sensitive to any psychopathology that may be occurring. Frequently there will have been bereavement due to the premature death of close relatives, particularly a parent. Unresolved bereavement may make it difficult for people to accept their own risks and make decisions on their own management. In addition, patients are sometimes unable to cope with their worries. Referral for formal counselling may resolve these problems. Of particular concern are those individuals who have prophylactic surgery because of excess anxiety but who, while being temporarily relieved, often return at a later date with further cancer phobic symptoms. A psychological assessment and counselling should be mandatory before prophylactic mastectomy.

25.12 PREDICTIVE GENETIC TESTING

The number of cancer susceptibilities that have been mapped by genetic linkage is steadily increasing. Linkage analysis and direct mutation analysis are now possible in theory for many different cancer susceptibilities (Table 25.4). This allows DNA analysis to be carried out and individuals with a susceptibility gene to be identified before the devel-

opment of the disease. In late-onset genetic disease susceptibilities, there is a consensus view that children (here classified as those aged under 18 years) should not be tested, unless there is to be a therapeutic intervention or change in management. However, some cancer susceptibilities do require screening during childhood; for instance, screening for familial polyposis coli usually starts in early teenage years by sigmoidoscopy. DNA testing before this time will allow half the individuals to avoid having this invasive procedure. Testing would therefore seem entirely reasonable, particularly as preventive treatment by prophylactic surgery has been demonstrated as being a successful cancer prevention. The value of testing for other cancer susceptibilities, where the role of screening and prevention is unknown, is more debatable. Many of the issues that have been discussed at length in relation to testing for other adult onset genetic diseases, such as Huntington's chorea where prevention is not possible, are relevant. It has been demonstrated that using a set protocol for individuals having predictive testing for Huntington's chorea helps to minimize the problems experienced and allows the individual to have time to decide if they really want the test and for what reason [24].

There may be many reasons why individuals may wish to have a predictive test. They may want to know if they have the gene before starting a family, or to make plans for their own future. Some wish to make choices concerning prophylactic surgery or participation in screening or chemoprevention studies.

Facing a high risk of breast cancer is particularly difficult for some women. Often there have been several deaths from the disease in the family, and since there is often a mother who had died when the patient was only in her teens, the memories can be particularly painful. Since there may already be a great deal of anxiety about the disease, it

Table 25.3 Screening protocols (for guidance only; different clinics may have individual minor alterations to this schema)

Disease	Screen	Age (years)
von Hippel–Lindau Affected	Annual: physical examination urine testing direct ophthalmoscopy fluorescein angiography 24 hr urinary VMA renal ultrasound 3 yearly: MRI brain CT kidneys (more frequent if multiple cysts)	
von Hippel–Lindau At-risk relatives	Annual: physical examination urine testing direct ophthalmoscopy fluorescein angiography 24 hr urinary VMA renal ultrasound 3 yearly: MRI brain CT kidneys (more frequent if multiple cysts) 5 yearly: MRI brain	5 upwards 5 upwards 10 upwards until 60 20 until 65 15 to 40 20 to 65 40–60
Familial polyposis Affected	Offer total colectomy with ileorectal anastomosis	Teenager (see below)
	Annual rectal stump screening (if conserved in surgery)	
	Upper gastrointestinal endoscopy 3 yearly (annually if polyps found)	20 upwards
Familial polyposis At-risk relatives	Offer genetic analysis if possible	11 upwards (polyps are rare before this age) to 40
	Annual sigmoidoscopy	Perform colonoscopy when polyps found on sigmoidoscopy and arrange colectomy
Gorlin's syndrome Affected (at-risk children usually have abnormal skull or spine X-rays by 5 years)	Annual dermatological examination	Infants upwards
	Six-monthly orthopantomogram for jaw cysts	
	Examination of infants for signs of medulloblastoma (some advocate MRI **but not** CT due to radiosensitivity)	

Table 25.3 Continued

MEN Type 2	Offer genetic screening if possible if positive perform prophylactic thyroidectomy	5
	Plasma calcium, phosphate and parathormone	8–70
	Pentagastrin test	
	Thyroid ultrasound	
	Abdominal ultrasound and CT	
	24 hr urinary VMA	
MEN 1	5 yearly:	5 upwards
	symptom enquiry (dyspepsia, diarrhoea, renal colic, fits, amenorrhoea, galactorrhoea)	
	Examination	
	serum calcium parathormone renal function pituitary hormones (PL, GH, ACTH, FSH, TSH) pancreatic hormones (gastrin, VIP, glucagon, neurotensin, somatostatin, pancreatic polypeptide)	
	lateral skull X-ray for pituitary size or MRI for pituitary adenomas	
Wilms tumour At-risk individuals	3 monthly: renal ultrasound	Birth–8 years
	6 monthly: renal ultrasound	8–12 years
Retinoblastoma (siblings and offspring of affected)	Offer genetic screening if possible	
	Monthly retinal examination without anaesthetic	Birth–3 months
	3 monthly retinal examination under anaesthetic	3 months until 2 years
	4 monthly retinal examination under anaesthetic	2–3 years
	6 monthly retinal examination without anaesthetic	3–5 years
	Annual retinal examination without anaesthetic	5–11 years
	Annual examination for sarcoma	Early teens for life

367

Table 25.3 Continued

Disease	Screen	Age (years)
Li–Fraumeni	Annual breast examination	18–60 years
	?MRI (under investigation)	
	Annual examination	Lifelong
NF 1 Affected	Annual: Examination Visual field assessement	Lifelong
NF 2 At risk relatives	Offer genetic screening if possible	
	Annual: Examination Ophthalmoscopy for congenital cataracts	Childhood
	Annual audiometry Brain-stem audiotory-evoked potentials 3 yearly MRI brain	10–40
Lynch I syndrome	5 yearly colonoscopy (3 yearly if polyps are found)	25 upwards
Lynch II syndrome	5 yearly colonoscopy (3 yearly if polyps are found)	25 upwards
	Annual pelvic examination and ovarian and endometrial ultrasound and CA125	35 upwards
	Some screen for other cancers in kindred such as skin and urothelial malignancy	35 upwards
	Annual: mammography	35 upwards. Its use depends on amount of breast cancer in family
Muir–Torré syndrome	5 yearly colonoscopy (3 yearly if polyps are found)	25 upwards
Turcot's syndrome	5 yearly colonoscopy (3 yearly if polyps are found)	20 upwards
Colon cancer in a single relative aged <45 years	5 yearly colonoscopy (3 yearly if polyps are found)	25–30 upwards
Familial melanoma	Annual: skin examination	Teenager upwards
Breast/ovarian syndrome	Annual mammography	35 upwards or 5 years younger than youngest case (not less than 25)
	Annual pelvic examination transvaginal ultrasound CA125	35 upwards

Table 25.3 Continued

Familial breast cancer	Annual mammography	35 upwards or 5 years younger than youngest case (not less than 25)
Familial ovarian cancer	Annual pelvic examination transvaginal ultrasound CA125	30 upwards
Familial prostate cancer	Annual: serum prostate specific antigen	50 upwards or 5 years younger than youngest case (minimum age 40)
	digital rectal examination	
Familial testicular cancer	Regular testicular self examination	Late teens –50

Table 25.4 Location of and status of testing for cancer predisposition genes

Disease	Location	Mutation analysis
Breast ovarian	17q21	Not yet available[1]
Familial breast cancer	13q12	Not yet available
von Hippel–Lindau	3p25	YES for *VHL*
Familial adenomatous polyposis	5q21	YES for *APC*
Gorlin's syndrome	9q	Not yet available
Multiple endocrine neoplasia Type 2	10q11.2	YES for *RET*
Multiple endocrine neoplasia Type 1	11q	Not yet available
Wilms tumour	11p13	YES for *WT1*
Retinoblastoma	13q14	YES for *RB1*
Li–Fraumeni	17p13	YES for *TP53*
Neurofibromatosis I	17q11.2	YES for *NF1*
Neurofibromatosis II	22q11.2 to q21.1	YES for *NF2*
Lynch syndrome I	2p22	YES for *hMSH2*
Lynch syndrome II	3p21	YES for *hMLH1*

[1] This will become available for high-risk families during 1996.

may be very traumatic to find that the chance of having the gene for early breast cancer is high. It is therefore recommended that a formal psychological protocol is followed when offering predictive testing for all cancer predisposition genes.

The genetic testing procedure has several phases. Initially, the pros and cons and accuracy of the test are explained to the patient. These are the differences a positive and negative test result would make to the cancer risk if the gene being tested is indeed the cause of the cancers in the family, the ending of uncertainty, and the provision of more data on which to base decisions about clinical management and lifestyle. Potential disadvantages are psychological morbidity (although many clients are already very anxious) and the insurance implications. In the UK, all results of genetic tests currently have to be declared in the same way as any other medical test when seeking insurance. At present, the insurance companies do not actively request that these tests are performed. In certain instances, testing can be advantageous since some individuals in families are denied critical illness insurance to cover a cancer diagnosis. A negative test in such individuals may enable them to obtain insurance, although then of course, the urgency for the insurance may be removed.

There is a concurrent psychological assessment with the first counselling session. The client is then given a period of reflection (usually a minimum of 1 month) to decide whether or not to have the test, and if they decide to proceed, they are seen again to discuss their reasons for wishing to do so. It is only then that the blood sample for testing is collected after written consent. The disclosure session is carefully planned so that the client knows how long they will have to wait for the result and they are advised to bring a supportive person to the consultation when the result is given. Following this, they are seen at suitable intervals to ensure that they are not having any psychological problems.

25.13 GENETIC HETEROGENEITY

The number of families that can have predictive testing is limited by the degree of genetic heterogeneity, i.e. when more than one locus may cause the same condition. For instance, approximately half the breast cancer families tested for linkage to *BRCA*1 in fact have another gene. Each family becomes an experiment in itself, as linkage must be established in that particular family if predictive testing is to be carried out. The family needs to be large so that there is at least a 95% likelihood of linkage. Most families at the moment are not suitable for linkage predictive testing, and patients are often disappointed that they are unable to have the test. Now that *BRCA*1 is cloned [25] the

number of families that can be tested will increase, since direct mutation analysis of an affected individual will be used to confirm a *BRCA*1 mutation in a family.

However, mutation analysis is more labour intensive, particularly when the gene is large and mutations can occur at many different sites within the gene in different families, as is the case with *BRCA*1. The procedure involves testing a sample of DNA extracted from blood collected from an affected individual in the family and mutation analysis is carried out (as described in Chapter 26). Once the cancer-causing mutation in that family is identified, other members of the family can then be tested to see whether or not they carry the specific mutation in the cancer-predisposition gene.

REFERENCES

1. Claus, E.B., Risch, N.J. and Thompson, W.D. (1991) Genetic analysis of breast cancer in the cancer and steroid hormone study. *Am. J. Hum. Genet.*, **48**, 232–42.
2. Ponder, B.A.J. (1994) Setting up and running a familial cancer clinic. *Br. Med. Bull.*, **50**, 732–45.
3. Harper, P.S. (1988) In *Practical Genetic Counselling*, 3rd edn, Wright, Butterworth & Co., pp. 3–17.
4. Bennett, R.L., Steinhaus, K.A., Uhrich, S.B. *et al.* (1995) Recommendations for standardized human pedigree nomenclature. *Am. J. Hum. Genet.*, **56**, 745–52.
5. St John, D.V.B., McDermott, F.T., Hopper, V.L., Debney, E.A., Johnson, W.R. and Hughes, E.S.R. (1993) Cancer risks in relatives of patients with common colorectal cancer. *Ann. Intern. Med.*, **118**, 785–90.
6. Murday, V.A. and Slack, J. (1989) Inherited disorders associated with colorectal cancer. *Cancer Surv.*, **8**, 139–59.
7. Croyle, R.T., Sun, T.-C. and Louie, T.H. (1993) Psychological minimization of cholesterol test results: moderators of appraisal in college students and community residents. *Health Psychol.*, **12**, 503–7.

8. Kelly, P.T. (1992) Informational needs of individuals and families with hereditary cancers. *Semin. Oncol. Nursing*, **8**(4), 288–92.

9. Evans, D.G.R., Burnell, L.D., Hopwood, P. and Howell, A. (1993) Perception of risk in women with a family history of breast cancer. *Br. J. Cancer*, **67**, 612–14.

10. Green, C.H. and Brown, R.A. (1978) Counting lives. *J. Occupational Accidents*, **2**, 55.

11. Sorensen, J.R., Swazey, J.P. and Scotch, N.A. (1981) Reproductive past, reproductive futures: genetic counselling and its effectiveness. Birth defects: original article series, 17, 4, New York. pp1–19.

12. Leonard, C., Chase, G. and Childs, B. (1972) Genetic counselling, a consumer's view. *N. Engl. J. Med.*, **287**, 433–9.

13. Josten, D.M., Evans, A.M. and Love, R.R. (1985) The cancer prevention clinic: a service program for cancer-prone families. *J. Psychosoc. Oncol.*, **3**, 5–20.

14. Merz, J.F. and Fisdhoff B. (1990) Informed consent does not mean rational consent. *J. Legal Med.*, **11**, 321–50.

15. Lerman, C., Daly, M., Masny, A. and Balshem, A. (1994) Attitudes about genetic testing for breast-ovarian cancer susceptibility. *J. Clin. Oncol.*, **12**, 843–50.

16. Guedeney, C. and Mendel, G. (1973) *L'Angoisse Atomique et les Centres Nucleaires.* Payot, Paris.

17. Evers-Kiebooms, G., Cassiman, J.-J., Van der Berghe, H. and d'Ydewalle, G. (eds) (1987) *Genetic Risk, Risk Perception and Decision Making.* Alan R. Liss, Inc., New York.

18. Vlek, C. (1987) Risk assessment, risk perception and decision making about courses of action involving genetic risk: an overview of concepts and methods. *March of Dimes Birth Defects Foundation*, **23**(2), 171–207.

19. Wilkie, P.A. (1992) *Genetic counselling and adult polycystic kidney disease: patients' knowledge, perceptions and understanding.* PhD Thesis, Stirling University.

20. Chase, G.A., Faden, R.R., Holtzman, N.A. *et al.* (1986) Assessment of risk by pregnant women: implications for genetic counseling and education. *Soc. Biol.*, **33**(1–2), 57–64.

21. Kash, K.M., Holland, J.C., Halper, M.S. and Miller, D.G. (1991) Psychological distress and surveillance behaviors of women with a family history of breast cancer. *J Natl Cancer Inst.*, **84**, 24–30.

22. Polednak, A.P., Lane, D.S. and Burg, M.A. (1991) Risk perception, family history and use of breast cancer screening tests. *Cancer Detect. Prevent.*, **15**(4), 257–63.

23. McNeil, B.J., Pauker, S.G., Sox, H.C. Jr and Tversky, A. (1982) On the elicitation of preferences for alternative therapies. *N. Engl. J. Med.*, **306**, 1259–62.

24. Tyler, A., Ball, D., Craufurd, D. on behalf of the United Kingdom Huntington's Disease Prediction Consortium (1992) Presymptomatic testing for Huntington's Disease in the United Kingdom. *Br. Med. J.*, **304**, 1593–6.

25. Miki, Y., Swensen, J., Shattuck-Eidens, D., *et al.* (1994) A strong candidate for the breast and ovarian cancer susceptibility gene, BRCA1. *Science*, **266**, 66–71.

371

Chapter 26

Screening for mutations in cancer predisposition genes

CHRISTOPHER G. MATHEW

26.1 INTRODUCTION

This chapter is concerned with bringing the fruits of research into the inherited cancer syndromes to the diagnostic table. Once the gene for a particular syndrome has been mapped or cloned, the information can be used to provide presymptomatic testing for families affected with the disorder. If the predisposing gene has been localized by genetic linkage (see Chapter 2) but has not yet been cloned, an indirect test can often be provided by analysing DNA from the family with DNA polymorphisms to determine which allele (or form) of the marker is linked to it. Once the gene has been cloned (Chapter 3), a direct test can generally be done by screening family members for mutations in the gene.

The amount of work involved in finding the causative mutation in a particular family by direct mutation testing will depend on the size and complexity of the relevant gene, and on the degree of heterogeneity of its mutations. If there are a limited number of relatively common mutations in the gene, simple diagnostic assays which make use of the polymerase chain reaction (PCR) [1] can be set up to test for specific mutations in the index case of each new family referred for screening. An example of this is multiple endocrine neoplasia type 2 (MEN 2, Chapter 6), in which mutations are clustered in the cysteine-rich region of the *RET* oncogene. If, however, almost every family has a different mutation, then the coding and regulatory regions of the gene will have to be scanned for novel mutations using more sophisticated and time-consuming techniques. New developments in both diagnostic and scanning methods for mutation detection have been reviewed recently [2].

The starting point for genetic screening in inherited cancer syndromes should, of course, be determination of the correct clinical diagnosis using well-established clinical, biochemical and cytogenetic tests, before elaborate molecular technology is deployed to find the mutation. However, as the genes associated with predisposition to the common cancers are defined, molecular tests will begin to be used to establish whether a family history of a site-specific cancer is indeed caused by an inherited mutation.

Genetic Predisposition to Cancer. Edited by R.A. Eeles, B.A.J. Ponder, D.F. Easton and A. Horwich. Published in 1996 by Chapman & Hall, London.
0 412 56580 3

26.2 INDIRECT TESTING FOR THE MUTATION

An indirect test for the predisposing gene using DNA polymorphisms will obviously be needed if the chromosomal location of the gene is known, but the gene has not been cloned. It may also be required if the cloned gene is very large, and the technical or financial resources required to locate the causative mutation are not available. The use of genetic linkage analysis and DNA polymorphisms to locate cancer genes has been discussed in Chapter 2, but several principles should be adhered to in the application of this approach in a diagnostic setting.

The first of these is that there should be some evidence that the cancer in the family is linked to the markers which are being used for presymptomatic testing. Many of the syndromes described in this book are genetically heterogeneous, with two or more different genes at different chromosomal locations being associated with the same clinical phenotype. For example, the predisposing gene in about one-third of families with early-onset inherited breast cancer is not linked to the *BRCA*1 locus on chromosome 17q. The degree of statistical support required before the *BRCA*1 markers can be used for predictive testing is discussed in Chapter 15.

The second principle is that the degree of error from meiotic recombination between the DNA markers used and the disease gene should be very small, preferably of the order of 1% or less. This can be achieved if tightly linked markers on either side of the disease gene are used, since the probability of a double recombination event occurring between two closely linked markers is extremely small. If the disease gene has been cloned, use of a single intragenic marker will usually be sufficient, as the probability of intragenic recombination between the marker and the mutation is very small in most genes.

On a practical level, markers should be chosen which are highly informative and which can be analysed by PCR. The polymorphisms which are composed of repeats of the dinucleotide sequence CA are ubiquitous in the human genome, show a high degree of heterozygosity, and are typed by PCR [3,4]. Analysis of two or three of these markers in a family will generally be sufficient to find at least one which is informative.

The use of linked markers for predictive testing is now widespread. For example, this approach was applied to presymptomatic testing for MEN 2 in combination with biochemical screening data prior to the cloning of the gene [5].

26.3 DIAGNOSTIC TESTS FOR KNOWN MUTATIONS

Although some disease-causing mutations involve gross deletions or rearrangements of DNA, the majority are either substitutions of a single base or small alterations such as the deletion of one or a few bases of the gene sequence. Several different methods are commonly used to detect such mutations, all of which are based on PCR amplification of the region of the gene which contains the mutation.

26.3.1 BAND SHIFT ASSAY

If the mutation is a deletion or insertion of one or more bases, a small segment of the gene – including the site of the mutation – can be amplified by PCR, and the mutated allele detected by gel electrophoresis because of its altered mobility. Separation of 1 bp size differences will usually require incorporation of a radioactive label into the PCR product, followed by electrophoresis on a large denaturing polyacrylamide gel and autoradiography. Differences of two or more base pairs can generally be resolved on non-denaturing polyacrylamide gels, and the DNA fragments detected by staining with ethidium bromide.

ARTIFICIAL RESTRICTION SITE ASSAY

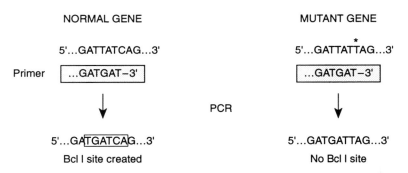

NORMAL GENE   MUTANT GENE

5'...GATTATCAG...3'   5'...GATTATTAG...3'

Primer | ...GATGAT–3' | | ...GATGAT–3' |

PCR

5'...GATGATCAG...3'   5'...GATGATTAG...3'

Bcl I site created   No Bcl I site

Fig. 26.1 Detection of the Q13X mutation (C→T*) in the Fanconi anaemia group C gene by creation of an artificial BclI restriction site adjacent to the mutation.

26.3.2 RESTRICTION SITE ANALYSIS

Restriction enzymes cut DNA at sequence-specific sites. If a mutation occurs within a recognition site for a particular restriction enzyme, the enzyme will no longer cut the DNA at this point. Conversely, the mutation may create a new cutting site. In either event, digestion of PCR product from the region of the mutation with the appropriate enzyme will produce fragments of a different size if the mutation is present. If the mutation does not happen to occur within a restriction site, PCR can often be used to create a restriction site in the PCR product adjacent to the position of the mutation [6]. This is done by synthesizing a PCR primer adjacent to the mutation with a sequence which is slightly different from the normal sequence, and which introduces a new restriction site into the PCR product (see Figure 26.1).

26.3.3 ALLELE-SPECIFIC OLIGONUCLEOTIDE ASSAY

In this technique, the PCR product is spotted onto a nylon or nitrocellulose membrane which is then incubated with a radioactively-labelled oligonucleotide sequence of about 18 bases, corresponding to either the normal or the mutant sequence [7,8]. The short oligonucleotide probes, or allele-specific oligonucleotides (ASOs), will only bind to their exact complementary sequence, provided that the temperature and salt concentration of the solution used for the incubation are carefully controlled. Binding of the mutant or normal ASO to the various patient samples on the strip is then detected by autoradiography. The oligonucleotide can also be labelled with a non-radioactive tag such as biotin [8]. This method is quite convenient for testing for several different mutations in the same region of the gene, since the membrane can be incubated with a succession of ASOs which are specific for different mutations. It has also been modified to enable testing of smaller numbers of samples for an extensive series of mutations by spotting many different ASOs onto the membrane, and hybridizing labelled PCR product from the patient to it [9].

26.3.4 ALLELE-SPECIFIC PRIMING

The allele-specific priming method (also called the ARMS method), utilizes the exquisite specificity of the PCR priming process to

ALLELE-SPECIFIC PRIMING

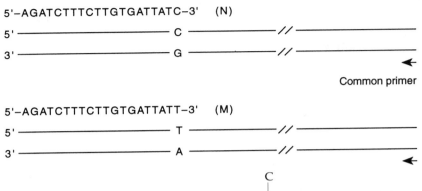

Fig. 26.2 Scheme for the detection of the Q13X mutation (G in top DNA strand has mutated to A shown in bottom DNA strand) by allele-specific priming. In practice, it is sometimes necessary to introduce an additional mismatch between the primer and the normal sequence to ensure that the mutant primer does not amplify from the normal DNA sequence. (N), primer for normal sequence; (M), primer for mutant sequence.

effect allele-specific priming of normal or mutant sequences [10]. The allele-specific primer (ASP) is so designed that its 3′ end is located exactly at the site of the mutation. PCR amplification will occur between this primer and a 'common' primer (C), some distance away on the other side of the mutation, only if the sequence at the 3′ end of the ASP matches the sequence of the sample DNA at this point. Thus two ASPs are made – one which will only prime off the normal sequence (N), and one which will prime off a particular mutant sequence (M). Two separate PCRs are then carried out on each sample (N→C and M→C), and the PCR products detected by gel electrophoresis. The principle of the ASP method is illustrated in Figure 26.2. Since no reaction products will be seen with the M primer in a sample which does not have the mutation, a pair of control primers from a different genetic locus is added to each reaction to check for failure of the PCR for trivial technical reasons.

The ASP method can be used to test for several different mutations simultaneously, by designing the primers so that the lengths of the PCR products are different for each of the mutations. A further advantage of the method is that it does not involve restriction enzyme digestion or time-consuming hybridization and detection steps. A successful and widely used ASP method has been established for population screening for multiple mutations in the cystic fibrosis gene [11], and should be generally applicable for repetitive testing for multiple mutations in any gene of interest.

26.4 SCANNING FOR UNKNOWN MUTATIONS

A variety of methods to scan for unknown mutations are available (reviewed in [2, 12]) and the choice will be governed by the size and complexity of the gene to be screened, the technical skills and laboratory equipment available, and the degree of sensitivity required. Some of the PCR methods commonly used to screen for mutations which alter one or a few nucleotides will be described. Their strengths and weaknesses are summarized in Table 26.1

Table 26.1 Comparison of methods for mutation scanning

	Size (bp)[1]	Sensitivity (%)	Simplicity	Remarks
Single-stranded conformational polymorphism	150–300	80–90	+++	
Heteroduplex analysis	up to 400	Unknown	+++	
Denaturing gradient gel electrophoresis	up to 600	>95	++	Temperature-controlled electrophoresis tank
Chemical cleavage method	up to 1700	100	+	Toxic chemicals used Localises mutation

[1] Optimum size of DNA fragment which can be scanned at the quoted sensitivity.

26.4.1 SINGLE-STRANDED CONFORMATION POLYMORPHISM (SSCP)

This technique relies upon the fact that, under non-denaturing conditions, single-stranded DNA molecules will fold into unique conformations which are determined by their nucleotide sequence [13]. The difference in secondary structure induced by a single base change is often sufficient to cause a measurable change in the electrophoretic mobility of the DNA. This phenomenon has been exploited by Orita and his co-workers to devise a rapid and simple method to screen for mutations in short DNA fragments [14]. One of the pair of PCR primers is radioactively labelled, the DNA fragment of interest is amplified by PCR, and the products are then electrophoresed on a non-denaturing polyacrylamide gel and detected by autoradiography. The shift in mobility caused by a single base substitution in the Fanconi anaemia group C gene is shown in Figure 26.3. The method can also be used in a non-radioactive format, in which the DNA fragments are detected by ethidium bromide staining [15].

The great advantage of the SSCP method is its simplicity. This makes it ideal for scanning a large number of samples for unknown mutations. Its chief disadvantage is that it is only suitable for scanning DNA fragments of about 150–250 bp in length, since its sensitivity of mutation detection falls off rapidly in longer PCR products. In one study, 97% of mutations were detected in a 155 bp fragment, falling to 58% in a product of 420 bp [16]. The size of fragment screened can be extended by digestion of a larger PCR product into two or three smaller fragments with a restriction enzyme before electrophoresis, but partial digestion products and an increasingly complex gel pattern limit the usefulness of this approach. The conditions of electrophoresis also influence sensitivity; the inclusion of glycerol in the gel, or electrophoresis at 4°C, may allow or prevent the detection of a particular mutation. Some workers therefore recommend using two different sets of electrophoretic conditions for screening, but this substantially increases the workload. The factors affecting the sensitivity of SSCP have been reviewed recently [17]. A further disadvantage of SSCP, in common with most methods for mutation screening, is that it does not localize the site of the mutation. Thus it may be necessary to sequence the entire fragment to find the change.

In spite of these caveats, SSCP is justifiably an extremely popular method which has detected a vast number of mutations in a wide variety of genes.

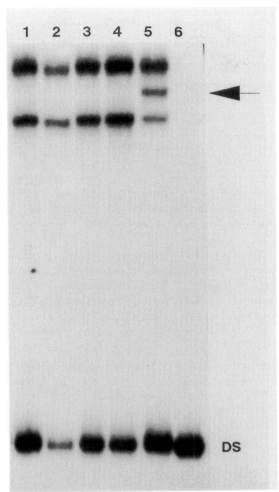

Fig. 26.3 Single-stranded conformation polymorphism detection of the Q13X mutation as a band shift (lane 5, indicated by arrowhead). DS, double-stranded DNA. Lane 6, control double-stranded DNA only. Other lanes (1–4) contain two bands (in addition to that from DS-DNA). Each corresponds to one of the single strands of DNA from the denatured PCR product.

26.4.2 HETERODUPLEX ANALYSIS (HA)

This method is based upon the observation that a hybrid between two single-stranded DNA molecules with sequences which differ from each other by a single nucleotide (heter-

oduplex) has an altered conformation, which may be detected as a reduction in electrophoretic mobility on non-denaturing gels [18, 19]. The formation of heteroduplexes after PCR is encouraged by a brief denaturation step, followed by slow cooling at room temperature. The DNA is then electrophoresed in a non-denaturing gel of either polyacrylamide or Hydrolink (AT Biochem), and stained with ethidium bromide. HA has been reported to detect single base substitutions in DNA fragments of up to 420 bp [18], but a systematic study of the sensitivity of this method is not yet available. Improved resolution of heteroduplexes from homoduplexes has been reported by inclusion of 10% urea in the gel matrix. The method is very simple to perform, and has been combined with SSCP analysis to improve the detection of mutations in the *TP*53 gene in human tumours [20].

A disadvantage of the HA method is that it would not detect a mutation for which the patient was homozygous, since no heteroduplex would be formed. This would only be a problem in recessive disorders since, in an autosomal dominant condition, the wild-type allele would always be present. This problem can be circumvented by mixing wild-type DNA with the patient's DNA before denaturation.

26.4.3 DENATURING GRADIENT GEL ELECTROPHORESIS (DGGE)

If a DNA fragment is electrophoresed at high temperature in a polyacrylamide gel which contains increasing concentrations of denaturants, it will become partially or completely denatured at some point. This will produce a sharp reduction in its electrophoretic mobility. Fischer and Lerman [21] were able to show that two DNA fragments which differed from each other by only a single base were generally denatured at different positions in the gradient, and could therefore be resolved by DGGE. However, base changes which occurred in the highest temperature melting domain did not cause a mobility shift because the strands had separated at that point. The sensitivity of the DGGE technique has been greatly improved by the attachment of a GC-rich sequence (known as a GC-clamp) to the end of the DNA fragment during PCR [22], which then serves as the last melting domain. Sensitive detection is also dependent on the use of computer programs to predict theoretical melting profiles for the sequence which is to be scanned for mutations.

Once suitable conditions have been established for the target region, mutations in DNA fragments of up to 600 bp can be detected rapidly, with a sensitivity of about 95% [12]. A further advantage is that the DNA is detected by ethidium bromide staining of the gel. Disadvantages are the development work required to establish suitable conditions for the gradient, the need for a gel electrophoresis apparatus which allows uniform heating of the gel, and the fact that the mutation is not localized precisely within the DNA fragment being scanned. A detailed protocol for the DGGE technique is available [23].

26.4.4 CHEMICAL CLEAVAGE METHOD (CCM)

This method is based upon the susceptibility of mismatched bases in a heteroduplex to modification by chemicals [24]. DNA from the test sample and a radioactively-labelled control is mixed, denatured, and allowed to form a heteroduplex. Incubation with hydroxylamine or osmium tetroxide results in modification of mismatched cytosines or thymines respectively, which are then cleaved with piperidine. The cleavage product produced by the mismatch is then detected by electrophoresis and autoradiography. If the ends of both strands of the wild-type DNA are labelled, mutations of adenine and guanine will also be detected as a mismatched T or C on the other strand. PCR amplification of the wild-type and control DNA prior to heteroduplex formation allowed this method to be applied to rapid mutation scanning in human genes [25]. A non-isotopic version of CCM has been developed, in which cleavage products are detected by silver staining [26]. Multiple cleavage products can be detected simultaneously by labelling PCR products from four different target fragments with fluorescent dyes of four different colours, and electrophoresis on an automated DNA sequencer [27].

CCM has three important advantages over most other methods of scanning for novel mutations. First, it is very sensitive, with a mutation detection rate approaching 100% if both DNA strands are labelled or stained [26, 28]. Second, it enables much longer segments of DNA to be scanned than the other methods, with successful detection reported in fragments of up to 2 kb in length [26]. Third, the approximate site of the mutation can be established from the size of the cleavage product, thus avoiding the need for extensive DNA sequencing to characterize it. Its disadvantages are the additional steps required for the chemical modification and cleavage, and the toxicity of the compounds used.

26.4.5 DIRECT SEQUENCING

All of the mutation scanning methods described above are designed to establish whether or not a mutation is present in the target region. The final step in all cases will be DNA sequencing of the fragment in order to establish the precise nature of the mutation. This is generally done by direct sequencing, in which PCR products are sequenced by the Sanger dideoxy chain termination method [29] without prior cloning in sequencing

378

vectors. The DNA can be sequenced from a double-stranded product, but a single-stranded template provides clearer and therefore more accurate sequence data. This can be obtained by biotinylation of one of the PCR primers, followed by capture of the PCR product on an avidin-coated magnetic bead, and degradation of the non-biotinylated strand with alkali [30]. Alternatively, the PCR product can be reamplified with one of the two PCR primers at a concentration 100-fold higher than that of the other. This second round of amplification produces a great excess of one strand, and is known as asymmetric PCR [31].

DNA sequencing is also, of course, the most sensitive and specific method that can be used for mutation scanning. However, it is too labour intensive for a primary scan of multiple samples unless costly equipment for automated fluorescent sequencing is available.

26.4.6 THE TARGET MOLECULE: GENOMIC DNA OR mRNA?

The target material for mutation scanning can either be genomic DNA or mRNA. If mRNA is used, it is first reverse-transcribed into complementary DNA (cDNA), and part or all of the coding sequence of the gene of interest is then amplified by PCR (RT–PCR). This approach is potentially very efficient, since large segments of the coding sequence can be scanned after a single PCR reaction, whereas the analysis of genomic DNA requires multiple PCRs from the constituent exons of the gene. It also does not require a knowledge of the genomic structure of the gene, or of intron sequence at the exon boundaries. However, this information will be needed to characterize mutations which give rise to aberrant splicing of the primary transcript. The RT–PCR method is more generally applicable than might be supposed, since the great sensitivity of PCR permits

amplification of mRNA from genes which are expressed at extremely low levels – a phenomenon referred to as 'illegitimate transcription' [32]. Thus, for example, dystrophin mRNA has been amplified from peripheral blood lymphocytes in order to detect mutations in patients with Duchenne muscular dystrophy [33]. Disadvantages of RT–PCR are that it will not detect mutations which result in a failure of transcription of the relevant gene (null alleles), and the production by RT–PCR of alternatively spliced transcripts which have no pathological significance may create diversions for the investigator. A helpful counter to the alternative splicing problem is to analyse a batch of control samples when first setting up the RT–PCR, and to analyse all test samples in duplicate.

The use of genomic DNA as the starting material for mutation scanning requires a knowledge of the genomic structure of the gene of interest, and enough of its intron sequence to allow amplification of each exon and its associated splice sites. Also, the highly interrupted nature of the coding sequence of most genes means that a rather large number of PCRs have to be set up and scanned. However, analysis of genomic DNA will detect all classes of mutation, and archival tissue such as paraffin-embedded tissue sections can be used for the analysis.

26.5 WHICH METHOD TO CHOOSE?

It would not be surprising if a new investigator felt somewhat overwhelmed by the variety of mutation scanning methods that are available. The choice of method should be based on the size of the coding region of the gene to be scanned, and on the complexity of its exon structure. The *TP53* gene, for example, has a coding sequence of 1200 bp, and is composed of 11 exons. Scanning of all 11 exons by SSCP analysis can be achieved in 9–10 PCRs (some of the *TP53* gene's introns are very small), and would probably detect 80–90% of mutations. Thus, SSCP analysis would be suitable if relatively large numbers of samples had to be screened, and if 100% sensitivity of mutation detection was not required. DGGE may offer marginally higher sensitivity [12], but would require a greater initial effort in establishing suitable conditions for efficient mutation detection. If 100% detection was needed, the chemical cleavage method would have to be used. A comparison of these three methods in scanning the *TP53* gene for mutations indicated a similar sensitivity for SSCP and constant denaturing gel electrophoresis (CDGE, a modification of DGGE) and a higher sensitivity for CCM [28].

If larger and more complex genes are to be scanned, the use of methods such as SSCP and HA are inappropriate. For example, analysis of the 8500 bp coding sequence of the APC gene, which is mutated in familial adenomatous polyposis, required 14 PCRs to scan exons 1–14, and a further 23 PCRs to scan the remaining 6500 bp of coding sequence in exon 15 by SSCP [34]. This heroic effort must have been very costly both in terms of reagents and of staff time. A more economical alternative would have been to use the chemical cleavage method to scan the large exon 15 in four overlapping PCRs. The remaining 14 exons could be scanned in two PCRs by RT–PCR and CCM, if the APC gene is expressed at low levels in peripheral blood lymphocytes.

An interesting new development in mutation scanning is the design of assays which detect a particular class of mutant allele. The protein truncation test (PTT) scans genes for mutations which cause premature termination of translation of the gene product [35]. In this assay, *in vitro* transcription of RNA is coupled with translation, to produce shortened peptides which are then detected by protein electrophoresis. PTT is particularly suited to scanning the *APC* gene for muta-

tions [36], since over 95% of mutations in this gene result in premature termination of translation.

26.6 WHAT IS A MUTATION?

The final, and very important, aspect of mutation analysis to be considered is the interpretation of the results of the scan. Some mutations would obviously be sufficient to inactivate a gene. A deletion of a single nucleotide from the coding sequence, for example, would alter the reading-frame of the mRNA and produce a 'scrambled' amino acid sequence from that point. Mutations which create a premature translation stop codon would lead to a truncated peptide, and those which alter the highly conserved RNA splice signals at exon boundaries would result in loss of that exon from the mRNA.

Missense mutations, which change a single amino acid, are more difficult to interpret. The usual rule about such mutations is that if they cause a non-conservative amino acid substitution (such as a charge change), and are not found in a panel of samples from normal controls, then they are likely to be causative. However, we have observed missense mutations in the Fanconi anaemia group C gene (Chapter 10) which met these criteria, and in which the wild-type sequence was conserved in the homologous gene in the mouse, but which were then shown not to segregate with the disease phenotype in the affected family. Thus, in the absence of a functional test for the gene product, it may be difficult to establish whether a missense mutation is a polymorphism or a pathological change. Its credentials may be strengthened by demonstrating that it is not present in a substantial number (conventionally 100 samples) of control individuals from a similar ethnic background to the index case. Mutations in introns or in untranslated regions of the gene should be treated with even greater scepticism.

ACKNOWLEDGEMENTS

Research in the author's laboratory is supported by the Medical Research Council (UK), the Muscular Dystrophy Group, and the Generation Trust. The SSCP gel photograph in Figure 26.3 was provided by Ian Pearson.

REFERENCES

1. Saiki, R.K., Gelfand, D.H., Stoffel, S. *et al.* (1988) Primer-directed enzymatic amplification of DNA with a thermostable DNA polymerase. *Science*, **239**, 487–91.
2. Dianzani, I., Camaschella, C., Ponzone, A. and Cotton, R.G.H. (1993) Dilemmas and progress in mutation detection. *Trends Genet.*, **9** (12), 403–5.
3. Weber, J.L. and May, P.E. (1989) Abundant class of human DNA polymorphisms which can be typed using the polymerase chain reaction. *Am. J. Hum. Genet.*, **44**, 388–96.
4. Litt, M. and Luty, J.A. (1989) A hypervariable microsatellite revealed by in vitro amplification of a dinucleotide repeat within the cardiac muscle actin gene. *Am. J. Hum. Genet.*, **44**, 397–401.
5. Mathew, C.G.P., Easton, D.F., Nakamura, Y. *et al.* (1991) Presymptomatic screening for multiple endocrine neoplasia type 2A with linked DNA markers. *Lancet*, **337**, 7–11.
6. Haliassos, A., Chomel, J., Tesson, A. *et al.* (1989) Modification of enzymatically amplified DNA for the detection of point mutations. *Nucleic Acids Res.*, **17**, 3606.
7. Conner, B.J., Reyes, A.A., Morin, C. *et al.* (1983) Detection of sickle cell β^s-globin allele by hybridization with synthetic oligonucleotides. *Proc. Natl Acad. Sci. USA*, **80**, 278–82.
8. Saiki, R.K., Bugawan, T.L., Horn, G.T. *et al.* (1986) Analysis of enzymatically amplified β-globin and HLA-DQα DNA with allele-specific oligonucleotide probes. *Nature*, **324**, 163–6.
9. Saiki, R.K., Walsh, P.S., Levenson, C.H. and Erlich, H.A. (1989) Genetic analysis of amplified DNA with immobilized sequence-specific oligonucleotide probes. *Proc. Natl Acad. Sci. USA*, **86**, 6230–4.
10. Newton, C.R., Graham, A., Heptinstall, L.E. *et al.* (1989) Analysis of any point mutation in DNA. The amplification refractory mutation system (ARMS). *Nucleic Acids Res.*, **17**, 2503–17.
11. Ferrie, M., Schwarz, M.J., Robertson, N.H. *et al.* (1992) Development, multiplexing, and application of ARMS tests for common mutations in the CFTR gene. *Am. J. Hum. Genet.*, **51**, 251–62.
12. Grompe, M. (1993) The rapid detection of unknown mutations in nucleic acids. *Nature Genet.*, **5**, 111–17.
13. Orita, M., Iwahana, H., Kanazawa, H. *et al.* (1989) Detection of polymorphisms of human DNA by gel electrophoresis as single-stranded conformation polymorphisms. *Proc. Natl Acad. Sci. USA*, **86**, 2766–70.
14. Orita, M., Suzuki, Y., Sekiya, T. and Hayashi, K. (1989) Rapid and sensitive detection of point mutations and DNA polymorphisms using the polymerase chain reaction. *Genomics*, **5**, 874–9.
15. Yap, E.P.H. and McGee, J.O'D. (1993) Nonisotopic discontinuous phase single strand conformation polymorphism (DP-SSCP): genetic profiling of D-loop of human mitochondrial (mt) DNA. *Nucleic Acids Res.*, **21** (17), 4155.
16. Sheffield, V.C., Beck, J.S., Kwitek, A.E. *et al.* (1993) The sensitivity of single-strand conformation polymorphism analysis for the detection of single base substitutions. *Genomics*, **16**, 325–32.
17. Hayashi, K. and Yandell, D.W. (1993) How sensitive is PCR–SSCP? *Hum. Mutat.*, **2**, 338–46.
18. Keen, J., Lester, D., Inglehearn, C. *et al.* (1991) Rapid detection of single base mismatches as heteroduplexes on Hydrolink gels. *Trends Genet.*, **7**, 5.
19. White, M.B., Carvalho, M., Derse, D. *et al.* (1992) Detecting single base substitutions as heteroduplex polymorphisms. *Genomics*, **12**, 301–6.
20. Soto, D. and Sukumar, S. (1992) Improved detection of mutations in the p53 gene in human tumors as single-stranded conformation polymorphs and double-stranded heteroduplex DNA. *PCR Methods and Applications*, **2**, 96–8.

21. Fischer, S.G. and Lerman, L.S. (1983) DNA fragments differing by single-base pair substitutions are separated in denaturing gradient gels: correspondence with melting theory. *Proc. Natl Acad. Sci. USA*, **80**, 1579–83.

22. Sheffield, V.C., Cox, D.R., Lerman, L.S. and Myers, R.M. (1989) Attachment of a 40-base-pair G+C-rich sequence (GC-clamp) to genomic DNA fragments by the polymerase chain reaction results in improved detection of single-base changes. *Proc. Natl Acad. Sci. USA*, **86**, 232–6.

23. Dlouhy, S.R., Wheeler, P., Trofatter, J. *et al.* (1991) Detection of point mutations by denaturing-gradient gel electrophoresis, in *Methods in Molecular Biology*, **vol. 9**, *Protocols in Human Molecular Genetics*, (ed. C. Mathew), Humana Press, Clifton, NJ, pp. 95–110.

24. Cotton, R.G., Rodrigues, N.R. and Campbell, R.D. (1988) Reactivity of cytosine and thymine in single-base pair mismatches with hydroxylamine and osmium tetroxide and its application to the study of mutations. *Proc. Natl Acad. Sci. USA*, **85**, 4397–401.

25. Montandon, A.J., Green, P.M., Giannelli, F. and Bentley, D. (1989) Direct detection of point mutations by mismatch analysis: application to haemophilia B. *Nucleic Acids Res.*, **17**, 3347–58.

26. Saleeba, J.A., Ramus, S.J. and Cotton, R.G.H. (1992) Complete mutation detection using Unlabeled Chemical Cleavage. *Hum. Mutat.*, **1**, 63–9.

27. Haris, I.I., Green, P.M., Bentley, D.R. and Giannelli, F. (1994) Mutation detection by fluorescent chemical cleavage: application to haemophilia B. *PCR Methods and Applications*, **3**, 268–71.

28. Condie, A., Eeles, R., Borresen, A.-L. *et al.* (1993) Detection of point mutations in the p53 gene: comparison of single-strand conformation polymorphism, constant denaturant gel electrophoresis, and hydroxylamine and osmium tetroxide techniques. *Hum. Mutat.*, **2**, 58–66.

29. Sanger, F., Nicklen, S. and Coulsen, A.R. (1977) DNA sequencing with chain-terminating inhibitors. *Proc. Natl Acad. Sci. USA*, **74**, 5463–7.

30. Hultman, T., Stahl, S., Hornes, E. and Uhlen, M. (1989) Direct solid phase sequencing of genomic and plasmid DNA using magnetic beads as solid support. *Nucleic Acids Res.*, **17**, 4937–46.

31. Gyllensten, U.B. and Erlich, H.A. (1988) Generation of single-stranded DNA by the polymerase chain reaction and its application to direct sequencing of the HLA-DQA locus. *Proc. Natl Acad. Sci. USA*, **85**, 7652–6.

32. Chelly, J., Concordet, J.P., Kaplan, J.C. and Kahn, A. (1989) Illegitimate transcription: transcription of any gene in any cell type. *Proc. Natl Acad. Sci. USA*, **86**, 2617–21.

33. Roberts, R.G., Bobrow, M. and Bentley, D.R. (1992) Point mutations in the dystrophin gene. *Proc. Natl Acad. Sci. USA*, **89**, 2331–5.

34. Varesco, L., Gismondi, V., James, R. *et al.* (1993) Identification of APC gene mutations in Italian adenomatous polyposis coli patients by PCR–SSCP analysis. *Am. J. Hum. Genet.*, **52**, 280–5.

35. Roest, P.A., Roberts, R.G., Sugino, S. *et al.* (1993) Protein truncation test (PTT) for rapid detection of translation-terminating mutations. *Hum. Molec. Genet.*, **2**, 1719–21.

36. Powell, S.M., Peterson, G.M., Krush, A.J. *et al.* (1993) Molecular diagnosis of familial adenomatous polyposis. *N. Engl. J. Med.*, **329**, 1982–7.

Chapter 27

The ethics of testing for cancer-predisposition genes

GARETH EVANS and RODNEY HARRIS

27.1 INTRODUCTION

The recent advances in molecular genetics have uncovered new ethical dilemmas in cancer genetics as vexed and almost certainly more complex than the disease which has up until now provoked the most debate: Huntington's disease. Many genes that predispose to cancer have no effect until well into adult life and, as with Huntington's, important issues arise about predictive genetic tests in fetal, childhood and adult life. Unlike Huntington's there are sometimes options which may prevent, or at least alter the course of the disease. Nonetheless, there are hereditary cancers where little or no effective screening or treatment is possible, even when pre-symptomatic testing shows an individual to carry a cancer predisposing gene. Many of the lessons that have been learned from study of Huntington's can be applied to predictive testing for cancer-predisposition genes [1].

27.2 CANCER-PREDISPOSITION GENES AND TESTING IN CHILDHOOD

For the purposes of this chapter we have divided these genes into those in which there is an identifiable phenotype (at least in a proportion of cases) and those in which there is no phenotype, but only the end result of a particular cancer. In phenotypic conditions the diagnosis can be made in a single individual, whereas in many cancer syndromes a clear familial aggregation is required for diagnosis. In recessive conditions such as Bloom's or ataxia telangiectasia the phenotype is usually clinically evident without predictive testing. This may also be the case in neurofibromatosis type 1 when the pigmentary disturbance and neurofibromas are nearly always expressed by 5 years of age [2] and the need for predictive testing is thus minimal. However in familial adenomatous polyposis (FAP), neurofibromatosis type 2 (NF2) and von Hippel–Lindau disease (vHL) the phenotype is variable and diagnostic features may not be present until well into adult life [3–5]. In such conditions individuals at 50% prior risk are usually screened for signs which may require mild (indirect ophthalmoscopy with mydriasis, magnetic resonance image (MRI) scanning of the brain) to considerable invasiveness (sigmoidoscopy/colonoscopy).

Some of these tests could be described as

Genetic Predisposition to Cancer. Edited by R.A. Eeles, B.A.J. Ponder, D.F. Easton and A. Horwich. Published in 1996 by Chapman & Hall, London.
0 412 56580 3

Table 27.1 Cancer-predisposition genes

Identifiable phenotype	Inheritance	No phenotype	Inheritance
Familial adenomatous polyposis	AD	Lynch type I	AD
Gorlin's syndrome	AD	Lynch type II	AD
Neurofibromatosis 1 and 2	AD	Familial breast	AD
Multiple endocrine neoplasia	AD	Breast–ovarian	AD
von Hippel–Lindau	AD	Li–Fraumeni	AD
Ataxia telangiectasia (A-T)	AR	A-T carrier	AD
Bloom's syndrome	AR		
Xeroderma pigmentosa	AR		
Dysplastic naevus syndrome	AD		

AD, autosomal dominant; AR, autosomal recessive.

being beneficial to at-risk individuals in that they might find premalignant adenomatous polyps (FAP), vestibular schwannomas (NF2) or retinal angiomas (VHL) which could be treated and prevent further disability. Others, such as congenital hypertrophy of the retinal pigment epithelium (CHRPE in FAP), posterior lenticular opacities (NF2) and pancreatic cysts in (VHL) would merely indicate that person had the gene without there being any immediate clinical benefit to the individual. Unlike many DNA predictive tests these clinical predictions do not give the same level of reassurance if they are favourable. Performing these tests has not been subjected to anywhere near the same ethical scrutiny as DNA predictive tests. Clinicians undertake such tests and clients who have them should be fully aware of the genetic implications of a positive test. It is all too easy, for example, to send a client to a busy ophthalmology clinic where they are casually told that they have the FAP gene because CHRPE is found, without adequate and immediate back-up in terms of follow-up and genetic counselling.

There is, therefore, a right **not** to know. While it may be argued that individuals at risk of one of the conditions with a phenotype (Table 27.1) are benefited in that there is something that can be done for their condition, it may be many years before they require any intervention. In the same way as the vast majority of geneticists would not perform a predictive test on a child at risk of Huntington's [6], even in the phenotypic conditions there are ages at which even apparently non-invasive tests such as ophthalmoscopy should not be used. For instance, very few geneticists in the UK would advocate DNA testing of a 1-year-old child with a 50% risk of FAP because the cancer risk at this age is minimal and the psychological problems for the parent–child relationship are considerable. It would, as suggested above, be all too easy to forget that a simple eye test may have the same predictive value.

However, most of the phenotypic cancer-predisposing conditions can sometimes result in tumour formation in childhood, and this decides when screening should be offered both to detect potentially harmful tumours, and also to identify 'benign' disease markers (e.g. CHRPE). Table 27.2 shows the probable earliest reported instance of a cancer or other harmful neoplasm for each condition and the overall risk in childhood.

In the UK, most centres offering DNA tests would build these into the initial work-up for the disorder. For instance, if screening was commenced at 12 years for FAP, the DNA test would be offered in conjunction with ophthalmoscopy and dental screening.

Table 27.2   Implications of various dominant cancer syndromes in childhood

Disease	Tumours	Probable earliest tumour reported	Risk in childhood (%)	Recommended starting age for screening
Familial adenomatous polyposis	Adenomas, bowel cancer	First year ?4 years, 7 years	80 <1	10–16 years
Neurofibromatosis 2	Schwannomas, meningiomas	First year (meningioma)	30	Birth
von Hippel–Lindau	Haemangioblastoma, renal carcinoma	1–2 years (retinal)	15	5 years
Multiple endocrine neoplasia 1	Parathyroid, insulinoma, gastrinoma	5 years	5	5 years
Multiple endocrine neoplasia 2A	Medullary thyroid, cancer, parathyroid, phaeochromocytoma	3 years	2–5	3–4 years
Multiple endocrine neoplasia 2B	As in MEN 2A except parathyroid	Neonates	>50	Birth
Li–Fraumeni	Sarcoma (bone/soft tissue), adrenal, leukaemia, breast cancer, gliomas, ?others	First year	30	First year
BRCA1	Breast and ovary carcinoma	>16 years	<0.1	30–35 years
Lynch I	Colorectum	>16 years	<0.1	25–35 years
Lynch II	Colorectum, breast, endometrium, ovary	>16 years	<0.1	25–35 years

Nevertheless, there are families in which huge pressure is exerted by the parents to have the DNA test earlier. In deciding when to use a DNA test one should assess the balance between benefit and damage to the **child**, and not the potential for relief of anxiety in the parents. If a screening programme starts at 12 years of age with sigmoidoscopy or colonoscopy, there is a clear benefit for 50% of children who are shown by DNA tests not to have the gene, as they will have to undergo fewer if any invasive tests. In contrast, at 1 year of age the potential for benefit is unclear while there is potential for harm, particularly if one child in the family is stigmatized from infancy as 'affected' and another is 'unaffected'. Nonetheless, colorectal cancer has been reported even under the age of 10 years and

hepatoblastoma is also a potential risk in infancy with little possibility of effective screening.

In balancing these various difficulties, most centres in the UK would still offer the DNA tests at the time of initial screening and most parents with sympathetic counselling will accept this timing of the test. Earlier testing may well be offered in occasional families where an individual clinician deems this to be psychologically beneficial.

The situation in the USA is fundamentally different; in some centres testing in infancy is the norm. Indeed, at the recent Leeds Castle Polyposis meeting in Copenhagen (1993), the consensus was that ethical decisions on timing should be discussed in each country as it would be impossible to impose a single international policy.

Timing of the DNA tests in the other conditions in which there is a distinctive recognizable phenotype again depends on weighing up the benefits. It could be argued that DNA testing does not differ from other tests which are also predictive – cataracts at birth in NF2, or high calcitonin in MEN at 4 years of age. It could also be argued that if the clinical investigations are non-invasive, there is no harm to the unaffected child in delaying DNA testing until a time at which they can participate in the decision. Because some conditions may occur in childhood, clinical screening and repeated hospitalization of children unnecessarily could be avoided by early DNA testing if they are found not to have the gene. So-called non-invasive tests such as MRI scans can actually be very traumatic, for example, if they require a general anaesthetic to keep a child still. Repeated blood tests are also unpleasant for children. While the debate should not really be centred on cost, there is the potential cost saving of **not** performing expensive screening on those who do not have the gene. Overall, most centres in the UK would, therefore, offer the tests at the time of the initial screen. However even using commencement of screening can be troublesome. It is important to examine newborn infants for cataracts in NF2 as these may threaten vision [3]. Nonetheless, only 10% of individuals present in the first decade when screening can be confined to a simple annual physical examination [7]. More intense screening for vestibular schwannomas (acoustic neuromas) with brainstem-evoked responses or MRI scans should probably commence at puberty, although shortage of scanners may preclude using MRI more than a few times. Should we, therefore, delay DNA testing until 16 years of age or an age at which the individual can make a decision for themselves? While the MRI scan is a predictive test it has an immediate benefit in diagnosing a tumour which can be managed optimally. The DNA

test will only say that the individual has the gene (or not) when tumours, particularly in late onset families, may not arise for decades. In NF2 there is a possible argument for testing at any age including birth, but equally that individual may have no features of the condition until they are 40. The decision on timing of DNA predictive testing could therefore, be left to the individual clinician treating each NF2 family considering each on its own merits (age at onset, etc.) (see Table 27.3).

27.2.1 NON-PHENOTYPIC CANCER SYNDROMES

The debate about testing in childhood is potentially easier where the risk of a child being affected is close to zero. This is the case in the Lynch cancer family syndromes and in those that carry a *BRCA1* gene mutation. There are few potential benefits of testing an 8-year-old girl for the *BRCA1* gene, as she will have little cancer risk until she is 30 years old. It could be argued that there is a potential for prevention by hormonal manipulation (delay of puberty, early first pregnancy), but these are unproven and are highly contentious. Gene therapy administered in childhood may one day help prevent cancer in these families, but as this is not yet possible, there can be little benefit to a child in having a predictive test for the *BRCA1* gene; moreover, the situation is similar for Huntington's disease [8]. Many young adults would prefer to live with the relative uncertainty (40–45% risk) of whether they were going to develop breast cancer rather than be faced with an 80–90% lifetime risk in the absence of definitive preventive or curative measures. There is also the problem of insurance. Common cancer predisposition can only be classified as dominant in a very few families. Insurance companies are currently unlikely to load or refuse the policy as they would for someone whose parent has Huntington's disease. However, if the results

Table 27.3 Guidelines for timing of DNA predictive tests

Disease	Age (years) of		
	Earliest screen	Intensive screening	DNA testing
Familial adenomatous polyposis	10	16	10–16
Neurofibromatosis 2	Birth	10–12	Birth
			or 10
			or 18+
von Hippel–Lindau	5	15	5
			or 15
			or 18+
Multiple endocrine neoplasia 1	5	5	5
			or 18+
Multiple endocrine neoplasia 2A	3–4	3–4	3–4
			or 18+
Multiple endocrine neoplasia 2B	1	1	Birth
Li–Fraumeni	First year	None yet agreed	Birth??
			18+
BRCA1	30	30	18+
Lynch I	25–35	35	18+
Lynch II	25–35	35	18+

of a test in childhood showed an inherited mutation in the *BRCA1* gene, this would almost certainly have to be disclosed on an insurance application, leading to refusal or heavy loading.

(a) Genetic and other screening for common cancers

All of the conditions described so far have the potential benefit of early detection of tumours by screening at-risk individuals. With benign tumours this allows optimal management and may be life-saving; with cancers, there is a real hope of improving morbidity and mortality. Screening programmes for the phenotypic conditions are well established and have been shown to be beneficial [3, 5, 10–12]. The situation is less clear with common cancer predisposition. In the US and some other countries, population screening is advocated for bowel and breast cancer from a relatively early age. Screening for breast cancer is now accepted in the UK only

after 50 years [13], with no general acceptance for bowel cancer at any age. However, targeted screening is offered by many for breast [14], bowel [15] and ovarian cancer [16]. While the benefits of early screening in breast cancer are still not clear even in high-risk groups, evidence of benefit is now emerging for both the ovary [16] and bowel [17].

It is not the purpose of this chapter to define whether a screening programme is suitable for a specific condition. However, when discussing predictive testing the nature of screening for a specific disorder is relevant. Negative screening at a particular age may in itself substantially reduce the risk of that individual having inherited the family gene fault [3, 5, 12]. Alterations in an established screening programme dependent on the result of a DNA test may also need to be discussed. This may involve more active screening with a bad predictive outcome, or relaxing or stopping screening altogether in those at low risk. Individuals who are accustomed to being screened for a condition for which there is still a relatively high population risk (breast, bowel or ovarian cancer), may wish to continue as before. The efficacy of any screening programme also needs to be made clear to someone considering undergoing a predictive test. It is unlikely that many women at 40% risk of breast cancer would accept prophylactic mastectomy [18], but faced with an 80% risk would they still be happy with a screening programme which is yet to be proven to be beneficial? Positive DNA predictive tests may substantially alter the current practice of screening. This has already led to early thyroidectomy in MEN 2 and may well lead to colectomy and prophylactic mastectomy in familial bowel and breast cancer.

27.3 ADULT DNA PREDICTIVE TESTS

27.3.1 THE RIGHT TO KNOW

The ethicists argue that it is every individual's right to know any information relevant to themselves, particularly if others (health care workers) are already party to it [19]. There are various reasons why someone may want to know if they have inherited the family gene fault [20].

1. To make decisions concerning having children
2. To have certainty
3. To plan appropriate action (e.g. prophylactic surgery)
4. To inform children and/or partner
5. To make provisions for the future
6. To help science

Where a predictive test is possible in adulthood, and when this is of physical or probable psychological benefit to an individual, the test should be offered after adequate counselling.

However, there are instances when an individual's 'right to know' may interfere with another individual's 'right **not** to know' [21]. Such a situation would occur if someone whose grandparent had a cancer-predisposing syndrome wanted a test when their relevant parent who was still clinically unaffected did not. In this situation the autonomy of one individual is in conflict with another. The situation is simpler when there is real physical benefit in knowing that they have the gene fault. For instance, denial of a predictive test in FAP could be extended to denying endoscopic screening as, if this were positive, it too would inform the unwilling parent of their genetic status. Clearly where there is clinical benefit the wishes of the offspring should prevail. The converse of this is in a condition where no treatment was possible, such as Huntington's, where it is now very easy to do a simple DNA predictive test which may be of marginal benefit to an adult offspring, but a devastating and unwanted blow to the parent if positive [21]. Therefore, the clinician must weigh up the conflicts in autonomy to decide whether it is appropriate to offer tests in these circumstances. In future, these decisions may involve the advice of medical ethicists.

(a) Disclosure

Another contentious area is the disclosure of information to an individual in a family who is at risk, when the affected individual specifically does not want this to happen. Again, the ethicist would argue that it is the duty of people in this situation to inform their relatives [19]. If the clinician were to disclose the information this would be a breach of confidentiality. However, there is also a possibly stronger duty to the at-risk individual who could have a life-saving procedure denied them by lack of this knowledge. DNA tests may further complicate the issue as it may be necessary to use the DNA sample from the unwilling affected relative either in linkage analysis or in a mutation study, to allow a predictive test on the at-risk relative. Although at-risk individuals may have a right to important relevant clinical information, do they also have the right to specific information from their unwilling relative's DNA? [22].

Disclosure may take another form, for instance, a child and his/her adoptive parents hearing of genetic disease in the biological family. This may be quite common in cancer-predisposing syndromes, because either the nature of the predisposition, or the disease itself does not arise until later in the natural parent. After adequate consultation with social services, disclosure of the likely genetic predisposition and with it the possibility of DNA tests may well be indicated [23].

27.4 THE RIGHT *NOT* TO KNOW

We have already pointed out potential areas of conflict in families, when the right of one individual to know may conflict with the right of a relative not to know. This has been described with regard to testing in childhood and also when an offspring's result would reveal a parent's genotype. However, there are several other reasons why a DNA predictive test may be refused [20].

1. Because a positive result would be too difficult to live with could not cope with a bad result.
2. The test does not predict when the disease will appear.
3. Preference to live in uncertainty.
4. Fear of increasing the risk to children.
5. Problems at work and with insurance.
6. A positive result would impose too great a burden on partner/family.
7. Negative tests generate guilt feelings in sibling relationships.

All of these reasons are applicable to a DNA predictive test for cancer predisposi-

tion, although unlike Huntington's, screening and prophylactic surgery may detect the disease earlier when it may be curable altogether. However, the Li–Fraumeni syndrome poses almost identical quandaries to Huntington's. Li–Fraumeni syndrome causes malignancies which may appear in childhood or more commonly in adult life. The range and number of tumours and sites make screening or removal of all at-risk tissues impossible. While early diagnosis may allow cure of a particular primary, many go on to develop further primaries and 90% will have developed a malignancy by 50 years of age [24]. A decision to opt for a predictive test in Li–Fraumeni should therefore, be preceded by counselling, as is advocated for Huntington's [25, 26].

After counselling most people at risk of Huntington's (which is effectively untreatable at present) do not opt for a predictive test [20, 25]. In contrast, in conditions like FAP, predictive testing is more acceptable because there are clear benefits which follow knowledge about one's genetic status. However, many people with predisposition to cancers for which screening or treatment is of arguable benefit may not want to know. Although those working in the cancer genetics field may have the impression that there is enthusiasm for predictive tests, one should be cautious because in the early stages, as with Huntington's, a highly motivated self-referred population volunteers itself. Such tests offered on a less selected or population basis may prove less acceptable. Many people may also be happy to be screened for their 40% risk of a cancer and prefer to continue with screening rather than have a predictive test. As occurred in Huntington's, it is important that the effects of counselling and predictive testing on the psychological well-being of each individual is carefully studied [27]. Follow-up of 'favourable' test results is also important, because even here there may be an adverse reaction based upon the well-recognized 'survivor syndrome' [28].

27.4.1 PRENATAL TESTING

It is not yet clear what level of demand there will be for prenatal testing in the cancer-predisposing syndromes. Some work has been done on type 1 neurofibromatosis, suggesting that in spite of couples expressing an interest in prenatal tests, few would contemplate termination [29]. This is reflected in the fairly low uptake of these tests when offered [30]. It is likely that decisions will depend on the experience within the particular family. Thus, severe conditions like NF2 may have a high take up rate and more manageable conditions like FAP a low rate.

Prenatal testing again touches on the rights of minors not to know should a positive test not be followed by termination. In Huntington's, a prenatal test is usually offered only if the couple intend to terminate should the test result be unfavourable [6]. When the prenatal test is limited to 'exclusion' the fetus, 25% risk may be reduced to a very low risk or be shown to have the same risk as the parent (50%). When, subsequently, the parent develops for example early-onset breast cancer, this would imply that the fetus also carried the gene and the child would carry the burden of knowledge through life. Prenatal tests should probably be undertaken only if there is a clear wish to terminate high-risk pregnancies, or in the future when this will allow early intervention which will be beneficial to the resultant child.

27.4.2 RESEARCH SAMPLES

Ethical problems arise in connection with samples taken for research which are subsequently used for prediction. Individuals at risk of a cancer syndrome may be tested as part of research into linkage in families or have blood taken 'for research' when attending family history clinics for screening. If individuals in these circumstances are fully aware of the possible outcome of this research then there may not be a problem when a predictive 'result' is arrived at. However, many will be unaware of the implications of a positive test result. It is unwise to store DNA on 'at-risk' individuals unless informed consent is given or the samples are anonymously coded and used for research purposes only [31]. Blood from unaffected relatives adds little information in late-onset disease unless specific questions about non-penetrance are being asked. In this situation the gene defect is known and the at-risk relative should be approached again for sampling on the understanding that the sample will be coded and there will be no result, or that there will be a proper predictive test with attendant counselling. Ideally, informed consent should be obtained with the first sample, there will then be no need for a repeat venepuncture.

27.4.3 TESTING WITHOUT SPECIFIC CONSENT

It is important to distinguish between screening for existing disease and genetic screening with its implications for the individuals and their relatives. A predictive test may be done incidentally while in hospital for related or even unrelated problems [1]. For example, a woman undergoing a laparoscopy for an ovarian cyst found on scan, may have blood taken for tests like the biomarker CA125, but a request may also be made for DNA diagnosis. This is not appropriate without consent.

The extreme sensitivity of the PCR test raises the prospect of illicit testing [19] as it is now possible to perform DNA tests on saliva samples. These could, for example, be carried out on residual traces on a glass someone had just drunk from. Employers and others could thus obtain information about the genetic status of unsuspecting individuals.

27.4.4 POPULATION SCREENING

The major aim of a population screen would be to identify the up to 50% of new germline mutations which occur in the cancer-predisposition syndromes [2, 3]. At present, population screening for cancers by genetic tests is impractical although it is an area for potential ethical problems in the future and these are being addressed by the Nuffield working party [32]. Population screening is impractical because of the variety of mutations within any of the cancer-predisposition genes. There is no simple test, or small number of tests, which could be performed on each gene on a population basis. Once more, informed consent would be mandatory should population screening for cancer predisposition become possible.

27.4.5 INSURANCE

The implications of genetic testing on personal insurance has recently received extensive attention in the medical and lay press [8, 33]. In the UK, the main concern is about the consequences of such testing on the eligibility for life assurance. Insurance companies are not currently asking for DNA tests as they do for HIV tests, but may do so in the future. Indeed, a recent article points out the usefulness of such tests for life assurance underwriting [34]. As in Huntington's disease, if the genetic nature of the condition is well enough defined, individuals may be unable to obtain insurance because they are at 50% risk, irrespective of DNA tests [8]. This may prompt those at risk to request testing in the hope that their 50%

prior risk will be reduced to the point of being able to obtain insurance. However, this was not found to be a particularly important reason for opting for a test in a recent study [35].

Insurance companies are understandably concerned about the possibility that someone who receives a high-risk result will obtain a policy with a high pay out either for life insurance or critical illness insurance to cover the development of cancer. They are also concerned about competition from other companies if they were not to discriminate and had to increase payments to ordinary risk individuals to cover their costs. Nonetheless, the companies want to avoid unnecessary discrimination and any attendant adverse publicity which may lead to legislation.

In the US and other countries without national health services, the main concern is about health insurance where a positive predictive test would have great relevance, although predictive genetic tests are rarely able to determine the time at which someone will become ill. In the US most health insurance is purchased on a group basis by employers, and the unemployed or low-income groups are often not insured. There is no obligation on an employer to insure a high-risk employee who would raise their costs. Thus 31–36 million people in the US have no health insurance [33]. Eventually, legislation is likely in order to prevent discrimination because insurers appear not to be prepared to pay, for example, for a FAP test, thus denying those on lower incomes the opportunity for testing in the first place.

The duty of the clinician is to ensure that there are no untoward pressures on an individual, to accept or refuse genetic tests and clarification, perhaps with legalisation or state indemnity may be required. Insurance matters are a legitimate concern during the process of pre-test counselling.

27.5 SUMMARY

The purpose of this chapter has been to highlight the ethical issues that arise in connection with DNA predictive tests. The primary duty of the clinician/counsellor is to do no harm (non-beneficence) [21]. The secondary aim is for the test to be of some benefit (beneficence). Clearly, each cancer-predisposition syndrome will have to be considered on its own merits with counselling on the implications of testing in pregnancy, childhood and adulthood for the individual and family requesting, or being offered testing. A full support service should be in place with follow-up not only of unfavourable results, but also of good predictive information.

REFERENCES

1. Harper, P. (1992) Ethical issues in genetic testing for Huntington's disease: lessons for the study of familial cancers. *Dis. Markers*, **10**, 185–8.
2. Huson, S.M., Harper, P.S. and Compston, D.A.S. (1988) Von Recklinghausen neurofibromatosis. *Brain*, **111**, 1355–81.
3. Evans, D.G.R., Huson, S., Donnai, D. *et al.* (1992) A clinical study of type 2 neurofibromatosis. *Q. J. Med.*, **84**, 603–18.
4. Evans, D.G.R., Guy, S.P., Armstrong, J. *et al.* (1993) Non penetrance and late appearance of polyps in families with familial adenomatous polyposis. *Gut*, **34**, 1389–93.
5. Maher, E.R., Iselius, L., Yates, J.R.W. *et al.* (1991) Von Hippel Lindau disease: a genetic study. *J. Med. Genet.*, **28**, 443–7.
6. Turner, D. (1992) Ethical considerations in the social context of Huntington disease. *Dis. Markers*, **10**, 171–83.
7. Evans, D.G.R., Huson, S.M., Donnai, D. *et al.* (1992) A genetic study of type 2 neurofibromatosis: II Guidelines for genetic counselling. *J. Med. Genet.*, **29**, 847–52.
8. Harper, P.S. (1993) Insurance and genetic testing. *Lancet*, **341**, 224–7.
9. Easton, D.F., Bishop, D.T., Ford, D. *et al.* (1993) Genetic linkage analysis in familial breast and ovarian cancer: results from 214 families. *Am. J. Hum. Genet.*, **52**, 678–701.
10. Ponder, B.A.J., Coffey, R. and Gagel, R.F. (1988) Risk estimation and screening in families of patients with medullary thyroid carcinoma. *Lancet*, **i**, 397–401.
11. Thakker, R.V. (1993) The molecular genetics of the multiple endocrine neoplasia syndromes. *Clin. Endocrinol.*, **38**, 1–14.
12. Burn, J., Chapman, P., Delhanty, J. *et al.* (1991) The UK Northern Region Genetic register for familial adenomatous polyposis coli: use of age of onset, congenital hypertrophy of the retinal pigment epithelium, and DNA markers in risk calculation. *J. Med. Genet.*, **28**, 289–96.
13. *Breast Cancer Screening: Forrest Report* (1988) HMSO, London.
14. Evans, D.G.R., Fentiman, I.S., McPherson, K., Asbury, D., Ponder, B.A.J. and Howell, A. (1993) Familial breast cancer. *Br. Med. J.*, **308**, 183–7.
15. Dunlop, M.G. (1992) Screening for large bowel neoplasms in individuals with a family history of colorectal cancer. *Br. J. Surg.*, **79**, 488–94.
16. Bourne, T.H., Campbell, S. and Reynolds, K.M. (1993) Screening for early familial ovarian cancer with transvaginal ultrasonography and colour flow imaging. *Br. Med. J.*, **306**, 1025–9.
17. Mandel, J.S., Bond, J.H. and Church, T.R. (1993) Reducing mortality from colorectal cancer by screening for faecal occult blood. *N. Engl. J. Med.*, **328**, 1365–71.
18. Evans, D.G.R., Donnai, D., Ribiero, G. and Warrell, D (1992) Ovarian cancer family and prophylactic choices. *J. Med. Genet.*, **29**, 416–18.
19. Harris, J. (1992) The use of information (autonomy and confidentiality). *Dis. Markers*, **10**, 195–8.
20. Wolff, G. and Walter, W. (1992) Attitudes of at risk persons for Huntington disease toward predictive genetic testing. *Birth Defects Original Article Series*, **28 (1)**, 119–26.
21. de Wert, G. (1992) Predictive testing for Huntington disease and the right not to know, some ethical reflections. *Birth Defects Original Article Series*, **28 (1)**, 133–8.

22. *Report of Committee on the Ethics of Gene Therapy.* (1992) HMSO, London.
23. Evans, G. (1992) Ethical issues: the geneticist's viewpoint. *Dis. Markers*, **10**, 199–203.
24. Garber, J.E., Goldstein, A.M. Kantor, A.F. *et al.* (1991) Follow-up study of twenty-four families with Li – Fraumeni syndrome. *Cancer Res.*, **51**, 6094–7.
25. Craufurd, D., Kerzin-Storrer, L., Dodge, A. and Harris, R. (1989) Uptake of presymptomatic predictive testing for Huntington's disease. *Lancet*, **ii**, 603–5.
26. Ethical issues policy statement on Huntington's disease molecular genetic predictive test. (1990) *J. Med. Genet.*, **27**, 34–8.
27. Craufurd, D. and Harris, R. (1986) Ethics of predictive testing for Huntington's chorea: the need for more information. *Br. Med. J.*, **293**, 249–51.
28. Demyttenaere, K., Evers-Kiebooms, G. and Decruyenaere, M. (1992) Pitfalls in counselling for predictive testing in Huntington disease. *Birth Defects Original Article Series*, **28 (1)**, 105–11.
29. Benjamin, C.M., Colley, A., Donnai, D. *et al.* (1993) Neurofibromatosis type 1 (NF1): knowledge, experience and reproductive decisions of affected individuals and families. *J. Med. Genet.*, **30**, 567–74.
30. Upadhyaya, M., Fryer, A., MacMillan, J., Broadhead, W., Huson, S.M. and Harper, P.S. (1992) Prenatal diagnosis and presymptomatic detection of neurofibromatosis type 1. *J. Med. Genet.*, **29**, 180–3.
31. Harper, P.S. (1993) Research samples from families with genetic disease: a proposed code of conduct. *Br. Med. J.*, **306**, 1391–4.
32. Nuffield Council On Bioethics (1993) Genetic screening ethical issues. Nuffield Bioethics, UK.
33. Ostrer, H., Allen, W., Crandall, L.A. *et al.* (1993) Insurance and genetic testing: where are we now? *Am. J. Hum. Genet.*, **52**, 565–77.
34. Brett, P. and Fischer, E.P. (1993) Effects on life insurance of genetic testing. *The Actuary*, **10 (3)**, 11-12.
35. Tyler, A., Morris, M., Lazarou, L., Meredith, L., Myring J. and Harper, P.S. (1992) Presymptomatic testing for Huntington's disease in Wales 1987–90. *Br. J. Psychiatr.*, **161**, 481–8.

Glossary

Allele: alternative sequences at a locus (can be coding or non-coding).

Alpha (α): the proportion of families linked to a particular locus.

Alternative splicing: alternative forms of mRNA produced by splicing at different points in heterologous nuclear RNA.

Alu: a short interspersed repeat about 300 bp long homologous to 5′ and 3′ ends of 7SL RNA. Conserved across all primates.

Antisense: a nucleotide sequence complementary to the coding sequence (sense strand).

Apoptosis: an active mechanism of cell death in which DNA degradation and nuclear destruction precede loss of plasma membrane integrity and cell necrosis.

Autosomal: on a chromosome which is not a sex chromosome (X or Y).

Bayesian analysis: a method of calculating posterior probability from prior probability.

Candidate gene: a gene that is considered to be a contender for the cause of a disease.

cDNA: DNA complementary to RNA and synthesized from it by reverse transcription.

Centimorgan (cM): the distance over which the probability of recombination is 1%.

Centromere: specific DNA sequences at the join of the p and q arms of a chromosome which attach it to the mitotic spindle.

Cloning: the generation of multiple identical copies of a DNA sequence by replication in a suitable vector.

Codon: a triplet of nucleotides coding for one amino acid.

Constitutional: present in every cell of the body.

Contiguous gene syndrome: a syndrome with several phenotypic features which is due to an alteration (e.g. large deletion) affecting more than one tightly linked gene.

Cosmid: a vector that replicates like a plasmid but can be packaged *in vitro* into λ phage coats.

C-terminal: the 3′ end of the gene.

Cytogenetics: analysis of chromosome structure.

Deletion: loss of a segment of a chromosome or base pair(s) in a gene.

Dominant: a disorder in which only one allele at a locus is needed for a phenotypic effect.

Dominant oncogene: an oncogene which only has to be altered in one allele at a locus to have an oncogenic effect.

Epistasis: where more than one genetic alteration is required to cause strong susceptibility ('gene–gene' interaction).

Exon: transcribed sequence not spliced out of mature RNAs.

Frameshift: a deletion or insertion that results in a shift in the reading of sets of three bases (codons). This usually results in a stop codon being created downstream.

Gene: DNA sequence which becomes transcribed and then translated into protein.

Genome: genetic component of a cell.

Genotype: the hereditary information encoded by nucleic acid.

Germline: in the DNA of every cell and inherited from the parents.

Haplotype: the sequence of alleles along a chromosome arm.

Hardy–Weinberg equilibrium: the genotypic probabilities which occur in a random mating population.

Hemizygous: only one parental copy of the gene is present (usually in a tumour).

Heterogeneity: where several genes can each independently cause the same disease phenotype.

Heterozygous: the alleles at a locus differ.

Homogeneity: a disease entity is only due to one gene.

Homologous: areas of the genome which have similar sequences.

Homozygous: the alleles at a locus are identical.

Hotspot: a site in a gene that is commonly mutated.

Hybridization: the base-pairing of complementary single strands of nucleic acid that leads to a double stranded molecule.

Imprinting: where parental origin affects the expression of a gene.

Intron: transcribed sequences spliced out of mature RNA.

Karyotype: the chromosomal composition of a cell.

Kilobase (kb): 1000 bases.

Kindred: a family (also termed a pedigree).

Library: collection of different cDNAs or genomic DNA fragments propagated in a cloning vector.

Linkage: co-segregation of two genetic loci (because they lie close together on a chromosome) at greater frequency than would be expected by chance.

Linkage disequilibrium: association between a disease and a marker allele, or two marker alleles, due to founder effects in closed populations.

Locus (pl. loci): position on a chromosome.

LOD Score: a measure of the evidence for linkage. Logarithm to the base 10 of the ratio of the probability of the observed data given linkage divided by the probability of the observed data given no linkage. LOD score of >3 is often taken as convincing evidence for linkage.

Loss of heterozygosity (LOH): loss of one allele at a heterozygous locus reducing it to hemizygosity.

Mapping: physical mapping: a map based on actual distances in base pairs between loci.

Genetic mapping: a map where distances between loci are based on recombination frequency.

Microsatellites: runs of short repeat sequences such as dinucleotide repeats (CACACA), tri- or tetra-nucleotide repeats.

Minisatellites: runs of longer repeat sequences such as VNTRs (variable number of tandem repeats).

Missense: a mutation where one base pair is replaced by another.

Mitotic recombination: recombination occurring during mitosis.

Mosaic: the presence of different genotypes in the germline.

mRNA: messenger RNA the product of DNA transcription and splicing that serves as a template for protein translation.

Mutation: an alteration in DNA sequence.

Non-disjunction: failure of chromatid sequences to separate during mitosis.

Nonsense: an alteration in DNA sequence resulting in the formation of a stop codon which results in premature termination of translation into protein.

Northern analysis: technique to identify RNA molecules to analyse gene expression.

N-terminal: the 5′ end of a gene.

Open reading frame (ORF): a sequence of translatable codons not interrupted by stop codons (codes for a polypeptide).

p arm: the short arm of a chromosome.

Pedigree: a family tree.

Penetrance: the chance that a disease will occur as the result of the presence of a predisposing mutation.

Phage: a virus that replicates in bacteria.

Phase: the ability to determine the pattern of inheritance of markers unambiguously.

Phenocopy: an individual who has the disease but does not have the disease-predisposing mutation (i.e. a sporadic case).

Phenotype: the physical or biochemical effect of the genotype (e.g. occurrence of a certain type of cancer).

Plasmid: a double-stranded circle of DNA capable of being anonymously replicated in bacteria.

Pleiotropy: where several phenotypic features are caused by the same mutation.

Point mutation: substitution of one base by another.

Polymerase chain reaction (PCR): an *in vitro* method that uses enzyme synthesis to exponentially amplify DNA sequences.

Polymorphism: alternative forms of a DNA sequence occurring naturally in a population.

Posterior probability: for example the probability that the person will have the predisposing mutation given all the information available, including age of the individual and number and type of affected relatives.

Prior probability: the chance that the individual at risk has the predisposition gene (calculated from the chance that the gene is present in the family and the position of the individual in the pedigree).

Proband: the initially ascertained case in a pedigree.

Probe: a short, specific DNA sequence with a marker label (e.g. radioactivity) that can be used to detect complementary sequences in 'test' DNA.

Pulse field gel electrophoresis: electrophoresis during which the orientation of the electric field is altered in time. It separates large pieces of DNA of up to 2000 kb.

q arm: the long arm of a chromosome.

Recessive: a disorder in which the gene can only exert a phenotypic effect if both alleles are altered.

Recessive oncogene: tumour suppressor gene; both alleles at a locus have to be altered to have an oncogenic effect.

Recombination: crossing over at meiosis resulting in the formation of a different haplotype.

Restriction fragment length polymorphism (RFLP): a polymorphism in the size of restriction fragments after cutting by a bacterial enzyme due to sequence differences between alleles at cutting sites.

Segregation: co-inheritance, e.g. of a disease and a genetic marker.

Somatic cell hybrid: formed by fusing the cells from two different species or by fusing the cells of one species with microcells of another that contain one or a few donor chromosomes. A cell line is then established which contains a set of donor chromosomes.

Southern analysis: a technique of fixing DNA to a nylon membrane. Usually the DNA is digested with a restriction enzyme and the DNA fragments are separated by electrophoresis, denatured and transferred by blotting on to a nylon membrane. A labelled probe will hybridize to a complementary sequence on the membrane.

Splice acceptor site: boundary between intron and exon at the 3' end of the exon.

Splice donor site: boundary between intron and exon at the 5' end of the exon.

Sporadic: a cancer case occurring in a person who is not a mutation carrier.

Stop codon: a codon which codes to end the translation of the coding sequence into protein.

Susceptible: an at-risk individual.

Telomere: either end of the chromosome.

Theta (θ): the recombination fraction.

Transcription: conversion of DNA into RNA.

Transition: conversion of a purine base into another purine or pyrimidine into a pyrimidine.

Translation: conversion of RNA into protein.

Translocation: the attachment of part of one chromosome arm on to another.

Transversion: conversion of a purine base into a pyrimidine or vice versa.

Tumour suppressor gene: see 'Recessive oncogene'.

Vector: an independently replicated DNA molecule into which specific DNA sequence can be integrated and replicated.

Western analysis: a technique for analysing proteins

5': the end of the gene from which transcription starts.

3': the end of the gene at which transcription ends.

Index

Page numbers in *italics* refer to figures and page numbers in **bold** refer to tables

397